D1294649

Handbook of Effective Psychotherapy

THE PLENUM BEHAVIOR THERAPY SERIES
Series Editor: Nathan H. Azrin

ANXIETY MANAGEMENT TRAINING
A Behavior Therapy
Richard M. Suinn

BEHAVIORAL TREATMENT OF ALCOHOL PROBLEMS
Individualized Therapy and Controlled Drinking
Mark B. Sobell and Linda C. Sobell

COGNITIVE-BEHAVIOR MODIFICATION
An Integrative Approach
Donald H. Meichenbaum

HANDBOOK OF EFFECTIVE PSYCHOTHERAPY
Edited by Thomas R. Giles

PHOBIC AND OBSESSIVE-COMPULSIVE DISORDERS
Theory, Research, and Practice
Paul M. G. Emmelkamp

THE TOKEN ECONOMY
A Review and Evaluation
Alan E. Kazdin

Handbook of Effective Psychotherapy

Edited by

Thomas R. Giles

Associates in Managed Care
Denver, Colorado

PLENUM PRESS • NEW YORK AND LONDON

Library of Congress Cataloging-in-Publication Data

Handbook of effective psychotherapy / edited by Thomas R. Giles.
p. cm. -- (The Plenum behavior therapy series)
Includes bibliographical references and index.
ISBN 0-306-44428-3
1. Psychotherapy--Handbooks, manuals, etc. I. Giles, Thomas R.
II. Series: Plenum behavior therapy series.
[DNLM: 1. Psychotherapy--handbooks. WM 34 H2355 1993]
RC456.H35 1993
616.89'14--dc20
DNLM/DLC
for Library of Congress 93-23996
CIP

ISBN 0-306-44428-3

A Division of Plenum Publishing Corporation
233 Spring Street, New York, N.Y. 10013

Printed in the United States of America

To my parents
JACK AND MARIAN GILES
and to my mentors
FREDERICK J. TODD, Ph.D., and JOSEPH WOLPE, M.D.

Contributors

Francis R. Abueg • Behavioral Science Division, National Center to PTSD, Palo Alto VAMC, Palo Alto, California 94304.

John P. Allen • National Institute on Alcohol Abuse and Alcoholism, Rockville, Maryland 20857.

David H. Barlow • Center for Stress and Anxiety Disorders, State University of New York-Albany, Albany, New York 12203.

Dudley David Blake • Clinical Laboratory and Education Division, National Center for PTSD, Palo Alto, California 94304.

Joan Busner • Rockland Children's Psychiatric Center, Orangeburg, New York and College of Physicians and Surgeons of Columbia University, New York, New York 10027.

Cheryl Carmin • St. Louis University Medical Center, Division of Behavioral Medicine, St. Louis, Missouri 63104.

Patricia Chamberlin • Oregon Social Learning Center, Eugene, Oregon 97401.

Guylaine Côté • Center for Stress and Anxiety Disorders, State University of New York-Albany, Albany, New York 12203.

T. J. Dishion • Oregon Social Learning Center, Eugene, Oregon 97401.

Robert Elliott • Department of Psychology, University of Toledo, Toledo, Ohio, 43606.

H. J. Eysenck • Institute of Psychiatry, University of London, London, England.

Thomas R. Giles • Associates in Managed Care, 10200 East Girard Avenue, Suite C-356, Denver, Colorado 80231.

Shirley M. Glynn • West Los Angeles VA Medical Center (Brentwood Division) and University of California, Los Angeles, Los Angeles, California 90073.

Richard G. Heimberg • Center for Stress and Anxiety Disorders, State University of New York-Albany, Albany, New York 12205.

Craig S. Holt • Iowa City VA Medical Center, Iowa City, Iowa 52246.

Debra A. Hope • Department of Psychology, University of Nebraska-Lincoln, Lincoln, Nebraska 68588-0308.

Stuart L. Kaplan • Rockland Children's Psychiatric Center, Orangeburg, New York and College of Physicians and Surgeons of Columbia University, New York, New York 10027.

Terrence M. Keane • Behavioral Science Division, National Center for PTSD, Boston VAMC, Boston, Massachusetts 02130.

Judy Lam • School of Social Work, Boston University, Boston, Massachusetts 02215.

Harold Leitenberg • Department of Psychology, Unviversity of Vermont, Burlington, Vermont 05405.

Marsha M. Linehan • Department of Psychology, University of Washington, Seattle, Washington 98195.

John R. Lutzker • Department of Psychology, Lee College of Judaism, Los Angeles, California 90077.

Margaret E. Mattson • National Institute on Alcohol Abuse and Alcoholism, Rockville, Maryland 20857.

Kim Meuser • Department of Psychiatry, Medical College of Pennsylvania at Eastern Pennsylvanis Psychiatric Institute, Philadelphia, Pennsylvania 19129.

Dan M. Neims • University of Denver, Denver, Colorado 80222.

G. R. Patterson • Oregon Social Learning Center, Eugene, Oregon 97401.

Jacqueline B. Persons • Department of Psychiatry, University of California, San Francisco, California 94143.

Gene Pekarik • Department of Psychology, Washburn University, Topeka, Kansas 66621.

C. Alec Pollard • St. Louis University Medical Center, Division of Behavioral Medicine, St. Louis, Missouri 63104.

Elizabeth M. Prial • University of Denver, Denver, Colorado 80222.

David A. Shapiro • 17 Churchill Avenue, North York, Ontario M2N 122, Canada.

Laurence Shapiro • St. Louis University Medical Center, Division of Behavioral Medicine, St. Louis, Missouri 63104.

Tristram Smith • Department of Psychology, University of California, Los Angeles, Los Angeles, California 90024-1563.

Gail Steketee • School of Social Work, Boston University, Boston, Massachusetts 02215.

William B. Stiles • Department of Psychology, Miami Univesity, Oxford, Ohio 45056.

Ralph M. Turner • Center for Research on Adolescents and Families, Temple University, and Department of Psychiatry, Temple University School of Medicine, Philadelphia, Pennsylvania 19140.

Darren A. Tutek • Department of Psychology, University of Washington, Seattle, Washington 98195.

Steven H. Woodward • Clinical Laboratory and Education Division, National Center for PTSD, Palo Alto, California 94304.

Preface

Handbook of Effective Psychotherapy is the culmination of 15 years of personal interest in the area of psychotherapy outcome research. In my view, this is one of the most interesting and crucial areas in the field: it has relevance across disparate clinical disciplines and orientations; it provides a measure of how far the field has progressed in its efforts to improve the effectiveness of psychotherapeutic intervention; and it provides an ongoing measure of how readily clinicians adapt to scientific indications in state-of-the-art care.

Regrettably, as several of the chapters in this volume indicate, there is a vast chasm between what is known about the best available treatments and what is applied as the usual standard of care. On the most basic level there appears to be a significant number of clinicians who remain reluctant to acknowledge that scientific study can add to their ability to aid the emotionally distressed. I hope that this handbook, with its many delineations of empirically supported treatments, will do something to remedy this state of affairs.

There is, of course, another subgroup of clinicians who values the results of research but believes that all therapies, because of "unspecified" mechanisms, yield roughly equivalent results. Despite more than a decade of experience with this reaction, I remain surprised that others still hold to this position given the published research findings of the last 30 years. I hope that some members of this subgroup will be sufficiently persuaded by the chapters in this handbook to experiment with the procedures identified herein to be the most effective. Whenever I read yet another article assuming the equivalence argument, however (and these are still being published by the score), I realize that this issue is so emotionally charged that no amount of research will be persuasive to all.

There is yet another subgroup that is receptive to what has been demonstrated by empirical study but that is unsure of the findings presented in the literature or where to go to obtain them. This subgroup, which, along with clinicians and academicians includes managed mental health care companies, administrators, chief executive officers, human services directors, and other policymakers should find this handbook of use. The chapters on specific disorders, while cautious as to the methodological limits of the findings and studies reviewed, provide a direction for disorder-driven care that stands to improve upon the outcomes usually observed.

The handbook is organized into three sections. The first part includes two general reviews. Eysenck first reviews the demonstrated efficacy of the traditional psychotherapies. The second review, written by my co-authors and me, provides an appendix of more than 100 studies indicating that certain types of directive treatment interventions result in outcomes superior to those observed with more traditional forms of care.

The next section is a compilation of reviews indicating which treatments appear to get the best outcomes, organized by disorder. These chapters provide the essence of the handbook.

The final section represents an attempt to acknowledge that the advances in research cited in Parts I and II have been accompanied by controversy and by the discovery of numerous areas in which the field can still improve. Pekarik's chapter, for example, while acknowledging the superior efficacy of cognitive and behavioral interventions, points out that these therapies have consistently overlooked various phenomena from the consumer preference literature. These oversights have adversely affected the outcomes of these varieties of care. At my request, Elliott, Stiles, and Shapiro provide a counterpoint to the thesis of my own chapters and to that of a number of the disorder-specific chapters. Among other things, this counterargument points to methodological weaknesses in the research, Rosenthal effects, and other possible research biases. As an additional attempt to provide a forum for the expression of countervailing points of view, a chapter on the merits of integrationism was invited. In this chapter, while also acknowledging the proven efficacy of cognitive and behavioral techniques, Turner argues that the contributions from other theorists may still lend substantial value and additional effectiveness to what are currently recognized as the most effective forms of care.

As this handbook will make clear, it is very difficult to take a stand on the comparative effectiveness of virtually any technique, orientation, or procedure without exciting adverse passions and charges of bias. Ironically, my experience as editor indicated that, if anything, the authors of the disorder-specific chapters took great pains to avoid anything but a conservative and cautious approach. I was interested to observe that, in more than half of the chapters, the authors did not at first specifically identify a treatment of choice despite their having presented research findings that justified a preference. I became so intrigued with this phenomenon that I began an informal survey of the authors' reticence. Their stated reasons included a fear of "retaliation" or criticism, as has been observed frequently, from traditionally oriented colleagues; the conservative influence of scientific training and philosophy of science; and a general distaste for anything that could be construed as an unreasoned championship of a "cause," regardless of the degree to which the authors believed their arguments were indeed correct. Perhaps John Allen, the first author of the chapter on the treatment of alcoholism, spoke best for the authors with his reply: "We do not wish to condemn the field of practice, much as it concerns us."

Since completing this handbook, I have left the directorship of a managed care company in order to start my own consulting firm. As such, I am most interested in the reaction to this volume by readership. Correspondence can be sent to me at the following address:

THOMAS R. GILES, Psy.D.
President
Associates in Managed Care
10200 East Girard Avenue
Suite C-356
Denver, Colorado 80231

Acknowledgments

After reading an article on psychotherapy outcome that I published in *The Behavior Therapist*, Dr. Nathan Azrin called to suggest that I expand the topic into an edited handbook. I am very grateful to Dr. Azrin for his suggestion and for his subsequent editorial support. I am also grateful to Drs. Alan Gross and Arthur Freeman, former editors of the journal, for encouraging me to write the article in the first place.

I am indebted to Joe Strahan, Dr. Randy Cox, and Mark Johnson, former executives of MCC Managed Behavioral Care, Inc., for their support of my work as Executive Director while I was employed by this firm. I am especially grateful to Mark Johnson for allowing me four hours a week—for several consecutive months—away from the office to complete this handbook.

Until one actually undertakes a project of this sort, it is difficult to realize the amount of time and effort it requires. Eliot Werner, Executive Editor for Medical and Social Sciences, and Herman Makler, Senior Production Editor for Plenum, provided much aid with this process. Their courtesy and efficiency made it all endurable, and I am happy to be able to extend my gratitude for their work.

Contents

I. REVIEWS OF THE OUTCOME LITERATURE

II. THE MOST EFFECTIVE TREATMENTS BY DISORDER

III. CRITICAL COMMENTARY

I

REVIEWS OF THE OUTCOME LITERATURE

1

Forty Years On

The Outcome Problem in Psychotherapy Revisited

H. J. Eysenck

Introduction

The problem of the effectiveness of psychotherapy has to be considered in the broad context of the agonizingly slow shift from common sense to science. The famous physicist Eddington used to give the example of the two tables: the one common sense recognizes—solid, having weight, reflecting light, with a flat surface and sturdy legs; the other as seen by science, constituted of empty space in which innumerable molecules dance their gavotte, electrons spinning around nuclei in never-ending circles. Common sense has told us much about physics, and we could not exist without that knowledge. We walk, run, and jump by keeping at bay the forces of gravity. We throw spears, shoot arrows, kick footballs, smash tennis balls with great accuracy, taking into account wind strength and direction, air pressure, and many other physical variables. We build igloos and tipis, we construct temples and palaces, all without the guidance of science. Even animals cope with nature most successfully; tigers jump, gazelles flee, monkeys climb—they all go their way by learning in the hard school of life.

The same is true of psychology. If we could not guess the motives of our friends and enemies, anticipate the behavior of our nearest and dearest, know about love and lust, hatred and despair, fun and laughter, how could we live in society, get on with other people, form communes, create nations? Our cognitions, without any scientific contribution, are often uncannily correct, and frequently anticipate later scientific discoveries. Galen 2,000 years ago laid the foundation of modern personality theory by describing the "four temperaments"; Plato anticipated Freud's ego, superego, and id in his fable of the charioteer and the good and the bad horse; Cicero described the difference between "state" and "trait" anxiety. The great German poet Goethe laid down quite clearly the basic law of behavior therapy when he said: "To heal psychic ailments, the understanding avails nothing, reasoning little, time much, but resolute action everything." And to prove it, he used desensitization, relaxation, and flooding with response prevention to cure

---

H. J. Eysenck • Institute of Psychiatry, University of London, London SE5 8AF England

Handbook of Effective Psychotherapy, edited by Thomas R. Giles. Plenum Press, New York, 1993.

his own neuroses (Eysenck, 1990b). And did not Maimonides apply instrumental conditioning to education 800 years before Skinner, while Maconochie used a token economy on prisoners in the middle of the last century, and very successfully, too? (Eysenck, 1972).

Two thousand years ago, Seneca pointed out that "*plura faciunt homines e consuctudine quam e ratione*" (People act more from habit than from reason), neatly anticipating William James's chapter on habit. Another hint that commonsense psychology is not without merit comes from the testimony of poets, dramatists, and writers who have distilled such knowledge in the form of poems, plays, and novels. Shakespeare, Sophocles, Goethe, Corneille, Dante, and Cervantes must have had some insight into human psychology, even if not based on scientific data collected under controlled conditions—not as reliable as experimental results, but perhaps more relevant to their everyday concerns. Hermeneutics has tried to follow the same path, without much success.

If we are such wonderful psychologists and physicists, why do we need science? The answer, of course, is that while we are often right, we also are often wrong. The world does not rest on the back of a giant elephant that stands on a giant tortoise, as the ancient Egyptians thought. The earth is not flat, nor does the sun circle round it. "Eye of newt and toe of frog, wool of bat and tongue of dog" are not going to cure our ailments, and prayer will not fulfill our wishes. Our psychological diagnoses are often faulty, with disastrous consequences. We have no idea of how to deal with criminals and psychopaths, and our educational failures are notorious. We do best where reward and punishment give immediate results, but elsewhere we surely need all the help science can give us.

How little science may be needed is shown by the fact that chimpanzees have discovered the healing properties of certain plants, sharing this discovery with humans (Sears, 1990). How much we need science is shown by the fact that a famous drug like diazepam has no effect other than placebo (Shapiro, Struening, Shapiro, & Milcarek, 1983). We are often misled into thinking that an effect occurs because we feel it ought to—thus class size between 20 and 40 should influence scholastic achievement but does not (Glass & Smith, 1979).

Given the wide spread of anxiety, depression, tenseness, guilt feelings, and other neurotic symptoms, it would be strange if society had not discovered methods of alleviating the resulting misery. And, indeed, we had witch doctors, shamans, priests, teachers, gurus, and other social agents trying to deal with psychological states thousands of years before psychiatry became a (putative) science. In addition, friends, relatives, prostitutes, and even strangers are often drawn into the circle of neurotic illness and are made to listen, advise, and commiserate; has not psychotherapy been called "the prostitution of friendship"? I have no doubt that all these helpers, and the methods they use, have been of immense utility; if they had not, it is unlikely that they would be so universal in their application, and so sought out by sufferers.

This "commonsense therapy" lies at the core of what has become known as "spontaneous recovery," that is, the fact that neurotic sufferers with even severe symptoms of anxiety, depression, phobias, and the like tend to recover without psychiatric help within a year or two (Eysenck, 1952). This recovery is not spontaneous in the sense of being uncaused; it happens because of events occurring over time, the events being the commonsense therapeutic interventions sought out by the sufferers.

This spontaneous recovery involves a kind of placebo therapy, in the sense that the therapy does not contain any ingredients deriving from a scientific theory of neurosis and is not applied by trained practitioners. Like all placebos, it can nevertheless be very powerful in its effect, particularly because it does in fact include important ingredients similar to, or even identical with, those contained in theory-derived behavior therapy. I will go into this point in detail later on; here let me merely note that "placebo" treatment in psychotherapy is not as straightforward a concept as it is in physical medicine (Meyer, 1990). As I shall argue later, commonsense therapy, placebo treatment, and psychotherapy all contain elements of behavior therapy which make them, in effect, successful as treatments, however unplanned this admixture may be (Eysenck, 1980).

It would follow that all types of psychological treatment are likely to be successful, but that none can be called scientific unless it is (1) based on a properly tested theory and (2) has effects clearly superior to spontaneous remission or placebo treatment (Eysenck, 1952).

Is Psychotherapy Effective?

Fifty years ago, it was widely believed and taught that psychoanalysis was the only acceptable method of treatment for neurotic patients, being the only method that concerned itself with *causes* rather than merely with *symptoms*; that symptomatic treatment might be superficially successful, but that it would soon be followed by a recurrence of symptoms, or symptom substitution; that "deep," "psychodynamic," and long-lasting investigations by trained psychoanalysts were required to produce stable and long-lasting cures; and that such cures could only be effected by analysts who had themselves been psychoanalyzed. Diagnoses and cures might be helped by administering psychodynamically oriented projection tests, like the Rorschach or the Thematic Apperception Test; the emphasis of both tests and treatment was on unconscious causes, transference phenomena, and early childhood experiences reconstructed through analysis of dreams and through other types of "dynamic" evidence.

Few knowledgeable psychologists and psychiatrists would now deny that there was no objective evidence for any of these beliefs. There were no clinical studies comparing the progress of neurotic patients under psychoanalysis with that of similar patients receiving no treatment or placebo treatment; it was often suggested that it would be unethical to withhold such obvious beneficial treatment as psychoanalysis from patients, disregarding the fact that of all the people suffering from severe neurotic illness in the United States, less than 0.01% would in fact receive psychoanalytic treatment! The superiority of psychoanalysis was simply assumed on the basis of pseudoscientific arguments, not empirical evidence. It was often suggested that the cases treated and described by Freud provided such evidence, but apart from the obvious point that there were no controls involved in his work, and no follow-ups, it is now well known that Freud was very economical with the truth—as far as description of his famous cases is concerned—and that the alleged cures in fact were not cures at all (Eysenck, 1985a). Thus, the famous "Wolf Man" was not in fact cured but continued with the selfsame symptoms, from which Freud claimed to have relieved him, for the next 60 years of his life, being under constant treatment during this time (Obholzer, 1982)! Similarly, the famous "cure" of Anna O. by Breuer, which was supposed to constitute the beginnings of psychoanalytic treatment, was shown by historians to have been a misdiagnosis and the cure a fraud (Thornton, 1983). Anna O. was not a hysteric but suffered from tuberculous meningitis, and she lived in a hospital for many years with the selfsame symptoms (Hirschmueller, 1989). The "Rat Man" was far from a therapeutic success as claimed, and Freud's process notes deviate notably from his final account (Mahony, 1986). It would be difficult to adduce these and other cases treated by Freud as evidence of psychoanalytic successes (Eysenck, 1985a).

Outcomes, then, were being completely disregarded, and the only kind of clinical studies being done were concerned with problems internal to the analytic process, it being assumed that psychoanalysis was not only the best but the only method of treatment. It seemed to me from the beginning that this was entirely the wrong way to look at the whole problem of psychotherapy (Eysenck, 1990a). Both from the theoretical and the practical points of view, the outcome problem was the most important and critical of all; if psychoanalysis, or psychotherapy in general, which was then as it is now largely based on Freudian assumptions, did not in fact do better than placebo treatments or no treatment at all, then clearly the theory on which it is based was wrong. Similarly, if there were no positive effects of psychoanalysis as a therapy, then it would be completely unethical to apply this method to patients, to charge them money for such treatment, or to train therapists in these unsuccessful methods. The practical importance of the issue will be clear without any great discussion, but the theoretical implications have been debated for a long time, and it has been asserted that even if the therapy itself does not work, the theory might nevertheless be correct. I took it for granted that if a treatment method based on theory does not work, then this suggests that the theory itself must be faulty. Grunbaum (1979, 1984) has argued the case in considerable detail and has come to a very similar conclusion. I will return to this point presently.

There were some dissenting voices asking for empirical evidence and looking critically at such comparative studies as were available (e.g., Denker, 1946; Landis, 1937; Salter, 1952; Wilder, 1945; Zubin, 1953). In 1952, I carried out an analysis of all the published material concerning recovery from neurotic illness after psychoanalysis, after psychotherapy, or after no treatment of a psychiatric nature at all (Eysenck, 1952); the results were published in an article which has been referred to as "the most influential evaluation of psychotherapy" (Kazdin, 1978, p. 33). In this article (Eysenck, 1952), I examined a number of outcome studies that primarily evaluated treatment of neurotic patients. I attempted to assess the effects of psychotherapy by comparing its outcome with an estimate of improvements in patients that occur in the absence of therapy. I concluded that approximately 67% of seriously ill patients recover within 2 years, even in the absence of formal psychotherapy. If we regard this figure as an approximate baseline against which treatment can be evaluated, then we can compare therapy outcome with it, and I found a cure rate of approximately the same magnitude. Thus, remissions with no treatment ("spontaneous remission") occur as often as recovery with psychotherapy or psychoanalysis. This is still apparently true (Svartberg & Stiles, 1991).

I took up the topic of effectiveness again in 1960 and in 1965, summarizing the large number of articles that had appeared, partly as a consequence of stressing the importance of the outcome problem. The results were not very dissimilar to my previous analysis, and more recent work has not disproved my assertion.

Arguments about Effectiveness

In these articles about the effectiveness of psychotherapy, I made a number of other points, which have not always been considered by critics. I emphasized the need for carefully controlled therapy research that not only takes into account spontaneous remission, but also controls for nonspecific treatment effects, that is, the inclusion of placebo treatment in assessment. I also pointed out that showing therapy to be superior to no treatment is not sufficient to demonstrate that any particular technique or ingredient of therapy is effective; nonspecific treatment effects, such as attending treatment or meeting with the therapist, would still have to be ruled out to argue for specific benefits of treatment (Eysenck, 1966). Arguments pro and con were taken up by many contributors, whose points of view are summarized by Kazdin (1978) and Schorr (1984). It would not be useful to take up these arguments here again, but it may be worthwhile to look at more recent surveys of the burgeoning literature and to see to what extent more recent studies have validated or invalidated my original conclusions.

Before turning to this task, however, I will consider the degree to which psychoanalysts have responded to the widespread criticism voiced concerning the efficacy of their treatment. Following the principle that criticism should be directed at what is regarded as the best, rather than the worst, project in the area, I will look at the Menninger Clinic project (Kernberg, 1972, 1973), a lavishly financed study published after 18 years of work. The aim of the project was to "explore changes brought about in patients by psychoanalytically oriented psychotherapies and psychoanalysis" (Kernberg, 1972, p. 3). Forty-two adult neurotic patients were studied, those in psychoanalytic therapy receiving an average of 835 hours of treatment, and those in psychoanalytically oriented psychotherapy receiving an average of 289 hours. A detailed criticism of the project has been made by Rachman and Wilson (1980). Listing such obvious faults as contamination, nonrandom allocation, and absence of any control, the authors of the Menninger report themselves admit that the most severe limitation of their study was its "lack of formal experimental design" (Kernberg, 1972, p. 76). They point out that it was not possible:

> (I) To list the variables needed to test the theories;
> (II) To have methods of quantification of the variables, preferably existing scales which would have adequate reliability and validity;
> (III) To be able to choose and provide controlled conditions which would rule out alternative explanations for the results;
> (IV) To state the hypotheses to be tested; or finally,
> (V) To conduct the research according to the design. (Kernberg, 1972, p. 75)

As Rachman and Wilson correctly point out,

> This astonishing conclusion can have few equals . . . one is left with a study that is so flawed as to preclude any conclusions whatsoever. Whilst the honesty of this self-appraisal is highly commendable, one cannot help wondering how the authors succeeded in persuading large and reputable foundations to provide them with financial support extending over many years. How does one persuade a foundation to uphold research which, in the words of the authors themselves, lacks a formal experimental design, or methods of quantification, or hypotheses? And which cannot be conducted "according to the design"? (Rachman & Wilson, 1980, p. 73)

(Over a million dollars was spent on the project, at a time when this was a considerable amount of money!)

Did this waste of time and money induce in the authors of the report a suitable feeling of humility? Malan (1976, p. 21) states: "When I met Dr. Kernberg at the meeting of the Society for Psychotherapy Research in Philadelphia, in 1973, he said that the problem of measuring outcome on psychodynamic criteria was essentially solved, and I could only agree with him." It is difficult not to resort to a quotation: "*Quem Jupiter vult perdere dementat prius*" (Whom Jupiter wants to destroy, he first renders mad). Clearly, psychoanalysts have learned nothing and forgotten nothing! They have no intention of submitting their beliefs to any kind of empirical scrutiny; they prefer assertion to demonstration. Anyone seriously interested in this topic ought to read the detailed critique by Rachman and Wilson (1980) to discover how far intellectual vacuity can go.

Am I being too hard in my interpretation? As Anthony Storr, one of the best known psychoanalysts in England, wrote in 1966 (as quoted by Wood, 1990):

> The American Psychoanalytic Association, who might be supposed to be prejudiced in favour of their own speciality, undertook a survey to test the efficacy of psychoanalysis. The results obtained were so disappointing that they were withheld from publication. . . . The evidence that psychoanalysis cures anyone of anything is so shaky as to be practically non-existent.

The Present Position

How true are the conclusions I drew in the early 1950s at the present time? Rachman and Wilson (1980) have provided us with to date the best and most honest survey of the literature, and it is reassuring that their verdict is not so very different from the one I arrived at 30 years before their survey appeared. A quotation makes clear their overall evaluation:

> The need for strict evaluation of the effects of various forms of therapy arises from several observations. In the first place, there is clear evidence of a substantial remission; as a result any therapeutic procedure must be shown to be superior to "non-professional" processes of change. Closely allied to this point is the wide range of therapeutic procedures currently on offer and the competing and often exclusive claims for effectiveness. The lengthy business of separating the wheat from the chaff can only be accomplished by the introduction of strict and rational forms of evaluation. One important function of strict evaluation would be to root out those ineffective or even harmful methods that are being recommended. The availability of incisive methods of evaluation might have averted the sorry episode during which coma treatment was given to a large number of hopeful but undiscriminating patients.
>
> The occurrence of spontaneous remissions of neurotic disorders provided a foundation stone for Eysenck's (1952) skeptical evaluation of the case for psychotherapy. His analysis of the admittedly insufficient data at the time led Eysenck to accept as the best available estimate the figure that roughly two-thirds of all neurotic disorders will remit spontaneously within 2 years of onset. Our review of the evidence that has accumulated during the past 25 years does not put us in a position to revise Eysenck's original estimate, but there is a strong case for refining his estimate for each of a group of different neurotic disorders; the early assumption of uniformity of spontaneous remission rates among different disorders is increasingly difficult to defend.

Given the widespread occurrence of spontaneous remissions, and it is difficult to see how they can any longer be denied, the claims made for the specific value of particular forms of psychotherapy begin to look exaggerated. It comes as a surprise to find how meagre is the evidence to support the wide-ranging claims made or implied by psychoanalytic therapists. The lengthy descriptions of spectacular improvements achieved in particular cases are outnumbered by the descriptions of patients whose analyses appear to be interminable. More important, however, is the rarity of any form of controlled evaluation of the effects of psychoanalysis. We are unaware of any methodical study of this kind which has taken adequate account of spontaneous changes or, more importantly, of the contribution of non-specific therapeutic influences such as placebo effects, expectancy, and so on. In view of the ambitiousness, scope, and influence of psychoanalysis, one might be inclined to recommend to one's scientific colleagues an attitude of continuing patience, but for the fact that insufficient progress has been made in either acknowledging the need for stringent scientific evaluations or in establishing criteria of outcome that are even half-way satisfactory. One suspects, however, that consumer groups will prove to be far less patient when they finally undertake an examination of the evidence on which the claims of psychoanalytic effectiveness now rest. (Rachman & Wilson, 1980, p. 259)

The rather negative evaluation of psychoanalysis, and indeed other forms of psychotherapy, to which Rachman and Wilson are finally forced contrasts spectacularly with conclusions arrived at by authors like Bergin (1971), Bergin and Lambert (1978), Lambert (1976), and Luborsky, Singer, and Luborsky (1975). The latter, in a memorable phrase, summarized their comparative studies of psychotherapies in the quotation "Everyone has won, and all must have prizes." This quote illustrates the "Alice in Wonderland" atmosphere of the psychotherapy field, as do the equally optimistic conclusions of Bergin and his colleagues.

Looking at Meta-Analysis

Where Luborsky, Bergin, and Lambert at least pretend to some kind of scientific objectivity, a much praised book by Smith, Glass, and Miller (1980) provides the seeds of its own destruction, without requiring any aid from outside critics. The contents of this book, which essentially aims at a meta-analysis of all published studies to date, amount to an essential contradiction of the conclusions I drew in 1952 and which were virtually unchanged in the review by Rachman and Wilson (1980). To illustrate this argument, let me quote the general conclusions drawn by Smith *et al.* (1980) from their data. They assert that

Psychotherapy is beneficial, consistently so and in many different ways. Its benefits are on a par with other expensive ambitious interventions, such as schooling and medicine. The benefits of psychotherapy are not permanent, but then little is. (p. 183, italics in original)

They go on to say

The evidence overwhelmingly supports the efficacy of psychotherapy . . . psychotherapy benefits people of all ages as reliably as schooling educates them, medicine cures them, or business turns a profit. (p. 183)

Apparently, psychotherapy sometimes seeks the same goals as education and medicine, and when it does, psychotherapy performs commendably well:

> We are suggesting no less than that psychotherapists have a legitimate, though not exclusive, claim, substantiated by controlled research, of those roles in society, whether privately or publicly endowed, whose responsibility is to restore to health the sick, the suffering, the alienated, and the disaffected. (p. 183)

Smith *et al.* then go on to repeat the Luborsky *et al.* view that

> Different types of psychotherapy (verbal or behavioral); psychodynamic, client-centered, or systematic desensitization) do not produce different types or degrees of benefit. (p. 184)

Allied to this odd conclusion is another one, to wit, that

> *Differences in how psychotherapy is conducted, whether in groups or individually, by experienced or novice therapists, for long or short periods of time, and the like make very little difference in how beneficial it is.* (p. 188, italics in original)

Actually, the data presented in Table 5–1 of Smith *et al.* completely contradict their own conclusions; for instance, they found average effect sizes of 0.28 for undifferentiated counseling and of 0.14 for reality therapy, with figures like 1.82 for hypnotherapy and 2.38 for cognitive therapies. These figures do not suggest equality of effectiveness! The authors also fail to note a very important conclusion from the same table; that is, placebo treatment (effect size 0.56) is as effective as Gestalt therapy (0.64), client-centered therapy (0.62), or psychodynamic therapy (0.69). Clearly, their own conclusions force us to argue that all the vaunted effects of psychotherapy are simply placebo effects (a conclusion also arrived at in the much more meaningful analysis carried out by Prioleau, Murdoch, and Brody, 1983). It is curious that almost none of the reviewers of the book saw this obvious contradiction between data and conclusions or commented on the devastating effects this contradiction must have on the claims for efficacy of psychotherapy.

Much the same must be said about the final conclusion of the book, which states that the effectiveness of therapy has little to do with the experience of the therapist or the length of treatment. If that is true, then, clearly, claims by psychoanalysts that their discipline requires a lengthy training period and a lengthy time to establish and then resolve transference relations are completely unjustified. Obviously, therapists should have just one hour's training and treatment should be one hour's duration; according to Smith *et al.* (1980), these restrictions should make no difference to the outcome! As in *Alice in Wonderland,* we should apparently follow the practice of The Red Queen to believe as many as six impossible things before breakfast. To believe the conclusions of Smith *et al.* would certainly constitute good practice for that.

Smith *et al.*, curiously enough, do discover that behavior therapy is more effective than psychotherapy, but they try to argue this conclusion out of existence with a rather specious argument. Eysenck and Martin (1987), who have discussed this question in some detail, have come to the conclusion that not only is a learning theory of neurosis the only scientific theory available at present but the methods of treatment to which it gives rise are the only ones more effective than no treatment or placebo treatment. Thus, the spontaneous remission objection does not apply to behavior therapy; Rachman and Hodgson's (1980) book presents an excellent example of the treatment of obsessive-compulsive behavior. The failure of psychotherapy to achieve a similar status, alas, does not seem to have reduced the ardor with which many therapists still proclaim its virtues and foist it on innocent victims.

Wittmann and Matt (1986) carried out a meta-analysis of German studies of psychotherapy and its effectiveness. Their results, which coincided with the true interpretation of the Smith *et al.* data, showed that "not everybody has won, therefore not all must have prizes" (p. 35); in particular, "therapies with behavioral orientation show the highest effects" (p. 35).

This general superiority of behavioral over "dynamic" types of therapy is well recognized (e.g., Giles, 1983a, 1983b, 1990). It is also found in the fields of criminality and psychopathy, where comparisons of the two types of therapies have been done. Andrews *et al.* (1980) conclude their analysis of published work by saying that "appropriate types of service . . . involve the use of behavioral and social learning principles of interpersonal influence, skill enhancement, and cognitive change. Specifically, they include modeling, graduated practice, rehearsal, role playing, reinforcement, resource provision, and detailed verbal guidance and explanation" (p. 375). Andrews *et al.* also point out that "traditional psychodynamic and nondirective client-centered therapies are to be avoided within general samples of offenders" (p. 376). Note that even with this group of clients, where little was expected, a 53% reduction in recidivism was achieved! This is a remarkable outcome in what is usually a disaster area.

The Importance of Theory

I would like to look in some detail at some of the consequences of the conclusions drawn by Luborsky *et al.*, Bergin, and Smith *et al.* from their analyses, faulty as these are. First, take the argument that all types of therapy are equally effective, and that this proves the correctness of the views of those who support the effectiveness of psychotherapeutic research and the theories on which this effectiveness is based. If it is true that different methods of psychotherapy (let us call them $T_1, T_2, T_3 \ldots T_n$) have indeed been shown to be equally effective in reducing or abolishing the neurotic illnesses for which they have been recommended, then it should be obvious that such an outcome would not support the hypotheses or theories (let us call them $H_1, H_2, H_3 \ldots H_n$) on which the treatments were based, but would completely disprove them. Consider psychoanalysis as T_1. This is based on H_1, which asserts that only psychoanalytic methods can produce a proper cure, and that all other methods must inevitably fail to do so. But according to Luborsky *et al.*, $T_2, T_3 \ldots T_n$ are equally successful as T_1; this clearly demonstrates that H_1 is incorrect, because it predicted the opposite, namely, that $T_2, T_3 \ldots T_n$ would have no effect or, at most, a markedly weaker effect than T_1.

Much the same can be said for all the other types of treatment—client-centered, Gestalt, primary therapy, and the like. They are all based on specific hypotheses which assert that the respective methods of treatment should be superior to all others; if they are not, then surely the theories themselves cannot be correct. If it can also be shown that placebo treatments are as effective as genuine treatments, then it should become plain that the outcome of all these studies must be that it is nonspecific factors, such as discussing one's troubles with a friendly person, receiving advice, relieving one's tensions through receiving positive reactions, and so forth, which are effective in mediating therapeutic success, rather than the specific methods derived from the various theories in question. If indeed all have won, and all must have prizes, then that surely spells the definite rebuttal to all the theories psychotherapists have fought so earnestly to elaborate and establish. I have elsewhere discussed "the place of theory in a world of facts" (Eysenck, 1985d), agreeing with Kurt Lewin that "there is nothing as practical as a good theory," and with Kant that "practice without theory is blind, theory without practice is lame." On this one point I agree with Freud; for a therapy to deserve the term "scientific," it must be based on a sound theory, with proper academic and experimental support (Eysenck, 1985d). No such experimental support, of course, has ever been forthcoming for Freudian theories (Eysenck & Wilson, 1973). As Gossop (1981) has shown, there really is no such theory other than the conditioning theory developed by Pavlov, Watson, and Wolpe, which I have lately refined and restated (Eysenck, 1976b, 1977, 1979, 1982, 1987a, 1987b; Eysenck & Kelley, 1987; Eysenck & Rachman, 1965). Such a restatement was clearly necessary because of the many well-justified criticisms which had been leveled at the Watson–Mowrer version of Pavlovian theory.

The major changes I made were as follows: (1) replacing Pavlovian conditioning A by Pavlovian conditioning B (Grant, 1964) as the fundamental basis of neurosis acquisition and (2) using genetic factors and "preparedness" in addition to conditioning as the fundamental building blocks of a natural science theory of neurosis and of treatment (Eysenck, 1986, 1987b; Eysenck & Beech, 1971; Eysenck & Martin, 1987).

This renovated theory, relying on the concept of "incubation" of conditional fear responses (Eysenck, 1985b), is in principle able to cope with all the known facts of neurosis genesis and treatment; it also makes it possible to accommodate the known facts of psychotherapy effectiveness, placebo treatment, and spontaneous remission (Eysenck, 1980). Per contra, psychoanalytic and dynamic theories have followed the course of a *degenerative* research program, rather than a *progressive* one like behavior therapy (Lakatos, 1970). As Smith *et al.* discovered to their discomfort, behavior therapy fared better than psychotherapy—a finding they tried to discredit by some contrafactual arguments.

The Question of Spontaneous Remission

Second, I will look at the foundation of Bergin and Lambert's (1978) critique of my original work, namely, that my original suggestion of a spontaneous remission rate of about two-thirds is much too high. As Bergin and Lambert say, "*It can be noted that the two-thirds estimate is not only unrepresentative but is actually the most unrealistic figure for describing the spontaneous remission rate or even rates for minimal treatment outcomes*" (p. 147, italics in original).

My estimate was based on data published by Landis (1937) and Denker (1946), which gave an estimate of spontaneous remission effects of something like two-thirds; Bergin (1971) compiled a table containing 14 studies and provided percentage improvement rates for each. The rates vary from 0% to 56% and "the median rate appears to be in the vicinity of 30%!" Although his figures "have their weaknesses," Bergin nevertheless felt that "they are the best available to date" and that they rest "upon a much more solid base" than the Landis–Denker data. In the face of such a large discrepancy, which is obviously vital in coming to any conclusions, it is essential to study the figures and arguments in detail. This has been done very carefully by Rachman and Wilson (1980), and the reader is referred to their discussion. I will only quote brief excerpts to illustrate the essential dishonesty of the Bergin and Lambert argument:

> Before commencing the close examination of what Bergin presents as the best available data, two points should be borne in mind. In the first place it seems to be a curious procedure in which one rediscovers data and then calculates a median rate of improvement, while ignoring the data on which the original argument was based. The new data (actually some of them are chronologically older than those of Landis–Denker) should have been considered in conjunction with, or at least in the light of, the existing information. The second point is that although Bergin considered some new evidence, he missed a number of studies more pertinent to the question of spontaneous recovery rates. His estimate of a 30% spontaneous recovery rate is based on the fourteen studies which are incorporated in Table 8 of this work. It will be noticed that the list omits some of the studies discussed earlier in this chapter, which antedate Bergin's review. (p. 41)

Rachman and Wilson give a list of the 14 studies cited in Bergin's review and then go on to a detailed discussion of each.

They demonstrate that several of the studies described are completely irrelevant to the issue, because they do not deal with neurotic disorders at all, give no figures which could be interpreted, or are not concerned with spontaneous remission! Their devastating critique should be read by anyone interested in this very important issue.

Negative Effects of Psychotherapy

If a therapist (whether teacher, friend, priest, psychoanalyst, or witch doctor) helps a sufferer by incorporating certain attitudes into therapy—reassurance, advice, help, warmth of personal reaction, encouraging an increase in autonomy—then it would seem to follow that harm may be done to the sufferer if these affirming attitudes are withheld (as in classical psychoanalysis). Mays and Franks (1985) and Strupp, Hadley, and Gomes-Schwartz (1977) have amply documented the fact that psychoanalysis, in particular, and dynamic therapies, in general, can indeed have disastrous results and worsen the state of neurotic patients (I have tried to explain this negative effect in theoretical terms; Eysenck, 1985c). It is curious that these facts are seldom if ever mentioned in the current literature in psychiatry or clinical psychology.

Altogether, it may be said that textbooks in psychotherapy fail to give an accurate picture of the situation. Howarth (1989) reviewed 10 recent texts in this field and finds that they do not show any interest in questioning or even asserting the value of the products they discuss.

> I looked carefully but in vain . . . for any reference to evaluation, assessment, cure, termination, outcome or any other word which might indicate a concern for the effect of their interventions on the clients. . . . The impression created by [these] books is appalling. But it is not extraordinary since the same characteristics are shown in approximately 90 per cent of the volumes dealing with psychotherapy, counselling and social work which are currently on sale at any good bookstore. (p. 150)

Howarth explains this odd state of affairs on the basis of two false beliefs:

> The first is the common belief that psychotherapists can learn from experience. Given the lack of specificity of the effects of psychotherapy, this is unlikely to be the case, but some reviewers go further than this, and present evidence that psychotherapists do not learn from experience. The second of these false beliefs is that scientific evaluation is not appropriate for procedures which deal with existential (or some other such phrase) rather than factual matters. They require, it is suggested, a phenomenological or hermeneutic approach. This excuse is worse than the primary fault, since it assumes that clients should be interested in their own constructional reality and not in the effects which they have on other people, nor in more objective measures of their well-being. It would be very difficult to convince the clients themselves of this. (pp. 150–151)

Ignorance and complete disregard for the lack of evidence for positive effects, and for the well-authenticated presence of negative effects, are thus endemic in modern clinical psychology (Eysenck, 1990b).

Psychosomatic Effects of Psychotherapy

Yet both the beneficial effects of behavior therapy and the negative effects of dynamic psychotherapy extend well beyond the field of neurosis and take in psychosomatic disorders and even the most serious medical diseases like cancer and coronary heart disease (CHD) (Eysenck, 1991). Grossarth-Maticek and Eysenck (1991) and Eysenck and Grossarth-Maticek (1991) have shown that behavior therapy directed toward increasing the autonomy of healthy people who are cancer-prone or CHD-prone can lessen dramatically their mortality rates. They have also shown that terminally ill cancer patients can be helped by the same kind of therapy to prolong life by almost 100% (i.e., doubling life expectancy), compared with nontherapy controls. What are the effects of psychoanalysis under similar circumstances?

Grossarth-Maticek and Eysenck (1990) investigated the effect of orthodox psychoanalytic treatment on the eventual probability of death from cancer and coronary heart disease in healthy probands treated by psychoanalysis for over 2 years, probands who broke off psychoanalytic treatment after less than 2 years, and various control groups. At 7-year follow-up, psychoanalysis was found to have had a significantly *negative* effect on survival. The effects were distinctly of a dose–response kind, being more negative the longer the psychoanalytic treatment. Table 1.1 shows the resulting mortality data. Probands were divided at the beginning of the study into a cancer-prone type (Type 1), a CHD-prone type (Type 2), and two healthy types (Type 3 and Type 4) (Eysenck, 1988, 1989; Grossarth-Maticek, Eysenck, & Vetter, 1988).

Probands were asked whether treatment had increased or decreased their autonomy. Table 1.2 shows the results; it appears that decreasing autonomy, which is a characteristic feature of psychoanalysis, had a very negative effect, while treatment which uncharacteristically increased autonomy had little effect either way. (Many psychoanalysts use methods and aim at results which are quite at variance with Freudian intentions.)

These results, while touched upon only briefly here, are of great importance. Subjective improvement in neurotic patients is difficult to operationalize and measure objectively; mortality is both more important and more objective, and to see the effectiveness of behavior therapy for positive outcome and the effectiveness of psychoanalysis for negative outcome so clearly demonstrated adds verisimilitude to our findings on psychological effects.

How is it possible that psychoanalysis can have such devastating effects? Remember that *stress* plays an important part in liability to cancer and CHD and shortens the life of patients so affected (Eysenck, 1991). As psychoanalysts themselves have stated, their treatment constitutes an enormous psychological stress for the first few years, the hope being that amelioration or cure will happen sometime in the (indefinite) future. But terminally ill patients do not have infinite time, so the stressful effects of psychoanalysis are the only ones they are likely to

Table 1.1. Mortality of Therapy and Control Groups

Therapy	Status	Type	1	Type	2	Type	3	Type	4
			%		%		%		%
1. Up to 2 years of	Cancer	11	7.1	4	4.6	5	4.8	1	100.0
psychoanalysis,	CHD	7	4.5	5	5.8	6	5.7	0	0
then terminated.	Other	7	4.5	5	5.8	6	5.7	0	0
	Living	129	83.7	72	83.7	87	83.6	0	0
	Omitted	8	4.9	4	4.4	5	4.5	0	
	Total	162		90		109		1	
			%		%		%		%
2. Psychoanalysis for	Cancer	9	9.3	3	6.5	8	7.7	1	33.3
longer than 2 yrs.,	CHD	8	8.2	6	13.0	8	7.7	1	33.3
not terminated.	Other	8	8.2	5	10.8	7	6.7	1	33.3
	Living	72	74.2	32	69.5	81	77.8	0	0
	Omitted	5	14.9	0	0	4	3.7	0	0
	Total	102		46		108		3	
			%		%		%		%
3. Control group for	Cancer	2	1.3	1	1.2	0	0	0	0
Group 1, matched	CHD	1	0.6	2	2.4	0	0	0	0
on age, sex, type	Other	3	1.9	2	2.4	3	2.7	0	0
and amount of	Living	149	96.1	80	94.1	100	95.2	1	100.0
smoking.	Omitted	7	4.3	5	5.5	5	4.6	0	0
	Total	162		90		109		1	
			%		%		%		%
4. Control group for	Cancer	1	1	1	2.2	0	0	0	0
Group 2, matched	CHD	1	1	1	2.2	1	0.9	0	0
on age, sex, type	Other	1	1	3	6.6	5	4.6	0	0
and amount of	Living	94	96.9	40	88.8	98	95.1	3	100.0
smoking.	Omitted	5	4.9	1	2.1	5	4.6	0	0
	Total	102		46		108		3	
			%		%		%		%
5. Control group for	Cancer	1	0.6	1	0.5	0	0	1	0.9
Groups 1 and 2	CHD	2	1.2	2	1.0	1	0.9	0	0
combined, matched	Other	5	2.9	5	2.7	2	1.8	2	1.8
on age, sex, and	Living	166	95.4	180	95.7	107	96.4	107	97.3
cigarette consump-	Omitted	13	6.9	9	46.6	10	8.3	6	5.2
tion.	Total	187		197		121		116	

Note. From Grossarth-Maticek & Eysenck, 1990.

Table 1.2. Mortality of Groups Treated with Psychoanalysis, Depending on Whether the Treatment Increased or Decreased Autonomy

	Type	1	Type	2	Type	3	Type	4
N		32		20		34		1
Increasing autonomy		%		%		%		%
Cancer	1	3.2	0	0	0	0	0	0
CHD	1	3.2	1	10	1	3	0	0
Other	1	3.2	1	10	1	3	1	100
Living	28	90.3	8	80	31	93.9	0	0
Omitted	1	3.1	0	0	1	2.9	0	0
N		70		36		74		2
Decreasing autonomy		%		%		%		%
Cancer	8	12.1	3	8.3	88	11.2	1	50
CHD	7	10.6	5	13.9	7	9.9	1	50
Other	7	10.6	4	11.1	6	8.4	0	0
Living	44	66.7	24	66.7	50	70.4	0	0
Omitted	4	5.7	0	0	3	4.1	0	0

Note. From Grossarth-Maticek & Eysenck, 1990.

experience. Healthy cancer-prone or CHD-prone probands experience the added stress and may develop illness as a consequence long before the alleged beneficial effects emerge—if ever. The widespread use of psychoanalysis for cancer victims in Germany is unethical and completely contraindicated; it should be illegal to administer a "treatment" which has been shown to lead to highly undesirable consequences.

Psychotherapy And Behavior Therapy: A Reconciliation?

Attempts have been made to reconcile behavioral and psychodynamic principles, resulting in a form of "broad-spectrum" therapy (Lazarus, 1966) embodying some variant of eclecticism (Lazarus, 1967). I have condemned such a mishmash of theories as being counterproductive (Eysenck, 1970); if one theory is right, the other must be wrong, and combining the two does not seem sensible (Eysenck, 1986, 1987a).

A similar point relates to the recent emergence of cognitive psychotherapy, or cognitive-behavior therapy. This term raises two questions:

1. Is cognitive-behavior therapy different from classical behavior therapy by incorporating cognitive components? Eysenck and Martin (1987) have argued that cognition is one kind of behavior, and that conditioning paradigms since Pavlov have always incorporated cognitions as important aspects of the processes involved. Thus, adding the term "cognitive" to "behavior therapy" is redundant.

2. The other question is whether the alleged addition of cognitive methods to behavioral intervention produces effects which are demonstrably better than would be achieved by traditional methods alone. Latimer and Sweet (1984) looked into the literature to resolve this question; their answer was in the negative:

> Cognitive therapy is an evolutionary rather than a revolutionary development in the field of behavior therapy. It is unique only in its greater emphasis on one

> class of behavior—cognitions. Several innovative therapeutic methods have been spawned as a result of this shift in emphasis, but these have not been demonstrated to be efficacious in the treatment of populations. Cognitive therapy as actually practiced usually involves a variety of methods including behavioral procedures of established efficacy. Most of the claims made in support of cognitive therapy are based on studies employing these cognitive-behavioral methods. It remains to be demonstrated either that the new cognitive therapy procedures make a significant contribution to therapeutic outcome or that existing behavioral methods are rendered more effective when conceptualized in cognitive terms. The widespread adoption of cognitive treatment procedures is unwarranted on the basis of existing outcome data involving clinical populations. (p. 21)

On both accounts we may conclude, then, that traditional methods of behavior therapy, embodying cognitive behaviors, are quite adequate for the purpose of treatment and do not require specific additions labeled "cognitive." Additions should always be justified by empirical studies demonstrating an increase of effectiveness over appropriate behavioral studies *not* including the specific cognitive methods alleged to improve therapeutic effectiveness.

Conclusions

This section recapitulates the arguments presented in preceding sections. I find that while there is good agreement that commonsense methods of trying to help emotionally disturbed people (neurotics) are effective (spontaneous remission), psychotherapy, placebo treatment and psychoanalysis do equally well, and may do better. (Certain experimental arrangements, such as waiting-list nontreatment, make it unlikely that clients will seek the lay help that would normally lead to spontaneous remission, because they are waiting hopefully for "proper" therapy. This should not count as a control representing spontaneous remission.)

Psychotherapy, particularly psychoanalysis, can have powerful negative effects, making the patient worse rather than better, both psychologically and physically. Such negative effects should always be borne in mind and should make the use of psychoanalysis and dynamic methods of treatment unacceptable on ethical grounds.

Behavior therapy, which significantly outperforms spontaneous remission, placebo treatment, and psychotherapy, is the method of choice for neurotic disorders of all kinds. It always contains cognitive elements, and the explicit stress on such elements has never been shown to improve the effects of classical behavior therapy.

The only effective theory of neurotic disorders, underlying behavioral methods of treatment, is one based on conditioning principles; these principles, which have changed dramatically from the days of early pioneers like Watson, now incorporate cognitive factors as well as other changes in traditional behavioristic principles. Critics of behavior therapy and its underlying theoretical foundations should take these changes into account and cease flogging a dead horse (Eysenck & Martin, 1984).

Psychotherapy, and the dynamic theories on which it is based, is an example of a "degenerating program shift"; behavior therapy, and the conditioning theory on which it is based, is an example of a "developing program shift." Behavior therapy is becoming a paradigm of theory and practice in psychotherapy (Eysenck, 1986). It is no longer a dogma, but a case of applied science (Eysenck, 1976a).

References

Andrews, D. A., Zinger, I., Hoge, R. D., Bonta, J., Gendreau, P., & Cullen, F. T. (1990). Does correctional treatment work? A clinically relevant and psychologically informed meta-analysis. *Criminology, 28*, 369–404.

Bergin, A. E. (1971). The evaluation of therapeutic outcomes. In A. E. Bergin & S. L. Garfield (Eds.), *Handbook of psychotherapy and behavior change: An empirical analysis* (pp. 217–270). New York: Wiley.

Bergin, A. E., & Lambert, M. J. (1978). The evaluation of therapeutic outcomes. In S. L. Garfield & A. E. Bergin (Eds.), *Handbook of psychotherapy and behavior change: An empirical analysis* (2nd ed., pp. 139–190). New York: Wiley.

Breschmer, B. (1980). In one word: Not from experience. *Beta Psychologia, 45*, 223–241.

Denker, P. G. (1946). Results of treatment of psychoneurosis by the general practitioner. A follow-up study of 500 cases. *New York State Journal of Medicine, 46*, 2164–2166.

Eysenck, H. J. (1952). The effects of psychotherapy: An evaluation. *Journal of Consulting Psychology, 16*, 319–327.

Eysenck, H. J. (1960). The effects of psychotherapy. In H. J. Eysenck (Ed.), *Handbook of abnormal psychology: An experimental approach* (pp. 697–721). London: Pitman Medical Publishing.

Eysenck, H. J. (1965). The effects of psychotherapy. *International Journal of Psychiatry, 1*, 99–144.

Eysenck, H. J. (1966). *The effects of psychotherapy*. New York: International Science Press.

Eysenck, H. J. (1970). A mish-mash of theories. *International Journal of Psychiatry, 9*, 140–146.

Eysenck, H. J. (1972). *Psychology is about people*. London: Allan Lane.

Eysenck, H. J. (1976a). Behaviour therapy—dogma or applied science? In M. P. Feldman & A. Broadbent (Eds.), *The theoretical and experimental foundations of behaviour therapy* (pp. 333–363). London: Wiley.

Eysenck, H. J. (1976b). The learning theory model of neurosis—a new approach. *Behaviour Research and Therapy, 14*, 251–267.

Eysenck, H. J. (1977). *You and neurosis*. London: Maurice Temple Smith.

Eysenck, H. J. (1979). The conditioning model of neurosis. *Behavioral and Brain Sciences, 2*, 155–199.

Eysenck, H. J. (1980). A unified theory of psychotherapy, behavior therapy and spontaneous remission. *Zeitschrift fur Psychologie, 188*, 43–56.

Eysenck, H. J. (1982). Neobehavioristic (S–R) theory. In G. T. Wilson & C. M. Franks (Eds.), *Contemporary behavior therapy* (pp. 205–276). New York: Guilford.

Eysenck, H. J. (1985a). *Decline and fall of the Freudian empire*. London: Viking.

Eysenck, H. J. (1985b). Incubation theory of fear/anxiety. In B. Reiss and R. R. Boutzin (Eds.), *Theoretical issues in behavior therapy* (pp. 83–105). New York: Academic Press.

Eysenck, H. J. (1985c). Negative outcome in psychotherapy: The need for a theoretical framework. In D. T. Mays & C. M. Franks (Eds.), *Negative outcome in psychotherapy* (pp. 267–277). New York: Springer.

Eysenck, H. J. (1985d). The place of theory in a world of facts. In K. B. Madsen & L. P. Mos (Eds.), *Annals of theoretical psychology* (pp. 17–114).

Eysenck, H. J. (1988). Psychotherapy to behavior therapy: A paradigm shift. In D. B. Fishman, F. Rutgers, & C. Franks (Eds.), *Paradigms in behavior therapy: Present and promise* (pp. 45–76). New York: Springer.

Eysenck, H. J. (1987a). Behavior therapy. In H. J. Eysenck & I. Martin (Eds.), *Theoretical foundations of behavior therapy* (pp. 3–36). New York: Plenum.

Eysenck, H. J. (1987b). The role of heredity, environment and "preparedness" in the genesis of neurosis. In H. J. Eysenck & I. Martin (Eds.), *Theoretical foundations of behavior therapy* (pp. 379–402). New York: Plenum.

Eysenck, H. J. (1988). The respective importance of personality, cigarette smoking and interaction effects for the genesis of cancer and coronary heart disease. *Personality and individual differences, 9*, 453–464.

Eysenck, H. J. (1989). Prevention of cancer and coronary heart disease, and reduction in the cost of the National Health Service. *Journal of Social, Political and Economic Studies, 14*, 25–47.

Eysenck, H. J. (1990a). Maverick psychologist. In E. Walker (Ed.), *History of clinical psychology in autobiography* (p. 39–86). Pacific Grove, CA: Brooks/Cole.

Eysenck, H. J. (1990b). *Rebel with a cause*. London: Allen.

Eysenck, H. J. (1991). *Smoking, personality and stress: Psychosocial factors in the prevention of cancer and coronary heart disease*. New York: Springer Verlag.

Eysenck, H. J., & Beech, H. R. (1971). Counter conditioning and related methods. In A. E. Bergin & S. L. Garfield (Eds.), *Handbook of psychotherapy and behavior change: An empirical analysis* (pp. 543–611). New York: Wiley.

Eysenck, H. J., & Grossarth-Maticek, R. (1991). Creative novation behaviour therapy as a prophylactic treatment for cancer and coronary heart disease—II. Effects of treatment. *Behaviour Research and Therapy, 29*, 17–31.

Eysenck, H. J., & Kelley, M. J. (1987). The interaction of neurohormones with Pavlovian A and Pavlovian B conditioning in the causation of neurosis, extinction and incubation of anxiety. In A. Davey (Ed.), *Cognitive processes and pavlovian conditioning* (pp. 251–286). London: Wiley.

Eysenck, H. J., & Martin, E. (Eds.). (1987). *Theoretical foundations of behavior therapy*. New York: Plenum.

Eysenck, H. J., & Rachman, S. (1965). *Causes and cures of neurosis*. London: Routledge & Kegan Paul.

Eysenck, H. J., & Wilson, G. D. (1973). *The experimental study of Freudian theories*. London: Methuen.

Giles, T. R. (1983a). Probable superiority of behavioral interventions—I. Traditional comparative outcome. *Journal of Behavior Therapy and Experimental Psychiatry, 14*, 29–32.

Giles, T. R. (1983b). Probable superiority of behavioral interventions—II. Empirical status of the equivalence of therapies hypothesis. *Journal of Behavior Therapy and Experimental Psychiatry, 14*, 189–196.

Giles, T. R. (1990). Bias against behavior therapy in outcome reviews: Who speaks for the patient? *Behavior Therapist, 19*, 86–90.

Glass, G. V., & Smith, M. L. (1979). Meta-analysis of research on class size and achievement. *Educational evolution and policy analysis, 1*, 2–16.

Gossop, M. (1981). *Theories of neurosis*. New York: Springer.

Grossarth-Maticek, R., & Eysenck, H. J. (1990). Prophylactic effects of psychoanalysis on cancer-prone and coronary heart disease-prone probands, as compared with control groups and behavior therapy groups. *Journal of Behavior Therapy and Experimental Psychiatry, 21*, 91–99.

Grossarth-Maticek, R., & Eysenck, H. J. (1991). Creative novation behaviour therapy as a prophylactic treatment for cancer and coronary heart disease—I. Description of treatment. *Behaviour Research and Therapy, 29*, 1–16.

Grossarth-Maticek, R., Eysenck, H. J., & Vetter, H. (1988). Personality type, smoking habit and their interaction as predictors of cancer and coronary heart disease. *Personality and Individual Differences, 9*, 479–495.

Grunbaum, A. (1979). Epistemological liabilities of the clinical appraisal of psychoanalytic theory. *Psychoanalysis and Contemporary Thought, 2*, 451–526.

Grunbaum, A. (1984). *The foundations of psychoanalysis: A philosophical critique*. London: University of California Press.

Hirschmueller, A. (1989). *The life and work of Josef Breuer*. New York: University Press.

Howarth, I. (1989). Psychotherapy: Who benefits? *The Psychologist, 2*, 150–152.

Kazdin, A. E. (1978). *History of behavior modification*. Baltimore, University Park Press.

Kernberg, O. (1972). Psychotherapy and psychoanalysis: Final report of the Menninger Foundation Psychotherapy Research Project. *Bulletin of the Menninger Clinic, 36*, 1 and 2.

Kernberg, O. (1973). Summary and conclusions of psychotherapy and psychoanalysis: Final Report of the Menninger Foundation's Psychotherapy Research Project. *International Journal of Psychobiology, 11*, 62–77.

Lakatos, I. (1970). Falsification and the methodology of scientific research programs. In I. Lakatos & A. Musgrove (Eds.), *Criticism and the growth of knowledge* (pp. 143–174). New York: Cambridge University Press.

Lambert, M. (1976). Spontaneous remission in adult neurotic disorders. *Psychological Bulletin, 83*, 107–119.

Landis, C. (1937). A statistical evaluation of psychotherapeutic methods. In L. E. Hinsie (Ed.), *Concepts and problems of psychotherapy* (pp. 118–132). New York: Columbia University Press.

Latimer, P. R., & Sweet, A. A. (1984). Cognitive versus behavioral procedures in cognitive behavior therapy: A critical review of the evidence. *Journal of Behavior Therapy and Experimental Psychiatry, 15*, 9–22.

Lazarus, A. A. (1966). Broad-spectrum behaviour therapy and the treatment of agoraphobia. *Behaviour Research and Therapy, 4*, 95–97.

Luborsky, L., Singer, B., & Luborsky, L. (1975). Comparative studies of psychotherapies: Is it true that "everyone has won and all must have prizes"? *Archives of General Psychiatry, 32*, 995–1008.

Mahony, P. J. (1986). *Freud and the rat man.* New Haven: Yale University Press.

Malan, D. H. (1976). *The frontier of brief psychotherapy.* New York: Plenum Press.

Mays, D. T., & Franks, C. M. (1985). *Negative outcome in psychotherapy.* New York: Springer.

Meyer, A. E. (1990). Eine taxonomie der bisherigen psychotherapieforschung. *Zeitschrift fur klinische psychologie, 19*, 287–291.

Obholzer, K. (1982). *The wolf-man: Sixty years later.* London: Routledge & Kegan Paul.

Prioleau, L., Murdoch, M., & Brody, N. (1983). An analysis of psychotherapy versus placebo. *Behavioral and Brain Sciences, 6*, 275–285.

Rachman, S., & Hodgson, R. (1980). *Obsessions and compulsions.* Englewood Cliffs, NJ: Prentice-Hall.

Rachman, S. J., & Wilson, G. T. (1980). *The effects of psychological therapy.* London: Pergamon Press.

Salter, A. (1952). *The case against psychoanalysis.* New York: Holt.

Schorr, A. (1984). *Die Verhaltenstherapie.* Weinkeim: Beltz.

Sears, L. (1990). The chimpanzee's medicine chest. *New Scientist, 4*, 42–44.

Shapiro, A. K., Struening, E. L., Shapiro, E., & Milcarek, B. I. (1983). Diazepam: How much better than placebo? *Journal of Psychiatric Research, 17*, 51–73.

Smith, M. L., Glass, G. V., & Miller, T. I. (1980). *The benefits of psychotherapy.* Baltimore: Johns Hopkins University Press.

Strupp, H. H., Hadley, S. W., & Gomes-Schwarts, B. (1977). *Psychotherapy for better or worse: The problem of negative effects.* New York: Aronson.

Svartberg, M., & Stiles, T. C. (1991). Comparative effects of short-term psychodynamic psychotherapy: A meta-analysis. *Journal of Consulting and Clinical Psychology*, 59, 704–714.

Thornton, E. N. (1983). *Freud and cocaine: The Freudian fallacy.* London: Bland and Briggs.

Wilder, J. (1945). Facts and figures on psychotherapy. *Journal of Clinical Psychotherapy, 7*, 311–347.

Wittmann, W., & Matt, G. E. (1986). Meta-Analyse ab Integration von Forschungsergebnissen am beispiel deutschsprachiger Arbeiten zur Effektivitat von Psychotherapie. *Psychologische Rundschau, 37*, 20–40.

Wood, J. (1990, August). The naked truth. *Weekend Guardian*, pp. 25–26.

Zubin, J. (1953). Evaluation of therapeutic outcome in mental disorders. *Journal of Nervous and Mental Diseases, 117*, 95–111.

2

The Relative Efficacy of Prescriptive Techniques

Thomas R. Giles, Daniel M. Neims, and Elizabeth M. Prial

Much of the available research on psychotherapy outcome has been characterized by puzzling and counterintuitive findings, termed *dose-paradox* in a former review (Giles, 1993). For example, results of inpatient mental health treatment fail to surpass, and are often inferior to, results obtained from partial care or other less restrictive treatments (Kiesler, 1982). This paradox also appears to be the case in the treatment of substance abuse (Miller, 1991; Miller & Hester, 1986). Insight-oriented therapy appears to produce results which are independent of the length of its administration (Rachman & Wilson, 1980). Although not as uniform an effect, paraprofessionals tend to attain results roughly equal to those of highly experienced professionals (Strupp & Hadley, 1979; Zilbergeld, 1983).

Another source of perplexity in this area has been the collection of studies and reviews reporting little outcome distinction between various types of treatment. This has led many experts to support the supposition that all therapies yield equal results (e.g., Bergin & Lambert, 1978; Frank, 1973, 1978; Garfield, 1976, 1980; Glass & Smith, 1978; Kazdin, 1979; Lambert 1979; Lambert, Shapiro, & Bergin, 1986; Llewelyn & Hume, 1979; Luborsky, Singer, & Luborsky, 1975; Luborsky & Spence, 1978; Ryle, 1984; Smith & Glass, 1977; Stiles, Shapiro, & Elliot, 1986; Strupp, 1978, 1981; Wachtel, 1977; see also Beutler *et al.*, 1991; Persons, 1991; see Giles, 1983a, for a review).

As a counterpoint, this chapter will attempt to demonstrate that the comparative argument for prescriptive forms of care, especially those of a behavioral or cognitive-behavioral nature, is more robust than is inferred by the equivalence literature. The greater efficiency of prescriptive therapies—compared to traditional treatments as defined below—provides the first and most obvious example of this outcome. Also, as many of the chapters in this handbook demonstrate, there is a fairly substantive body of research indicating that these therapies have

Thomas R. Giles • Associates in Managed Care, Denver, Colorado 80231. **Daniel M. Neims** and **Elizabeth M. Prial** • University of Denver, Denver Colorado.

Handbook of Effective Psychotherapy, edited by Thomas R. Giles. Plenum Press, New York, 1993.

additional outcome advantages across a multitude of disorders. This literature is bolstered by the current review, which proceeds in the following order: single-case studies, placebo trials, meta-analyses, and interorientation comparisons.

Single-Case Studies

Increased sophistication in experimental designs (Barlow & Hersen, 1984; Kazdin, 1986) caused select "single-case" methodologies (typically using multiple-baseline designs) to stand on firmer ground with regard to inferential support for treatment-specific effects. In addition to threats to internal validity (see Kazdin, 1986), the number and heterogeneity of cases play an important role in fortifying or weakening such inferential support. *Specific treatment effects run contrary to the role of attentional variables upon which equivalence relies* (Giles, 1983b). Turner and Ascher (1979a) provide an example of this by their within-subjects analyses of stimulus control treatment for severe sleep-onset insomnia. Figure 2.1 exemplifies findings indicating treatment effects independent from those of attentional variables alone.

Specific effects of directive therapies have been indicated in single-case studies concerning disorders such as agoraphobia (e.g., Agras, Leitenberg, & Barlow, 1968; Ascher, 1981), reactive depression (e.g., Eisler & Hersen, 1973), marital discord (e.g., Bornstein, 1981; Jacobson, 1977), bulimia (e.g., Giles, Young, & Young, 1985; Rosen & Leitenberg, 1982), sexual deviations (e.g., Alford, Webster, & Sanders, 1980; Barlow, Leitenberg, & Agras, 1969; Marks & Gelder, 1967), compulsive rituals (e.g., Mills, Agras, Barlow, & Mills, 1973), enuresis (e.g., Miller, 1973), tension headache (e.g., Epstein, Hersen, & Hemphill, 1974), depression (e.g., McKnight, Nelson, Hayes, & Jarrett, 1984), insomnia (e.g., Turner & Ascher, 1979b), incestuous behavior (e.g., Harbart, Barlow, Hersen, & Austin, 1974), social skills training (e.g., Bellack, Hersen, & Turner, 1976), schizophrenic delusional verbal behavior (e.g., Wincze, Leitenberg, & Agras, 1972), trychotilomania (Bernard, Kratchowill, & Keefauver, 1983), simple phobia (e.g., Leitenberg, Agras, Thompson, & Wright, 1968; Liberman & Smith, 1972), tics (e.g., Azrin & Petersen, 1989), childhood posttraumatic disorders (e.g., Saigh, 1987), oppositional disorders (e.g., Mace, Page, Ivancic, & O'Brien, 1986; Ramp, Ulrich, & Dulaney, 1971), alcoholism (e.g., Miller, Hersen, Eisler, & Watts, 1974), and obesity (Mann, 1972).

Attention/Placebo Comparisons

The equivalence hypothesis designates nonspecific effects (such as attention or empathy) as the means by which therapeutic progress occurs. Thus, directive treatment effects should not surpass those of placebo or other treatments which fully include nonspecific mechanisms. Studies which have tested this hypothesis include comparisons of different treatments within and between orientations, dismantling designs, constructive designs, and formal comparisons with placebo controls.

With the caveat that the equilibration of treatment is difficult (Kazdin & Wilcoxon, 1976), an earlier, brief review of placebo comparisons (Giles, 1983b) reported that directive interventions exceeded nonspecific effects in research inclusive of the following disorders: agoraphobia (e.g., Foa, Jameson, Turner, & Payne, 1980; Mathews, Gelder, & Johnson, 1981; Stern & Marks, 1973), primary insomnia (e.g., Ascher & Turner, 1980; Lawrence & Tokartz, 1976; Steinmark & Borkovec, 1974; Turner & Ascher, 1979b), marital discord (e.g., Jacobsen, 1978), sexual dysfunctions (e.g., Marks, 1978; Mathews *et al.*, 1976), obsessive–compulsive disorders (e.g., Foa, Steketee, & Milby, 1980; Marks, 1978; Milby & Meredith, 1980; Rachman & Hodgson, 1980), unipolar depression (e.g.,. DeRubeis & Hollon, 1981; McLean & Hakstian, 1979), Type A behavior (e.g., Friedman *et al.*, 1982), stutter-

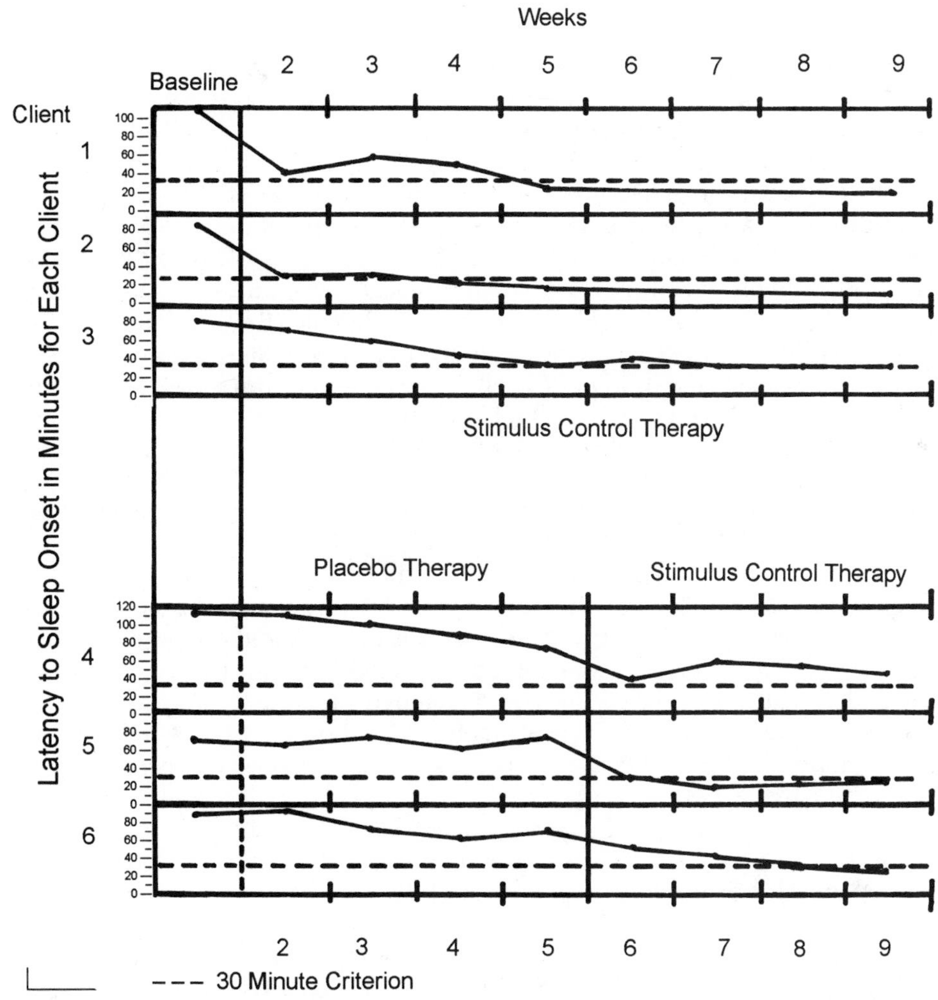

Figure 2.1. Mean latency to sleep onset per week for the 9 weeks of the study is shown for the 6 clients. Clients 4, 5, and 6 were placed in the placebo condition. At week 6, clients 4, 5, and 6 were placed in the stimulus control condition, while clients 1, 2, and 3 were maintained in the stimulus control therapy. (From "A Within Subject Analysis of Stimulus Control Therapy with Severe Sleep-Onset Insomnia" by R. Turner and M. Ascher, 1979. *Behaviour Research and Therapy, 17,* 86. Reprinted by permission from Pergamon Press.)

ing (e.g., Azrin, Nunn, & Frantz, 1980), problem drinking (e.g., Azrin, 1976; Hedberg & Cambell, 1974; Hunt & Azrin, 1973; Miller, 1982; Miller & Munoz, 1982), social skills deficits in psychiatric inpatients (e.g., Goldsmith & McFall, 1975; Schaefer & Martin, 1966), dysmenorrhea (e.g., Chesney & Tasto, 1975), simple phobia (e.g., Biran & Wilson, 1980; Gillan & Rachman, 1974; Moses & Hollandsworth, 1981; Paul, 1966), tension headaches (e.g., Kondo & Canter, 1977; Phillips, 1978), obesity (e.g., Harmatz & Lapuc, 1968; Levitz & Stunkard, 1974; Wollersheim, 1970), enuresis (e.g.,McConaghy, 1969), hyperactivity (e.g., Christensen & Sprague, 1973; Wulpert & Dries, 1977), chronic pain (e.g., Ritchie, 1976), and in the management of autism (e.g., Rimland, 1977).

This earlier review did not include all of the extant literature supportive of a possible superiority of prescriptive treatment to attention/placebo, and the number of relevant studies has continued to enlarge. For example, in a meta-analytic review by Lerner & Clum (1990) of 69 studies, behavioral interventions were shown to yield effect sizes significantly greater than placebo. Chapters in the present handbook review much of the literature by disorder, reaching the same conclusions. For an additional sample of such studies, see Blanchard *et al.* (1990); Butler, Fannell, Robson, and Gelder (1991); Cappe and Alden (1986); Carr-Kaffashan and Woolfolk (1979); Chambless, Foa, Groves, and Goldstein (1982); Christensen, Hadzi-Pavlovic, Andrews, and Mattick (1987); Denney and Rupert (1977); Durham and Turvey (1987); Gatchel, Hatch, Maynard, Turns, and Taunton-Blackwood (1979); Goldstein, Niaura, Follick, and Abrams (1989); Halonen and Passman (1985); Holyroyd, Nash, Pingel, Cordingley, and Jerome (1991); Jacobson (1977); Keefe *et al.* (1990); Klosko, Barlow, Tassinari, and Cerny (1990); Lacks, Bertelson, Gans, and Kunkel (1983); Lent, Russell, and Zamostny (1981); Lick and Heffler (1977); Lindsay, Gamsu, McLaughlin, Hood, and Espie (1987); Lipsky, Kassinove, and Miller (1980); Margolin and Weiss (1978); Marshall (1985); McClusky, Milby, and Switzer (1991); Morin and Azrin (1988); O'Leary and Beach (1990); Ost (1988); Power *et al.* (1990); Slutsky and Allen (1978); Spence and Marzillier (1981); Turner and Ascher (1979b); Turner and Clancy (1988).

Comparative studies of traditional psychotherapies have often been unable to demonstrate superiority to nonspecific effects. Such results are congruous with the equivalence hypothesis (e.g., Prioleau, Murdock, & Brody, 1983; Strupp & Hadley, 1979). A recent review of psychotherapy outcome for depression, for example, concluded that traditional psychotherapy, though superior to no treatment, was equivalent to attention/placebo (Hollon, Shelton, & Loosen, 1991). Directive (usually cognitive) therapies, however, were indicated in this review to be superior to nonspecific therapy effects.

Meta-Analytic Studies

While granting the susceptibility of meta-analysis to methodological deficiencies and experimenter bias (Searles, 1985; Wilson & Rachman, 1983), we include some of this literature due to its indications—heretofore inadequately acknowledged—in favor of directive (again, usually behavioral or cognitive-behavioral) techniques (see Chapter 19, this volume, by Elliott, Stiles, and Shapiro for a discussion of meta-analytic studies supportive of equivalence). For example, systematic desensitization was found more effective than other therapies in the first meta-analysis (Smith & Glass, 1977). Smith, Glass, and Miller (1980) examined well-controlled studies in one of several ad hoc analyses. These authors divided outcome measures into "psychological" and "less tractable" classes, finding that behavioral therapies were superior for psychological measures such as fear–anxiety, self-esteem, global assessment, personality traits, and vocational–personal development (the subsequent methodology by which Smith and colleagues arrived at "equivalence" has been severely criticized—see Wilson and Rachman, 1983).

In a vein similar to that of Smith and Glass, Shapiro and Shapiro's (1982) meta-analysis also found in favor of directive techniques. Andrews and Harvey (1981) meta-analyzed Smith and Glass's (1977) studies addressing "psychoneurotic" cases. While reporting that psychotherapy yielded effect sizes significantly greater than those of no-treatment controls, the authors also found that effect sizes from directive (behavioral) therapies were significantly greater than those of psychotherapy.

Two meta-analytic reviews across disorders in children and adolescents (Casey & Berman, 1985; Weisz, Weiss, Alicke, & Klotz, 1987) also found behavioral and cognitive-behavioral procedures to be most efficacious. To quote Weisz *et al.* (1987, p. 542), "behavioral treatments proved superior to non-behavioral treatments regardless of client age, therapist experience, or treated problem."

Searles's (1985) reanalysis of Andrews and Harvey's (1981) data showed that the effect size of behavioral therapy was 300% greater than that of psychotherapy. His reexamination of Shapiro and Shapiro's (1982) meta-analysis indicated that, "the composition of the sample demonstrates that the support for Smith and Glass was more apparent than real since the dynamic and humanistic approaches accounted for only 5% of the data base while behavioral and cognitive therapies comprised the remaining 95%" (p. 460). Revisiting Landman and Dawes's (1982) paper entitled "Psychotherapy Outcome: Smith and Glass' Conclusions Stand Up under Scrutiny," Searles reported that 90% of the comparisons utilized prescriptive interventions. According to Searles (1985), the effect size of these interventions was 450% greater than the effect size of psychotherapy. Searles concluded that "when quality of study is associated with a meta-analysis, the large effect sizes obtained are almost exclusively a function of the positive outcomes of behaviorally-oriented approaches" (p. 460).

Bowers and Clum's (1988) meta-analysis reported that behavior therapy was superior to controls for attention/placebo. As indicated, this contrasts with the equivalence of traditional psychotherapy to attention/placebo in the meta-analysis by Prioleau *et al.* (1983).

Dobson's (1989) meta-analysis of cognitive therapy for depression found it to be superior to pharmacotherapy, behavior therapy, and other psychotherapies. Steinbrueck, Maxwell, and Howard (1983), in a meta-analysis of 56 outcome studies, found psychotherapy to be superior to drug therapy for the treatment of unipolar depression in adults. Of the psychological therapies reviewed in this analysis, 97% utilized one variant or another of directive technique. A meta-analysis of behavior therapy and tricyclic medication (Christensen *et al.*, 1987) for obsessive–compulsive disorder showed that both were "significantly superior to nonspecific treatment programs" (p. 701).

Finally, Svartberg and Stiles (1991) used meta-analysis to compare short-term dynamic psychotherapy (STPP) with alternative (usually behavioral or cognitive-behavioral) psychotherapies (AP). These investigators found that

> STPP was . . . inferior to AP at posttreatment, and even more so at 1-year follow-up. STPP was inferior to AP in treating depression and, in particular, to cognitive-behavioral therapy for major depression. As research quality increased . . . STPP increased its overall inferiority to AP on a series of clinically relevant variables. (p. 704)

Interorientation Comparisons

In this chapter, we have used the term "traditional" to describe therapies that typically persist for a long period of time (months or years), address symptoms indirectly, target general personality change, orient toward historical events, and prescribe interventions which are primarily interpretive, cathartic, reflective, nondirective, confrontive, and/or transferential. We have used "directive" or "prescriptive" to describe treatments that are usually, or to a large extent, goal and present oriented, behaviorally specific, symptom focused, guided by empirical findings, advice-giving, educational, collaborative, and aimed toward the resolution or amelioration of symptoms in briefer periods of time (typically 1–20 hours of outpatient visits—Giles, 1983b). Several studies (e.g., Sloane, Staples, Cristol, Yorkston, & Whipple, 1975) have indicated that these two general types of treatment can be distinguished by blind viewers listening to taped therapy sessions.

The original interorientation review (Luborsky, Singer, & Luborsky, 1975) indicated that 6 of 19 significant differences favored behavioral over traditional techniques (the rest were tie scores). Since then, the available literature has expanded considerably. A more recent review (Giles, 1983b) located 52 studies demonstrating significant differences between treatments. All 52 favored directive (usually behavioral or cognitive-behavioral) techniques. Since then, several dozen additional studies have been located. Two of these favored traditional therapies (Johnson & Greenberg, 1985; Snyder, Wills, & Grady-Fletcher, 1991). The remaining 50 or so of these additional studies reported a superiority of directive interventions. A complete list of 105 studies reporting outcome superiority is available in the Appendix.

The unit of comparison in this research was the study itself (as opposed to a dependent-measure comparison as in Luborsky *et al.*, 1975). Studies in the first review (Giles, 1983b) were taken from papers presented at conventions as well as from articles, dissertations, and unpublished manuscripts across clinical and analogue populations. Articles referenced in the Appendix after the first review were taken primarily from refereed journals. Although each article in the Appendix is numbered, the total number is somewhat inflated because several of the studies listed were follow-ups to previously cited research (e.g., Falloon, McGill, Boyd, & Pederson, 1987; Falloon & Pederson, 1985; Paul, 1966, 1967).

The consistency and breadth of these findings indicate that some directive treatments yield superior outcome in comparison to traditional psychotherapies. The equivalence hypothesis appears to have been negated by both the number and the distribution of the significant-difference studies reported in this section.

Discussion

Psychotherapy outcome has frequently been associated with controversy and bitter debate. The present chapter, perhaps especially with reference to the "box score" results listed here, provides a perspective disfavoring the equivalence hypothesis. In this regard we wish to anticipate, discuss, and defend a number of possible objections to these points of view:

1. *"Box scores" and meta-analyses equate methodologically poor with methodologically superior studies, invite selectivity in study review, and generally make impossible the correct interpretation of conflicting results.* This criticism would be more telling were it not for the consistency and uniformity of results, perhaps especially with regard to the interorientation comparisons.

2. *Box scores, meta-analyses, and psychotherapy–placebo reviews tell us nothing about the efficacy of specific interventions for specific problems.* A review of the Appendix will reveal that a number of studies directly address this question. There are, for example, two dozen studies comparing directive with traditional intervention for the treatment of schizophrenia and unipolar depression, all of which favor directive techniques. (Also see in the Appendix studies on conduct/ oppositional disorder, enuresis, panic disorder, and so forth showing the same result.) When available research is reviewed by specific disorder, as indicated by the chapters in this handbook, prescriptive treatments again appear to have a significant advantage over traditional psychotherapies.

3. *The comparative research indicating a superiority of directive treatments is marred by serious methodological deficiencies.* The design of a methodologically "perfect" comparative outcome study between orientations is a complicated matter (e.g., Kazdin, 1986; Kazdin & Bass, 1989), involving much time and expense (Kazdin & Wilson, 1980; Rachman & Wilson, 1980). Constructive and dismantling designs may offer more feasible alternatives (Kazdin & Wilson, 1980).

Nevertheless, due to the diversity of both the available literature and its methodological problems, it would be problematic to discount the present conclusions based solely upon methodological grounds. It should also be noted that much of this research is quite methodologically sophisticated and that, as Searles (1985) demonstrated, greater methodological strength is more likely to be associated with the superiority of directive techniques.

4. *The research showing superiority of directive therapies has been conducted primarily with analogue subject populations suffering from nonclinical disturbances.* This criticism was summarized in an article in the *American Psychologist* by Stiles, Shapiro, and Elliott (1986):

> Some behaviorally oriented researchers . . . appear to believe . . . that behavioral therapies have been shown in comparative studies to be differentially effective. The overwhelming majority of investigations, however, are laboratory analogues using brief treatments with student volunteers who present only minor difficulties . . . thus, a substantial body of evidence and opinion points to the conclusion that the outcomes of different psychotherapies with clinical populations are equivalent. (p. 166)

It should be noted that the equivalence hypothesis is inclusive of analogue research and that consistent, significant differences with analogue subjects provide at least a limited means of negation. Inspection of the reference list and Appendix, however, will indicate that this criticism is not valid. The Appendix (and the handbook chapters) references studies on schizophrenia, unipolar depression, borderline personality disorder, self-lethal inpatients, bulimia nervosa, severe conduct disorder, panic disorder, mental health center outpatients, obsessive–compulsive disorder, and so forth.

5. *The results in favor of directive treatments were obtained due to a confound of experimenter bias.* Rosenthal effects have been hypothesized to explain results such as those reported in the Appendix. This is an important caveat and one upon which we devote somewhat greater attention below.

Using an inferential determination of therapist allegiance, Robinson, Berman, and Neimeyer (1990) meta-analyzed outcome research on psychotherapy for the treatment of depression. The results in this meta-analysis were no longer significantly in favor of directive intervention once the effect of therapist allegiance was statistically controlled.

This inferential methodology may have led to confusing results. Loizeaux (1991) assessed confirmation bias in behavioral versus cognitive treatment outcome research by *directly assessing* therapist allegiance via questionnaire. Therapist allegiance was an insignificant factor in these comparisons.

Some of the studies in the Appendix (e.g., Gunderson *et al.*, 1984; Morrison & Shapiro, 1987) found in favor of directive treatments despite the fact that the researchers were traditionalists. Paul (1967) found a superiority of desensitization over insight treatment for speech anxiety, both posttreatment and at long-term follow-up, despite the fact that the insight-oriented psychotherapists implemented the behavioral technique.

A study reporting the superiority of prescriptive over exploratory therapy (Morrison & Shapiro, 1987) reported that the prescriptive therapy was more credible to subjects. The higher credibility ratings, however, appeared *subsequent* to therapy, exerting no apparent pretreatment influence. To quote the authors:

> Consistent with previous, analogue findings, the present data suggest that cognitive/behavioural treatments are particularly credible to clients. However, regression analysis showed that statistical control for this expectancy difference only slightly attenuated the treatment effect, whereas statistical control for the treatment effect abolished the expectancy effect. These results do not support the proposition that differential outcomes of psychotherapy are due to differential arousal of positive outcome expectations . . . by credibility differences among treatments. Credibility differences appear secondary to the treatment effect rather than its cause. (p. 60)

The alleged experimenter confound would also have to account for the reported superiority of behavioral interventions in the meta-analytic findings cited above, the findings on directive treatment versus placebo comparisons, and the available dismantling and constructive designs in which experimenter bias would seem to be more difficult to suspect.

If our dismissal of equivalence is empirically justified, then the field must face a number of troubling ethical issues associated with the historical—and current—underutilization of comparatively effective psychotherapies. These issues are further addressed in Chapter 20 of this handbook.

References

Agras, W. S., Leitenburg, H., & Barlow, D. H. (1968). Social reinforcement in the modification of agoraphobia. *Archives of General Psychiatry, 19,* 423–427.

Alford, G. S., Webster, J. S., & Sanders, S. H. (1980). Covert aversion of two interrelated deviant sexual practices: Obscene phone calling and exhibitionism. A single case analysis. *Behavior Therapy, 11,* 13–25.

Andrews, G., & Harvey, R. (1981). Does psychotherapy benefit patients? *Archives of General Psychology, 38,* 1203–1208.

Ascher, M. (1981). Employing paradoxical intention in the treatment of agoraphobia. *Behaviour Research and Therapy, 19,* 533–542.

Ascher, M., & Turner, R. (1980). A comparison of two methods for the administration of paradoxical intention. *Behaviour Research and Therapy, 18,* 121–126.

Azrin, N. H. (1976). Improvements in the community-reinforcement approach to alcoholism. *Behaviour Research and Therapy, 14,* 339–348.

Azrin, N. H., Nunn, R., & Frantz, S. (1980). Habit reversal versus negative practice treatment of nervous tics. *Behavior Therapy, 11,* 169–178.

Azrin, N. H., & Peterson, A. L. (1989). Reduction of an eye tic by controlled blinking. *Behavior Therapy, 20,* 467–473.

Barlow, D. H. (1981). On the relation of clinical research to clinical practice: Current issues, new directions. *Journal of Consulting and Clinical Psychology, 49,* 147–155.

Barlow, D. H., & Hersen, M. (1984). *Single case experimental designs. Strategies for studying behavior change* (2nd ed.). Elmsford, NY: Pergamon Press.

Barlow, D. H., Leitenburg, H., & Agras, W. (1969). Experimental control of sexual deviation through manipulation of the noxious scene in covert sensitization. *Journal of Abnormal Psychology, 74,* 596–601.

Bellack, A. S., Hersen, M., & Turner, S. M. (1976). Generalization effects of social skills training in chronic schizophrenics: An experimental analysis. *Behaviour Research and Therapy, 14,* 391–398.

Bergin, A., & Lambert, M. (1978). The evaluation of therapeutic outcomes. In S. Garfield & A. Bergin (Eds.), *Handbook of psychotherapy* and behavior change (2nd ed., pp. 16–37). New York: Wiley.

Bernard, M. E., Kratchowill, T. R., & Keefauver, L. W. (1983). The effects of rational-emotive therapy and self-instructional training on chronic hair pulling. *Cognitive Therapy and Research, 7,* 273–279.

Beutler, L., Engle, D., Mohr, D., Daldrup, R. Bergan, J., Meredith, K., & Merry, W. (1991). Predictors of differential response to cognitive, experiential, and self-directed psychotherapeutic procedure. *Journal of Consulting and Clinical Psychology, 59,* 333–340.

Biran, M., & Wilson, G. (1980, November). *Participant modeling versus cognitive restructuring in the treatment of phobic disorders.* Paper presented at the annual meeting of the Association for the Advancement of Behavior Therapy, New York.

Blanchard, E., Appelbaum, K., Radnitz, C., Michultka, D., Morrill, B., Kirsch, C., Hillhouse, J., Evans, D., Guarier, P., Attanasio, V., Andrasik, F., Jallard, J., & Dentinger, M. (1990). Placebo-controlled evaluation of abbreviated progressive muscle relaxation and of relaxation combined with cognitive therapy in the treatment of tension headache. *Journal of Consulting and Clinical Psychology, 58,* 210–215.

Bornstein, P. (1981, November). *Behavioral communications treatment of marital discord.* Paper presented at the annual meeting of the Association for the Advancement of Behavior Therapy, Toronto.

Bowers, T., & Clum, G. (1988). Relative contribution of specific and nonspecific treatment effects: Meta-analysis of placebo-controlled behavior therapy research. *Psychological Bulletin, 103,* 315–323.

Butler, G., Fannell, M., Robson, P., & Gelder, M. (1991). Comparison of behavior therapy and cognitive behavior therapy in the treatment of generalized anxiety disorder. *Journal of Consulting and Clinical Psychology, 59,* 167–175.

Cappe, R. F., & Alden, L. E. (1986). A comparison of treatment strategies for clients functionally impaired by extreme shyness and social avoidance. *Journal of Consulting and Clinical Psychology, 54,* 796–801.

Carr-Kaffashan, L., & Woolfolk, R. L. (1979). Active and placebo effects in treatment of moderate and severe insomnia. *Journal of Consulting and Clinical Psychology, 47,* 1072–1080.

Casey, R., & Berman, J. (1985). The outcome of psychotherapy with children. *Psychological Bulletin, 98,* 388–400.

Chambless, D. L., Foa, E. B., Groves, G. A., & Goldstein, A. J. (1982). Exposure and communications training in the treatment of agoraphobia. *Behaviour Research and Therapy, 20,* 219–231.

Chesney, M., & Tasto, D. (1975). The effectiveness of behavior modification with spasmodic and congestive dysmenorrhea. *Behaviour Research and Therapy, 13*, 242–253.

Christensen, D., & Sprague, R. (1973). Reduction of hyperactive behavior by conditioning procedures done and combined with methylphenidate (Ritalin). *Behaviour Research and Therapy, 11*, 331–334.

Christensen, H., Hadzi-Pavlovic, D., Andrews, G., & Mattick, R. (1987). Behavior therapy and tricyclic medication in the treatment of obsessive compulsive disorder: A quantitative review. *Journal of Consulting and Clinical Psychology, 55*, 701–711.

Denney, D. R., & Rupert, P. A. (1977). Desensitization and self-control in the treatment of test anxiety. *Journal of Counseling Psychology, 24*, 272–280.

DeRubeis, R., & Hollon, S. (1981). Behavioral treatment of affective disorders. In L. Michelson, M. Hersen, & S. Turner (Eds.), *Future perspectives in behavior therapy*. New York: Plenum.

Dobson, K. (1989). A meta-analysis of the efficacy of cognitive therapy for depression. *Journal of Consulting and Clinical Psychology, 57*, 414–419.

Durham, R. C., & Turvey, A. A. (1987). Cognitive therapy versus behavior therapy in the treatment of chronic general anxiety. *Behaviour Research and Therapy, 25*, 229–234.

Eisler, R., & Hersen, M. (1973, August). *The A-B design: Effects of token economy on behavioral and subjective measures in neurotic depression*. Paper presented at the American Psychological Association convention, Montreal.

Epstein, L., Hersen, M., & Hemphill, D. (1974). Music feedback as a treatment for tension headache: An experimental case study. *Journal of Behavior Therapy and Experimental Psychiatry, 5*, 59–63.

Falloon, I., McGill, C., Boyd, J., & Pederson, J. (1987). Family management in the prevention of morbidity of schizophrenia: Social outcome of a two-year longitudinal study. *Psychological Medicine, 17*, 59–66.

Fallon, I., & Pederson, J. (1985). Family management in the prevention of morbidity: The adjustment of the family. *British Journal of Psychiatry, 147*, 156–163.

Foa, E., Jameson, J., Turner, R., & Payne, L. (1980). Massed versus spaced exposure sessions in the treatment of agoraphobia. *Behaviour Research and Therapy, 18*, 333–338.

Foa, E., Steketee, G., & Milby, J. (1980). Differential effects of exposure and response prevention in obsessive-compulsive washers. *Journal of Consulting and Clinical Psychology, 48*, 71–79.

Frank, J. D. (1973). *Persuasion and healing*. Baltimore: Johns Hopkins University Press.

Frank, J. D. (1978). Psychotherapy: Contemporary trends in the United States. *Psychotherapy and Psychosomatics, 29*, 13–18.

Friedman, M., Threson, C., Gill, J., Ulmer, D., Thompson, L., Powell, L., Price, V., Elek, S., Rabin, D., Breall, W., Praget, G., Dixon, T., Bourg, E., Levy, R., & Tasto, D. (1982). Feasibility of altering type A behavior pattern after myocardial infarction. *Circulation, 66*, 83–92.

Garfield, S. (1976). All roads lead to Rome. *Contemporary Psychology, 21*, 328–329.

Garfield, S. (1980). Psychotherapy: A forty year appraisal. *American Psychologist, 36*, 174–183.

Gatchel, R. J., Hatch, J. P., Maynard, A., Turns, R., & Taunton-Blackwood, A. (1979). Comparison of heart rate biofeedback, false biofeedback, and systematic desensitization in reducing speech anxiety: Short- and long-term effectiveness. *Journal of Consulting and Clinical Psychology, 47*, 620–622.

Giles, T. R. (1983a). Probable superiority of behavioral interventions—I: Traditional comparative outcome. *Journal of Behavior Therapy and Experimental Psychiatry, 14*, 29–32.

Giles, T. R. (1983b). Probable superiority of behavioral interventions—II: Empirical status of the equivalence of therapies hypothesis. *Journal of Behavior Therapy and Experimental Psychiatry, 14*, 189–196.

Giles, T. R. (1984). Probable superiority of behavioral interventions—III: Some obstacles to acceptance of findings. *Journal of Behavior Therapy and Experimental Psychiatry, 15*, 23–26.

Giles, T. R. (1989, August). *Ethical considerations in managed mental health care systems*. Paper presented at the American Psychological Association convention, New Orleans.

Giles, T. R. (1990a). Bias against behavior therapy in outcome reviews: Who speaks for the patient? *Behavior Therapist, 19*, 86–90.

Giles, T. R. (1990b). Underutilization of effective psychotherapy: Managed mental health care and other forces of change. *Behavior Therapist, 19*, 107–110.

Giles, T. R. (1993). *Managed mental health care: A guide for practitioners, employers, and hospital administrators*. New York: Allyn and Bacon.

Giles, T. R. (1991). Managed mental health care and effective psychotherapy: A step in the right direction? *Journal of Behavior Therapy and Experimental Psychiatry, 22*, 86–88.

Giles, T. R., & Hom, P. (1987, November). *New evidence on comparative efficacy of directive psychotherapy.* Paper presented at the Association for the Advancement of Behavior Therapy convention, Boston.

Giles, T. R., Young, R. R., & Young, D. E. (1985). Case studies and clinical replication series: Behavioral treatment of severe bulimia. *Therapy, 16,* 393–405.

Gillan, P., & Rachman, S. (1974). An experimental investigation of behavior therapy in phobic patients. *British Journal of Psychiatry, 124,* 932–401.

Glass, G., & Smith, M. (1978). Reply to Eysenck, *American Psychologist, 33,* 517–519.

Goldsmith, J., & McFall, R. (1975). Development and evaluation of an interpersonal skill-training program for psychiatric inpatients. *Journal of Abnormal Psychology, 84,* 51–58.

Goldstein, M. G., Niaura, R., Follick, M. J., & Abrams, D. B. (1989). Effects of behavioral skills training and schedule of nicotine gum administration on smoking cessation. *American Journal of Psychiatry, 146,* 56–60.

Halonen, J. S., & Passman, R. H. (1985). Relaxation training and expectation in the treatment of postpartum distress. *Journal of Consulting and Clinical Psychology, 53,* 839–845.

Harbart, T., Barlow, D., Hersen, M., & Austin, J. (1974). Measurement and modification of incestuous behavior. *Psychology Report, 34,* 79–86.

Harmatz, M., & Lapuc, P. (1968). Behavior modification of overeating in a psychiatric population. *Journal of Consulting and Clinical Psychology, 32,* 583–587.

Hedberg, A., & Campbell, L. (1974). A comparison of four behavioral treatments of alcoholism. *Journal of Behavior Therapy and Experimental Psychiatry, 5,* 251–256.

Hollon, S., Shelton, R., & Loosen, P. (1991). Cognitive therapy and pharmacotherapy for depression. *Journal of Consulting and Clinical Psychology, 59,* 88–99.

Holyrod, K. A., Nash, J. M., Pingel, J. D., Cordingley, G. E., & Jerome, A. (1991). A comparison of pharmacological (amitriptyline HCL) and non-pharmacological (cognitive-behavioral) therapies for chronic tension headaches. *Journal of Consulting and Clinical Psychology, 59,* 387–393.

Hunt, G., & Azrin, N. (1973). The community-reinforcement approach to alcoholism. *Behaviour Research and Therapy, 11,* 91–104.

Jacobson, N. (1977). Training couples to solve their marital problems. *International Journal of Family Counseling, 4,* 22–31.

Jacobson, N. (1978). Specific and non-specific factors in the effectiveness of a behavioral approach to the treatment of marital discord. *Journal of Consulting and Clinical Psychology, 45,* 442–452.

Johnson, S. M., & Greenberg, L. S. (1985). Differential effects of experiential and problem-solving interventions in resolving marital conflict. *Journal of Consulting and Clinical Psychology, 53,* 175–184.

Kazdin, A. E. (1979). Fictions, factions, and functions of behavior therapy. *Behavior Therapy, 10,* 629–654.

Kazdin, A. E. (1986). Comparative outcome studies of psychotherapy: Methodological issues and strategies. *Journal of Consulting and Clinical Psychology, 54,* 95–105.

Kazdin, A. E., & Bass, D. (1989). Power to detect differences between alternative treatments in comparative psychotherapy outcome. *Journal of Consulting and Clinical Psychology, 57,* 138–147.

Kazdin, A. E., & Wilcoxon, L. A. (1976). Systematic desensitization and non-specific treatment effects: A methodological evaluation. *Psychological Bulletin, 83,* 729–758.

Kazdin, A. E., & Wilson, G. (1980). *Evaluation of behavior therapy.* Lincoln: University of Nebraska Press.

Keefe, F. J., Caldwell, D. S., Williams, D. A., Gil, K. M., Mitchell, D., Robertson, C., Martinez, S., Nunley, J., Beckham, J. C., & Helms, M. (1990). Pain coping skills training in the management of osteoarthritic pain-II: Follow-up results. *Behavior Therapy, 21,* 435–447.

Kiesler, C. (1982). Public and professional myths about mental hospitalization. *American Psychologist, 37,* 1323–1339.

Klosko, J., Barlow, D., Tassinari, R., & Cerny, J. (1990). A comparison of alprazolam and behavior therapy in the treatment of panic disorder. *Journal of Consulting and Clinical Psychology, 58,* 77–84.

Kondo, C., & Canter, A. (1977). True and false electromyographic feedback: Effect on tension headache. *Journal of Abnormal Psychology, 86,* 93–100.

Lacks, P., Bertleson, A. D., Gans, L., & Kunkel, J. (1983). The effectiveness of three behavioral treatments for different degrees of sleep onset insomnia. *Behavior Therapy, 14,* 593–605.

Lambert, M. (1979). *The effects of psychotherapy.* Montreal: Eden Press.

Lambert, M., Shapiro, D., & Bergin, A. (1986). The effectiveness of psychotherapy. In S. Garfield & A. Bergin (Eds.), *Handbook of psychotherapy and behavior change* (3rd ed., pp. 157–211). New York: Wiley.

Landman, J., & Dawes, R. (1982). Psychotherapy outcome: Smith and Glass' conclusions stand up under scrutiny. *American Psychologist, 37*, 504–516.

Lawrence, P., & Tokarz, T. (1976, November). *A comparison of relaxation and stimulus control treatments for insomnia*. Paper presented at the annual meeting of the Association for the Advancement of Behavior Therapy, New York.

Leitenberg, H., Agras, W. S., Thomson, L. E., & Wright, D. E. (1968). Feedback in behavior modification: An experimental analysis in two phobic cases. *Journal of Applied Behavior Analysis, 1*, 131–137.

Lent, R. W., Russell, R. K., & Zamostny, K. P. (1981). Comparison of cue-controlled desensitization, rational restructuring, and a credible placebo in the treatment of speech anxiety. *Journal of Consulting and Clinical Psychology, 49*, 608–610.

Levitz, L., & Stunkard, A. (1974). A therapeutic coalition for obesity: Behavior modification and patient self-help. *American Journal of Psychiatry, 131*, 423–427.

Liberman, R. P., & Smith, V. (1972). A multiple baseline study of systematic desensitization in a patient with multiple phobias. *Behavior Therapy, 3*, 597–603.

Lick, J. R., & Heffler, D. (1977). Relaxation training and attention placebo in the treatment of severe insomnia. *Journal of Consulting and Clinical Psychology, 45*, 153–161.

Lindsay, W. R., Gamsu, C. V., McLaughlin, E., Hood, E. M., & Espie, C. A. (1987). A controlled trial of treatments for generalized anxiety. *British Journal of Clinical Psychology, 26*, 3–15.

Lipsky, M., Kassinove, H., & Miller, N. (1980). Effects of rational-emotive therapy, rational role reversal, and rational-emotive imagery on the emotional adjustment of community mental health center patients. *Journal of Consulting and Clinical Psychology, 48*, 366–374.

Llewelyn, F., & Hume, W. (1979). Patient's view of therapy. *British Journal of Medical Psychology, 52*, 29–35.

Loizeaux, A. (1991). *Confirmation bias in behavioral and cognitive treatment outcome research*. Unpublished doctoral dissertation, University of Denver.

Luborsky, L., Singer, B., & Luborsky, L. (1975). Comparative studies of psychotherapies. *Archives of General Psychiatry, 32*, 995–1008.

Luborsky, L., & Spence, D. (1978). Quantitative research on psychoanalytic therapy. In S. Garfield & A. Bergin (Eds.), *Handbook of psychotherapy and behavior change* (2nd ed.). New York: Wiley.

Mace, C., Page, T., Ivancic, M., & O'Brien, S. (1986). Analysis of environmental determinants of aggression and disruption in mentally retarded children. *Applied Research in Mental Retardation, 7*, 203–211.

Mann, R. (1972). The behavior therapeutic use of contingency contracting to control an adult behavior problem: Weight control. *Journal of Applied Behavior Analysis, 5*, 99–109.

Margolin, G., & Weiss, R. L. (1978). Comparative evaluation of therapeutic components associated with behavioral marital treatments. *Journal of Consulting and Clinical Psychology, 46*, 1476–1486.

Marks, I. (1978). Behavioral psychotherapy of adult neurosis. In S. Garfield & A. Bergin (Eds.), *Handbook of psychotherapy and behavior change* (2nd ed.), New York: Wiley.

Marks, I. (1982). Toward an empirical clinical science. Behavioral psychotherapy in the 1980's. *Behavior Therapy, 13*, 63–81.

Marks, I., & Gelder, M. (1967). Transvestism and fetishism: Clinical and psychological changes during foradic aversion. *British Journal of Psychiatry, 113*, 711–729.

Marshall, W. L. (1985). The effect of variable exposure in flooding therapy. *Behavior Therapy, 15*, 117–135.

Mathews, A., Gelder, M., & Johnson, D. (1981). *Agoraphobia: Nature and treatment*. New York: Guilford.

Mathews, A., Whitehead, A., Hackman, A., Julier, D., Bancroft, J., Goth, D., & Shaw, P. (1976). The behavioral treatment of sexual inadequacy: A comparative study. *Behaviour Research and Therapy, 14*, 427–430.

McClusky, H., Milby, J., & Switzer, P. (1991). Efficacy of behavioral versus triazolam treatment in persistent sleep-onset insomnia. *American Journal of Psychiatry, 148*, 121–126.

McConaghy, N. (1969). A controlled trial of imipramine, amphetamine, pad-and-bell conditioning, and random awakening in the treatment of nocturnal enuresis. *Medical Journal of Australia, 2*, 237–239.

McKnight, D. L., Nelson, R. O., Hayes, S. C., & Jarret, R. B. (1984). Importance of treating individually assessed response classes in the amelioration of depression. *Behavior Therapy, 15*, 315–335.

McLean, P., & Hakstian, A. (1979). Clinical depression Comparative efficacy of outpatient treatments. *Journal of Consulting and Clinical Psychology, 47*, 818–836.

Milby, J., & Meredith, R. (1980). Obsessive-compulsive disorders. In R. Daitzman (Ed.), *Clinical behavior therapy and behavior modification*. New York: Garland.

Miller, N. (1991). Emergent treatment concepts and techniques. *Annual Review of Addictions Research and Treatment, 1*, 1–14.

Miller, P. M., (1973). An experimental analysis of retention control training in the treatment of nocturnal enuresis in two institutionalized adolescents. *Behavior Therapy, 4*, 288–294.

Miller, P., Hersen, M., Eister, R., & Watt, J. (1974). Contingent reinforcement of lowered blood alcohol levels in outpatient chronic alcoholics. *Behaviour Research and Therapy, 12*, 261–263.

Miller, W. (1982). Treating problem drinkers: What works? *Behavior Therapy, 5*, 15–18.

Miller, W., & Hester, R. (1986). Inpatient alcoholism treatment: Who benefits? *American Psychologist, 41*, 794–805.

Miller, W., & Munoz, R. (1982). *How to control your drinking*. Albuquerque: University of New Mexico Press.

Mills, L., Agras, W., Barlow, D., & Mills, J. (1973). Compulsive rituals treated by response prevention: An experimental analysis. *Archives of General Psychiatry, 28*, 524–529.

Morin, C. M., & Azrin, N. H. (1988). Behavioral and cognitive treatments in geriatric insomnia. *Journal of Consulting and Clinical Psychology, 56*, 748–753.

Moses, A., & Hollandsworth, J. (1981, November). *Relative effectiveness of education alone versus stress inoculation training in the treatment of dental phobia*. Paper presented at the annual meeting of the Association for Advancement of Behavior Therapy, Toronto.

O'Leary, K. D., & Beach, S. R. H. (1990). Marital therapy: A viable treatment for depression and marital discord. *American Journal of Psychiatry, 147*, 183–186.

Ost, L. (1988). Applied relaxation versus progressive relaxation in the treatment of panic disorder. *Behaviour Research and Therapy, 26*, 13–22.

Paul, G. (1966). *Insight versus desensitization in psychotherapy*. Stanford, CA: Stanford University Press.

Paul, G. (1967). Outcome research in psychotherapy. *Journal of Consulting and Clinical Psychology, 31*, 109–118.

Persons, J. (1991). Psychotherapy outcome studies do not accurately represent current models of psychotherapy: A proposed remedy. *American Psychologist, 46*, 99–106.

Philips, C. (1978). Tension headache: Theoretical problems. *Behaviour Research and Therapy, 16*, 249–261.

Power, K. G., Simpson, R. J., Swanson, V., Wallace, L. A., Feistner, A. T. C., & Sharp, D. (1990). A comparison of therapy, diazepam, and placebo, alone and in combination, for treatment of generalized anxiety disorder. *Journal of Anxiety Disorders, 4*, 267–292.

Prioleau, L., Murdock, M., & Brody, N. (1983). An analysis of psychotherapy versus placebo studies. *Behavioral and Brain Sciences, 6*, 275–310.

Rachman, S., & Hodgson, R. (1980). *Obsessions and compulsions*. Englewood Cliffs, NJ: Prentice Hall.

Rachman, S., & Wilson, G. (1980). *The effects of psychological therapy*. London: Pergamon Press.

Ramp, E., Ulrich, R., & Dulaney, S. (1971). Delayed time out as a procedure for reducing disruptive classroom behavior: A case study. *Journal of Applied Behavior Analysis, 4*, 235–239.

Rimland, B. (1977). Comparative effects of treatment on child's behavior (drugs, therapies, schooling, and several non-treatment events). *Institute for Child Behavior Research, Publication 34*.

Ritchie, R. (1976). A token economy system for changing controlling behavior in chronic pain patients. *Journal of Behavior Therapy and Experimental Psychiatry, 7*, 341–343.

Robinson, L., Berman, J., & Neimeyer (1990). Psychotherapy for the treatment of depression: A comprehensive review of controlled outcome research. *Psychological Bulletin, 108*, 30–49.

Rosen, J., & Leitenberg, H. (1982). Bulimia nervosa: Treatment with exposure and response prevention. *Behavior Therapy, 13*, 117–124.

Ryle, A. (1984). How can we compare different psychotherapies: Why are they all effective? *British Journal of Medical Psychology, 57*, 261–264.

Saigh, P. (1987). In vivo flooding of childhood post-traumatic stress disorders: A systematic replication. *Professional School Psychology, 2*, 133–144.

Schaefer, H., & Martin, P. (1966). Behavioral therapy for "apathy" of hospitalized schizophrenics. *Psychological Bulletin, 19*, 1147–1158.

Searles, J. (1985). A methodological critique of psychotherapy outcome meta-analysis. *Behaviour Research and Therapy, 23*, 453–463.

Shapiro, D., & Shapiro, D. (1982). Meta-analysis of comparative therapy outcome studies: A replication and refinement. *Psychological Bulletin, 92*, 581–604.

Sloane, R., Staples, F., Cristol, A., Yorkston, N., & Whipple, K. (1975). *Psychotherapy versus behavior therapy*. Cambridge: Harvard University Press.

Slutsky, J. M., & Allen, G. J. (1978). Influence of contextual cues on the efficacy of desensitization and a credible placebo in alleviating public speaking anxiety. *Journal of Consulting and Clinical Psychology, 46*, 119–125.

Smith, M., & Glass, G. (1977). Meta-analysis of psychotherapy outcome studies. *American Psychologist, 132*, 752–760.

Smith, M., Glass, G., & Miller, T. (1980). *Benefits of psychotherapy*. Baltimore: Johns Hopkins University Press.

Snyder, D. K., Wills, R. M., & Grady-Fletcher, A. (1991). Long-term effectiveness of behavioral versus insight-oriented marital therapy: A four year follow-up study. *Journal of Consulting and Clinical Psychology, 59*, 138–141.

Spence, S. H., & Marzillier, J. S. (1981). Social skills training with adolescent male offenders: Short-term, long-term, and generalized effects. *Behaviour Research and Therapy, 9*, 349–368.

Steinbrueck, S., Maxwell, S., & Howard, G. (1983). A meta-analysis of psychotherapy and drug therapy in the treatment of unipolar depression with adults. *Journal of Consulting and Clinical Psychology, 51*, 856–863.

Steinmark, S., & Borkovec, T. (1974). Active and placebo treatment effects of moderate insomnia under counter-demand and positive demand instructions. *Journal of Abnormal Psychology, 83*, 157–163.

Stern, R., & Marks, I. (1973). Brief and prolonged flooding. *Archives of General Psychiatry, 28*, 278–276.

Stiles, W., Shapiro, D., & Elliot, R. (1986). Are all psychotherapies equivalent? *American Psychologist, 41*, 165–180.

Strupp, H. (1978). Psychotherapy research and practice: An overview. In S. Garfield & A. Bergin (Eds.), *Handbook of psychotherapy and behavior change* (2nd ed.). New York: Wiley.

Strupp, H. (1981). *Clinical trials and psychotherapy*. Paper presented at the Seventh Annual Temple University Conference on Behavior Therapy, Philadelphia.

Strupp, H. H., & Hadley, S. W. (1979). A model of mental health and therapeutic outcomes: With special reference to negative effects in psychotherapy. *American Psychologist, 32*, 187–196.

Svartberg, M., & Stiles, T. (1991). Comparative effects of short-term psychodynamic psychotherapy: A meta-analysis. *Journal of Consulting and Clinical Psychology, 59*, 704–714.

Turner, J. A., & Clancy, S. (1988). Comparison of operant behavioral and cognitive behavioral group treatment for chronic low back pain. *Journal of Consulting and Clinical Psychology, 56*, 261–266.

Turner, R., & Ascher, M. (1979a). A within subject analysis of stimulus control therapy with severe sleep-onset insomnia. *Behaviour Research and Therapy, 17*, 107–112.

Turner, R., & Ascher, M. (1979b). Controlled comparison of progressive relaxation, stimulus control, and paradoxical intention therapies for insomnia. *Journal of Consulting and Clinical Psychology, 47*, 500–508.

Wachtel, P. (1977). *Psychoanalysis and behavior therapy*. New York: Basic Books.

Weisz, J., Weiss, B., Alicke, M., & Klotz, M. (1987). Effectiveness of psychotherapy with children and adolescents: A meta-analysis for clinicians. *Journal of Consulting and Clinical Psychology, 55*, 542–549.

Wilson, G., & Rachman, S. (1983). Meta-analysis and the evaluation of psychotherapy outcome: Limitations and liabilities. *Journal of Consulting and Clinical Psychology, 51*, 54–64.

Wincze, J. P., Leitenberg, H., & Agras, W. S. (1972). The effects of token reinforcement and feedback on the delusional verbal behavior of chronic paranoid schizophrenics. *Journal of Applied Behavior Analysis, 5*, 247–262.

Wollersheim, P. (1970). Effectiveness of group therapy based on learning principles in the treatment of overweight women. *Journal of Abnormal Psychology, 76*, 462–474.

Wulpert, M., & Dries, R. (1977). The relative efficacy of methylphenidate (Ritalin) and behavior modification in the treatment of a hyperactive child. *Journal of Applied Behavior Analysis, 10*, 21–31.

Zilbergeld, B. (1983). *The shrinking of America*. New York: Little, Brown.

Appendix: Comparative Studies Showing Superiority of Directive Psychotherapies

1. Alexander, J., & Parsons, B. (1973). Short-term behavioral intervention with delinquent families. *Journal of Abnormal Psychology, 81*, 21–31.

2. Argyle, M., Bryant, B., & Trower, P. (1974). Social skills training and psychotherapy: A comparative study. *Psychological Medicine, 4*, 435–443.
3. Azrin, N., Naster, B., & Jones, R. (1973). Reciprocity counseling: A rapid learning-based procedure for marital counseling. *Behaviour Research and Therapy, 11*, 365–382.
4. Bellack, A., Hersen, M., & Himmelhock, J. (1983). A comparison of social skills training, pharmacology, and psychotherapy for depression. *Behaviour Research and Therapy, 21*, 101–107.
5. Beutler, L. E., Engle, D., Mohr, D., Daldrup, R. J., Bergan, J., Meredith, K,. & Merry, W. (1991). Predictors of differential response to cognitive, experiential, and self-directed psychotherapeutic procedures. *Journal of Consulting and Clinical Psychology, 59*, 333–340.
6. Beutler, L. E., & Mitchell, R. (1981). Differential psychotherapy outcome among depressed and impulsive patients as a function of analytic and experiential treatment procedures. *Psychiatry, 44*, 297–306.
7. Blowers, C., Cobb, J., & Mathews, A. (1987). Generalized anxiety: A controlled treatment study. *Behaviour Research and Therapy, 25*, 493–562.
8. Borkovec, T. D., Mathews, A. M., Chambers, A., Embrahimi, S., Lytle, R., & Nelson, R. (1987). The effects of relaxation training with cognitive or non-directive therapy and the role of relaxation-induced anxiety in the treatment of generalized anxiety. *Journal of Consulting and Clinical Psychology, 55*, 883–888.
9. Boudewuns, P., & Hyer, L. (1990). Physiological response to combat memories and preliminary treatment outcomes in Vietnam veteran PTSD patients treated with direct therapeutic exposure. *Behavior Therapy, 21*, 63–87.
10. Chaney, E. F., O'Leary, M. R., & Marlatt, G. A. (1978). Skill training with alcoholics. *Journal of Counseling and Clinical Psychology, 46*, 1092–1104.
11. Cooper, J., Gelder, M., & Marks, I. (1965). Results of behavior therapy in 77 psychiatric patients. *British Medical Journal, 1*, 1222–1225.
12. Cooper, N. D., & Clum, G. A. (1989). Imaginal flooding as a supplementary treatment for PTSD in combat veterans: A controlled study. *Behavior Therapy, 20*, 381–391.
13. Covi, L., & Lipman, R. (1987). Cognitive-behavioral group psychotherapy combined with imipramine in major depression. *Psychopharmacological Bulletin, 23*, 173–176.
14. Crowe, M. (1978). Conjoint marital therapy: A controlled outcome study. *Psychological Medicine, 8*, 623–636.
15. De Jong, R., Treiber, R., & Henrich, G. (1986). Effectiveness of two psychological treatments for inpatients with severe and chronic depression. *Cognitive Therapy and Research, 10*, 645–663.
16. DeLeon, G., & Mandell, W. (1966). A comparison of conditioning and psychotherapy in the treatment of functional enuresis. *Journal of Consulting and Clinical Psychology, 22*, 326–330.
17. DiLoreto, A. (1971). *Comparative psychotherapy; An experimental analysis.* Chicago, IL: Aldine.
18. Dworkin, S. H., & Kerr, B. A. (1987). Comparison of interventions for women experiencing body image problems. *Journal of Counseling Psychology, 34*, 136–140.
19. Eriksen, L., Bjornstad, S., & Gotestam, K. G. (1986). Social skills training in groups for alcoholics: One-year treatment outcome for groups and individuals. *Addictive Behaviors, 11*, 309–329.
20. Fairburn, C. G., Kirk, J., O'Conner, M., & Cooper, M. J. (1986). A comparison of two psychological treatments for bulimia nervosa. *Behaviour Research and Therapy, 24*, 629–643.
21. Falloon, I., McGill, C., Boyd, J., & Pederson, J. (1987). Family management in the prevention of morbidity of schizophrenia: Social outcome of a two group longitudinal study. *Psychological Medicine, 17*, 59–66.
22. Falloon, I., & Pederson, J. (1985). Family management in the prevention of morbidity of schizophrenia; The adjustment of the family. *British Journal of Psychiatry, 147*, 156–163.
23. Feldman, M., & MacCullock, M. (1971). *Homosexual behavior: Therapy and assessment.* Oxford, England: Pergamon Press.
24. Fisher, R. (1974). The effect of two group counseling methods on perceptual congruence in married pairs. *Dissertation Abstracts International, 35*, 885A.
25. Foa, E., Rothbaum, B. Riggs, D., & Murdock, T. (1991). Treatment of posttraumatic stress disorder in rape victims: A comparison between cognitive-behavioral procedures and counseling. *Journal of Counseling and Clinical Psychology, 59*, 715–753.
26. Gallagher, D. E., & Thompson, L. W. (1982). Treatment of major depressive disorder in older adult outpatients with brief psychotherapies. *Psychotherapy: Theory, Research, and Practice, 19*, 482–490.
27. Gelder, M., Bancroft, J., Gath, D., Johnston, D., Mathews, A., & Shaw, P. (1973). Specific and non-specific factors in behavior therapy. *British Journal of Psychiatry, 123*, 445–462.

28. Gelder, M., & Marks, I. (1968). A cross-over study of desensitization in phobias. *British Journal of Psychiatry, 114*, 323–328.
29. Gelder, M., Marks, I., & Wolff, H. (1967). Desensitization and psychotherapy in the treatment of phobic states: A controlled inquiry. *British Journal of Psychiatry, 113*, 53–73.
30. Giles, T., McMullin, R., & Turner, R. (1982, November). *Outcome of cognitive restructuring with mental health center outpatients*. Paper presented at the annual meeting of the Association for the Advancement of Behavior Therapy, Los Angeles.
31. Gillan, P., & Rachman, S. (1974). An experimental investigation of behavior therapy in phobic patients. *British Journal of Psychiatry, 124*, 392–401.
32. Glagower, F., Fremouw, W., & McCrosky, J. (1978). A component analysis of cognitive restructuring. *Cognitive Research and Therapy, 2*, 241–254.
33. Graff, R. W., Whitehead, G. I., & LeCompte, M. (1986). Group treatment with divorced women using cognitive-behavioral and supportive insight methods. *Journal of Counseling Psychology, 33*, 276–281.
34. Gunderson, J. G., Frank, A. F., Katz, H. M., Vannicelli, M. L., Frosch, J. P., & Knapp, P. H. (1984). Effects of psychotherapy in schizophrenia: A comparative outcome of two forms of treatment. *Schizophrenia Bulletin, 10*, 564–598.
35. Harmatz, M., & Lapue, P. (1968). Behavior modification of over-eating in a psychiatric population. *Journal of Consulting and Clinical Psychology, 32*, 583–587.
36. Hartlage, L. (1970). Subprofessional therapists' use of reinforcement vs. traditional psychotherapeutic techniques with schizophrenia. *Journal of Consulting and Clinical Psychology, 34*, 181–183.
37. Heimberg, R., Dodge, C., Hope, D., Kennedy, C., Zollo, L., & Becker, R. (1990). Cognitive-behavioral group treatment for social phobia: Comparison with a credible placebo control. *Cognitive Therapy and Research, 14*, 1–23.
38. Hersen, M., Bellack, A. S., Himmelhoch, J. M., & Thase, M. E. (1984). Effects of social skills training, amitriptyline, and psychotherapy in unipolar depressed women. *Behavior Therapy, 15*, 21–40.
39. Hoffart, A., & Martinsen, E. (1991). Exposure-based integrated vs. pure psychodynamic treatment of agoraphobic patients. *Psychotherapy, 27*, 210–218.
40. Hogarty, G., Anderson, C., Deiss, D., Kornblith, S., Greenwald, D., Jauna, C., & Madonia, M. (1986). Family psychoeducation, social skills training, and maintenance chemotherapy I: One year of a controlled study of relapse and expressed emotion. *Archives of General Psychiatry, 43*, 633–642.
41. Hogarty, G., Anderson, C., & Rekj, D. (1987). Family psychoeducation, social skills treatment, and medication in schizophrenia: The long and short of it. *Psychopharmacology Bulletin, 23*, 12–13.
42. Humphrey, J. (1966). *Behavior therapy with children: An experimental evaluation*. Unpublished doctoral dissertation, University of London.
43. Kazdin, A. E., Bass, D., Siegel, T., & Thomas, C. (1989). Cognitive-behavioral therapy and relationship therapy in the treatment of children referred for anti-social behavior. *Journal of Consulting and Clinical Psychology, 57*, 522–535.
44. Kazdin, A. E., Esveldt-Dawson, K., French, N. H., & Unis, A. S. (1987). Problem-solving skills training and relationship therapy in the treatment of antisocial child behavior. *Journal of Consulting and Clinical Psychology, 55*, 76–85.
45. Kendall, P. C., Reber, M., McLeer, S., Epps, J., & Ronan, K. (1990). Cognitive-behavioral treatment of conduct-disordered children. *Cognitive Therapy and Research, 8*, 121–125.
46. King, G., Armitage, S., & Tilton, J. (1960). A therapeutic approach to schizophrenics of extreme pathology: An operant-interpersonal method. *Journal of Abnormal Social Psychology, 61*, 276–286.
47. Kirkley, B. G., Schneider, J. A., Agras, W. S., & Bachman, J. A. (1985). Comparisons of two group treatments for bulimia. *Journal of Consulting and Clinical Psychology, 53*, 43–48.
48. Klein, N., Alexander, J., & Parsons, B. (1977). Impact of family systems intervention on recidivism and sibling delinquency. *Journal of Consulting and Clinical Psychology, 45*, 469–474.
49. LaPointe, K. A., & Rimm, D. (1980). Cognitive, assertive, and insight-oriented group therapies in the treatment of reactive depression in women. *Psychotherapy: Theory, Research, and Practice, 17*, 312–321.
50. Lazarus, A. (1961). Group therapy of phobic disorders by systematic desensitization. *Journal of Abnormal Social Psychology, 63*, 504–510.

51. Lerner, M. S., & Clum, G. A. (1990). Treatment of suicide ideators: A problem-solving approach. *Behavior Therapy, 21*, 403–411.
52. Levene, H., Breger, L., & Patterson, V. (1972). A training program in brief psychotherapy. *American Journal of Psychotherapy, 26*, 90–100.
53. Levis, D., & Carerra, R. (1967). Effects of ten hours of implosive therapy in the treatment of outpatients: A preliminary report. *Journal of Abnormal Psychology, 72*, 504–508.
54. Liberman, R., & Eckman, T. (1981). Behavior therapy vs. insight-oriented therapy for repeated suicide attemptors. *Archives of General Psychiatry, 38*, 1126–1130.
55. Liberman, R., Levine, J., Wheeler, E., Sanders, N., & Wallace, C. (1976). Experimental evaluation of marital group therapy: Behavioral vs. interaction-insight formats. *Acta Psychiatrica Scandinavica*, (Suppl. 266), *27*, 99–115.
56. Linehan, M., Armstrong, H., Scaree, A., & Allman, D. (1988). *Comprehensive behavioral treatment for suicidal behaviors and borderline personality disorder I: Outcome*. Unpublished manuscript, University of Washington, Seattle.
57. Maes, W., & Heimann, R. (1970). *The comparison of three approaches to the reduction of test anxiety in high school students*. Unpublished manuscript, Arizona State University, Tucson.
58. Margolin, G., & Weiss, R. (1978). Comparative evaluation of therapeutic components associated with behavioral marital treatments. *Journal of Consulting and Clinical Psychology, 46*, 1476–1486.
59. Mazadas, N., & Duehn, W. (1977). Stimulus modeling videotape for marital counseling: Method and application. *Journal of Marriage and Family Counseling, 3*, 35–42.
60. McLean, P., & Hakstian, A. (1979). Clinical depression: Comparative efficacy of outpatient treatments. *Journal of Consulting and Clinical Psychology, 47*, 323–330.
61. McLean, P., & Hakstian, A. (1990). Relative endurance of unipolar depression treatment effects: Longitudinal follow-up. *Journal of Consulting and Clinical Psychology, 58*, 482–488.
62. McLean, P., Ogston, K., & Graver, L. (1973). A behavioural approach to the treatment of depression. *Journal of Behaviour Therapy and Experimental Psychiatry, 4*, 323–330.
63. Michelson, L., Mannarino, A. P., Marchione, K. E., Stern, M., Figuera, J., & Beck, S. (1983). A comparative outcome study of behavioral social-skills training, interpersonal-problem-solving, and non-directive control treatments with child psychiatric outpatients. *Behaviour Research and Therapy, 21*, 546–556.
64. Miller, I. W., Norman, W. H., & Keitner, G. I. (1989). Cognitive-behavioral treatment of depressed inpatients: Six- and twelve-month follow-up. *American Journal of Psychiatry, 146*, 1274–1279.
65. Miller, I. W., Norman, W. H., Keitner, G. I., Bishop, S. B., & Dow, M. G. (1989). Cognitive-behavioral treatment of depressed inpatients. *Behavior Therapy, 20*, 25–47.
66. Moreno, A. (1981). The treatment of obsessive-compulsive disorders: An outcome study. In W. Minsel & W. Herff (Eds.), *Research on psychotherapeutic approaches*. New York: Peter Lang.
67. Moreno, A. (1983). *Experimental analysis of comparative psychotherapy*. Unpublished manuscript, Universidad Complutense de Madrid.
68. Morris, N. (1978). A group self-instruction method for the treatment of depressed outpatients. *Dissertation Abstracts International, 38*, 4473–4474A.
69. Morrison, L. A., & Shapiro, D. A. (1987). Expectancy and outcome in prescriptive vs. exploratory psychotherapy. *British Journal of Clinical Psychology, 26*, 59–60.
70. Ney, P., Palvesky, A., & Markely, J. (1971). Relative effectiveness of operant conditioning and play therapy in childhood schizophrenia. *Journal of Autism and Childhood Schizophrenia, 1*, 337–349.
71. Nezu, A. M. (1986). Efficacy of a social problem-solving therapy approach for unipolar depression. *Journal of Consulting and Clinical Psychology, 54*, 196–202.
72. Novick, J. (1966). Symptomatic treatment of acquired and persistent enuresis. *Journal of Abnormal Psychology, 77*, 363–368.
73. Obler, M. (1973). Systematic desensitization in sexual disorders. *Journal of Behaviour Therapy and Experimental Psychiatry, 4*, 93–101.
74. Oei, T. P. S., & Jackson, P. (1980). Long-term effects of group and individual social skills training with alcoholics. *Addictive Behaviors, 5*, 129–136.
75. Oei, T. P. S., & Jackson, P. R. (1982). Social skills and cognitive-behavioral approaches to the treatment of problem drinking. *Journal of Studies on Alcohol, 43*, 532–547.
76. Ollendick, T. H., & Hersen, M. (1979). Social skills training for juvenile delinquents. *Behaviour Research and Therapy, 17*, 547–554.

77. Olson, R., Ganiey, R., Devine, V., & Dorsey, G. (1981). Long-term effects of behavioral vs. insight-oriented therapy with inpatient alcoholics. *Journal of Consulting and Clinical Psychology, 49*, 866–877.
78. Patsiokas, A. T., & Clum, G. A. (1985). Effects of psychotherapeutic strategies in the treatment of suicide attemptors. *Psychotherapy, 22*, 281–290.
79. Patterson, G. R., Chamberlain, P., & Reid, J. B. (1982). A comparative evaluation of a parent-training program. *Behavior Therapy, 13*, 638–650.
80. Patterson, V., Levene, H., & Breger, L. (1971). Treatment and training outcomes with two time-limited therapies. *Archives of General Psychiatry, 25*, 161–167.
81. Paul, G. (1966). *Insight vs. desensitization in psychotherapy*. Stanford, CA: Stanford University Press.
82. Paul, G. (1967). Insight vs. desensitization in psychotherapy two years after termination. *Journal of Consulting and Clinical Psychology, 31*, 333–348.
83. Paul, G., & Lentz, R. (1977). *Psychological treatment of chronic mental patients: Mileu vs. social learning programs*. Cambridge, MA: Harvard University Press.
84. Paulsen, K., Rimm, D., Woodburn, L., & Rimm, S. (1977). A self-control approach to inefficient spending. *Journal of Consulting and Clinical Psychology, 45*, 433–435.
85. Penick, S., Filion, R., Fox, S., & Stunkard, A. (1971). Behavior modification in the treatment of obesity. *Psychosomatic Medicine, 33*, 49–55.
86. Pomerleau, O., Pertschuck, M., Adking, D., & Brady, J. (1976, December). *Comparison of behavioral and traditional treatment for problem drinking*. Paper presented at the annual meeting of the Association for the Advancement of Behavior Therapy, New York.
87. Riley, A. J., & Riley, E. J. (1978). A controlled study to evaluate directed masturbation in the management of primary orgasmic failure in women. *British Journal of Psychiatry, 133*, 404–409.
88. Rimland, B. (1977). Comparative effects of treatment on child's behavior (drugs, therapies, schooling, and several non-treatment events). *Institute of Childhood and Behavioral Research, Publication 34*.
89. Roskies, E., Kearney, H., Sperack, M., Surkis, A., Cohen, C., & Gilman, S. (1979). Generalizability and durability of treatment effects in an intervention program for coronary prone (Type A) managers. *Journal of Behavioral Medicine, 2*, 195–207.
90. Salkovskis, P. M., Atha, C., & Storer, D. (1990). Cognitive-behavioural problem solving in the treatment of patients who repeatedly attempt suicide: A controlled trial. *British Journal of Psychiatry, 157*, 871–876.
91. Schefft, B. K., & Kanfer, F. H. (1987). The utility of a process model in therapy: A comparative study of treatment effects. *Behavior Therapy, 2*, 113–134.
92. Schwartz, J., & Bellack, A. S. (1975). A comparison of a token economy with standard inpatient treatment. *Journal of Consulting and Clinical Psychology, 43*, 107–108.
93. Shaw, B. (1977). Comparison of cognitive therapy and behavior therapy in the treatment of depression. *Journal of Consulting and Clinical Psychology, 45*, 543–551.
94. Sisson, R. W., & Azrin, N. H. (1986). Family-member involvement to initiate and promote treatment of problem drinkers. *Journal of Behaviour Therapy and Experimental Psychiatry, 17*(1), 15–21.
95. Sloane, R., Staples, F., Cristol, A., Yorkston, N., & Whipple, K. (1975). *Psychotherapy vs. behavior therapy*. Cambridge, MA: Harvard University Press.
96. Sokol-Kessler, B., & Beck, A. (1987). Cognitive approaches to panic disorder: Theory and therapy. In S. Rachman & J. Maser (Eds.), *Panic: Psychological Perspectives*. Hillsdale, NJ: Lawrence Erlbaum.
97. Solyom, L., Shugar, R., Bryntwick, S., & Solyom, C. (1973). Treatment of fear of flying. *American Journal of Psychiatry, 130*, 423–427.
98. Steuer, J. L., Mintz, J., Hammen, C. L., Hill, M. A., Jarvik, L. F., McCarley, T., Motoike, P., & Rosen, R. (1984). Cognitive-behavioral and psychodynamic group psychotherapy in treatment of geriatric depression. *Journal of Consulting and Clinical Psychology, 52*, 180–189.
99. Szapoczinik, J., Rio, A., Murray, E., Cohen, R., Scopetta, M., Vasquez, A. R., Heruis, O., Posada, V., & Kurtines, W. (1989). Structural family vs. psychodynamic child therapy for problematic hispanic boys. *Journal of Consulting and Clinical Psychology, 57*, 571–578.
100. Tavormina, J. (1975). Relative effectiveness of behavior and reflective group counseling with parents of mentally retarded children. *Journal of Consulting and Clinical Psychology, 43*, 22–31.

101. Telch, C. F., & Telch, M. J. (1968). Group coping skills instruction and supportive group therapy for cancer patients: A comparison of strategies. *Journal of Consulting and Clinical Psychology, 54*, 802–808.
102. Townsend, R., House, J., & Addario, D. (1975). A comparison of biofeedback mediated relaxation and group therapy in the treatment of chronic anxiety. *American Journal of Psychology, 132*, 598–601.
103. Turner, R. W., Ward, M. F., & Turner, D. J. (1979). Behavioral treatment for depression: An evaluation of therapeutic components. *Journal of Clinical Psychology, 35*, 166–175.
104. Werry, J., & Cohrssen, J. (1965). Enuresis: An etiologic and therapeutic study. *Journal of Pediatrics, 67*, 423–431.
105. Wollersheim, J. (1970). Effectiveness of group therapy based on learning principles in the treatment of overweight women. *Journal of Abnormal Psychology, 76*, 462–474.

II

THE MOST EFFECTIVE TREATMENTS BY DISORDER

3

Outcomes and Methodological Issues Relating to Treatment of Antisocial Children

G. R. Patterson, T. J. Dishion, and Patricia Chamberlain

Introduction

This chapter is divided into four main sections. The introduction covers a very brief history of the first organized efforts to treat children's problems. It also includes information from epidemiological studies of conduct disorders in children. The second section consists of a summary of two of the primary theories that currently inform the majority of the treatment and prevention studies for antisocial children. These include parent training therapy and variants of social skills training that may emphasize a variety of skill deficits ranging from poor peer relations to anger control and deficits in cognitive processes.

The third section contains a review of the data from outcome studies that have used random assignment designs and that have included pre- and posttreatment observation data collected in the home, from court records, or from teachers' ratings (if teachers were uninformed about the design).

The fourth section includes an outline of a two-parameter model for evaluating treatment outcome. Presumably, all measures of treatment outcome are biased in some sense. The extensive research on mothers' biases in rating their sons is evaluated as a case in point. Because of the biases, the model includes converging measures collected pre- and postintervention. The two parameters in the model consist of the termination scores (intercept) and rate-of-change scores (slope). The

G. R. Patterson, T. J. Dishion, and **Patricia Chamberlain** • Oregon Social Learning Center, Eugene, Oregon 97401.

Handbook of Effective Psychotherapy, edited by Thomas R. Giles. Plenum Press, New York, 1993.

differential utilities for these two parameters in evaluating treatment outcome and future child adjustment are discussed.

Prevalence

There are several very different ways of referring to antisocial problem behaviors. A trait approach views antisocial acts as falling along a continuum varying from relatively trivial acts (e.g., disobedience, temper tantrums) to more severe forms (e.g., physical assault) (Patterson, 1982). There are also individual differences in the frequency with which these acts are performed. The data show that the more frequently the child performs antisocial acts the more likely the child is to also perform more extreme forms of the behavior. The best description of the antisocial trait would be based on reports from multiple agents from both the home and the school. It has been shown that the distribution of scores from this composite is normal (Capaldi & Patterson, 1989). In this continuous distribution, the more extreme the trait score the greater the risk for pathological outcomes such as age of first arrest (Patterson, Crosby, & Vuchinich, 1992), delinquent behavior (Patterson, Capaldi, & Bank, 1991) and substance abuse (Dishion, 1992). In all of these studies the relationship is linear; there is no particular threshold where increases in the antisocial score are accompanied by a nonlinear increment for risk.

The other approach is to arbitrarily set a threshold for antisocial behaviors and determine that all those who score beyond that point are clinical cases (e.g., a categorical approach). If one follows a medical strategy, the categorical approach makes sense in that it immediately identifies those cases in need of treatment. It also provides a convenient means for counting the number of cases in a community (i.e., an epidemiological perspective). For example, the DSM-III selects a set of 13 relatively severe antisocial behaviors (e.g., stealing, lying, assault, cruelty, weapon use) and stipulates that the child belongs in the category if the child displays three or more of the problems and if they have persisted for at least 6 months.

Perhaps the best known study using the categorical approach was the Isle of Wight study conducted by Rutter, Tizard, and Whitmore (1970). This large-scale survey of parent and teacher ratings of 10- and 11-year-olds provided the basis for selecting 271 children who seemed definitely at risk. These children were then studied intensively by psychiatric interviews with the child and the parents and teachers. The study showed that 3.6% of the boys and 0.9% of the girls were conduct disordered. In fact, 60.5% of all boys with psychiatric problems were conduct disordered.

The even more systematic study by Offord, Boyle, and Racine (1991) was based on all children born between January 1, 1966, and January 1, 1978, whose usual place of residence was in the province of Ontario. Each child aged 4 to 16 years was described by teachers, parents, and self-report. Scores were weighted based on the scores' previous demonstrated ability to differentiate among diagnoses by child psychiatrists. The weighted composite score showed that 6.5% of the 4- to 11-year-old boys would be classified as conduct disordered, compared to 1.8% of the girls in the same age group. The comparable rates for 12- to 16-year-olds were 10.4% and 4.1% respectively.

Certainly there is nothing intrinsically wrong with using arbitrary categories to provide a rough estimate of prevalence. If the antisocial trait is really on a continuous distribution, however, then arbitrarily taking the upper 10% of the distribution means that we are simply ignoring the fact that the other 40% above the median are also likely to represent problems both to themselves and to the community.

Most clinical operations that provide treatment for children find that at least half of the referrals are for problems of aggression. If we expand the category to include all forms of externalizing problems (e.g., hyperactivity), then two-thirds to three-fourths of the referrals fit this category. Wolff (1967) studied referrals to a child psychiatry department and found that about 47% of referrals for younger children (ages 2 to 5) involved aggression or oppositional problems. For older children these problems accounted for 74% of all referrals.

Early Beginnings

When Beers founded the National Committee on Mental Hygiene in 1908, the stated goal for the movement included the prevention of insanity and delinquency (Kanner, 1950). By 1922, the National Committee had become firmly committed to establishing child guidance clinics. The clinics were based on a team approach; ideally, each team comprised a psychiatrist, a social worker, and a psychologist. Each member of the team was assigned a different role in the treatment of children. Up until the mid-1950s, the treatment of choice in these clinics was psychodynamic (Kessler, 1966). The core of treatment emphasized the therapist–child relationship. Most of the treatment included intensive psychotherapy with the parents in an effort to alter their relationship with the child. Release of emotion, particularly in the context of play, was given a good deal of the emphasis. The implicit goal was to help the child achieve some insight about the nature of the conflicts that produced the adjustment problems (Kessler, 1966). This point of view remains a dominant one, characterizing much of the treatment provided by the mental health establishment for antisocial children. For example, these same concepts and techniques characterized the day-care program for problem children described by Grizenko and Sayegh (1990).

From this perspective, the child's inner conflicts and cognitive distortions cause the aggressive behavior. The dynamic theories emphasize different sources of conflict, but essentially they agree that the basic source of children's inner conflicts is their anxiety-provoking interactions with family members, particularly their parents. This orientation assumes that the essential problem is "in" the child. The strategy in treatment is to reduce the conflicts that drive the problem behaviors and to strengthen the ego control mechanisms. If these changes are made, the aggressive symptoms go into remission.

Levitt (1971) reviewed the outcome studies for a variety of children's problem behaviors and concluded that the case for these treatments remained to be proven. To our knowledge there have been no adequately controlled studies in the last two decades that used random assignment and pre- and posttreatment measures based on court records or observation. In effect, there is no adequate basis for evaluating the psychodynamic approach to the treatment of antisocial children. This is most unfortunate because, at the community level, this is probably the treatment approach most frequently applied to these children. One component of this early approach, relationship therapy, has been used as a placebo condition in several controlled studies; it produced no significant changes in the child's observed behavior or in court records of antisocial behavior.

Later Beginnings: The 1960s and 1970s

During the 1960s and 1970s, developments in experimental psychology and child psychiatry led to major innovations in the treatment of antisocial children. B. F. Skinner's *Science and Human Behavior* (1953) had a profound influence on a small group of investigators who were studying children's aggressive behavior. A series of laboratory studies and efforts to intervene led to the development of what might be characterized as a contingency theory of children's aggression. This in turn led to the development of the early forms of parent training therapy (PTT).

The 1960s also witnessed a major revolution within the general field of psychotherapy. Young psychiatrists of various persuasions were moving away from the psychoanalytic emphasis on daily sessions stretching over years to forms of short-term treatment. Among these professionals were the founders of the new structural family therapies (Minuchin, 1974) and strategic family therapy (Haley, 1976). This orientation has become the dominant form of treatment for families, including some families of antisocial children.

Early Forms of Contingency Theory

What Cairns (1979) identified as second-generation social learning theories generated a basis for the development of PTT. Both the theory of aggression and the intervention techniques are still developing.

Most or all of the early investigators were strongly influenced by Skinner, and they adopted an operant framework for thinking about how aggression is learned and performed. From this perspective, aggressive behaviors are directly produced by reinforcing contingencies supplied by the social environment (e.g., siblings, peers, and parents) (Bandura & Walters, 1963). The fact that children also learn by merely observing others' behavior (imitation) immeasurably speeds up the process of socialization. However, what the child elects to do is presumably based on the reinforcing contingencies offered by the social environment. From this viewpoint, the problem is not in the child, but in the contingencies supplied by the social environment.

Later developments in this model suggested that the anger, social cognitions, low self-esteem, and negative attributions so readily noted in the behavior of the problem child were secondary products of the training process (Patterson, 1982). Presumably, changing any one of these conditions without also altering the contingencies for aggressive behavior would not produce reduction in aggressive symptoms. In both the early and the current versions of PTT, changing the contingencies is viewed as a necessary, but not sufficient, condition for bringing about remission of the core symptoms.

The question was soon raised as to whether reinforcers could be used to increase aggressive behaviors. What are the reinforcers in the natural environment? It seemed counterintuitive that anyone in the child's world would intentionally reinforce such behaviors. The laboratory studies carried out in the early 1960s clearly identified a variety of positive reinforcers (e.g., approval, money, candy, points) as potential reinforcers for aggressive responses (e.g., hitting a rubber clown). The carefully crafted studies also showed that having another child model the responses could reliably increase the rate of these analogue aggressive behaviors (Bandura, 1973). There were several problems with this analogue theory; chief among them was the fact that these reinforcers were not the primary contingencies controlling children's aggressive behavior in their natural environment. Observation studies showed that in certain settings the victim inadvertently supplied positive reinforcers for aggression (e.g., the aggressor gets the desired toy, the victim cries) (Patterson, Littman, & Bricker, 1967). In the home, however, the crucial contingencies for aggression seemed to involve negative reinforcement (escape conditioning) rather than positive reinforcement (Patterson, 1982).

These new ideas about aggression were first applied to the treatment of problem children by Wahler, Winkle, Peterson, and Morrison (1965) and then by Hawkins, Peterson, Schweid, and Bijou (1966), Patterson and Brodsky (1966), and Hanf (1968). Most of these studies employed pre- and posttreatment observation data collected in the home to evaluate treatment outcome. The early studies demonstrated that the therapist skills could be taught and applied to clinical samples (Fleischman, 1981) and transplanted to new communities (Fleischman & Szykula, 1981).

According to Patterson and Narrett (1990), accurate feedback from observation data collected in homes and classrooms made it possible to quickly identify those components that were not working. For example, placing aggressive behavior on extinction and reinforcing competing responses proved ineffective for clinical cases. Presumably, the reduction in rate for aggressive behavior requires the use of an effective punishment and reinforcement for prosocial behaviors.

An Empirically Based Theory of Aggression

The early successes in training parents to change the behavior of their own out-of-control children were accompanied by a growing interest in building an empirically based theory of children's aggression. The key idea was that families who provided faulty contingencies would produce children who were not only antisocial, but also very likely lacking in social skills (Patterson, 1982). Observations in the home showed that the parents in these families tend to be highly irritable, as do all the other family members (Patterson, 1982; Snyder, 1977). In two clinical samples both the target child and his siblings tended to be more irritable with each other than did children from normal families, but the parents were significantly more irritable only with the problem child (Patterson, 1984). The children in these families *quickly learned that an aversive counterattack often paid off* (i.e., the family member who initiates the aversive intrusion backs off following a counterattack). Such a three-step arrangement (aversive intrusion–child counterattack–other withdraw) is an example of negative reinforcement or escape conditioning. These contingencies form a significant correlation between the antecedent behavior of the family member and the coercive reaction of the target child.

Individual differences in coerciveness in the home are determined by the strength of the connection between these antecedents and the child's coercive reaction and the density with which these controlling stimuli occur in the home. Several small-scale experiments described by Patterson (1982) showed that only a few presentations of negative reinforcement produced profound changes in the child's coerciveness. Snyder and Patterson (1986) showed that in the home such an arrangement is followed by an increase in the probability of the child's coercive reaction given that the same controlling stimulus was presented at a later point in time. Snyder and Patterson (1993) also showed that in the home the covariation between the relative rate of coercive child behavior and the relative rate of payoffs for these behaviors was a startling .73! The child's social behavior matches the payoffs provided by the social environment.

In effect, the family members in chaotic families operate in such a way as to maximize short-term gains and, in doing so, increase the likelihood of future misery. They natter and threaten at high rates, but usually fail to follow through. The scoldings and occasional beatings only make things worse (Patterson, 1982), and parents' failure to use contingent positive reinforcers means they do not function as a mutual support system for growth and development.

The core of PTT still includes a focus on changing parents' noncontingent reactions by (1) increasing their use of positive support for prosocial behaviors such as compliance and cooperation and (2) increasing their use of effective punishment for deviant behaviors when they do occur.

By the mid-1970s there were noticeable shifts within social learning theory. A number of investigators began to emphasize the bidirectional nature of the parent–child relationship. Others began to see that the context in which the family was embedded seemed to determine the contingencies observed in the home. Wahler (1980) identified the isolation of the mother as a significant factor in determining the interaction of child and mother. Patterson (1983) and Wahler and Dumas (1987) demonstrated how daily variations in stress impact daily variations in maternal irritability. Still other investigators showed that parental depression, antisocial trait, and social disadvantage all seemed to function as determinants for ineffective parenting practices.

Patterson, Reid, and Dishion (1992) presented a detailed description of this expanded theory of children's antisocial behavior. One of the primary assumptions of this fourth-generation social learning theory is that family management skills control the contingencies that govern antisocial behavior. Ineffective parental discipline and monitoring practices, for example, are thought to control the reinforcers available for antisocial behavior. If this is true, then measures of parental discipline and monitoring practices should account for much of the variance in measures of child antisocial behavior. Forgatch (1991) summarized the findings from three different samples in which multimethod, multiagent indicators were used to define each of the three constructs in the parenting model. The findings from the structural equation models for three at-risk samples are summarized in Figure 3.1. The fit between the data set and the *a priori* clinical model was acceptable for each sample. The measures of parenting practices accounted for 30% to 50% of the variance in the criterion measures of child antisocial behavior.

Of course, the correlations do not establish the causal status of parenting practices. Experimental manipulations are prerequisites for acceptance of any theory about child aggression. Three such experiments have been carried out; each set of findings is consistent with the idea of a causal status of parent discipline practices (Dishion, Patterson, & Kavanagh, in press; Forgatch, 1991; Forgatch & Toobert, 1979).

As noted earlier, the assumption is that contextual variables, such as stress, social disadvantage, divorce, or parental depression, and the antisocial trait all disrupt family processes. Patterson, Reid, and Dishion (1992) summarized findings showing that a mediational model provided an appropriate fit for each of the contextual variables. In the mediational model the impact of the contextual variable on child adjustment is mediated through its effect on parenting practices.

A study of social disadvantage by Larzelere and Patterson (1990) is presented in Figure 3.2. The effect of the contextual variable social disadvantage on later delinquency is almost entirely mediated through the measures of parenting practices. This model is a replication of earlier work by Laub and Sampson (1988).

Contextual variables are extremely important in two senses: (1) they are helpful in defining which families are at risk for disrupted family management practices, and (2) they define some of the primary sources of parental resistance during treatment (Patterson & Chamberlain, in press). These studies are reviewed in separate sections of this chapter.

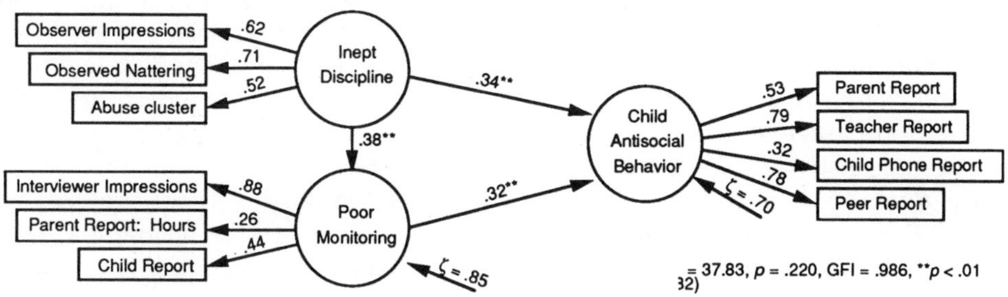

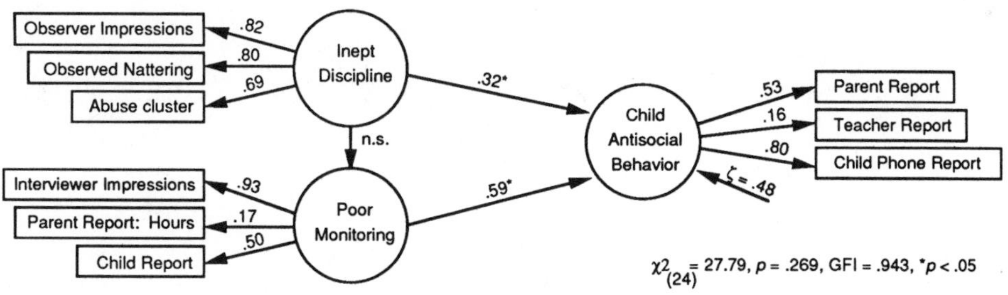

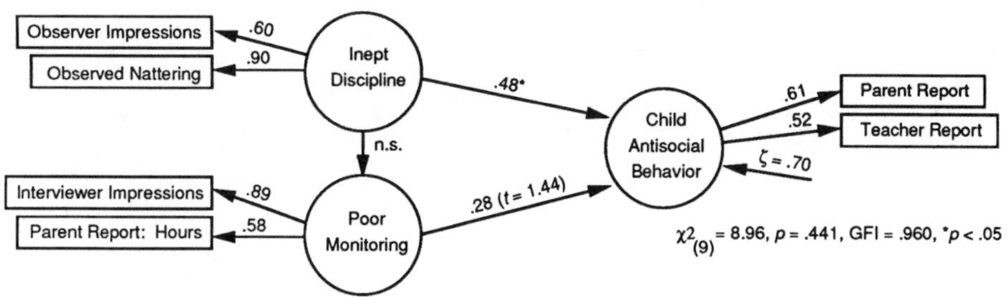

Figure 3.1. Two replications of the parenting practices model (from Forgatch, 1991).

Primary Theories

Parent Training Therapy

Although variations of PTT exist, most are based on a similar set of well-prescribed principles. There are, however, systematic differences in the types of skills, which vary somewhat depending on the age of the child. We discuss in a separate section the series of efforts that has considerably strengthened PTT in the last decade.

Hanf's (1968) application of PTT to preschoolers and younger children begins with a heavy emphasis on positive interactions between the mother and the child. This point is also heavily underscored in the work by Webster-Stratton (1984) and Forehand and McMahon (1981). Parents are trained to use such techniques as distraction, selective attention, and ignoring to reduce child conduct problems. Time-out is used for problems such as hitting or temper tantrums. There is a general emphasis on skills that enhance closeness between parent and child and parent emotional availability. The work with these younger children and their parents does not generally require a high order of clinical skill and can be carried out in a relatively brief series of contacts (6 to 12 sessions). Most therapists view these families as the easiest and most successful one-third of their caseload.

For elementary-age children, more emphasis is placed on helping parents establish programs for contingent discipline and reinforcement. The targets of treatment reflect the child's newly acquired status as a student with increased community contacts. The focus is on having the parents work to improve the child's skills in self-maintenance, work, homework, and academics. In cases where there are serious or long-standing problems, the treatment usually includes a school-

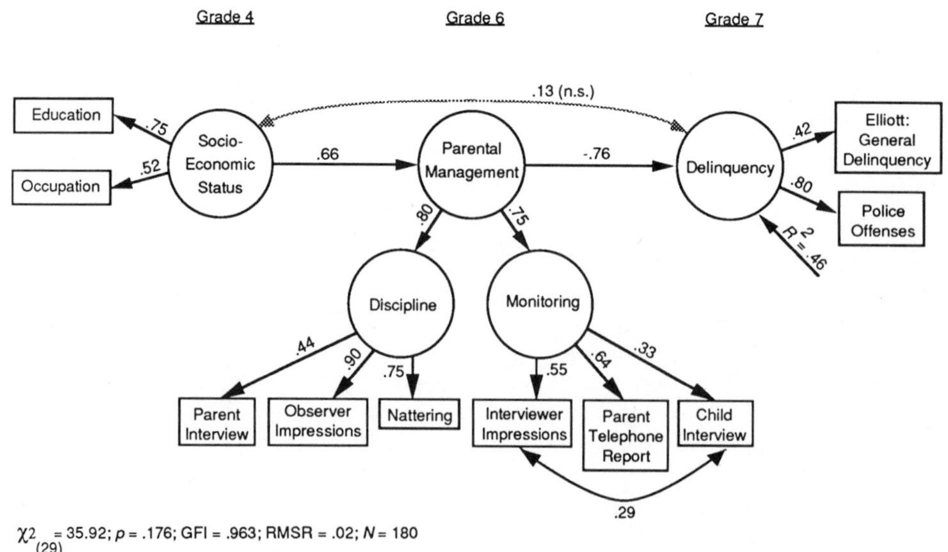

Figure 3.2. Structural equation method of the effects of socioeconomic status (SES) and parental management on early delinquency (from Larzelere & Patterson, 1990).

based intervention and monitoring component. The reason for this is that a substantial portion of these cases are academically retarded.

Daily incentive programs (contracts) are commonly used, and typical discipline methods endorsed include privilege removal and time-out. These procedures were presented by Fleischman and Horne (1979) and Patterson, Reid, Jones, and Conger (1975).

It is our distinct impression that the parents of these children are much more resistant during treatment; because they have been defeated so often, they have a thicket of defenses against confrontations with the child. These families are probably the one-third of therapists' caseload that most of them find difficult but with which they have some success. Therapists at the Oregon Social Learning Center find themselves consistently introducing enhancement components such as anger control, cognitive skill training, paradoxing, and reframing, to mention but a few.

For adolescents, parent supervision skills are emphasized. Poor supervision has been strongly linked with adolescent delinquency (e.g., Farrington, 1978; Laub & Sampson, 1988; Wilson, 1987), poor school achievement (e.g., Crouter, MacDermid, McHale, & Perry-Jenkins, 1990), fighting (Loeber & Dishion, 1984), lying (Stouthamer-Loeber & Loeber, 1986), drug use (Baumrind, 1991), and other antisocial and conduct problems (reviewed by Kazdin, 1985). Goldstein (1984) showed that the level of parental supervision was a better predictor of the likelihood of an adolescent having conduct problems than whether the adolescent lived in a one- or two-parent household.

Emphasis is placed on the parents' monitoring of the child's peer relationships and school performance. There is also a focus on teaching family problem solving, negotiation, and communication skills (e.g., Patterson & Forgatch, 1987, 1989). Contingency contracting is a major treatment component, and typical discipline methods include privilege removal and restitution through chores.

Although efforts to use PTT for chronic delinquents produced statistically significant results, the results suggest that this is not a viable approach to the problem. We review the findings in a section that follows.

A more practical approach to the problem of adolescent delinquency is the treatment foster care (TFC) model, which is now widely used in the United States for children and teenagers with a variety of presenting problems, such as abuse (Hawkins, Meadowcroft, Trout, & Luster, 1985) and medical fragility (Yost, Hochstadt, & Charles, 1988). The TFC program described here is aimed at delinquent and emotionally disturbed adolescents who are at risk for placement in or leaving institutions (Chamberlain, 1990; Chamberlain & Reid, 1991). This approach combines two models: social learning/interactional family treatment and family foster care.

In TFC, community families who are experienced with teenagers, have good parenting skills, and have a willingness to work as part of a treatment team are recruited. They are trained in behavior management strategies, including specific methods for teaching prosocial skills, discipline, problem solving, and contingent responding. One teenager is placed in each home. Their treatment plan consists of a minimum of five components, including:

1. A daily individualized at-home program implemented by the foster parents.
2. A school program monitored by teachers and followed through on by foster parents.

3. Individual therapy that focuses on changing the child's maladaptive cognitive-processing patterns.
4. PTT for the biological family.
5. Close monitoring and supervision of peer relationships.

Other components, such as specialized treatment (e.g., for substance abuse) or work-setting interventions, are added as needed. This multicomponent treatment plan is supervised and coordinated by a case manager who also maintains daily contact with the foster parents. The individual and family therapies are conducted by therapists who are thoroughly trained in the social learning approach.

In most cases the goal of the program is to have the adolescent return to live with his or her family. The typical placement length is 6 months. During that time it is the family therapist's job to teach the biological parents to improve their supervision, discipline, and reinforcement skills. The parents are given opportunities to practice these skills during weekend home visits. In order to program in generalization rather than leave it to chance, the parents are taught to use the same daily at-home program with their teenager that the foster parents are using. As treatment for the biological parents progresses, home visits are lengthened and implementation of the school program is transferred to them.

Preliminary evaluations of the social learning TFC program model are encouraging. Using a matched comparison design, Chamberlain (1990) examined incarceration rates for 32 chronic juvenile offenders who had been placed in TFC or in group homes or residential care. More TFC cases completed treatment, and fewer TFC cases were incarcerated at 1 year and at follow-up. Chamberlain and Reid (1991) reported a stronger test of the TFC model. They randomly assigned 9- to 18-year-olds who were leaving the state psychiatric hospital to TFC or treatment as usual in their communities. The TFC cases were placed outside of the hospital more frequently and more quickly than those in the control group; once placed outside of the hospital, TFC cases were more successful at continuing to live in an unlocked setting. Recently, investigators in several different settings have experimented with foster home placement as a prelude to returning children to their biological parents. This application of PTT looks promising. Three years from now we should have the results from Chamberlain's ongoing study; it will be the first systematic evaluation of the approach.

Family Systems Theory and Treatment

The relation between child development and a general systems theory has been articulated by a number of writers (e.g., Sameroff, 1989). In such a formulation, antisocial behavior is viewed as the logical outcome of a malfunction of the family system. Sameroff (1989) based his definition of a general system on the following principles:

1. The whole is greater than the sum of its parts.
2. A family system has a set point or equilibrium that it attempts to maintain. Perturbations from inside or outside the family, are met by efforts to shift internal structural relationships to meet these new demands. In a sense, the system is self-stabilizing.
3. The efforts to self-stabilize lead to a reorganization of the structure of the system.
4. The changes will emerge along hierarchical lines.

From the systems view, problem behaviors can best be understood by examining the family structure within which the problems occur. For example, how clearly defined are the boundaries between roles within the family? Are the structural relations between some roles more proximal or more distant than they should be? Are the boundaries too rigid or too diffuse? Are these structural flaws accompanied by repetitive sequences?

Treatment approaches focus on getting therapist's accepted within the system. Once involved, their goal is to interrupt the dysfunctional relation between the child's problem behaviors and the structures that produced them. The concomitant goal is to get the child to try some new behaviors while getting the family members to respond when they occur.

The therapy itself may introduce family enactments in which family members try a reversal of their usual roles. The enactments created by the therapist during the sessions bring the structural problems into dramatic focus and are a major vehicle for bringing about change (Minuchin, 1974). In addition, the systems-oriented family therapist works to change the family members' perceptions about each other's behavior by making frequent use of *reframe* statements. Paradoxes are used as a means of breaking up the repetitive nature of negative interaction sequences (Haley, 1976). Here, the therapist requests that family members "practice" the symptom as a means of teaching them that it can be controlled.

Minuchin and Montalvo (1967) described their groundbreaking efforts to apply some of these ideas to a small sample of delinquents living in the slums. They did not systematically evaluate outcome, but they clearly identified antisocial behavior as one of the early targets for this approach to intervention. Wells and Egan (1988) conducted the one systematic study that has been done with antisocial children; they showed that family systems therapy (FST) produces no changes in observed child compliance. A number of efforts to combine FST with PTT have suggested it may be a very useful adjunct. We review these studies in a separate section.

More Recent Innovations: The 1980s

Within the last decade, cognitive and developmental psychologists have contributed significantly to the treatment of antisocial children. Both emphasize that antisocial children lack critical social survival skills. The developmentalists, who see that these problem children almost invariably lack skills in forming relationships with members of the normal peer group, have carried out a long series of studies to determine whether social skills training (SST) will reduce antisocial behaviors. By contrast, cognitive psychologists, who showed that some crucial cognitive procedures have been disrupted in these problem children, have spent more than a decade developing intervention procedures designed to redress these omissions.

Social Skills Development: Peer Relations

Developmentalists such as Ladd and Asher (1985) showed that social skills training directly altered the interactions of withdrawn children with peer group members. This led to systematic efforts to develop standardized programs that could be applied to these problem children. Hops (1982) showed that these efforts were at least partially successful. Using observations and role-play tasks, Walker *et al.* (1983) showed that social skills interventions in the school can have positive effects on children's social behavior at school. Nevertheless, it is unclear to what extent such improvements relate to the conduct problems leading to referral for outpatient treatment. These promising results led to efforts to develop a similar technology that could be applied to antisocial boys.

Although intuitively appealing, the concept of replacing aggressive behavior with socially skilled behavior (Goldstein, Sprafkin, Gershaw, & Klein, 1980) has not been particularly successful. Studies have shown that role-play measures of social skill could be changed (Minkin *et al.*, 1976), but these changes tend not to generalize to other settings and are not accompanied by reductions in antisocial behavior (Spence & Marzillier, 1981).

Bierman, Miller, and Stabb (1987) showed in their programmatic studies that training was followed by increased positive and decreased negative interactions for target populations of rejected children. These significant changes in the experimental groups were not reflected by concomitant improvements in either teacher or peer group ratings! As Bierman's observation and intervention studies continued, she concluded that aggressive boys were *not* deficient in prosocial skills. The skills were present, but there was an increase in risk of a negative behavior occurring in subsequent interactions. When it did, it disrupted ongoing peer interactions. She concluded that social skill training alone was an insufficient treatment for antisocial children and that it must be accompanied by procedures that would reduce antisocial symptoms.

Social Cognitive Theory of Children's Aggression

Bandura (1978, 1985) took the position that children's perceptions and processing of their ongoing commerce with the social environment serve as the causal variables for social behavior. The perspective emphasizes the fact that children are not merely passive reactors to contingencies supplied by the social environment. Rather, their expectancies about the payoffs and negative sanctions are what govern their behavior. From this perspective, the problem lies not so much in the noncontingent social environment, but within the child. This, of course, has a major implication for treatment.

Some of the basis work in this area was drawn directly from cognitive theory by clinicians such as Spivack, Platt, and Shure (1976). Their position was that aggression and other forms of disruptive behavior were the outcomes of faulty cognitive processing. They demonstrated that laboratory measures of cognitive skills correlated significantly with teachers' ratings of child adjustment. For example, they found that problem children were less able to generate alternatives to problem solutions, less able to trace out the intermediate steps required to meet a goal, and less likely to accurately perceive the consequences of their behavior. Their studies moved on from the correlations to experimental interventions designed to demonstrate that improving the child's cognitive skills would result in improved classroom adjustment. Although the results from their early intervention studies could not be replicated, the work served as an impetus for many contemporary efforts to employ cognitive skills as components to enhance the impact of other procedures, such as PTT.

Dodge (1985, 1991) has carried out a decade of work that places disrupted cognitive processes directly in a social context; cognitive variables are used to build an empirically based theory of children's aggression. He takes the position that the child is not accurately processing the social cues generated during social interactions. The child's misperceptions about what is going on are exacerbated by a failure to consider a range of alternative reactions that might follow. Dodge carefully mapped out the correlation between aggressive behavior and several distortions in cognitive processes. His programmatic studies examine cognitive processes based on the child's responses to a series of vignettes. The vignettes reveal how the child encodes information about the reactions of other children (e.g., are relatively ambiguous behaviors perceived as threats? Are these misperceptions accompanied by negative attributions that in turn facilitate counterattacks to ward off the threat?). Several aspects of the formulation are similar to the earlier work by Spivack and his colleagues. For example, how likely is the child to search for alternative means for solving the problem, and does the child expect a favorable outcome if he or she initiates an aggressive response?

Several studies have shown low-level but significant correlations between the child's aggressive behavior in school and the cognitive-processing variables measured by the vignettes. According to Dodge (1991), the reason for the relatively low-order correlations is that they are based on faulty criterion measures of aggression. Typically, the aggression scores are the sum of two very different kinds of aggressive behavior. In his new formulation, *reactive* aggressive behaviors are accompanied by strong negative affect that reflects a history of violence and abuse. These prior experiences are strongly related to hypervigilance and negative attributions, which in turn elicit reactive aggression. *Proactive* aggression reflects a history of modeling for attack behavior and of positive and negative reinforcement for its occurrence. His data showed that proactive aggressive children were less likely to distort cognitive processing than were reactive aggressive children.

Cognitive-behavioral approaches to children's aggression have recently drawn heavily from the work of Dodge (e.g., Kendall, Ronan, & Epps, 1991; Pepler, King, & Byrd, 1991). The other important source of components for these innovations is based on the applied work of Meichenbaum and Goodman (1971) and their emphasis on teaching self-talk. Currently, there is not a single cognitive-behavioral theme.

In the section that follows we review studies evaluating the contribution of cognitive and social skills training components. In general, there is a good case to be made for adding either or both of these components to a treatment package. Nevertheless, there is no evidence to support the notion that either procedure is necessary or sufficient for the treatment of antisocial children.

Outcome Studies

We review here only those studies that use random comparison designs *and* include pre- and posttreatment measures such as court records, observation, or teacher ratings. The reasons for not including studies that rely primarily on parental report of treatment outcomes are detailed in a section that follows. We begin the review with PTT because it has received the most attention by investigators. In the second segment we focus on such alternative treatments as cognitive skills training, family systems therapy, and biochemical procedures as stand-alone treatments for antisocial behavior. In the third segment we review efforts to combine PTT with enhancement components.

Parent Training

Reviewers of the literature on the treatment of conduct problems have unanimously concluded that PTT produces the most consistent positive treatment effects for antisocial children (Dumas, 1989; Kazdin, 1987; McMahon & Wells, 1989). Based on our clinical experience, we hypothesize that younger problem children are easier to treat than older problem children because older children have a longer history of defeating their parents in discipline confrontations. The implication would be that the older the problem children, the more likely parents are to avoid attempts to confront or control them in any way.

An evaluation of treatment outcomes for the cases treated at the Oregon Social Learning Center (OSLC) was consistent with this hypothesis. In a reanalysis of clinical archival data from OSLC, Dishion (1984) compared the effectiveness of PTT with younger and older children. In this reanalysis, outcome was conceptualized as the extent of clinically significant change (Jacobsen, Follette, & Revenstorf, 1984). Comparing the means and standard deviations of the clinical sample and a normal (nonreferred) sample, cutoff points can be derived that indicate the extent to which a member of the clinical group is within the normal range following treatment. This, of course, is the goal of most clinical interventions. Home observation Total Aversive Behavior scores were used as the benchmark criterion of adjustment, with different cutoff points established for younger (3 years to 6½ years) and older (6½ years to 12 years) children. Comparing the outcome of 87 referred children to the home observation data for 63 nonreferred children (Reid, 1978), Dishion found that 36.6% of the children were within the normal range following treatment. Comparing younger with older children revealed dramatic differences in treatment outcome, with 63.2% of the younger children and 26.9% of the older children showing clinically significant improvement. In a discriminant functional analysis, several client characteristics (deviance at baseline, family chaos, parent psychopathology, and the child's age) were included as independent variables, discriminating between clinically improved and unimproved. Age of the child was the strongest (negative) predictor of treatment outcome: The younger the child, the more likely there was to be clinically significant improvement. The younger children also tended to have smaller families (mean 3.7) than the older referred children (mean 4.5).

A structural equation model based on more recently treated cases showed that the older the problem child, the less parental discipline improved from baseline to termination of PTT (Patterson & Stoolmiller, 1991). Less change in discipline was associated with poor treatment outcome (Forgatch, 1991). Forgatch employed changes in several indicators to define improved parental discipline (baseline to termination of treatment). The findings from Figure 3.3 are from a set of unpublished analyses. The data directly test the hypothesis that parents with older problem children have more difficulty improving their discipline practices (using contingent punishment). Parents of older problem children (11 to 12 years) had worse discipline practices during baseline and failed to show any improvement during the course of treatment.

Treatment Outcomes for Younger Antisocial Children

Forehand and his colleagues have documented in their programmatic studies the effectiveness of PTT for young oppositional children. They have articulated the correlations between changes in parental behavior and changes in noncompliance and have examined the contribution of contextual variables to these changes. Webster-Stratton (1984) carried out the first systematic comparison study for this age group that used both random assignment and pre- and posttreatment observation data. Families were assigned either to a PTT group that also included videotapes and other self-help materials or to a group that received only videotape materials; the groups were then compared to a wait-list control group. Both experimental groups showed significant changes in parent and child behavior on the observation data, but the control group did not show these changes. These effects were obtained for mildly disturbed, young (ages 6 to 8) children from essentially middle-class families.

Webster-Stratton, Kolpacoff, and Hollingsworth (1988) followed this major contribution to the field with a replication study of disturbed children referred to a university clinic because of oppositional problems. This also was a sample of young children (mean 4.5 years; range 3 to 8 years) from a wide range of socioeconomic levels. The 80 families were randomly assigned to three experimental groups (self-administered videotape-based, group discussion plus videotape materials, or group discussion alone) and a wait-list control condition. As before, the videotape and self-help materials detailed the PTT procedures. The pre- and posttreatment comparison data from the observations showed significant changes for all three experimental groups compared to the wait-list control group. There were no significant differences among the experimental groups. The replicated findings

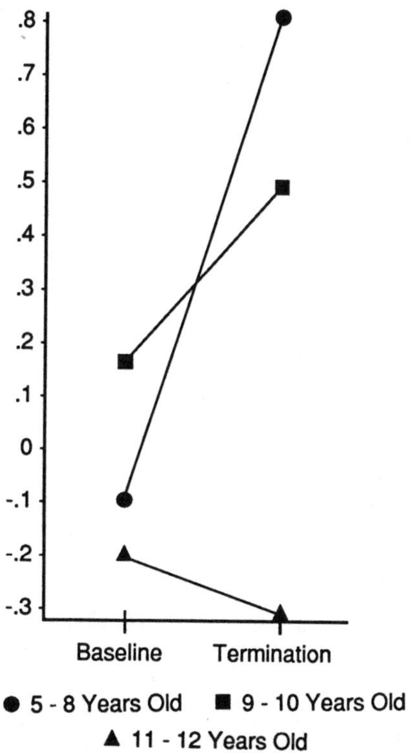

Figure 3.3. Changes in parental discipline as a function of the age of problem child.

strongly underscore the utility of self-administered parent training materials. The effects were maintained for two-thirds of the sample in a 1-year follow-up study (Webster-Stratton, Hollingsworth, & Kolpacoff, 1989). The study was further strengthened by data collected for a 3-year follow-up of the same treated sample (Webster-Stratton, 1990). During the follow-up, about 10% of the families sought additional treatment, 16% were in special education classes, and about 19% of the mothers and 15% of the fathers requested additional therapy. Twenty-six percent of the teachers reported significant behavior problems; about half of the mothers and fathers said they were still concerned about their child's problem behaviors. Children who remained maladjusted tended to be from single-parent, lower socioeconomic status families in which there was increased maternal depression and a family history of alcoholism and drug abuse.

Although there may be a slight advantage to using group discussion plus videotape materials, the finding that self-administered videotape materials are effective has major implications for treatment and prevention. A family that is not socioeconomically disadvantaged but does have a problem child seems to be the family of choice for the novice therapist.

Many therapists report that about one-third of their PTT cases move rapidly through therapy (in 6 to 18 hours) and are relatively easy to treat. We believe these cases are probably young and from lower-middle to middle-class families.

Interventions for Preadolescents

Older antisocial children typically require more treatment time (20 to 50 hours). Outcomes of PTT studies involving such children are less consistent in producing either clinical or statistical significance. Outcome studies that used unsystematic designs based on interventions with older children have failed to demonstrate significant changes in pre- and posttreatment observation comparisons (Eyberg & Johnson, 1974; Ferber, Keely, & Shemberg, 1974). Bernal, Klinnert, and Schultz (1980) used a large-scale systematic design based on a sample that included preadolescent antisocial children. Parent ratings indicated positive changes, but the pre- and posttreatment observation data showed no change for either the experimental group for the comparison (client-centered relationship-building) group. Treatment was limited to 10 sessions and was carried out by inexperienced therapists. The three studies that failed to find a significant outcome had three common characteristics: (1) they included some preadolescent problem children, (2) they consisted of time-limited treatment, and (3) the treatment was provided by inexperienced therapists.

We believe older antisocial children are more difficult to treat. Our case is considerably strengthened by Phillips (1984), who summarized the findings that resulted when the 12 treatment sessions used in the Eyberg and Johnson (1974) study were extended to roughly 20 hours. There was a significant improvement in pre- and posttreatment observation scores for the children referred for treatment. The level of experience of the staff may or may not be a factor, but the number of treatment sessions does play a critical role in treatment of older problem children. We also believe a high order of clinical skills is a significant factor for these cases, although there are no studies available that directly test this hypothesis. The reason for the omission probably lies in the difficulty of measuring clinical skills.

Phillips's (1984) finding that about 20 hours of treatment are necessary to bring about significant changes is in keeping with our own findings. At OSLC, the average length of treatment for PTT is around 20 hours and closer to 30 if it includes intensive work in the school and classroom.

Patterson, Chamberlain, and Reid (1982) conducted a comparison study in which 19 families referred for treatment received an average of 17 hours of treatment (range of 4 to 48 hours). The average age of the problem child was around 7 years (range of 3 to 11 years). The families were randomly assigned to experimental or comparison groups. The comparison families received an eclectic mix of treatments including structural family therapy, Adlerian, and behavioral components. The pre- and posttreatment comparison of home observation data showed significant changes for families in the experimental group and nonsignificant changes for families in the comparison group. In observations at termination, 33% of the problem children in the comparison group were functioning within the normal range, compared to 70% of the children in the experimental group. Parents' global ratings at termination showed that 25% in the comparison group thought the treatment was "very effective," compared to 90% of the parents in the experimental group.

Dishion *et al.* (in press) reported data for a random-assignment study of PTT with high-risk early adolescents ages 10–14 ($N = 119$). Families were randomly assigned to the following groups: (1) parent training only, (2) cognitive-behavioral training only, (3) parent training and cognitive-behavioral training, and (4) self-administered parent training materials only. Parents were seen in group sessions, and children in the social cognitive condition were treated in "teen groups." Families receiving self-administered materials only were provided with instructional videotapes and a newsletter containing the intervention information delivered in the other intervention conditions.

In one analysis, families involved in parent training were compared to those who received other forms of treatment. A treatment effect was found for boys, with those in the groups with a parent training component showing greater improvement in teacher ratings on antisocial behavior than those involved in the other treatment conditions. The effects were associated with improvement in maternal discipline reactions in a videotaped problem-solving session. Structural equation modeling was used to model treatment outcome. This model indicates that random assignment to parent training is associated with improvements in maternal discipline as well as the child's antisocial ratings.

Many of the families of these preadolescent problem children are difficult to treat and require the full range of clinical techniques. They probably constitute the one-third of the caseload that is tough to treat but satisfying in that the therapist is often able to point to some definite areas of progress.

Interventions for Adolescent Antisocial Youth

In every decade since the 1940s there has been at least one review on the lack of effectiveness of interventions for antisocial adolescents. Investigators have consistently been unable to find interventions based on well-designed, random-assignment studies for which the effects (1) persist during follow-up and (2) can be replicated.

In one of the best known efforts to intervene with families, Alexander and Parsons (1973) used a combination of PTT and family systems therapy (FST). The design is not exactly clear, but it seems that 86 families of adolescent offenders were referred by the juvenile court and also had complete file data. From these, 46 were randomly selected for the experimental procedures; 30 families were randomly assigned to either client-centered (19), or psychodynamic (11) treatment; and 10 families were randomly assigned to a wait-list control. From the description, it does not seem that at any given time a family could be at risk for assignment to four different groups. Recidivism rates were used to demonstrate a significantly better outcome for the families in the experimental group (26%) than for families in the client-centered (47%) or the psychodynamic (73%) group. This is very good news; unfortunately, the results are uninterpretable because there was no information given for baseline arrests in the four groups. It is extremely likely that the baseline frequency of police arrests would differ for the four groups. Studies with sample sizes of less than 10 or 20 per group seem particularly prone to this problem. The inability to balance baseline arrests for comparison groups was a crippling factor in the Arbuthnot and Gordon (1986) study. It was also a major difficulty in the earlier comparison studies carried out at OSLC (e.g., Wiltz & Patterson, 1974). With the small samples, it is unlikely that the baseline means were equal in the Alexander and Parsons study, and it is not clear what the outcome data mean. This is one of those extremely important studies we all want to believe; it is badly in need of replication.

During the last decade there were two large-scale efforts to intervene using techniques based on social learning principles. Kirigin, Braukman, Atwater, and Wolf (1982) showed that while the adolescents in their study were in a highly structured setting (token economy in a halfway house), there was a significant reduction in delinquent behavior and well-documented increases in prosocial behaviors. As shown by a national evaluation study of halfway houses (e.g., Achievement Place), the effect was quickly lost when the youths returned to their homes and to the communities that had originally referred them (Jones, Weinrott, & Howard, 1981).

Bank, Marlowe, Reid, Patterson, and Weinrott (1991) carried out a 3-year follow-up of a sample of adolescent chronic offenders randomly assigned to over 50 hours of either community treatment or PTT at OSLC. In many instances these extremely difficult cases required that our best therapy staff work in pairs. During intervention the PTT group showed significantly greater reduction than the comparison group in police offenses. The effects persisted during the 3-year follow-up, although there no longer was a significant difference between the two groups in police offenses. In effect, this massive effort to intervene accelerated the boys' dropping out of the crime process—one year earlier than they might otherwise have done. The experimental group also spent significantly less time in institutions. Unfortunately, because of the very high level of training and experience necessary for the therapists in this study, it cannot be said that these procedures should be adopted as a practical means for handling community-level problems of delinquency.

Alternative Treatment Approaches

In the section that follows, we briefly review the outcome studies that include cognitive, biosocial, social skills, and family systems approaches to the problem.

Contingency-Based Change in Social Skills. As noted earlier, efforts to train for peer relational skills outside of the classroom and then test for generalization have been successful. An alternative is to imbed the training in the classroom itself and increase social skills by direct manipulation of contingencies controlled by the teacher. Such approaches (e.g., the Good Behavior Game) have a history of reliably reducing antisocial behavior for entire classrooms (Barrish, Saunders, & Wolf, 1969; Medland & Stachnik, 1972). Moreover, the Good Behavior Game appears to be most effective with the most aggressive youths (Dolan *et al.*, in press). Consistent with the coercion model (Patterson, 1982; Patterson, Reid, & Dishion, 1992), effective interventions with antisocial children include alterations in the natural consequences provided for antisocial behavior.

As yet, no one has combined the effects of PTT with changes produced by altered classroom contingencies that focus on peer relational and academic skills. This is a study that certainly needs to be done.

Family Systems Therapy. A growing number of studies are using one or more components of FST in conjunction with PTT. By and large, this combination looks promising; we review the studies in a later section of this chapter. We have been able to find only one systematic evaluation of its effectiveness for antisocial problems (Wells & Egan, 1988). In this carefully designed study, 24 families were referred to a child psychiatry clinic. The cases were carefully screened. All of those accepted for the study had been diagnosed with oppositional disorder, and all had demonstrated at least 50% noncompliance in a brief (15-min) prestudy observation. The cases were randomly assigned to either PTT or an FST condition. The treatment was carried out by graduate students supervised by senior practitioners of PTT and FST. Each intern carried out both types of treatment.

There were no significant differences between the groups on pre- and post-treatment measures of parental depression, anxiety, or marital satisfaction. The observation data showed significant increases in parental use of rewards for the PTT group. There was also a significant increase in observed child compliance to commands for the PTT group.

More studies are needed before we can conclude that FST is an ineffective stand-alone treatment for antisocial children. The fact that FST has been effective with anorexic and asthmatic children suggests that it should also be carefully evaluated as a potential treatment for antisocial children.

Drug and Biosocial Treatment. Most of the studies that have used drug treatments with antisocial children seem to be clinical trials. In general, the field could be characterized as being in the presystematic stage—a necessary prelude for the design of large-scale comparison studies. In the systematic studies that have been completed, drug treatment has almost always been accompanied by some form of psychosocial intervention. We consider the use of drugs a form of biosocial treatment.

The literature on the use of drug treatment has been somewhat atheoretical and incidental. One would expect that the use of drugs to ameliorate antisocial behavior would be based on theories about the biological underpinnings of antisocial behavior. This is not the case. Lithium (DeLong & Aldeshof, 1987), neuroleptics (Campbell, Green, & Deutsch, 1985), and imipramine (Puig-Antich, 1982) have been used in children with conduct problems. The choice of drug treatment appears to be related to the comorbid symptoms of the clinical sample, and some success has been observed in reducing the antisocial behaviors as assessed via parent or treatment staff ratings.

There is a strong comorbidity between antisocial behavior and attention deficit disorders; therefore, methylphenidate is often used in youth with conduct problems. The treatment of choice for children showing the attention deficit syndrome is also methylphenidate, which reliably produces improvements in children's school behavior (Barkley, 1989; Pelham, Bender, Caddell, Booth, & Moorer, 1985). The consensus, however, is that stimulants are beneficial only when accompanied by child-management training for parents. To date, there are no data that conclusively indicate a synergistic effect for PTT and methylphenidate treatment (Barkley, 1989).

Quay (1990) and colleagues are investigating the possibility that there is a physiological predisposition toward conduct problems and attention deficits in children. Their goal is to link social experiences with the physiological predisposition in order to understand the biosocial processes leading to more extreme pathology in antisocial behavior. This could lead to a better understanding of the mechanism of drug action on behavior, as well as new strategies for drug treatment. The model arises out of Gray's notion of the behavioral activation (reward) and inhibition systems, which are assumed to be biological substrata underlying basic behavioral dispositions to seek rewards even under threat of punishment. These children are also more susceptible to escape conditioning of the sort suggested by coercion theory (Patterson, 1982). They are difficult to socialize and require tighter contingencies and more careful parenting (Quay, 1990). Some laboratory studies have confirmed that conduct-disordered children show response perseveration under laboratory experimental conditions where contingencies of reward and punishment are systematically manipulated (Daugherty & Quay, 1991; Shapiro, Quay, Hogan, & Schwartz, 1988). Other developmental investigators, working from a different theoretical perspective, have provided data suggesting that autonomic activity and hyperactivity and hyperactivity accompanied by antisocial behavior are highly prognostic of more serious criminality in late adolescence (Magnusson, 1988). A better understanding of physiological mechanisms that contribute to individual differences in responsiveness to environmental circumstances may lead to more comprehensive biosocial treatment strategies. We assume that such comprehensive strategies would be employed for individuals at extremely high risk for an antisocial lifestyle. Linking such developmental research with clinical outcome studies would lend some understanding of what, if any, physiological processes need attention in treatment and how they might be assessed.

Social Cognitive Skills Training. Much of the current effort to apply cognitive skills training (CST) to aggressive children is based on the primary prevention work of Spivack and Shure (1974). Among the most promising of these CST studies was the research program of John Lochman. Within a solid experimental design, Lochman, Burch, Curry, and Lampron (1984) compared several versions of an anger control intervention with a no-treatment control. The subjects were boys aged 9 to 12 years who had been identified by teachers as aggressive. Three versions of the intervention were analyzed: anger control only, anger control and goal setting, and goal setting only. The data revealed that the three cognitive behavioral interventions compared favorably with the no-treatment control in producing improvements in disruptive aggressive behavior in the classroom. Moreover, it appeared that a combination of anger control and goal setting (with teacher contingencies) was superior to the other three versions of cognitive-behavioral intervention. The extension of this study by Coie, Underwood, and Lochman

(1991) included 26 treatment sessions for a carefully screened sample of aggressive–rejected children in Grade 3. The intervention consisted of four components, one of which included an elaboration of the procedures employed by Lochman *et al.* (1984). The other three included social problem solving, group entry skills, and positive play training. The treatment has been applied to three cohorts. Although there is a trend toward significant changes in aggressive behavior, the overall results are not consistent. Coie's extensions of this work include PTT components.

Pepler, King, and Byrd (1991) also tested an intervention that was described as a social cognitively based social skills training program. The essential feature of the experimental design was random assignment to a wait-list control. They found that teacher ratings of improvements in externalizing and internalizing behavior were associated with social cognitive skills training. Parent ratings of these problem behaviors also improved. An examination of the extent to which the intervention produced improvements in social problem solving yielded mixed and weak findings. The treatment group was not different than the wait-list control group. The only light on the horizon was the fact that the wait-list control group did improve in social problem-solving skills when they eventually received treatment.

Other clinical investigators (Kazdin, Esveldt-Dawson, French, & Unis, 1987) have documented important treatment effects using a cognitive-behavioral intervention with aggressive inpatient children. The growing number of positive treatment effects with the cognitive-behavioral approach supports continued research and development.

One of the most interesting attempts to use a stand-alone procedure for treatment of antisocial children can be found in the application of Kohlberg's theory of moral reasoning (Arbuthnot & Gordon, 1986). The sample of 48 boys and girls (aged 13–17) was screened by teacher ratings on school adjustment. Those randomly assigned to the experimental condition received 4 or 5 months of weekly groups discussions on moral reasoning. Unfortunately, 50% of the sample was lost during follow-up. Although some of the findings for teacher ratings and court referral are suggestive, it is difficult to interpret the data because of the marked differences in baseline performance on several of the key variables.

The strongest case yet for the contribution to treatment of these problem children has been made by Kazdin and his colleagues in their work with children from an inpatient psychiatric setting (Kazdin *et al.*, 1987). The 56 children (ages 7 to 13) were being treated in a structured ward setting. They were randomly assigned to either a control group, individual general counseling (relationship-enhancing) sessions, or 20 problem-solving sessions. These were Spivak-type procedures in which the children practiced generating alternative solutions, taking the perspective of the other, and the like. At 1-year follow-up, the teachers' ratings showed a significant reduction in externalizing problems. The effects persisted through the follow-up period for the problem-solving group; the other two groups became worse. Kazdin is very conservative in his evaluation of these findings; he points out that although the results are statistically significant, there did not seem to be marked clinical changes in these children.

Although they did not employ systematic designs (random assignment, comparison group), there is one other study that should be mentioned here. Stanton, Todd, and Associates (1987) designed an FST approach that could be applied to families of drug abusers. They used behavioral techniques such as therapist incentives to get the families to come in for treatment and regular telephone calls between sessions to maintain contact. After strategic family therapy, the majority of the adolescents and their families reported improved functioning and reductions in drug use. The effects maintained but were somewhat diminished during follow-up.

It is too early to judge the potential for these procedures. We need more carefully designed studies like Kazdin's. It seems odd that so many investigators have adopted the strategy of using CST as an enhancement rather than test for its efficacy as a stand-alone component.

Enhancement of PTT

There have been no attempts to increase the effectiveness of PTT for older problem children by systematically adding academic and peer-relational skills training components. We see this as one line of studies urgently needed in the near future. To date, most of the enhancement studies have combined PTT with components for marital discord, maternal depression, FST, or CST.

Much of the PTT work in the 1970s included clinical efforts to cope with maternal depression and marital discord, but there were no systematic studies of what these components added to the overall effect. As shown in the review of enhancement studies by Miller and Prinz (1990), these studies are now occurring with greater frequency: for example, training the mother to more accurately synthesize her daily range of experience (Wahler & Barnes, 1988); and direct assistance in coping with parental distress, which seemed to enhance the impact of PTT (Forehand, Furey, & McMahon, 1984).

Brunk, Henggeler, and Whelan (1987) are three of the investigators who have expanded the focus to include all of the transactions within the family as well as those of the family with other crucial social units. They randomly assigned child-abusing families to standard PTT or to enhanced treatment. The pre- and posttreatment observation data showed stronger treatment effects for the enhanced group. These and other similar studies suggest that expanding the treatment focus to include components that impact parental stress, depression, marital conflict, and child peer-relational skills may significantly enhance PTT effects for families of antisocial boys. As Miller and Prinz (1990) pointed out, however, the efforts to date are not systematic enough to provide a basis for estimating effect sizes for these new components.

Even during the early stages of PTT development, it was apparent that a great deal might be gained by adding some ideas and procedures from FST (e.g., Attneave, 1969). For example, Alexander's work combines some elements of PTT with some elements of a systems approach. Compernolle *et al.* (1985) have made a systematic effort to incorporate the work of Minuchin and that of the OSLC group. Most practicing PTT therapists, particularly those working with older and more difficult children, are convinced that some features of FST are essential for effective interventions. The study by Kolko and Milan (1983) is a case in point. They studied three adolescents with school problems who were moderately out of control. They set up the usual school-based contract that was monitored by the parents. The multiple-baseline data suggested that they were having little success until they introduced *paradoxing* (e.g., the child was told to increase his truancy).

An increasing number of studies are combining contingency manipulations with cognitive skills training. Horn, Ialongo, Greenberg, Packard, and Smith-Winberry (1990) compared the two approaches with attention-deficit grade-school children; they found some indication of improved outcome when parent training and cognitive-behavioral approaches were combined. Kendall *et al.* (1991) described a series of programmatic studies that nicely combine contingency control by the therapist in a school setting with provision for teaching anger control plus cognitive skills. These procedures served as the model for the study by Kazdin *et al.* (1987). In their study, Kendall and colleagues applied the 20 treatment sessions to 29 black and hispanic children (ages 6 to 13) from a psychiatric facility. Each child was carefully screened and had received a diagnosis of conduct disorder. The children were randomly assigned to receive either the current psychiatric program or the cognitive-behavioral treatment. Both the teacher and the child self-report data showed significant effects in favor of the experimental group for increased self-control and prosocial behavior. Six-month follow-up showed that these effects did not persist; more to the point, there were no significant changes in antisocial behavior.

In general, there is very weak evidence that the two approaches yield synergistic effects (McMahon & Wells, 1989). A developmental data base is badly needed to guide clinical activity with conduct-disordered children from preschool through adolescence, with particular attention paid to the environmental and organismic factors needing attention at each age.

Resistance

One result of the prolonged warfare between parent and problem child is the parent's sense of having been defeated by the child. The thousands of failures during discipline confrontations lead the parent to feel both anger and anxiety at the thought of confronting the child one more time. We hypothesize that PTT encounters very strong avoidant behavior on the part of the parents as soon as they are placed in the position of having to impose rules, limits, or negative sanctions. The older the problem child, the stronger the avoidant behavior.

Avoidant behavior is reflected in the twin themes of "I can't" and "I won't" that we find throughout the treatment sessions (Patterson & Chamberlain, in press). The key role of these resistant behaviors is that they change the behavior of the therapist. Strong parental resistant behavior is experienced by therapists as aversive, and it literally drives them out of the therapy relationship.

For parents of aggressive/antisocial children, the determinants of parental resistance are thought to be influenced by two key factors: the dispositions that the parent(s) brings to the treatment sessions and the demands for change made by the therapist. Resistance to the therapist's suggestions for change occur both in the context of the therapist's face-to-face interactions with the parent, and in the parent's reactions to homework assignments given by the therapist.

Patterson and Chamberlain (in press) reported that for severely antisocial youngsters, the mean proportion of mothers' overtly resistant in-session statements was 6% to 10% of total statements, depending on the phase of treatment measured (i.e., at baseline, midtreatment, or termination, and fathers' was 6% to 9%. Chamberlain, Patterson, Reid, Forgatch, and Kavanagh (1984) found that the number of parental resistant statements in the first two sessions predicted which families would complete treatment and which would drop out.

The specific type of parental resistance expressed has been shown to relate to social and contextual factors in the family. For instance, Patterson and Chamberlain (in press) reported that maternal depression and antisocial scores at baseline were correlated with "I can't" but not with "I won't" statements at midtreatment. For fathers, baseline antisocial scores related to midtreatment "I can't" and "I won't," but depression correlated only with "I can't" statements. The age of the child appears related to the parent's homework completion rates: those parents with younger children being more successful.

For fathers, social disadvantage was related to all three forms of parental resistance measured. There is some longitudinal evidence that paternal social disadvantage may relate to the father's own antisocial tendencies (Elder, Caspi, & Downey, 1983). Data from our own studies showed that antisocial traits, social disadvantage, and depression all contributed significantly to parental resistance during all stages of PTT.

The mission of the therapist treating these families is to get parents to develop or improve a well-specified set of parenting skills. The amount of session time that is focused on these skills and concepts has been shown to relate to the level of case improvement and also to the amount of parental resistance that occurs (Forgatch, 1991). Patterson and Forgatch (1985) described this paradox for the therapist in an experimental test of the influence of therapist in-session behavior on client resistance. They showed that as the therapist talked about parenting skills or confronted the parent, there was a significant increase in the likelihood of parental resistance over the base rate. Decreases in therapist teaching and confronting were associated with decreases in client resistance.

In their face-to-face interactions, therapists who persistently focus on having parents improve their parenting skills are punished by the parents' resistant reactions. The effect is that these therapists are gradually influenced not to like, and finally to give up on, the family. Patterson and Chamberlain (in press) found that maternal and paternal rates of "I can't" statements and poor homework effort at midtreatment were associated with therapist ratings of not liking the parent at termination (*r*s ranged from .35 to .49, all significant at $p < .05$). Therapists' ratings of not liking were also related to mothers' (but not fathers') levels of "I won't" statements ($r = .44$) at midtreatment. The actual amount of session time spent talking about social learning topics was negatively related to the number of parental "I can't" statements during the closing phase of treatment. Furthermore, maternal rates of "I can't" at baseline predicted time spent on social learning topics at closing ($-.42$, $p < .001$). For both parents, success at homework was significantly correlated with the amount of session time spent on social learning.

Not surprisingly, the length of treatment is affected by the therapist's liking of the client, although the patterns of findings appear to be different for mothers and fathers. Patterson and Chamberlain (in press) hypothesized a curvilinear relationship between resistance and length of treatment. Because of Chamberlain *et al.*'s (1984) finding that clients who are most resistant tend to drop out of treatment before the fifth session, these cases were dropped from the analysis. The two forms of in-session resistance and homework in three phases of treatment were correlated to number of sessions. The only maternal resistant behavior that related to length of treatment was "I won't," which did not emerge until midtreatment ($-.24$; $p < .05$). More "I won't" statements from mothers were related to fewer sessions. Oddly, one form of fathers' resistance was related to longer treatment. Statements of "I can't" at midtreatment correlated .47 ($p < .001$) with number of sessions. Because of the high rate of absent fathers in the families studied, this effect was found for a sample of only 30 cases and should be interpreted with caution.

The therapist's ability to persist in teaching key skills in the face of the expressed helplessness of the parent and the therapist's own increasing discouragement or dislike appears to account for much of the variance in the success of treatment. Patterson (1985) articulated the need for a support system for the therapist to aid them in this effort.

A Model for Evaluating Treatment Outcomes

Treatment outcome studies should provide an empirical base for deciding whether one treatment works better than another. At the very least, they should inform us about whether a specific treatment is better than no treatment at all. The general model presented here assumes a two-step procedure. The first step is to identify the bias and validity of the pre-/posttreatment criterion measures used to evaluate outcome. The second step is to estimate the true change score from baseline to termination or, better yet, through follow-up. The primary hypothesis is that when biased and invalid criterion measures are used to estimate change, erroneous conclusions will be reached about what works and what does not. The implicit assumption is that this problem holds for a vast bulk of published work evaluating therapy for children.

We begin this section by defining what the target behaviors are for evaluating the outcome of treatment for antisocial children. We present a case for including multiple indicators for each problem behavior typically associated with the antisocial child. The reason for this is that any single measure of outcome is assumed to be biased. As a case in point, we review the studies relating to maternal bias in describing their problem children. We also present data that evaluate the validity of five outcome measures in predicting later child adjustment. Finally, we use the general model to evaluate the conclusion from meta-analysis of therapy outcomes that anything works as well as anything else.

What Behaviors to Target?

There is more to conduct-disordered children than just a set of antisocial symptoms (Patterson, Reid, & Dishion, 1992). Clinical studies typically describe antisocial boys as having myriad problems, including rejection by peers, academic failure, low self-esteem, depressed mood, substance abuse, and involvement with deviant peers. Structural equation modeling of the longitudinal Oregon Youth Study (OYS) has shown that, for many boys, these co-morbid symptoms have a common set of causes. The shared process is due to the nature of the antisocial symptoms themselves. When the antisocial acts are generalized to other settings (e.g., the school), the noncompliance, explosive temper tantrums, and refusal to accept negative feedback produce highly predictable reactions from the social environment. These behaviors cause many children in the normal peer group to reject the boy (most of the studies have been of boys). The boy's obdurate noncompliance includes spending little time on academic tasks, either in the classroom or on homework. The result is that he fails in school. These reactions from the social environment produce predictable reactions from the boy. His obvious failure leads him to become sad and to develop low self-esteem (Patterson & Capaldi, 1990; Patterson & Stoolmiller, 1991). Such experiences lead him to seek the islands of social support that do exist, which he finds in the deviant peer group (Dishion, Patterson, Stoolmiller, & Skinner, 1991). The effect over time is a steady unfolding of new problems and complications. The metaphor we use, "a cascade of effects," is summarized in Figure 3.4 (Patterson & Yoerger, 1993). It implies that *the more extreme the antisocial behavior, the more likely the child is to be characterized by a cascade of secondary problems.* One might say these problems are comorbid (i.e., they coexist), but this generally implies separate symptoms with separate causes. In the cascade model, a symptom in the sequence is a *cause* for the one that follows it: antisocial symptoms are a direct cause of school failure and an indirect cause of depressed mood. One direct cause of depressed mood is rejection by peers, another is school failure, and so forth.

A key assumption in the cascade model is that the process begins as soon as the problem child enters school. Tremblay (1988) showed that boys identified as antisocial in kindergarten were significantly more likely to be failing as early as Grade 3. Studies of the peer rejection process have shown that it takes only a few hours of interaction to set this process in motion. The implication for outcome evaluation studies is clear. By the age of 9 or 10, the antisocial symptoms will likely be accompanied by any or all of the following: school failure, peer rejection, and depressed mood. The implication is that for older children, both the treatment components and the outcome measures must target these concerns. On the other hand, one might be able to sidestep these concerns when working with younger children (ages 3 and 7 or 8). The cascade model was developed recently. In its wake comes the understanding that all of the outcome studies carried out previously failed to include components that directly addressed deficits in peer-relational and academic skills, or depressed mood. The next generation of outcome studies must include these as part of the treatment package, as the new generation of prevention studies has already done.

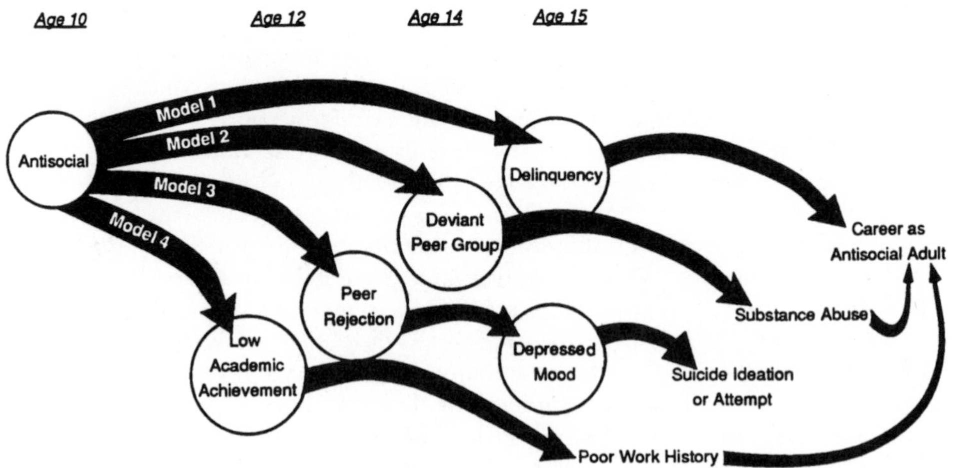

Figure 3.4. Cascade models.

Because PTT typically includes some components for tracking school adjustment and homework completion, there should be a significant generalization of effects from the home to the school. If the academic deficit is severe, however, this will probably not be sufficient, as demonstrated by the long-term follow-up of young oppositional children successfully treated by PTT (Forehand & MacMahon, 1981). In either case, the "ideal" assessment package would include variables that tap both home and school settings. Another characteristic of such an assessment package would be a provision for the use of observation data for both settings.

The use of observation data is thought to be a necessary, but not sufficient, basis for evaluating the treatment of antisocial children. This exalted status is based on the findings that suggest observation data is a relatively unbiased measure of change (Patterson, 1982). In a later section we will briefly review the data relating to the issue of bias in observation data. Our confidence in this type of data has been further bolstered by data showing that it can be effectively used to make long-term predictions about child adjustment. Using longitudinal data from the OYS, Bank and Patterson (1992) found that the path coefficients predicting later delinquency were roughly equivalent (each around .50) whether they were based on ratings from multiple agents (parents, teachers, peers, child) or observations from multiple settings (home, playground, classroom). Our confidence was further buttressed by the findings from a large-scale follow-up study of cases treated over the years at OSLC. The data showed that the observation-based Total Aversive Behavior (TAB) score could also predict long-term clinical adjustment (Prescott, 1991). The median follow-up interval for the 83 cases was about 10 years. A search of the records showed that the baseline TAB score obtained 10 years earlier correlated .201 ($p = .035$) with later adult police offenses. The observation score showed a correlation of .231 ($p = .018$) with the total pathology score from the Brief Symptom Inventory (Derogatis, 1975). The higher the level of observed deviancy in the home, the more likely the individuals will be to report 10 lyears later that they experienced a wide range of psychiatric symptoms. The TAB score also showed a borderline correlation of .19 ($p = .106$) with institutionalization as an adult.

Ideally, we collect data from multiple agents, including observers, with each agent sampling from different settings when evaluating outcome. One of the key assumptions underlying the developments in structural equation modeling has been the eminently reasonable notion that all measures typically employed in the social sciences are characterized by biases of some kind (Bentler, 1980). The bias issue is particularly significant in the analyses of change over time. Some agents seem more biased than others. If this is so, and if reports from only a single source are used, then it is conceivable that an estimate of treatment effectiveness is totally in error. In fact, we see the problem of analyzing agent bias in reporting changes in problem behavior as one of the key issues for the next generation of outcome studies.

We believe that parent, child, teacher, and peer data may each be characterized by a different set of biases in estimating a child's trait score. It is even more likely that each of these agents is differentially sensitive to change: some are biased to perceive change when it hasn't occurred (mothers), and others are biased to perceive no change when in fact it has occurred (e.g., the peer group in the Bierman *et al.*, 1987 study).

In this section, we briefly review the hypothesis that maternal ratings are strongly biased in several important ways. This discussion is also illustrative of what we expect to find when we examine bias in teachers' and fathers' ratings.

Mothers' biases seem to exist both in their descriptions of their children's traits and in their reports on improvements after treatment. The hypotheses to be examined are the following: (1) maternal bias is stronger in deviant samples than in normal samples (e.g., clinical or socially disadvantaged families); (2) the effect of the bias in clinical samples is also related to a lack of validity for these ratings; and (3) certain maternal traits are related significantly to false-positive errors in maternal ratings, while other traits are related to false-negative errors.

Maternal Bias in Rating Child Traits. A review of the 10 studies of parental ratings on the Child Behavior Checklist showed that mothers and fathers differed very little in their ability to predict such criteria as teachers' ratings or police arrest (Achenbach, McConaughy, & Howell, 1987). We suspect that a different situation holds when more deviant samples of parents are used as raters. Our hypothesis is that the more deviant the sample, the lower the convergence and validity of maternal ratings in predicting future adjustment. We also hypothesize that the maternal errors are selectively related to certain personality traits.

Our earliest efforts to model data from a severely disturbed clinical sample convinced us that it is more difficult to obtain convergence among family members' ratings in clinical samples than in nonclinical samples. When using the baseline data from a severely disturbed sample referred for treatment (Patterson & Chamberlain, 1988), it was difficult to obtain solid convergence on almost every construct we examined (see Table 3.1). The difficulty held across all agents, though the convergence seemed better for termination than for baseline data sets.

Both samples included boys and girls. The data from the clinical sample consisted of baseline measures of children ages 6 through 12 referred for treatment because of severe antisocial problems. For purposes of contrast, the comparable convergence data for the Grade 4 assessment from the OYS is shown below the

Table 3.1. Convergence Matrices for the Antisocial Trait

	Clinical sample			
OYS sample	Mother	Father	Teacher	Observer
Mother CBC[a]	—	.543***	.353***	.071
		(40)	(69)	(79)
Father CBC	.648***	—	.321*	−.212
	(132)		(39)	(79)
Teacher CBC	.406***	.420**	—	.053
	(196)	(142)		(70)
Observer[b]	.167**	.193**	.117*	—
		(142)	(206)	

Note. Figures in parentheses denote subsample sizes. OYS = Oregon Youth Study.
[a]The Child Behavior Checklist (CBC) was scored for our definition of antisocial behavior (see Capaldi & Patterson, 1989).
[b]Total Aversive Behavior (Capaldi & Patterson, 1989).
$^{*}p < .05$. $^{**}p < .01$. $^{***}p < .001$.

diagonal. These at-risk families were living in the four highest crime areas in the metropolitan area of Eugene–Springfield, Oregon. The details of the OYS sample and the psychometric properties for the scales were described by Capaldi and Patterson (1989).

In all six of the comparisons, the magnitude of the correlation from the OYS sample of at-risk families was higher than the comparable value for the clinical sample (i.e., the convergence was lower for the clinical sample than for the at-risk sample).

We propose that social disadvantage is another means for identifying samples that will be characterized by a lack of convergence for maternal ratings. West and Farrington (1973) found that the extent of the correlation between teachers' and parents' ratings varied as a function of social class. The convergence was lower for socially disadvantaged parents than it was for parents of middle-class families. They cited an earlier study by Glidewell, Gildea, Domke, and Kantor (1959), who found similar convergence. We consider this issue in a section that follows.

Although the poor convergence of maternal ratings in clinical or socially disadvantaged samples is a matter of some concern, the key issue is how valid those ratings are. They might not converge but still be a better predictor of future child adjustment than ratings by any other agent. To test this hypothesis, Jackson, Reid, Patterson, Schaughency, and Ray (1989) analyzed the OYS data collected at Grade 4 to predict police arrests during the ensuing 5 years. Mothers' ratings of sons were less predictive of later police arrests than were ratings by fathers or teachers. The correlations were .44 for teachers, .39 for fathers, and .23 for mothers.

We propose that the criterion variables used to evaluate outcomes should first be attempted for the clinical sample that is the target for the intervention. Do measures of this kind collected at termination effectively predict some relatively unbiased measures of future child adjustment? To provide a base for examining this hypothesis, a sample of 78 boys and girls (Patterson & Chamberlain, 1989) were followed up for 2 years after completion of PTT. Three relatively objective measures of child adjustment were selected: juvenile court records of police arrests, agency records of placement out of the home, and school records of discipline contacts. The convergence correlations among these indicators for the child adjustment construct are summarized in Table 3.2.

The covariation between arrest and out-of-home placement is quite strong (.421), but the school discipline variable shows only borderline (.220) correlation with arrest.

Five measures seemed to have a good deal of face validity: mothers', fathers',

Table 3.2. Convergence among Three Measures of Child Adjustment at 2-Year Follow-up

Criterion variable	Arrest	Placement	School discipline
Arrest	—		
Placement out of home	.421** (n = 78)	—	
School discipline contacts	.220* (n = 62)	.032 (n = 61)	—

*$p < .05$. **$p < .001$.

and teachers' ratings of antisocial behavior, observation TAB scores, and therapists' ratings of risk for future arrest (see Table 3.3). Mothers correlate somewhat with teachers and correlate well with fathers, as do therapists with fathers, but each agent is looking at a slightly different aspect of outcome. According to these data, the measures do not converge to form a coherent latent construct; rather, they resemble what we think of as a risk score.

How does an investigator choose among indicators when comparing treatment outcomes? We propose selecting one or more termination measures that are the most valid predictors of future adjustment. In the present context, we test the utility of ratings at termination of PTT by mothers, fathers, teachers, observers, and therapists for child adjustment measured 2 years later. The findings are summarized in Table 3.4. Of the five termination scores, only the one based on mothers' ratings showed no significant predictive validity. Each of the other indicators significantly predicted at least two of the three adjustment criteria. This suggests that three of the four variables may be used in a composite risk score. Presumably, a good score on each of the four indicators would mean a good prognosis for future adjustment; a very low score would indicate a poor prognosis.

Patterson and Reid (1984) reviewed four laboratory studies carried out at OSLC. They found that mothers of problem children were significantly overinclusive in categorizing child deviant behavior. They were more likely to classify as deviant those child behaviors perceived as neutral by others. Although it was not tested in those studied, we suspect that the tendency to be overly inclusive in classifying child deviancy correlates with maternal depression. A number of studies have shown that mothers of problem children tend to be more depressed than mothers of untroubled children (Forehand *et al.*, 1984; Patterson, 1980). Presumably, depressed mothers tend to make negative attributions not only about themselves but about their children and spouses as well. We hypothesize that depression is one of the important sources of bias in mothers' ratings of their children, particularly their sons.

Griest, Forehand, Wells, and McMahon (1980) carried out a study that relates to this hypothesis. They demonstrated that mothers' ratings of children covaried significantly with self-reported depression and anxiety. These theme was reiterated by Forehand *et al.* (1984), who showed that maternal ratings reflected maternal distress as much as observed child behavior did. These findings could also mean

Table 3.3. Intercorrelations among Termination Variables

	Mother CBC	Father CBC	Observation	Therapist	Teacher CBC
Mother CBC	—				
Father CBC	.449**	—			
	(32)				
Observation	.151	.118	—		
	(62)	(33)			
Therapist	−.024	.336*	−.084	—	
	(62)	(34)	(66)		
Teacher CBC	.263*	.114	.132	.139	—
	(50)	(27)	(51)	(52)	

Note. Figures in parentheses denote subsample sizes. CBC = Child Behavior Checklist.
$*p < .05$. $**p < .01$.

that having a deviant child increases maternal depression. Indeed, there is mounting evidence that the relation between maternal depression and child problem behavior is bidirectional (Forgatch & Patterson, in press).

Duncan, Patterson, Reid, and Bank (1992) refined the bias hypothesis further by demonstrating that maternal depression contributes to a particular kind of error in predicting future child adjustment. They used longitudinal data from the OYS to demonstrate a very subtle interaction between certain maternal personality traits and the *type of bias* reflected in maternal ratings of antisocial behavior in boys. They used mothers' ratings of their 10-year-old boys to predict police arrest in the next 5 years. The first hypothesis tested was that depressed mothers would tend to be overly inclusive in their ratings. This implies that maternal depression would be associated with high risk for false-positive errors in prediction of future arrest (i.e., the mothers see their sons as deviant, but this is not reflected in later arrest record). The second hypothesis tested was that maternal antisocial trait (measured by driving violations, MMPI scales 4 and 9, and substance abuse) would be at greater risk for false-negative errors of prediction (i.e., even though the boy was arrested, the mother had not previously seen him as being antisocial). The data provided strong support for both hypotheses.

In summary, the data now available support the hypothesis that the more at risk the sample, the less likely the maternal ratings of child adjustment are to be valid indicators of the level of child adjustment. This is paradoxical in that much of the fields of social development and child psychiatry are built on a foundation of maternal report data.

Maternal Bias Evaluating Treatment. It is hypothesized that maternal ratings are biased in a positive way when used to evaluate treatment outcome (i.e., mothers perceive improvement when none has occurred). Early publications evaluating the effect of PTT often commented that mothers perceived improvement even though none was reflected in the observation data (Atkeson & Forehand, 1978). In their review of 24 studies evaluating PTT, parent-reported change did not agree with observer-reported change in 22% of the studies. The problem is still with us today, as shown in the study by Knapp and Deluty (1989). Their observation data showed no significant changes in child behavior, but parent ratings of child behavior showed significant improvement. These parent ratings probably included fathers as well as mothers. Our hunch is that the act of seeking help may be

Table 3.4. Predicting Future Clinical Outcome

	2-year follow-up		
Prediction at termination	Out-of-home placement	Arrest (yes–no)	School discipline contacts
Mother CBC	.003 (62)	.139 (63)	.050 (52)
Father CBC	.331* (33)	.246[a] (34)	−.094 (25)
Observation (TAB)	−.068 (66)	.175[a] (67)	.43[a] (54)
Therapist rating	.439*** (66)	.277* (68)	−.045 (53)
Teacher CBC	.138 (51)	.286* (52)	.558*** (44)

Note. Figures in parentheses denote subsample sizes. CBC = Child Behavior Checklist. TAB = Total Aversive Behavior.
[a]$p < .10$. *$p < .05$. **$p < .01$. ***$p < .001$.

followed by a decrease in maternal depression, and then by the mother's perception of the problem child in a more positive light.

The most extreme example of this bias is found in studies where the mothers believed their children were receiving treatment when in fact none had occurred. This phenomenon occurred in a study by Collins (1966). After obtaining the initial parent ratings, the children in the study were to be assigned to one of several experimental conditions. Unbeknownst to the mothers, however, the scheduled treatment had been delayed, and Collins found it necessary to ask for a second set of ratings to reestablish his baseline estimates. The parents though their children had been receiving treatment, and their ratings reflected substantial improvement. Peed, Roberts, and Forehand (1974) and Pepler (1988) noted similar improvements from pre- to posttreatment ratings for wait-list control groups.

A parental bias to perceive improvement in problem children is certainly understandable; all parents hope for change. It seems also to be present in ratings from middle-class samples of mildly disturbed children. In a study by Sloane, Endo, Hawkes, and Jenkins (1991), the correlation between parents and observers was quite significant (.55, $p < .05$); the parent-report data identified 46% of the problem children as improving, while home observation data identified 33% as having improved.

We first encountered this problem in the early 1970s while designing a series of comparison studies. In a carefully crafted procedure, parents in the experimental (PTT) and placebo (parent-led discussion) groups were matched for expectancies for change (Walter & Gilmore, 1973). The pre- and posttreatment observation data showed that after 5 weeks, the families in the experimental group significantly improved, but those in the placebo group were slightly worse. The parents' global ratings showed that about two-thirds of the parents in the placebo group saw improvement, while virtually all of those in the PTT group perceived improvement. Despite the fact that the sample sizes were terribly small, we have come to believe that almost any form of treatment will produce global ratings of improvement in 60% of the families regardless of changes in the child's behavior.

The focus of this discussion has been exclusively on mothers. As we noted earlier, the reason for this is the richness of the available test data set. We suspect that mothers may be more biased in their ratings of improvement than teachers, fathers, or therapists, although the appropriate studies have not been carried out. We are convinced that teachers, fathers, and therapists are significantly biased too. In one small pilot study, we found that teachers rating children whose parents had been divorced and who had recently moved into the area underestimated the level of deviancy. If they did not know the child well, they did not want to rate the child as being deviant. While this situation may deserve some less pejorative term than bias, it does constitute a source of noise in convergence and predictive matrices.

Over the years, we have come to view the pre-/posttreatment estimates based on observation data as the golden standard. Our own preference in this matter is based on a series of methodology studies carried out in the 1970s and summarized by Patterson (1982). Studies carried out in Stonybrook, New York, and in Eugene showed it was possible to bias global ratings made by observers after home visits. The studies also showed, however, that the biases were not reflected in the molecular data they had coded. Programmatic studies were carried out at several centers to identify the impact of the observers' presence on social interactions in homes and classrooms. The studies left little doubt that the observers were noticed and responded to, but several approaches to the problem failed to demonstrate that the observers' presence significantly altered rates of observed deviant child behavior. This is not to say that there is *no* bias in observation data; the studies to date just failed to find it.

We presently believe that the TAB score is a less biased estimate of treatment change than, say, ratings by mothers for clinical samples. Another reason for emphasizing the value of observation data is that they seem to have a moderate level of validity. As shown earlier, observation data were significant predictors for school discipline problems and police arrests 2 years after termination of PTT, and for adult antisocial behavior some 10 years later.

Termination and Change Scores Are NOT the Same!

Up to this point, we have made a case for thinking of the criterion measures obtained at termination of treatment as a set of predictors for future child adjustment. Studies such as the one by Alexander and Parsons (1973) that give only termination scores are providing a valuable base for predicting outcomes (e.g., children arrested after treatment are more likely to be arrested later on). But we cannot simply look at a termination score and deduce from it who improved in treatment and who did not. Children who look good at termination might have looked even better prior to treatment. It is even conceivable that those who look terrible at termination were doing relatively well before the intervention (i.e., an iatrogenic effect).

To understand change, it is necessary to use the termination scores to calculate a difference score (e.g., the pre- and post-home observation designs used in the Webster-Stratton, 1984, study and most of the studies reviewed in this report). Before it can be said that one treatment works better than another, it must be demonstrated that the mean rate of change for one group differs from that of another.

It is true, of course, that change and termination scores are inextricably tied to each other as necessary dimensions for describing process. If you know where an individual started or ended up, and if you know the magnitude of change, then you have accounted for all the information in intraindividual growth.

A score describing rate of change is not necessarily correlated with the termination score. The individual who improves the most during treatment might very well still be the most poorly adjusted at termination. In the hypothetical cases shown in Figure 3.5, individual A is a case in point. Knowing about the rate of change, for example, does not necessarily tell us much about the termination score. If we wish to evaluate the magnitude of treatment effect, then it is the difference score that is of interest. If we wish to predict future adjustment, then the termination score is the measure of choice.

Rogosa, Brandt, and Zimowski (1982) pointed out that the simple difference score (e.g., termination minus baseline) is an unbiased estimate of true change. They attribute psychologist' reluctance to consider it as such the result of some confusion about concepts of regression to the mean, reliability, and errors of measurement. Our position is that the simple difference score is the ideal means for describing intraindividual changes during treatment. This is hardly news; ANOVA repeated measures have been the prime tool in the investigation of treatment outcomes. In this report, however, we are making a case for using multiple measures of change. Methods available now, such as latent growth models, are ideally suited to such a task.

It seems important, perhaps as a secondary issue, to know whether change measured at termination of PTT is a stable estimate of change that would be measured during follow-up. For the sample of teachers from the treated clinical sample (Patterson & Chamberlain, in press), the correlation was .633 ($p < .001$). This means that if we calculate the difference score based on the child's adjustment 1 year after intervention, the slope looks much as it did when we used that child's termination measure. The comparable stability correlation for mothers was .422 ($p < .01$); for the observed TAB score it was .520 ($p < .001$).

The changes being measured are not ephemeral. But is it possible to form a latent construct composed of change scores all measuring changes in therapy in the same way? Again, we suspect that it may not be possible to form such a construct when using data from more disturbed families. It may be that the family process is more chaotic in these extreme families, or perhaps there is a higher level of noise in the social judgments made about these families.

As shown in Table 3.5, data from two treated samples were used to derive multiple estimates of change. The at-risk sample consisted of preadolescent boys and girls referred for treatment because they were thought to be at significant risk for substance abuse (Dishion *et al.*, in press). The hypothesis tested was that the

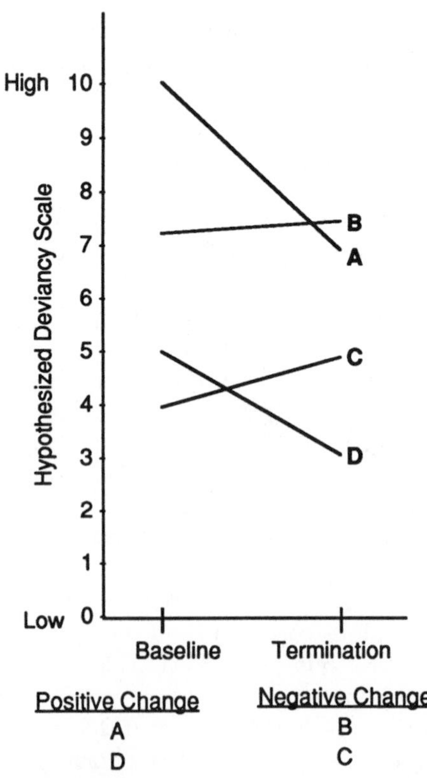

Figure 3.5. Intraindividual growth during intervention. Individuals A and D exhibit positive change; individuals B and C show negative change.

convergence among change scores would be significant for Dishion's less disturbed at-risk sample, but not significant for the more disadvantaged and disturbed clinical sample described earlier. Both samples contained boys and girls. The data from the at-risk sample are for parents (average mother and father ratings), while the data from the clinical sample contain ratings only from mothers. For the clinical sample, there is no support for the notion of a latent construct for measuring change; all of the convergence correlations were nonsignificant. For the at-risk sample, however, the convergence is moderately successful. The teacher estimates for intraindividual change scores correlated significantly with the other estimates of change.

Dishion *et al.* (in press) carried the analyses one step further, analyzing the data for boys and girls separately. None of the convergence correlations for girls were significant! The convergence for boys was significant, however. For example, the correlation between observers' and teachers' change scores was a robust .39. The implication of the findings are quite profound. For example, it is a distinct possibility that in evaluating preadolescent girls from an at-risk sample, one may obtain as many different answers to questions about improvement following treatment as there are criterion measures. For this subsample and this treatment, there simply is no single accurate measure of change. It seems that we must rely upon some type of multivariate averaging across change scores. We are faced with a similar choice for the extremely disadvantaged clinical sample. Again, there is no acceptable single measure of change. This means there is no way of precisely specifying the absolute magnitude of the treatment effect for such a group. The best we could do would be to add up the number of variables that reflected overall positive change and the number of variables that show no change or a negative slope. This is hardly a satisfying state of affairs, but it seems to apply to the very disturbed clinical sample and to Dishion's sample of treated girls.

We should eventually have solid information about which variables can be used to measure change in various samples of antisocial children. For example, it may be that therapists' ratings of improvement correlate well with the observation-based measure of change. It may be that we cannot rely on reports by any of the family members as a reliable measure of change for these more disturbed samples. The present data set suggests that for some subgroups, such as the boys from the Dishion studies, we will be able to be more precise in describing change during treatment. The increased precision rests on the fact that different agents agree on

Table 3.5. Correlations among Difference Scores[a] for Two Samples[b]

	Teacher CBC	Mother CBC	Observation TAB
Teacher CBC	—	.22* (.29)	.26* (.39)
Mother CBC	−.18	—	.10 (.13)
Observation TAB	.15	.18	—

Note. Figures in parentheses are for boys only. CBC = Child Behavior Checklist. TAB = Total Aversive Behavior.

[a]Termination-to-baseline measure

[b]At-risk sample above the diagonal; clinical sample below the diagonal.

$^{*}p < .05$.

the change that occurs. This means that we can build a latent construct—defined by a set of indicators used at baseline, termination, and follow-up—to define change. McArdle and Epstein (1987) described a latent growth model with several useful characteristics. Figure 3.6 shows some of the possible relations that can be explored. For example, we can ask if teacher scores collected at three points in time really load on the same concept. Are the factor loadings for the teacher ratings significant at all points in treatment? If so, we can assume all of the ratings reflect the same underlying construct. We can then ask if intraindividual growth curves defined by observers and teachers really define the same latent construct. Dishion is currently carrying out these analyses on the data set for boys.

We can now move to the question of what variables associated with treatment account for the differences in the intraindividual growth curves. Why do some boys improve but others get worse? We can introduce these variables as covariates measured at Time 1, and then determine the relative contribution of each in accounting for the individual differences in growth curves (McArdle & Epstein, 1987). We would assume, for example, that families who were randomly assigned to receive twice as much treatment would show greater changes. Similarly, the socially disadvantaged, more deviant problem children with disturbed parents would probably show less change (Patterson & Chamberlain, in press). Using a latent growth model, we can test the even more interesting proposition that changes in, say, parenting practices covary with the latent construct assessing changes in child adjustment. At this point in Dishion's study, his sample size is not quite large enough—150 subjects would be the minimum. Completing his replication study will take care of this problem.

Reinforcement Trap for Therapists

What are the implications for the fact that, for some extremely disturbed samples, different agents perceive change differently? One is that by selecting agents to report on change, investigators can use a random assignment and wait-list control design to obtain any effect that pleases them. If one wished to obtain strong positive outcome, then mothers should be selected as the reporting agents. The studies reviewed here suggest that any treatment for antisocial behavior that looks even remotely plausible to mothers can be expected to produce strong ratings of

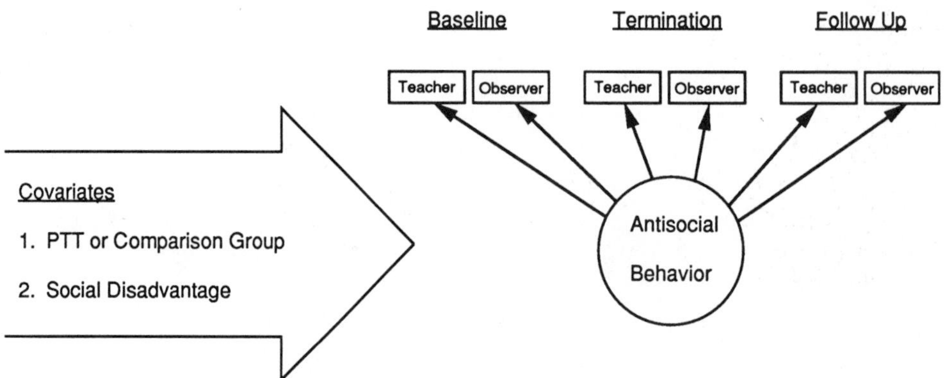

Figure 3.6. Latent growth model describing intraindividual growth during treatment.

positive change for the experimental group and little or no change for a wait-list control group. One might even replicate such findings many times as further proof of treatment efficacy (e.g., the review of Adlerian family counseling studies by Dinkmeyer, McCay, & Dinkmeyer, 1990). The positive results are forthcoming whether or not the child's behavior has changed; it may be that the child was actually helped by the treatment, but we cannot infer that from these kinds of data.

There is another, even more debilitating scenario that unfolds from this syllogism. Imagine a situation in which several hundred studies have been completed in an effort to determine which treatment for antisocial children is most effective. Let us say that most investigators have followed what seems to be a perfectly reasonable procedure; each used mothers' ratings as the key criterion variable in evaluating outcome. Let us also assume that if mothers believe their child is receiving some kind of treatment, they are preprogrammed to perceive improvement 60% to 70% of the time. The success rate holds regardless of what the treatment was. *It also holds even though the child did not actually receive any treatment.* By contrast, if the child actually did receive a beneficial treatment, then 70% to 90% of the mothers will rate the outcome as successful. A meta-analysis of these studies should show that everything other than wait-list control "works." It would also show that some things seem to work a little better than others, although the differences among treatment approaches are not all that large.

We believe this is precisely the problem with the conclusions reached by meta-analyses such as the one for child treatments reported by Casey and Berman (1985). We agree with Whalen and Henker (1991), who advocate the use of multiagent, multimethod indicators to evaluate treatment outcomes. We also believe that each indicator should be screened to evaluate both validity and bias before it is used as a measure of change.

Decades of effort to help children have resulted in the scores of treatments that are now being offered. Each of them appears like a shooting star on the horizon, accompanied by their charismatic leaders' glowing reports of success. They continue to be used even after they have been replaced by some new fad. In our desperate search for something that works, those of us who wish to help these children must learn each therapy. As Patterson and Narrett (1990) phrased it,

> Global ratings provide a feedback to therapists of an 80% success rate, even if the child makes no improvement. No matter what therapy is used, the same percentage of clients will show improvement on global ratings. Thus, each therapy remains immobilized, without chance of improvement. Old and new alike float like lost galleons on a Sargasso Sea of forgotten therapies. (p. 9)

Implications

At the most practical level, the most effective treatment for antisocial children seems to be some variant of parent training. It is too soon to say whether alternate stand-alone approaches, such as family systems, social cognitive, and social skills will be effective for these cases. There is a growing belief that one or more of these components, when added to PTT, significantly enhance the effect. It is probably safe to say that most of the major PTT studies have included all of these components for at least the last decade or two. It was not until the 1980s that the revised procedures were actually studied systematically. Consequently, most of the early treatment manuals are badly in need of revision. Which components are used for what? What are the clinical skills required to bring them into play?

Parent training therapy is most likely to have a demonstrated effect in reducing noncompliance and other antisocial symptoms for children between the ages of 3 and 8 (a very rough guess). We can expect about half of the children in this age group to function within the normal range (according to observation data) after treatment. Although PTT may produce statistically significant effects for older children (9–12 years old), only about 25% of them will be observed to function in the normal range.

It is not surprising that studies have demonstrated improved school adjustment following PTT; most of the programs include components for keeping the parents and school working together on academic skills. It is important to note, however, that long-term follow-up studies (like Forehand's) show that successfully treated children continued to show school problems some years later. These outcomes highlight the need to expand PTT and increase the emphasis on academic deficits. We believe a comparable follow-up study would show that many of the successfully treated cases would be having problems with peer relations or with forming intimate relationships in general. It seems clear that future developments in PTT must include stronger components to redress both of these skill deficits.

Another byproduct of PTT shown in several different studies is a reduction in maternal depression following successful completion of the program. There is some evidence that adding components that directly alter depression and marital discord would further enhance treatment outcomes.

The findings suggest that social disadvantage is a major risk factor for treatment outcome. The more socially disadvantaged the parents, the less likely treatment is to be effective. One set of studies showed that the reason for this lies in the increased resistance of the parents to the therapist's efforts to intervene. In effect, the aversive exchanges with the socially disadvantaged parents turn off the efforts of the therapist to help the family. In the same vein, there are now several well-controlled studies suggesting that written or videotaped presentations alone produce significant and long-lasting treatment outcomes for middle-class parents of younger children with relatively mild problems. One implication of these findings is that self-administered parent training materials may be particularly effective for this large segment of our population.

At this point, there are no treatments shown in systematic evaluations to produce long-term effects for antisocial adolescents. Major efforts to apply social learning-type procedures to these problem youth demonstrated that there were significant reductions in offense rates while the intervention was in place. In the years following intervention, however, the differences among the comparison groups were no longer significant. On theoretical grounds, the most promising approach for these individuals seems to be foster home placement. The clinical effects noted to date are startling. Well-controlled evaluation studies are currently under way, so future reviewers should be in a good position to evaluate this promising approach.

It is clear that, despite being the best current treatment for antisocial children, PTT is very costly. The addition of the necessary academic and social skills deficit components will make it even costlier. We must expand our perspective on this important societal problem. The cost of applying intervention procedures shown to be 100% effective would be too high. We must concentrate on preventing these problems before they are fully developed. At least three major programs (in Montreal, Eugene, and Baltimore) have been set up to determine the feasibility of preventing antisocial problems. All of these programs are well designed and employ carefully crafted assessment batteries. It is entirely possible that in 10 years, communities will have carefully evaluated prevention packages backed up by improved versions of PTT for younger antisocial children, and perhaps foster home placement for antisocial adolescents. This combination of prevention and treatment seems the most practical.

We have made a case for changing the way we think about studying treatment outcome. Thinking of outcome as a study of process or change over time introduces the necessity for assessing both intercept and slope. Presumably, only those measures that have previously been shown for that sample to significantly predict future child adjustment would be used to describe change. The study of outcome becomes the study of intraindividual growth. Structural equation models can then be used to describe not only the significance of these changes but also the contributions of key variables in accounting for these changes (e.g., experience level of therapist, time in treatment, social disadvantage, parental depression).

We introduced data showing that the more deviant the sample of families, the greater the risk that maternal ratings had neither convergent nor predictive validity. This simple fact was used to evaluate the hypothesis that "everything works": Investigators can obtain any outcome they wish simply by choosing the right measure of outcome.

ACKNOWLEDGMENTS. Support for this project was provided by Grant No. MH 37940 from the Center for Studies of Antisocial Behavior, NIMH, U.S. PHS; Grant No. DA 07031 from the National Institute of Drug Abuse, U.S. PHS; Grant No. MH 46690 from the Prevention Research Branch, NIMH, U.S. PHS; Grant No. MH 47458 from the Center for Studies of Violent Behavior and Traumatic Stress, NIMH, U.S. PHS; and Grant No. 90CW099401 from the Child Welfare Research and Demonstration Office, HDS, DHHS.

The authors are grateful to Kathy Jordan and Kristen Greenley for their careful scrubbing of the data.

References

Achenbach, T. M., McConaughy, S. H., & Howell, C. T. (1987). Child/adolescent behavioral and emotional problems: Implications of cross-informant correlations for situational specificity. *Psychological Bulletin, 101*, 213–232.

Alexander, J. F., & Parsons, B. V. (1973). Short-term behavioral intervention with delinquent families: Impact on family process and recidivism. *Journal of Abnormal Child Psychology, 81*, 219–225.

Arbuthnot, J., & Gordon, D. A. (1986). Behavioral and cognitive effects of a moral reasoning development intervention for high-risk behavior-disordered adolescents. *Journal of Consulting and Clinical Psychology, 54*, 208–216.

Atkeson, B. M., & Forehand, R. (1978). Parent behavioral training for problem children: An examination of studies using multiple outcome measures. *Journal of Abnormal Child Psychology, 6*, 449–460.

Attneave, C. L. (1969, July). *Innovations in outpatient therapy from a social learning perspective*. Position paper for Symposium on Mental Health in the Americas, Instituto Nacional de Neurologia, Mexzicao.

Bandura, A. (1973). *Aggression: A social learning analysis*. Englewood Cliffs, NJ: Prentice-Hall.

Bandura, A. (1978). The self system in reciprocal determinism. *American Psychologist, 33*, 344–358.

Bandura, A. (1985). Model of causality in social learning theory. In M. J. Mahoney & A. Freeman (Eds.), *Cognition and psychotherapy* (pp. 81–99). New York: Plenum.

Bandura, A., & Walters, R. H. (1963). *Social learning and personality development.* New York: Holt, Rinehart & Winston.

Bank, L., Marlowe, J. H., Reid, J. B., Patterson, G. R., & Weinrott, M. R. (1991). A comparative evaluation of parent training for families of chronic delinquents. *Journal of Abnormal Child Psychology, 19*, 15–33.

Bank, L., & Patterson, G. R. (1992). The use of structural equation modeling in combining data from different types of assessment. In J. Rosen & P. McReynolds (Eds.), *Advances in psychological assessment* (Vol. 8, pp. 41–74). New York: Plenum.

Barkley, R. A. (1989). Attention deficit-hyperactivity disorder. In E. J. Mash & R. A. Barkley (Eds.), *Treatment of childhood disorders* (pp. 39–72). New York: Guilford.

Barrish, H. H., Saunders, M., & Wolf, M. M. (1969). Good behavior game: Effects of individual contingencies for group consequences on disruptive behavior in a classroom. *Journal of Applied Behavior Analysis, 2*, 119–124.

Baumrind, D. (1991). Effective parenting during the early adolescent transition. In P. A. Cowan & E. M. Hetherington (Eds.), *Family transitions* (pp. 111–163). Hillsdale, NJ: Lawrence Erlbaum.

Bentler, P. M. (1980). Multivariate analyses with latent variables: Causal modeling. *Annual Review of Psychology, 31*, 419–456.

Bernal, M. E., Klinnert, M. D., & Schultz, L. A. (1980). Outcome evaluation of behavioral parent training and client-centered parent counseling for children with conduct problems. *Journal of Applied Behavioral Analysis, 13*, 677–691.

Bierman, K. L., Miller, C. L., & Stabb, S. D. (1987). Improving the social behavior and peer acceptance of rejected boys: Effects of social skill training with instructions and prohibitions. *Journal of Consulting and Clinical Psychology, 55*, 194–200.

Brunk, M. A., Henggeler, S. W., & Whelan, J. P. (1987). A comparison of multisystemic therapy and parent training in the brief treatment of child abuse and neglect. *Journal of Consulting and Clinical Psychology, 55*, 171–178.

Cairns, R. B. (1979). *Social development: The origins and plasticity of interchanges.* San Francisco, CA: Freeman.

Campbell, M., Green, W., & Deutsch, S. (1985). *Child and adolescent psychopharmacology.* Beverly Hills, CA: Sage.

Capaldi, D. M., & Patterson, G. R. (1989). *Psychometric properties of fourteen latent constructs from the Oregon Youth Study.* New York: Springer-Verlag.

Casey, R. J., & Berman, J. S. (1985). The outcome of psychotherapy with children. *Psychological Bulletin, 98*, 388–400.

Chamberlain, P. (1990). Comparative evaluation of Specialized Foster Care for seriously delinquent youths: A first step. *Community Alternatives: International Journal of Family Care, 2*(2), 21–36.

Chamberlain, P., Patterson, G. R., Reid, J. B., Forgatch, M. S., & Kavanagh, K. (1984). Observation of client resistance. *Behavior Therapy, 15*, 144–155.

Chamberlain, P., & Reid, J. B. (1991). Using a specialized foster care treatment model for children and adolescents leaving the state mental hospital. *Journal of Community Psychology, 19*, 266–276.

Coie, J., Underwood, D. M., & Lochman, J. T. (1991). Programmatic intervention with aggressive children in the school setting. In D. J. Pepler & K. H. Rubin (Eds.), *The development and treatment of childhood aggression* (pp. 389–410). Hillsdale, NJ: Lawrence Erlbaum.

Collins, R. C. (1966). *The treatment of disruptive behaviors by the employment of a partial milieu consistency program.* Unpublished doctoral dissertation, University of Oregon, Eugene.

Compernolle, T., Wiewauters, C., Laureyssen, L., DeCroo, L., De Vos, A., Vercruysse, B., Lesaffre, E., & Pyck, K. (1985). *Six sessions of social learning oriented structural family therapy improves the symptoms of attention deficit disorder (MBD) at home and in school.* Unpublished manuscript.

Crouter, A. C., MacDermid, S. M., McHale, S. M., & Perry-Jenkins, M. (1990). Parental monitoring and perceptions of children's school performance and conduct in dual- and single-earner families. *Developmental Psychology, 26*, 649–657.

Daugherty, T., Quay, H. C. (1991). Response perseveration and delayed responding in childhood behavior disorders. *Journal of Child Psychology, Psychiatry, and Allied Professions, 32*, 453–461.

DeLong, G. R., & Aldershof, A. L. (1987). Long-term experience with lithium treatment in childhood: Correlation with clinical diagnosis. *Journal of the American Academy of Child and Adolescent Psychiatry, 26*, 389–394.

Derogatis, L. R. (1975). *Brief symptom inventory*. Baltimore: Clinical Psychometric Research.

Dinkmeyer, D., Sr., McKay, G. D., & Dinkmeyer, D., Jr. (1990). Inaccuracy in STEP research reporting. *Canadian Journal of Counseling, 24*, 103–106.

Dishion, T. J. (1984). *Changing child social aggression within the context of the family: Factors predicting improvement in parent training*. Unpublished manuscript. (Available from the Oregon Social Learning Center, 207 E. 5th Ave., Suite 202, Eugene, OR 97401.)

Dishion, T. J. (1992, July). *Structural equation models for adolescent substance use*. Seminar conducted at the Oregon Social Learning Center, Eugene.

Dishion, T. J., & Patterson, G. R. (in press). A trait confluence model for the influence of peers on the trajectory of child antisocial behavior. In L. R. Huesmann (Ed.), *Current perspectives on aggressive behavior*. New York: Plenum.

Dishion, T. J., Patterson, G. R., & Kavanagh, K. (in press). An experimental test of the coercion model: Linking measurement theory and intervention. In J. McCord & R. Tremblay (Eds.), *The interaction of theory and practice: Experimental studies of intervention*. New York: Guilford.

Dishion, T. J., Patterson, G. R., Stoolmiller, M., & Skinner, M. L. (1991). Family, school, and behavioral antecedents to early adolescent involvement with antisocial peers. *Developmental Psychology, 27*, 172–180.

Dodge, K. (1985). Attributional bias in aggressive children. In P. C. Kendall (Ed.), *Advances in cognitive behavioral research and therapy* (Vol. 4, pp. 73–110). Orlando, FL: Academic Press.

Dodge, K. (1991). The structure and function of reactive and proactive aggression. In D. J. Pepler & K. H. Rubin (Eds.), *The development and treatment of childhood aggression* (pp. 201–218). Hillsdale, NJ: Lawrence Erlbaum.

Dolan, L. J., Kellam, S. G., Brown, C H., Werthamer-Larsson, L., Rebok, G. W., Mayer, L. S., Laudolff, J., Turkkan, J. S., Ford, C., & Wheeler, L. (in press). The short-term impact of two classroom-based preventative interventions on aggressive and shy behaviors and poor achievement. *Journal of Applied Developmental Psychology*.

Dumas, J. E. (1989). Treating antisocial behavior in children: Child and family approaches. *Clinical Psychology Review, 9*, 197–222.

Elder, G. H., Caspi, A., & Downey, G. (1983). Problem behavior in family relationships: A multigenerational analysis. In A. Sorensen, F. Weinert, & L. Sherrod (Eds.), *Human development: Interdisciplinary perspective* (pp. 93–118). Hillsdale, NJ: Lawrence Erlbaum.

Eyberg, S. M., & Johnson, S. M. (1974). Multiple assessment of behavior modification with families: Effects of contingency contracting and order of treated problems. *Journal of Consulting and Clinical Psychology, 42*, 594–606.

Farrington, D. P. (1978). The family backgrounds of aggressive youths. In L. A. Hersov, M. Berger, & D. Shaffer (Eds.), *Aggression and antisocial behavior in childhood and adolescence* (pp. 73–93). Oxford: Pergamon.

Ferber, H., Keely, S. M., & Shemberg, K. M. (1974). Training parents in behavior modification: Outcomes of and problems encountered in a program after Patterson's work. *Behavior Therapy, 5*, 415–419.

Fleischman, M. J. (1981). A replication of Patterson's "Interventions for boys with conduct problems." *Journal of Consulting and Clinical Psychology, 49*, 342–354.

Fleischman, M. J., & Horne, A. M. (1979). Working with families: A social learning approach. *Contemporary Psychology, 50*, 66–71.

Fleischman, M. J., & Szykula, S. (1981). A community setting replication of a social learning treatment for aggressive children. *Behavior Therapy, 12*, 115–122.

Forehand, R., Furey, W. M., & McMahon, R. J. (1984). The role of maternal distress in parent training program to modify child noncompliance. *Behavioral Psychotherapy, 12*, 93–108.

Forehand, R., & McMahon, R. (1981). *Helping the noncompliant child: A clinician's guide to parent training*. New York: Guilford.

Forgatch, M. S. (1991). The clinical science vortex: A developing theory of antisocial behavior. In D. J. Pepler & K. H. Rubin (Eds.), *The development and treatment of childhood aggression* (pp. 291–316). Hillsdale, NJ: Lawrence Erlbaum.

Forgatch, M. S., & Patterson, G. R. (in press). Divorce and boys' adjustment problems: Two paths with a single model. In E. M. Hetherington (Ed.), *Stress, coping, an resiliency in children and the family*. Hillsdale, NJ: Lawrence Erlbaum.

Forgatch, M. S., & Toobert, D. J. (1979). A cost-effective parent training program for use with normal preschool children. *Journal of Pediatric Psychology, 4*, 129–145.

Glidewell, J. C., Gildea, M. C., Domke, H. R., & Kantor, M. B. (1959). Behavior symptoms in children and adjustment in public school. *Human Organization, 18*, 123–130.

Goldstein, A. P., Sprafkin, R.P., Gershaw, N. J., & Klein, P. (1980). *Skill-streaming the adolescent: A structured learning approach to teaching prosocial skills*. Champaign, IL: Research Press.

Goldstein, H. S. (1984). Parental composition, supervision, and conduct problems in youths 12–17 years old. *Journal of the American Academy of Child Psychiatry, 23*, 679–684.

Griest, D. L., Forehand, R., Wells, K. C., & McMahon, R. J. (1980). An examination of differences between nonclinic and behavior-problem clinic-referred children and their mothers. *Journal of Abnormal Child Psychology, 89*, 497–500.

Grizenko, N., & Sayegh, L. (1990). Evaluation of the effectiveness of a psychodynamically oriented day treatment program for children with behaviour problems: A pilot study. *Canadian Journal of Psychiatry, 35*, 519–525.

Haley, J. (1976). *Problem solving therapy: New strategies for effective family therapy*. San Francisco, CA: Jossey-Bass.

Hanf, C. (1968, July). *Modification of mother–child controlling behavior during mother–child interactions in a controlled laboratory setting*. Paper presented at the regional meeting of the Association for Advancement of Behavior Therapy, Olympia, WA.

Hawkins, R. P., Meadowcroft, P., Trout, B. A., & Luster, W. C. (1985). Foster family-based treatment. *Journal of Clinical Child Psychology, 14*, 220–228.

Hawkins, R. P., Peterson, R. F., Schweid, E., & Bijou, S. W. (1966). Behavior therapy in the home: Amelioration of problem parent–child relations with the parent in a therapeutic role. *Journal of Experimental Child Psychology, 4*, 99–107.

Hops, H. (1982). Social skill training for socially isolated children. In P. Karoly & J. Steffen (Eds.), *Enhancing children's competencies* (pp. 211–242). New York: Gardner Press.

Horn, W. F., Ialongo, N., Greenberg, G., Packard, T., & Smith-Winberry, C. (1990). Additive effects of behavioral parent training and self-control therapy with attention deficit hyperactivity disordered children. *Journal of Clinical Child Psychology, 19*, 98–110.

Jackson, M. J., Reid, J. B., Patterson, G. R., Schaughency, E. A., & Ray, J. A. (1989, June). *Interrater reliability and validity of the child behavior checklist: Their relations to parent gender, family structure and age of child*. Paper presented at the conference of the Association for the Advancement of Behavior, San Francisco, CA.

Jacobsen, N. S., Follette, W. C., & Revenstorf, D. (1984). Psychotherapy outcome research: Methods for reporting variability and evaluating clinical significance. *Behavior Therapy, 15*, 336–352.

Jones, R. R., Weinrott, M. R., & Howard, J. R. (1981). *The national evaluation of the Teaching Family Model*. Final report to the Center for Studies of Antisocial and Violent Behavior, National Institute of Mental Health, Bethesda, MD. (Available from the Oregon Social Learning Center, 207 E. 5th Ave., Suite 202, Eugene, OR 97401.)

Kanner, L. (1950). *Child psychiatry* (2nd ed.). Springfield, IL: Charles Thomas.

Kazdin, A. E. (1985). *Treatment of antisocial behavior in children and adolescents*. Homewood, IL: Dorsey.

Kazdin, A. (1987). Treatment of antisocial behavior in children: Current status and future directions. *Psychological Bulletin, 102*, 187–203.

Kazdin, A. E., Esveldt-Dawson, K., French, H. H., & Unis, A. S. (1987). Problem-solving skills training and relationship therapy in the treatment of antisocial child behavior. *Journal of Consulting and Clinical Psychology, 55*, 76–85.

Kendall, P. C., Ronan, K. E., & Epps, J. (1991). Aggression in children and adolescents: Cognitive behavioral treatment perspectives. In D. J. Pepler & K. H. Rubin (Eds.), *The development and treatment of childhood aggression* (pp. 341–360). Hillsdale, NJ: Lawrence Erlbaum.

Kessler, J. W. (1966). *Psychopathology of childhood*. Englewood Cliffs, NJ: Prentice-Hall.

Kirigin, K. A., Braukman, C. J., Atwater, J. D., & Wolf, M. M. (1982). An evaluation of teaching (Family Achievement Place) group homes for juvenile offenders. *Journal of Applied Behavior Analysis, 15*, 11–16.

Knapp, P. A., & Deluty, R. H. (1989). Relative effectiveness of two behavioral parent training programs. *Journal of Clinical Child Psychology, 18*, 314–322.

Kolko, D. J., & Milan, M. A. (1983). Reframing and paradoxical instructions to overcome resistance in the treatment of delinquent youth: A multiple baseline analysis. *Journal of Consulting and Clinical Psychology, 51,* 655–666.

Ladd, G. W., & Asher, S. R. (1985). Social skills training and children's peer relations. In L. L'Abate & M. A. Milan (Eds.), *Handbook of social skills training and research* (pp. 219–244). New York: Wiley.

Larzelere, R. E., & Patterson, G. R. (1990). Parental management: Mediators of the effect of socio-economic status on early delinquency. *Criminology, 28,* 301–323.

Laub, J. H., & Sampson, R. J. (1988). Unraveling families and delinquency: A reanalysis of the Gluecks' data. *Criminology, 26,* 355–379.

Levitt, E. E. (1971). Research on psychotherapy with children. In A. E. Bergin & S. L. Garfield (Eds.), *Handbook of psychotherapy and behavior change* (pp. 474–494). New York: Wiley.

Lochman, J. E., Burch, P. R., Curry, J. F., & Lampron, L. B. (1984). Treatment and generalization effects of cognitive-behavioral and goal-setting interventions with aggressive boys. *Journal of Consulting and Clinical Psychology, 52,* 915–916.

Loeber, R., & Dishion, T. J. (1984). Boys who fight at home and in school: Family conditions influencing cross-setting consistency. *Journal of Consulting and Clinical Psychology, 52,* 759–768.

Magnusson, D. (1988). Aggressive, hyperactivity, and autonomic activity/reactivity in the development of social maladjustment. In D. Magnusson (Ed.), *Paths through life: Individual development from an interactional perspective* (pp. 153–175). Hillsdale, NJ: Lawrence Erlbaum.

McArdle, J. J., & Epstein, D. (1987). Latent growth curves within developmental structural equation models. *Child Development, 58,* 110–133.

McMahon, R. J., & Wells, K. C. (1989). Conduct disorders. In E. J. Mash & R. A. Barkley (Eds.), *Treatment of childhood disorders* (pp. 73–132). New York: Guilford.

Medland, M. B., Stachnik, T. J. (1972). Good behavior game: A replication and systematic analysis. *Journal of Applied Behavior Analysis, 5,* 45–51.

Meichenbaum, D. H., & Goodman, J. (1971). Training impulsive children to talk to themselves as a way of developing self-control. *Journal of Abnormal Child Psychology, 77,* 115–126.

Miller, G. E., & Prinz, R. J. (1990). Enhancement of social learning family interventions for childhood conduct disorders. *Psychological Bulletin, 108,* 291–307.

Minkin, N., Braukmann, C. J., Minkin, B. L., Timbers, G. D., Timbers, B. J., Fixsen, D. L., Phillips, E. L., & Wolf, M. M. (1976). The social validation and training of conversational skills. *Journal of Applied Behavior Analysis, 9,* 127–139.

Minuchin, S. (1974). *Families and family therapy.* Cambridge, MA: Harvard University Press.

Minuchin, S., & Montalvo, B. (1967). *Families of the slums.* New York: Basic Books.

Offord, D. R., Boyle, M. C., & Racine, Y. (1991). The epidemiology of antisocial behavior in childhood and adolescence. In D. Pepler & K. H. Rubin (Eds.), *The development and treatment of childhood aggression* (pp. 31–54). Hillsdale, NJ: Lawrence Erlbaum.

Patterson, G. R. (1980). Mothers: The unacknowledged victims. *Monographs of the Society for Research in Child Development, 45* (Serial No. 186).

Patterson, G. R. (1982). *A social learning approach to family intervention: III. Coercive family process.* Eugene, OR: Castalia.

Patterson, G. R. (1983). Stress: A change agent for family process. In G. Garmezy & M. Rutter (Eds.), *Stress, coping, and development in children* (pp. 235–264). New York: McGraw-Hill.

Patterson, G. R. (1984). Siblings: Fellow travelers in the coercive family process. In R. J. Blanchard & D. C. Blanchard (Eds.), *Advances in the study of aggression* (pp. 174–213). New York: Academic Press.

Patterson, G. R. (1985). Beyond technology: The next stage in development an empirical base for parent training. In L. L'Abate (Ed.), *Handbook of family psychology and therapy* (Vol. 2, pp. 1344–1379). Homewood, IL: Dorsey.

Patterson, G. R., & Brodsky, G. (1966). A behaviour modification programme for a child with multiple problem behaviours. *Journal of Child Psychology and Psychiatry, 7,* 277–295.

Patterson, G. R., & Capaldi, D. (1990). A mediational model for boys' depressed mood. In J. E. Rolf, A. Masten, D. Cicchetti, K. Neuchterlein, & S. Weintraub (Eds.), *Risk and protective factors in the development of psychopathology* (pp. 141–163). Boston, MA: Syndicate of the Press, University of Cambridge.

Patterson, G. R., Capaldi, D. M., & Bank, L. (1991). An early starter model for predicting delinquency. In D. J. Pepler & K. H. Rubin (Eds.), *The development and treatment of childhood aggression* (pp. 139–168). Hillsdale, NJ: Lawrence Erlbaum.

Patterson, G. R., & Chamberlain, P. (1988). Treatment process: A problem at three levels. In L. C. Wynne (Ed.), *State of the art in family therapy research: Controversies and recommendations* (pp. 189–223). New York: Family Process Press.

Patterson, G. R., & Chamberlain, P. (in press). A functional analysis of parent resistance during parent training. In H. Arkowitz (Ed.), *Why don't people change? New perspectives on resistance and noncompliance*. New York: Guilford.

Patterson, G. R., Chamberlain, P., & Reid, J. B. (1982). A comparative evaluation of parent training procedures. *Behavior Therapy, 13*, 638–651.

Patterson, G. R., Crosby, L., & Vuchinich, S. (1992). *Predicting risk for early police arrest. Journal of Quantitative Criminology, 8*, 335–355.

Patterson, G. R., Duncan, T., Reid, J. B., & Bank, L. (1992). *Systematic maternal errors in predicting sons' future arrests*. Manuscript submitted for publication.

Patterson, G. R., & Forgatch, M. S. (1985). Therapist behavior as a determinant for client resistance: A paradox for the behavior modifier. *Journal of Consulting and Clinical Psychology, 53*, 846–851.

Patterson, G. R., & Forgatch, M. S. (1987). *Parents and adolescents living together: I. The basics*. Eugene, OR: Castalia.

Patterson, G. R., & Forgatch, M. S. (1989). *Parents and adolescents living together: II. Family problem solving*. Eugene, OR: Castalia.

Patterson, G. R., Littman, R. A., & Bricker, W. (1967). Assertive behavior in children: A step toward a theory of aggression. *Monographs of the Society for Research in Child Development, 32*(5, Serial No. 113).

Patterson, G. R., & Narrett, C. M. (1990). The development of a reliable and valid treatment program for aggressive young children. *International Journal of Mental Health, 19*, 19–26.

Patterson, G. R., & Reid, J. B. (1984). Social interactional processes within the family: The study of moment-by-moment family transactions in which human social development is embedded. *Journal of Applied Developmental Psychology, 5*, 237–262.

Patterson, G. R., Reid, J. B., & Dishion, T. J. (1992). *A social learning approach: IV. Antisocial boys*. Eugene, OR: Castalia.

Patterson, G. R., Reid, J. B., Jones, R. R., & Conger, R. E. (1975). *A social learning approach: I. Families with aggressive children*. Eugene, OR: Castalia.

Patterson, G. R., & Stoolmiller, M. (1991). Replications of a dual failure model for boys' depressed mood. *Journal of Consulting and Clinical Psychology, 59*, 491–498.

Patterson, G. R., & Yoerger, K. (1993). Developmental models for delinquent behavior. In S. Hodgins (Ed.), *Mental disorder and crime* (pp. 140–172). Newbury Park, CA: Sage.

Peed, S., Roberts, M., & Forehand, R. (1977). Evaluation of the effectiveness of a standardized parent training program in altering the interaction of mothers and their noncompliant children. *Behavior Modification, 1*, 323–350.

Pelham, W. E., Bender, M. E., Caddell, J., Booth, S., & Moorer, S. H. (1985). Methylphenidate and children with attention disorder: Dose effects on classroom, academic and social behaviors. *Archives of General Psychiatry, 42*, 948–952.

Pepler, D. J. (1988, June). *A social-cognitively based skills training program for aggressive children*. Paper presented at the Earlscourt Symposium on Childhood Aggression, Toronto, Ontario.

Pepler, D. J., King, G., & Byrd, W. (1991). A social-cognitively based social skills training program for aggressive children. In D. J. Pepler & K. H. Rubin (Eds.), *The development and treatment of childhood aggression* (pp. 361–379). Hillsdale, NJ: Lawrence Erlbaum.

Phillips, S. B. (1984). *The effect of posttreatment interventions on long-term maintenance of behavioral family therapy*. Unpublished doctoral dissertation, University of Oregon, Eugene.

Prescott, A. (1991). *Early aversive social interaction in the family and later retrospective reports of physical child abuse*. Unpublished doctoral dissertation, University of Oregon, Eugene.

Puig-Antich, J. (1982). Major depression and conduct disorder in prepuberty. *Journal of the American Academy of Child Psychiatry, 21*, 118–128.

Quay, H. (1990, October). *Electrodermal responding, inhibition and reward-seeking in undersocialized aggressive conduct disorder*. Paper presented at the annual meeting of the American Academy of Child and Adolescent Psychiatry, Chicago, IL.

Reid, J. B. (Ed.). (1978). *A social learning approach to family intervention: II. Observation in home settings*. Eugene, OR: Castalia.

Rogosa, D., Brandt, D., & Zimowski, M. (1982). A growth curve approach to the measurement of change. *Psychological Bulletin, 92*, 726–748.

Rutter, M., Tizard, J., & Whitmore, K. (1970). *Education, health, and behavior*. London: Longmans.

Sameroff, A. J. (1989). Commentary: General systems and the regulation of development. In M. R. Gunnar & E. Thelen (Eds.), *Systems and development: The Minnesota Symposia on Child Psychology* (Vol. 22, pp. 219–230). Hillsdale, NJ: Lawrence Erlbaum.

Shapiro, S. K., Quay, H. C., Hogan, A. E., & Schwartz, K. P. (1988). Response perseveration and delayed responding in undersocialized aggressive conduct disorder. *Journal of Abnormal Psychology, 97*, 371–373.

Skinner, B. F. (1953). *Science and human behavior*. New York: The Free Press.

Sloane, H. N., Endo, G. T., Hawkes, T. W., & Jenson, W. R. (1991). Improving child compliance through self-instructional parent training materials. *Child and Family Behavior Therapy, 12*(4), 39–63.

Snyder, J. J. (1977). A reinforcement analysis of family interaction in problem and nonproblem families. *Journal of Abnormal Psychology, 86*, 528–535.

Snyder, J. J., & Patterson, G. R. (1986). The effects of consequences on patterns of social interaction: A quasiexperimental approach to reinforcement in natural interaction. *Child Development, 57*, 1257–1268.

Snyder, J. J., & Patterson, G. R. (1993). *The covariation between relative rate of occurrence and relative rate of pay offs for children's coercive behaviors*. Manuscript submitted for publication.

Spence, S. H., & Marzillier, J. S. (1981). Social skills training with adolescent male offenders—II. Short-term, long-term, and generalized effects. *Behaviour Research and Therapy, 19*, 349–368.

Spivack, G., Platt, J. J., & Shure, M. B. (1976). *Problem solving approaches to adjustment*. San Francisco, CA: Jossey-Bass.

Spivack, G., & Shure, M. B. (1974). *Social adjustment of young children: A cognitive approach to solving real-life problems*. San Francisco, CA: Jossey-Bass.

Stanton, M. D., Todd, T. C., & Associates (1987). *The family therapy of drug abuse and addiction*. New York: Guilford Press.

Stouthamer-Loeber, M., & Loeber, R. (1986). Boys who lie. *Journal of Abnormal Child Psychology, 14*, 551–564.

Tremblay, R. (1988, June). *Some findings from the Montreal Longitudinal Studies*. Paper presented at the Earlscourt Conference on Childhood Aggression, Toronto, Ontario.

Wahler, R. G. (1980). The insular mother: Her problems in parent–child treatment. *Journal of Applied Behavioral Analysis, 13*, 207–219.

Wahler, R., & Barnes, P. G. (1988, November). *Synthesis teaching as a supplement to parent training with troubled mothers*. Paper presented at the meeting of the Association for the Advancement of Behavior Therapy, New York.

Wahler, R. G., & Dumas, J. E. (1987). Stimulus class determinants of mother–child coercive exchanges in multidistressed families: Assessment and intervention. In J. D. Burchard & S. N. Burchard (Eds.), *Prevention of delinquent behavior* (pp. 190–219). Newbury Park, CA: Sage.

Wahler, R. G., Winkle, G. H., Peterson, R. F., & Morrison, D. C. (1965). Mothers as behavior therapists for their own children. *Behaviour Research and Therapy, 3*, 113–124.

Walker, H. M., McConnell, S., Walker, J., Clark, J. Y., Todis, B., Cohen, G., & Rankin, R. (1983). Initial analysis of the ACCEPTS curriculum: Efficacy of instructional and behavioral management procedures for improving the social adjustment of handicapped children. *Analysis and Intervention in Developmental Disabilities, 3*, 105–127.

Walter, H., & Gilmore, S. K. (1973). Placebo versus social learning effects in parent training procedures designed to alter the behaviors of aggressive boys. *Behavior Therapy, 4*, 361–371.

Webster-Stratton, C. (1984). Randomized trial of two parent training programs for families with conduct-disordered children. *Journal of Consulting and Clinical Psychology, 52*, 666–678.

Webster-Stratton, C. (1990). Long-term follow-up of families with young conduct problem children: From preschool to grade school. *Journal of Clinical Child Psychology, 19*, 144–149.

Webster-Stratton, C., Hollinsworth, T., & Kolpacoff, M. (1989). The long-term effectiveness and clinical significance of three cost-effective training programs for families with conduct-problem children. *Journal of Consulting and Clinical Psychology, 57*, 550–553.

Webster-Stratton, C., Kolpacoff, M., & Hollinsworth, T. (1988). Self-administered videotape therapy for families with conduct problem children: Comparison with two cost-effective treatments and a control group. *Journal of Consulting and Clinical Psychology, 56*, 558–566.

Wells, K. C., & Egan, J. (1988). Social learning and systems family therapy for childhood oppositional disorder: Comparative treatment outcome. *Comprehensive Psychiatry, 29*(2), 138–145.

West, D. J., & Farrington, D. T. (1973). *Who becomes delinquent?* London: Heinemann Educational Books.

Whalen, C. K., & Henker, B. (1991). Therapies for hyperactive children: Comparisons, combinations, and compromise. *Journal of Consulting and Clinical Psychology*, *59*, 126–137.

Wilson, H. (1987). Parental supervision re-examined. *British Journal of Criminology*, *27*(3), 215–301.

Wiltz, N. A., Jr., & Patterson, G. R. (1974). An evaluation of parent training procedures designed to alter inappropriate aggressive behavior of boys. *Behavior Therapy*, *5*, 215–221.

Wolff, S. (1967). Behavioural characteristics of primary school children referred to a psychiatric department. *British Journal of Psychiatry*, *113*, 885–893.

Yost, D. M., Hochstadt, N. J., & Charles, P. (1988). Medical foster care: Achieving permanency for seriously ill children. *Children Today*, *17*(5), 22–26.

4

Behavior Analysis for Developmental Disabilities

The Stages of Efficacy and Comparative Treatments

John R. Lutzker

Historical Overview

Developmental disabilities are generally considered to comprise mental retardation, autism, and cerebral palsy. This chapter focuses on mental retardation and autism because the large majority of behavioral treatment focuses on those two disabilities. Mental retardation involves impaired functioning in social, educational, intellectual, and adaptive behavior. Some forms of mental retardation have organic etiology that is understood, such as Down syndrome; other forms are clearly congenital with unknown etiology. Most forms are considered "familial," with the role of genes, organic trauma, and social/environmental factors being less clear. Systems of classification are based upon the degree of retardation, educability, and adaptive behavior. The total incidence of mental retardation in the United States is approximately 3% (Scheerenberger, 1971). Autism occurs in 1 of 2,500 children born in the United States (Schriebman, 1988).

In any historical overview of mental retardation, it becomes readily apparent that in looking prior to the twentieth century it is difficult to clearly distinguish between the history of mental retardation and the history of mental illness. A look at old photographs or paintings sometimes shows clear genetic anomalies of institutionalized individuals, indicating mental retardation. But, these individuals may have been residing in institutions that also housed people with mental illness. Thus, any historical overview can at times be describing what we might broadly conceive of as the history of mental retardation, deficiencies, disorders, and illness. Once the review is taken into the twentieth century, however, the distinctions become more discriminable and the focus narrows to true mental retardation.

John R. Lutzker • Department of Psychology, Lee College, University of Judaism, Los Angeles, California 90077.

Handbook of Effective Psychotherapy, edited by Thomas R. Giles. Plenum Press, New York, 1993.

The history of mental retardation is a contemporary recollection of sorts. Before the eighteenth century it appears as though there were few provisions made for persons with mental retardation. Throughout the centuries, depending on the country and the times, mental defectives were either scorned, persecuted, tortured, or killed, or were considered "gifted" and thus treated quite favorably. More often than not, however, negative treatment was the "mode o'day." For example, the great religious reformer Martin Luther believed that persons with mental illness were possessed by the devil, and he encouraged their execution. It has been reported that in the time of Calvin, individuals with retardation were thrown into rivers to drown, put into the woods for animals to attack, or thrown over cliffs. A consensus exists that the age of enlightenment in the care and training of persons with mental retardation began with the pioneering efforts of Jean Marc Gaspard Itard (1775–1838), a French physician working in a school for deaf persons in Paris (Ball, Seric, & Payne, 1971; Kanner, 1964).

Jean Marc Gaspard Itard

Itard was an otologist (a physician specializing in problems relating to the ear and hearing). Much of his work was influenced by the teaching model provided by his employer, Jacob Rodrigues Pereire, who operated a school for the deaf and was actively involved in their instruction. Itard is mostly known for his work with, and descriptions of, "the wild boy of Aveyron."

The boy, whom Itard named Victor, had been captured in the woods outside of Paris in 1799 and was assigned to Itard for treatment. The boy was thought to be 11 or 12 years old when he was brought to the school, apparently after living all or most of his life in the woods acting like, and living among, the animals. Victor possessed no receptive nor expressive language, was not toilet trained, wore no clothes, had eating habits (manners) resembling those of the animals of the woods, rejected all social contacts, and became aggressive (including growling) when approached by normal individuals. Of course, it would be inappropriate to summarily conclude that Victor had spent his entire life in the woods, because persons with profound mental retardation occasionally have been known to exhibit some or many of the behaviors demonstrated by Victor, even though these individuals have resided at home and/or in institutions. In any case, Victor provided a challenge to Itard, who felt that he had an opportunity to study the effect of environmental deprivation on intelligence (Ball *et al.*, 1971).

Clearly, Victor was a child with virtually total developmental deficits. What becomes apparent, however, in reviewing Itard's innovative teaching, is that Itard was one of the first (unlabeled) behaviorists, relying greatly on discrimination learning and other "modern" strategies. For example, one of Itard's early successes with Victor was teaching him to discriminate between hot and cold by having Victor bathe frequently.

Another example of Itard's foresighted approach is the "education plan" he set forth for Victor by outlining five aims. The aims included involving Victor in social life, "awakening his nervous sensibility," extending his range of ideas, giving him speech, and providing him with what today would be labeled as preacademic training. Thus, Itard provided Victor with a social education using strategies that closely resemble some of the best-known techniques of the late twentieth century, such as individual education plans.

Edouard Onesimus Seguin

Seguin was Itard's student. He imitated, and then embellished, some of Itard's techniques. Seguin was concerned with teaching persons with mental retardation adaptive behaviors, and some of his techniques closely resemble those used today in teaching adaptive social behavior. In order to facilitate learning and minimize distractions in the educational environment, Seguin taught his students in a drably furnished room. Also, he used an approach favored by many educators today, in that he utilized advanced children as models for less-advanced children. He was also opposed to the use of corporal punishment with institutionalized residents.

Samuel Gridley Howe

The first public institution in the United States was the Perkins Institution for the Blind, founded in 1832 in Watertown, Massachusetts, by Samuel Gridley Howe. In 1850, the experimental school of the Perkins Institute was separately incorporated as the Massachusetts School for Idiotic and Feeble-Minded Youth. In 1891, the school moved from its South Boston location to Waverley, Massachusetts, where it was named the Walter E. Fernald State School.

In Europe, the first government-sponsored German center for the care of "idiotic children" was opened in Mariaberg on May 1, 1847. In 1846, a small school was opened at Bath-on-the-Avon in Great Britain. In 1877, in Britain, William Weatherspoon Ireland published *On Idiocy and Imbecility*, the first well-organized and medically oriented book on mental deficiency.

One of the most important medical-genetic contributions of the nineteenth century was made by the British scientist John Langdon Haydon Down, who formally identified "the Mongolian type of idiocy," which was first called "mongolism" and is today known as Down syndrome. As it turned out, Down was initially misled by the features of persons with this genetic anomaly, believing that such persons had Mongolian blood (Down, 1876). Down later dropped that notion and presented three groupings to explain the etiology of "idiocy."

Nineteenth Century—Summary

The nineteenth century saw great changes in the treatment of individuals with mental impairments in the Western world. While we have come to discover that institutions can be quite problematic, in the nineteenth century they represented a major step forward. By 1888, at least 15 states in the United States had institutions for the feebleminded. Institutions proliferated until two factors came to light in this century. First, institutionalizing an individual for a lifetime is prohibitively expensive. Second, institutions themselves promote some of the very behavior that society deems unacceptable. Thus, deinstitutionalization, community reentry, and normalization have become the focus in the recent history of mental retardation.

The Twentieth Century

Two major developments in mental retardation occurred around the turn of the century. The first was a focus on eugenics, or heredity. The second was the development and validation of intelligence tests. This latter effort also allowed for a more sophisticated classification system to come into place.

Eugenics

The emphasis on eugenics has been called the "eugenics scare" (Kanner, 1964). Some of the pioneering work of Down, and others examining the role of heredity in human development, caused concern in many that, unchecked, people passing on genetic anomalies would produce large races of deformed, mentally subnormal people. In 1910, a study was conducted by Goddard (and published in 1912) in which he traced six generations of the Martin Kallikak family. Mr. Kallikak and a "feebleminded" barmaid bore illegitimate children, who bore children, and so on. Goddard produced evidence that the illegitimate side of Mr. Kallikak's family produced several hundred individuals with mental retardation over six generations. By contrast, Martin Kallikak married an upstanding colonial "maid," and the progeny from that side of the family over six generations produced judges, teachers, and other individuals respected by society.

Today we know that factors such as lifestyle, health, nutrition, education, and other sociological variables cannot be separated from the heredity factors in looking at a genealogy such as Martin Kallikak's. Nonetheless, in the early part of this century, the new discoveries in biology and genetics greatly favored the "nature" side of what came to be known by developmental psychologists as the "nature–nurture" controversy.

Despite the eugenics scare, several foresighted professionals were striving for improvements in the institutional environments. For example, in 1919, Walter E. Fernald called for

- early identification of retardation
- family visits to institutionalized persons
- home support systems and training manuals
- professional consultation
- legal provisions
- aftercare assistance for graduates of special education programs
- outpatient clinics

The provisions listed represented "treatment" in mental retardation, basically until 1964. Thus, although by 1926, sterilization laws had been passed in 23 states because of the concern over the "spread" of retardation, individuals such as Fernald were still able to press for progressive changes. Further innovations by Fernald and others included the establishment of farm colonies where higher-functioning persons with mental retardation could live or work.

Intelligence Testing

The other major emphasis affecting mental retardation after the turn of the century was intelligence testing. Although it is still controversial today, intelligence testing has been a major factor in shaping the direction that psychology and education have taken.

Although he was the pioneer of intelligence testing, Binet expressed concern and suggested caution when using intelligence tests to diagnose mental retardation without corresponding behavioral and clinical observations and socioeconomic considerations.

The work of Binet and Simon was translated into English in 1911 by Henry Goddard. In 1916, Lewis Terman, an American psychologist, further perfected and standardized the Binet–Simon Test. Terman set the following standards for I.Q. scores: 50–70, moron; 25–50, imbecile; less than 25, idiot. During the remainder of the twentieth century, more research in intelligence testing brought refinements of the early tests, new tests (such as the WISC and the WAIS and their revisions), and considerable arguments about the biasing features of tests. Nonetheless, there remains general agreement in psychology and education that intelligence tests, when appropriately and carefully administered (to the correct population for the test), continue to have a primary function in those fields.

The Great Lull

During the "great lull," described by Kanner (1964) as the period between 1910–1935, no new advances in treatment or education of the people with mental retardation came to light. More institutions were built in Europe and the United States, and more special education classes and programs came into being, but no great advances in philosophy, treatment, or training appeared.

During this period, work by Clifford Beers fostered the establishment of child guidance clinics. This "mental hygiene" movement had little impact on the retardation field.

A New Era in the Twentieth Century

In 1934, the great lull came to an end. The precipitating event was the discovery by Dr. Ivan A. Folling that phenylpyruvic acid oligophrenia as a metabolic disorder (phenylketonuria-PKU) could be considerably reversed by a diet low in certain protein intake. This was a major medical discovery, but only later did PKU testing become required before hospital discharge in the United States. Nonetheless, Folling's work seemed to rekindle scientific/educational concern over the care and treatment of individuals with mental retardation.

Although Folling's work produced some new movement, the Great Depression and World War II caused the field of mental retardation to take a back burner again in terms of any clearly measurable great studies or discoveries.

One of the major developments to occur after World War II was the founding of the National Association for Retarded Children (NARC). Beginning with a small group of concerned parents and professionals, the group grew into a major advocacy, lobbying, and scientific support organization of over 50,000 members. In the 1950s and 1960s, NARC was instrumental in bringing the issues of persons with mental retardation into the educational and legislative forefronts. Thus, NARC provided a model that parent groups could be formed in order to secure rights and opportunities for children with mental retardation.

The work of NARC in the 1950s set the framework for President John F. Kennedy's 1962 President's Panel on Mental Retardation. The work of the panel produced sweeping changes in law and funding. The enactment of PL 88-164 and PL 88-156 authorized the establishment and construction of research centers for the study of the causes, prevention, and treatment of retardation. These laws also provided for the development of university-affiliated facilities for training and service demonstrations and the development of community mental health centers.

Research and training was the focus of the 1960s; deinstitutionalization was the focus of the 1970s. Group homes and other community facilities became alternatives to state institutions. Many institutions either closed or were made smaller, often restricting their services to persons with severe and profound mental retardation and residents with severe multiple handicaps.

Treatment—Behavior Modification

Behavior modification and applied behavior analysis have become the treatment and training strategies in mental retardation and developmental disabilities, particularly autism. The historical landmarks covered thus far in this chapter have primarily been philosophical, custodial, or medical, but the most significant treatment breakthroughs came to be in the 1960s.

The foundations of behavior modification were laid in the laboratories of I. Pavlov and B. F. Skinner. But the work of these pioneer researchers had no measurable impact on treatment in mental retardation until 1949, when an article appeared in the *American Journal of Psychology* entitled "Operant Conditioning of a Vegetative Idiot." In this article, Fuller, a graduate student at Indiana University, described using warm sugared milk as a reinforcer to increase arm raising in an 18-year-old male with profound mental retardation. In Alan Kazdin's *History of Behavior Modification* (1978), Kazdin describes the impact of Fuller's work as ". . . a landmark because it showed operant responding in a human whose inability to learn anything had been assumed" (p. 246).

Not many advances in this extension of Skinner's operant technology to humans occurred during the 1950s. Ogden Lindsley and Skinner did some experiments at Metropolitan State Hospital and the Walter E. Fernald State School in Massachusetts, but the first dramatic breakthroughs came in the early 1960s in Seattle, Washington, and Anna, Illinois (Lutzker & Martin, 1981). On psychiatric wards in Anna, Ayllon and Azrin (1968) demonstrated that patients with schizophrenia could learn adaptive skills and show fewer psychiatric symptoms when they were motivated by a token reinforcement management program.

The Washington Monuments

In the meantime, at the University of Washington and Ranier School, Drs. Sidney Bijou and Jay Birnbrauer were using token reinforcement programs to control deviant behavior and improve academic performance in children with mental retardation (e.g., Zimmerman & Zimmerman, 1962). Researchers at Arizona State University shaped vocalizations in a 9-year-old girl who was mute. At the University of Washington, and later at the University of California, Los Angeles, Dr. O. Ivar Lovaas pioneered behavior modification treatment for children with severe autism.

A landmark case was reported by Wolf, Risley, and Mees (1964), who described the intensive use of behavior-change techniques with a child with autism named Dicky. At the time of referral Dicky was a 3-year-old boy. The child did not eat normally and lacked age-appropriate social and verbal behavior. Further, he engaged in severe tantrums and self-injurious behavior. Complicating the behavior problems was a medical problem, the need to wear corrective lenses following eye surgery for the removal of cataracts. If Dicky did not wear the glasses regularly he would go blind; yet he refused to wear the glasses. When adults tried to put the glasses on Dicky, he would immediately pull them off and often throw them. Primary positive reinforcement was the major component of the efforts to get Dicky to wear his glasses. Near the beginning of their efforts the experimenters reinforced Dicky by small bites of candy, cereal, or ice cream for wearing his glasses for just a few seconds. Gradually, the response requirement was lengthened in that he had to wear the glasses for longer periods in order to receive the edible reinforcers. After several days Dicky was wearing the glasses for several minutes at a time. By the end of this stage of his treatment (a little over 2 months), he was wearing his glasses 12 hours per day.

The method used to teach Dicky to wear his glasses, described in this historic report (Wolf *et al.*, 1964), is one of the first systematic examples of *positive primary reinforcement* and *shaping*, the reinforcement of successive approximations to a desired goal response.

Some of the earliest successes in the behavior-change field occurred in state hospitals and special education schools where large-scale token economies were employed. Among these were the education programs at Ranier School in Washington State (Bijou & Orlando, 1961) and the Cottage Program at Parsons State Hospital in Kansas (Lent & Spradlin, 1966).

In these programs children with mental retardation earned large numbers of points or tokens (plastic chips) each day for performing academic and self-help behaviors. They were able to trade the points in for a variety of differently priced "back-up" reinforcers. Systems such as these demonstrated the powerful utility of the contingent use of generalized conditioned reinforcers. Jones and Kazdin (1975) showed that mentally retarded children in a special education classroom could be gradually weaned from the tokens to a system of more natural reinforcers such as peer praise and activities.

Other Techniques

Self-injurious behavior is a severe problem for some children and adults with mental retardation. O. I. Lovaas was one of the pioneers in applying behavior-change strategies to the treatment of self-injurious behavior. In 1969, he and Simmons reported a comparison between extinction and painful electric shock punishment in treating self-injury in three children with severe mental retardation. Today, there is still little evidence to support any uniform theory of self-injurious behavior, but many have concluded that for whatever reasons self-injurious behavior appears in children, adult attention to it can contribute greatly to its maintenance and can often increase its rate of occurrence. With this as the undergirding philosophy behind their investigation, Lovaas and Simmons placed the children in rooms isolated from social contacts. The rates per minute of self-injurious behavior during these 90-min extinction sessions fell from almost 3,000 to zero over nine days. Thus, these researchers showed that an extinction protocol could be used to treat behavior problems of children with mental retardation. It should be noted, however, that the contingent shock stimuli worked much more efficiently than extinction in suppressing the highly problematic self-injurious behavior, but shock represents a host of ethical problems and there is little documentation that its use has long-term benefits (Lutzker, 1990).

Recently, after two decades of treatment of self-injurious biting in individuals with mental retardation or developmental disabilities, Hite and Vatterott (1991) concluded that differential reinforcement of other behavior coupled with social time-out or brief informational restraint was effective in reducing biting. This is compared to more restrictive procedures such as a variety of response-contingent stimulation techniques.

Stressing the critical role of assessment in treating self-injury, Iwata *et al.* (1990) determined that a demand is a primary antecedent for self-injury in children with developmental disabilities. That is, self-injury occurs more often in instructional sequences than in other situations, such as when a child is alone, receiving attention, or playing. Treatment was successful during demand conditions when the children were physically guided through compliance to instructions and blocked from engaging in self-injury.

One of the earliest reports of the successful use of a response-cost procedure describes point removal for the psychotic verbalizations of a 29-year-old woman with severe mental retardation who was a client in a sheltered workshop (Kazdin, 1979). Receiving points for work-oriented behavior had greatly increased the woman's performance, but her bizarre vocalizations were distracting to others and were not in her best interests in promoting normalization for her. Thus, a simple response-cost system was implemented whereby she lost points each time she engaged in these strange verbalizations. By the second week of treatment the problem had been virtually eliminated. A 15-week treatment showed maintenance of the treatment gains. Obviously, the back-up reinforcers for the points were so meaningful to the woman that when restricted access to them (as a function of point loss), she quickly changed her behavior.

In a study comparing response cost to aversive sound stimulation, Kazdin (1973) found response cost to be more effective in reducing speech disfluencies in 40 clients with mental retardation. Further, Kazdin (1973) had independent raters verify the superiority of the response-cost procedures.

Differential Reinforcement of Other Behavior (DRO) is a procedure whereby reinforcement strategies are used in combination with extinction in order to reduce the occurrences of unwanted behaviors. Usually done on a time-sampling basis, DRO involves reinforcing (with primary or conditioned reinforcers) *any* behavior other than the unwanted behavior. At any time the unwanted behavior is seen to occur, it is ignored. For example, a 52-year-old resident of a state school for individuals with mental retardation had a long history of exposing himself several times a day (Lutzker, 1974). This unfortunate habit precluded him from participating in off-ward habilitative activities both on and off the residence grounds. During at least 8 hours each day, ward staff members collected data every 10 min, noting whether or not the client was exposing himself. After 9 days of baseline data were collected, DRO treatment was begun. This involved the staff members continuing to check the client every 10 min. If he was not exposing himself, a staff member hugged him and said, "Good, your pants are on right." If at any time during each 10-min interval the client was exposing himself, he was completely ignored. This DRO procedure totally eliminated a long-standing maladaptive behavior problem after 30 treatment sessions. For the first time in his life the client was able to participate in a number of therapeutic and habilitative activities, such as attending occupational therapy sessions at the school, and cultural and sports events in the city.

The literature on DRO is replete with examples of its effectiveness in reducing a variety of behavior problems. For example, Repp and Dietz (1974) found it to be effective alone in some cases, and in combination with time-out in case involving four children with severe mental retardation who were self-injurious and aggressive. One child had a history of engaging in severe tantrums, self-mutilation, and biting others. The reinforcer was "M & M" candy, which was delivered contingent upon the absence of the target problem behaviors. Whenever the problem behavior occurred, this 12-year-old boy was restrained for 30 sec. This combined treatment program virtually eliminated these grossly maladaptive behaviors. Similar strategies were used with equal success with the other children. In another study, Repp, Deitz, and Speir (1974) reported the use of DRO (verbal praise) plus saying "no" for inappropriate behavior to reduce the stereotypical responding of three children with severe mental retardation. The single-subject, ABAB research design conclusively showed that saying "no" alone, without the DRO procedure, was ineffective in reducing the stereotypic behavior. Unfortunately, what cannot be determined is whether the DRO procedure alone would have produced the same effect as the DRO plus the verbal reprimand.

Looking at DRO across a number of behaviors and settings, Deitz, Repp, and Deitz (1976) found it useful in reducing hair twirling, hand biting, and thumb sucking in the residential bedrooms of two children with mental retardation and in the home living room of another. The disruptive classroom behavior of three children was also eliminated by using DRO.

Used in combination with social restitution, DRO (social praise) eliminated the assaultive and inappropriate sexual behavior of a 13-year-old male with Down syndrome (Polvinale & Lutzker, 1980). The adolescent, who lived at home and attended a public special education school, faced institutionalization because of his high rate of sexually aggressive behavior and public masturbation. After a very brief treatment phase that involved praise for appropriate behavior and repeated public apologies to others for inappropriate sexual behavior, the inappropriate sexual behavior was eliminated. During the course of treatment the adolescent also received a sex education program designed for special education students.

One advantage to DRO is the relative ease with which it can be applied. It is clearly a very useful treatment strategy that should be one of the first attempted when considering a behavior reduction treatment plan. This is because inherent in the procedure is positive reinforcement for appropriate behavior; thus, the extinction component cannot be considered very restrictive or aversive.

Response-contingent stimulation as a behavior reduction technique has had a variety of other labels, such as aversive conditioning, punishment, response-contingent punishment, and so forth. "Response-contingent stimulation" seems preferable because it is descriptively accurate and is not charged with emotional overtones. *Response-contingent stimulation* acts as a behavior reduction technique when a stimulus is added contingent upon a response (behavior) and there is a reduction in future frequencies of that response. The classic example of this technique, of course, is spanking. But spanking is only accurately described as a behavior reduction technique when it, in fact, reduces the future rate of the behavior that precedes it. Thus, as reinforcement is defined according to its effect on behavior (increases in), so are behavior reduction techniques defined according to their effects on behavior (decreasing it).

Most of the formal investigations of response-contingent stimulation have involved self-injurious behavior (SIB). This is because SIB is often severe and dangerous and resistant to various treatment modes. It is believed to occur in as much as 4% to 6% of children institutionalized with mental retardation.

In some clients, painful (but harmless) contingent electric shock has been shown to be successful in eliminating or greatly suppressing SIB (Lovaas & Simmons, 1969). Although some people are appalled at the thought of shocking children, it should be remembered that this is considered a treatment of last resort with the hope that reducing severe SIB will take clients away from the serious dangers posed to themselves, and then allow for the training of habilitative behaviors. Two issues, however, have precluded shock from being a panacea for the treatment of self-injury. First, its use is illegal in some states. Second, its effects seem to be quite varied. In some cases it seems to work exceedingly well to reduce rates of SIB; in other cases its effects seem transient or limited to highly discriminate settings or situations (Corte, Wolf, & Locke, 1971). Thus, by necessity, many other stimuli have been investigated as methods of reducing SIB.

Pulling neck hair, while not a technique to be strongly recommended, was shown to reduce SIB (Banks & Locke, 1966). Also, effective have been the use of aromatic ammonia (Tanner & Zeiler, 1975), air splints (Ball, Campbell, & Barkemeyer, 1980), and lemon juice (Sajwaj, Libet, & Agras, 1974) to suppress life-threatening rumination, and facial screening whereby a bib is placed over the client's head contingent upon SIB (Demetral & Lutzker, 1980; Lutzker, 1978; Singh, 1980; Zegiob, Alford, & House, 1978).

Finally, a procedure called *required relaxation* deserves mention. It was first described by Webster and Azrin (1973), who used the procedure to reduce the extremely agitated and disruptive behavior of several institutionalized clients with mental retardation. When extremely disruptive behavior occurred, clients individually were required to spend 2 hours being quiet on their own beds (relaxing). This procedure was effective in eliminating extremely disruptive behaviors that had previously been resistant to other treatment techniques.

Of course, all treatment procedures should be subjected to treatment plans that undergo professional and, when necessary, human rights committee reviews. Careful data collection procedures and, when possible, simple research designs, should be used in order to provide careful accountability and documentation of treatment effects. Further, habilitative skill-building programs should take precedence over behavior reduction programs; however, when problem behavior inhibits adaptive skill training, consideration for behavior reduction programs may be in order. When response-contingent stimulation is the treatment of choice, after less restrictive treatment alternatives have been tried or considered, special and careful attention to the rules of careful staff/parent/teacher training, accountability, and professional review is especially in order. That is, anyone taught to use these techniques must be trained and supervised to criterion levels of performance.

Consequences are very important in increasing or decreasing the frequencies of behaviors upon which the consequences are made contingent. On the other hand, also of great importance are the *antecedent* stimuli (events) that set the occasion for behavior to occur. When a response occurs in the presence of a particular stimulus, *stimulus control* has been produced. Stimulus control can be both a habilitation strategy, or it can be a problem that might need to be changed. For example, as a treatment strategy in teaching a child with mental retardation to verbalize a noun label describing a picture, say, a cow, we want the picture of the cow to set the occasion for the verbal response, "cow," which, if produced by the child, will be reinforced. An example of inappropriate stimulus control is what has been called in children with autism "overselectivity" (Lovaas, Schreibman, Koegel, & Rehm, 1971). That is, many children with autism have difficulty learning academic or preacademic tasks because they attend to irrelevant, highly specific stimuli, such as, perhaps, the handedness of the therapist or the teacher. In other words, a child might learn to name pictures held in the therapist's left hand. But, if the therapist (unknowingly) held the same picture in her right hand, or a new therapist held it in her hand, the child might fail to respond.

Cuvo and Davis (1980) identified multiple examples of stimulus control in facilitating the training of community-living skills. Specifically, they cited the advantages and disadvantages of verbal instruction, stating the response, asking questions, procedural descriptions, rules, and visual cues such as pictures, visual stimulation, and color cues. Also reviewed were manual gestures, modeling, role playing, and other physical prompts. These authors point out that all of these events, when properly adapted to the skill of the client to be trained, should be taken into consideration, along with the consequences to be used, in planning a community-living skills training program. For example, stimulus control using procedural descriptions was used by Cuvo, Jacobi, and Sipko (1981) to teach laundry skills to community-living candidates with mental retardation. Pictures and color cues have been used to teach nutritious meal planning to a mother with mental retardation who could not read and who was referred to treatment for child neglect because of her inability to provide nutritious meals to her daughter (Sarber, Halasz, Messmer, Bickett, & Lutzker, 1983). The experimenters taught the woman to identify pictures of foods according to their food groups by pairing each food group with a particular color. These are just two of countless examples of the arrangement of antecedent events and reinforcement (in these examples, *social* reinforcement) to produce the stimulus control that allowed clients to learn important community-living skills.

Several other aspects of stimulus control have been covered by Etzel and LeBlanc (1979). They have pointed out that professionals who are involved in teaching difficult-to-teach children should be aware of the multiplicity of stimulus control strategies available and should know how to choose the least complex, but still-effective, procedure. The first simple rule within this strategy is that the special education teacher or other mental retardation specialists should know what skills the child already possesses. The motivational system needs examination. Is the child having performance difficulties because of a lack of reinforcement? This may be the simplest level at which to produce change. The next consideration is if the child is engaging in behavior that is incompatible with the tasks that should be learned.

Another aspect of using stimulus control in teaching is the analysis and training of prerequisite skills. This might include attention training, learning to hold a pencil, and so on. Finally, of these aspects of stimulus control to consider, Etzel and LeBlanc (1979) have pointed to the analysis of the effects of instructions. Considerable research has been done in this area. For example, Miller and LeBlanc

(1973) found that minimal instruction was superior to detailed instructions. Instructions should be paced, and it has been determined that learning sessions should be "brisk" and that instructions should be continued even if the child tries to avoid following them (Plummer, Baer, & LeBlanc, 1977).

Innovations

Researchers in autism have, in recent years, strayed from the highly controlled, discrete trial training of the 1960s and 1970s to the use of more natural training situations (Wolery, Kirk, & Gast, 1985). As reinforcers for on-task behavior, Charlop, Kurtz, and Casey (1990) used stereotypy and delayed echolalia, other natural self-stimulatory behaviors, and aberrant behaviors for many children with autism. They found these unusual reinforcers to be superior to food in increasing on-task behavior. Further, use of these reinforcers in a contingent manner did not increase the frequency of the aberrant behavior during unstructured periods.

Time delay has been useful in increasing spontaneous language with children with autism (Charlop, Schreibman, & Thibodeau, 1985; Charlop & Walsh, 1986). This involves a 2-sec graduated time delay between the presentation of a stimulus and a model (by the experimenter, therapist, or teacher). After the model, such as, "crayon please," the child is reinforced with the item if she imitates the model. Using a multiple-baseline design across three children, Matson, Sevin, Fridley, and Love (1990) produced an increase in spontaneous language and generalization to novel stimuli 1 month after training.

Using task analysis, modeling, and social reinforcers, several researchers have taught a host of independent living skills, such as janitorial skills (Cuvo, Leaf, & Borakove, 1978), mending skills (Cronin & Cuvo, 1979), and apartment upkeep (Williams & Cuvo, 1986), to adults and young adults with mental retardation. Also, Zencius, Davis, and Cuvo (1990) used a personalized system of instruction to teach checking account skills to adults with mild disabilities.

In recent years attention has turned to more natural treatment procedures and to further insuring rights and choices for individuals with developmental disabilities. For example, Bannerman, Sheldon, Sherman, and Harchik (1990) have made the poignant case for the consideration of personal liberties whenever a behavioral treatment plan is developed. They note that most people without developmental disabilities sometimes choose to nap or eat too many doughnuts, instead of working or eating something more nutritious. Similarly, persons with developmental disabilities may need to be allowed these choices periodically.

This issue of choice was empirically demonstrated by Parsons and Reid (1990), who used an assessment procedure with persons with profound mental retardation that involved repeated, paired-item presentations for food and drink. Of particular interest was that caregiver predictions of which reinforcers the clients would choose were inaccurate. Use of the reinforcers "chosen" by the clients then increased adaptive skills when they were delivered (contingently) to the clients by the caregivers.

Another important issue that has been examined in recent years is the context of behavior. For example, Haring and Kennedy (1990) looked at the role of DRO and time-out in reducing the disruptive behavior of students with severe developmental disabilities. They found that DRO was effective when the context was demand and that time-out was effective when the context was a leisure situation. Thus, empirical data supported the experience of many parents and teachers that time-out is ineffective in situations in which demands are placed on children. In other words, time-out is more reinforcing than staying in a demand situation. Thus, the data from this research suggest that context must be considered in choosing procedures.

A life-threatening problem, failure to thrive, presents in a number of children with developmental disabilities. This feeding disorder has been successfully treated with activity reinforcers, time-out plus reinforcement, and negative reinforcement. It has been recommended that evaluation for children with feeding problems should further include an interdisciplinary approach with medical, nutritional, occupational therapy, and behavioral evaluation, and that parents must be included in training in mealtime and nonmealtime situations (O'Brien, Repp, Williams, & Christophersen, 1991).

Family satisfaction increases even though formal parent training can be burdensome for parents of children with developmental disabilities (Baker, Landen, & Kashima, 1991). Despite the strain of structured parent training, training may increase the likelihood of avoiding the need to place a child in a more restrictive setting.

To improve the likelihood of parents' generalizing newly learned skills and maintaining their skills over time, there has been a recent focus on programming for generalization. For example, Moran and Whitman (1991) added problem solving and self-monitoring to written materials, modeling, behavioral rehearsal, and verbal feedback in teaching behavior management skills to mothers of several children with autism. Maintenance of the mothers' new skills was shown over numerous follow-up sessions.

Generalization of parent and child behavior is most likely to occur if a comprehensive approach is provided to families (Singer & Irvin, 1989). This has recently been documented by Lutzker, Campbell, Harrold, and Kiesel (1992). They provided data from Project Ecosystems showing that placements did not occur in 200 families. Project Ecosystems provides an ecobehavioral approach to families with children with developmental disabilities at high risk for placement because of their severe behavioral excesses or deficits. The authors contend that the ecobehavioral approach used by Project Ecosystems reduces the probability of placement because of the multifaceted nature of the treatment. Project Ecosystems (Lutzker, Campbell, Newman, & Harrold, 1989) provides in-home, *in situ* parent training, stress reduction, behavioral pediatrics, and basic skills training.

Parent training involves contingency management, but it also focuses on affect (Lutzker, Megson, Webb, & Dachman, 1985) and activities. Stress reduction can be used for parents and children. For example, Kiesel, Lutzker, and Campbell (1989) used behavioral relaxation training (posturing) to reduce hyperventilation-preceded seizures in a child with profound mental retardation. Behavioral pediatrics involves feeding programs, treatment of medical fears (Lutzker, 1991), and compliance to medical regimens. Basic skills include toilet training, feeding, emergency skills, hygiene, and communication (Lutzker, 1991). Singer and Irvin (1989) detail similar approaches as essential in preventing placement and improving family satisfaction.

Pharmacology

Thorazine has been evaluated to treat severe behaviors of persons with developmental disabilities. Singh and Aman (1981) and Aman and White (1988) found that although self-injury and hyperactivity were reduced, irritability, lethargy, and social withdrawal increased. Haldol has been shown to have modest effects in children with autism (Aman, Teehan, White, Turbott, & Vaithianathan, 1989) and no effect in two self-injurious children (Durand, 1982; Luiselli, 1987). Some use of anxiolytics has been attempted with persons with developmental disabilities, but Gadow and Poling (1988) concluded that there is little evidence of any efficacy of these drugs. Some reduction of self-injury has been reported with the use of naltrexone, an opiate antagonist, but studies to date have used single subjects (Barrett, Feinstein, & Hole, 1989). Long-term follow-ups and larger-scale studies are clearly in order. Some clinical success was reported for the use of fenfluramine in children with autism (Geller, Ritvo, Freeman, & Yuwiler, 1982), but enthusiasm over the drug has greatly abated.

It seems rather evident that no medication can serve as a panacea in treating developmental disabilities. Some may aid in reducing activity levels, improving attention, or reducing serious behaviors such as self-injury; but it is also clear that the combined genetic, organic, biological, and environmental factors that limit the abilities of such persons prevent any medication from producing dramatic habilitative effects without skill development and behavior management.

Milieu

In a book comparing treatments, a chapter on developmental disabilities is unique because until the 1960s no definable, empirical, data-based treatments were reported. Since then, behavior modification/behavior analysis strategies remain the only empirical treatments. More broadly, what can be described as "milieu" has also received much discussion but little empirical documentation. This includes family support groups, advocacy, sheltered workshops and other vocational training, and special education (Turnbull & Turnbull, 1990). Such programs and approaches undoubtedly have great value, but like medications, these activities do not replace specific treatment strategies to improve skills or reduce dangerous behaviors. Behavior analysis procedures must still be used in workshop settings, families, and special education classrooms in order for these milieux to be effective.

Conclusions

Behavior analysis has produced considerable data showing skill development and reduction of severe behavior problems. The use of single-subject research designs provides evidence that behavioral treatment strategies are effective. These designs also allow comparisons among behavioral techniques, and they have been used, along with direct observation methods, to evaluate the effects of medication on behavior.

There are numerous reviews related to examining procedures and research aimed at some specific problems such as feeding disorders, self-injury, independent living, and so on. However, most empirical research in behavior analysis in developmental disabilities ranges from one to ten individuals with two or three being the likely mode. Part of the logic of behavior analysis is that confidence or believability is accomplished through replication, and this has occurred since the 1960s. However, good, long-term, large-number actuarial studies do not exist. It may be that funding and practicality keep such work from occurring. If this is the case, replication is essential; however, longer follow-up must become a goal in behavior analysis.

Perhaps the most encouraging innovations in recent research involve the study of context and the programming for generalization. The early research often limited behavioral assessment and treatment to temporarily proximate A-B-C's (antecedents, behaviors, consequences). The current attempt to look at context will necessarily expand this analysis to temporally less proximate antecedents and more varied antecedents. Is the situation one of demand? Was the child teased on the bus on the way to school? These are contextual variables that are beginning to be considered and will produce new innovations in the years ahead.

Similarly, multifaceted ecobehavioral approaches that are *in situ,* and that include parent generalization strategies, continue to appear more frequently in the literature. These approaches, also because of their empirical design, will continue to produce data that will document the efficacy of these approaches in treatment and habilitation in developmental disabilities.

ACKNOWLEDGMENTS. Appreciation is extended to Ronit Gershater and Sylvia Grinberg for their help in the preparation of this chapter.

References

Aman, M. G., Teehan, C. J., White, A. J., Turbott, S. H., & Vaithianathan, C. (1989). Haloperiodol treatment with chronically medicated residents: Dose effects on clinical behavior and reinforcement contingencies. *American Journal on Mental Retardation, 93*, 452–460.

Aman, M. G., & White, A. J. (1988). Thioridazine dose effects with reference to stereotypic behavior in mentally retarded residents. *Journal of Autism and Developmental Disorders, 18*, 355–366.

Ayllon, T., & Azrin, N. H. (1968). *The token economy*. New York: Appleton-Century-Crofts.

Baker, B. L., Landen, S. J., & Kashima, K. J. (1991). Effects of parent training on families of children with mental retardation: Increased burden or generalized benefit? *American Journal on Mental Retardation, 96*, 127–136.

Ball, T. S., Campbell, R. V., & Barkemeyer, R. (1980). Air-splints applied to control self-injurious finger sucking in profoundly retarded individuals: A case study. *Journal of Behavior Therapy and Experimental Psychiatry, 11*, 267–271.

Ball, T. S., Seric, K., & Payne, L. E. (1971). Long-term retention of self-help skill training in the profoundly retarded. *American Journal of Mental Deficiency, 76*, 378–382.

Banks, M. I., & Locke, B. J. (1966). Self-injurious stereotypes and mild punishment with retarded subjects (Working paper No. 123). Parsons, KS: Parsons State Hospital and Training Center, Parsons Research Project.

Bannerman, D. J., Sheldon, J. B., Sherman, J. A., & Harchik, A. E. (1990). Balancing the right to habilitation with the right to personal liberties: The rights of people with developmental disabilities to eat too many doughnuts and take a nap. *Journal of Applied Behavior Analysis, 23*, 79–90.

Barrett, R. P., Feinstein, C., & Hole, W. T. (1989). Effects of naloxone and naltrexone on self-injury: A double-blind, placebo controlled analysis. *American Journal of Mental Retardation, 93*, 644–651.

Bijou, S. W., & Orlando, R. (1961). Rapid development of multiple-schedule performances with retarded children. *Journal of the Experimental Analysis of Behavior, 4*, 7–16.

Charlop, M. H., Kurtz, P. F., & Casey, F. G. (1990). Using aberrant behaviors as reinforcers for autistic children. *Journal of Applied Behavior Analysis, 23*, 163–181.

Charlop, M. H., Schreibman, L., & Thibodeau, M. G. (1985). Increasing spontaneous verbal responding in autistic children using a time delay procedure. *Journal of Applied Behaviour Analysis, 18*, 155–166.

Charlop, M. H., & Walsh, M. E. (1986). Increasing autistic children's spontaneous verbalizations of affection: An assessment of time delay and peer modeling procedures. *Journal of Applied Behavior Analysis, 19*, 307–314.

Corte, H. E., Wolf, M. M., & Locke, B. J. (1971). A comparison of procedures for eliminating self-injurious behavior of retarded adolescents. *Journal of Applied Behavior Analysis, 4*, 201–213.

Cronin, R. A., & Cuvo, A. J. (1979). Teaching mending skills to mentally retarded adolescents. *Journal of Applied Behavior Analysis, 12*, 391–400.

Cuvo, A. J., & Davis, P. K. (1980, November). Teaching community living skills to mentally retarded persons: An examination of discriminative stimuli. In J. R. Lutzker (Chair), *Behavior Therapy in Rehabilitation*. Symposium presented at the meeting of the Association for the Advancement of Behavior Therapy, New York.

Cuvo, A. J., Jacobi, L., & Sipko, R. (1981). Teaching laundry skills to mentally retarded adults. *Education and Training of the Mentally Retarded, 16*, 54–64.

Cuvo, A. J., Leaf, R. B., & Borakove, L. S. (1978). Teaching janitorial skills to the mentally retarded: Acquisition, generalization, and maintenance. *Journal of Applied Behavior Analysis, 11*, 345–356.

Deitz, S. M., Repp, A. C., & Deitz, D. E. D. (1976). Reducing inappropriate classroom behavior of retarded students through three procedures of differential reinforcement. *Journal of Mental Deficiency Research, 20*, 155–170.

Demetral, G. D., & Lutzker, J. R. (1980). The parameters of facial screening in treating self-injurious behavior. *Behavior Research of Severe Developmental Disabilities, 1*, 261–277.

Down, J. L. H. (1876). On the education and training of the feeble-in-mind. London: Lewis and Company.

Durand, V. M. (1982). A behavioral/pharmacological intervention for the treatment of self-injurious behaviors. *Journal of Autism and Developmental Disorders, 12*, 243–251.

Etzel, B. C., & LeBlanc, J. M. (1979). The simplest treatment alternative: The law of parsimony applied to choosing appropriate instructional control and errorless-learning procedures for the difficult-to-teach child. *Journal of Autism and Development Disabilities, 9*, 361–382.

Fuller, P. R. (1949). Operant conditioning of a vegetative human organism. *American Journal of Psychology, 62*, 587–590.

Gadow, K. D., & Poling, A. D. (1988). *Pharmacotherapy and mental retardation*. Boston: Little, Brown.

Geller, E., Ritvo, E. R., Freeman, B. J., & Yuwiler, A. (1982). Preliminary observations on the effect of fenfluramine on blood serotonin and symptoms in three autistic boys. *New England Journal of Medicine, 307*, 165-169.

Haring, T. G., & Kennedy, C. H. (1990). Contextual control of problem behavior in students with severe disabilities. *Journal of Applied Behavior Analysis, 23*, 235–244.

Hite, M. G., & Vatterott, M. K. (1991). Two decades of treatment for self-injurious biting in individuals with mental retardation or developmental disabilities: A treatment-focused review of the literature. *Journal of Developmental and Physical Disabilities, 3*, 81–113.

Iwata, B. A., Pace, G. M., Kalsher, M. J., Cowdery, G. E., Edwards, & Cataldo, M. F. (1990). Experimental analysis and extinction of self-injurious escape behavior. *Journal of Applied Behavior Analysis, 23*, 11–27.

Jones, R. T., & Kazdin, A. E. (1975). Programming response maintenance after withdrawing token reinforcement. *Behavior Therapy, 6*, 153–164.

Kanner, L. (1964). *A history of the care and study of the mentally retarded*. Springfield, IL: Charles C. Thomas.

Kazdin, A. E. (1973). The effect of response cost and aversive stimulation in suppressing punished and non-punished speech disfluencies. *Behavior Therapy, 4*, 73–82.

Kazdin, A. E. (1978). *History of behavior modification*. Baltimore: University Park Press.

Kazdin, A. E. (1979). Therapy outcome questions requiring control of credibility and treatment—generated expectancies. *Behavior Therapist, 10*, 81–93.

Kiesel, K. B., Lutzker, J. R., & Campbell, R. V. (1989). Behavioral relaxation training to reduce hyperventilation and seizures in a profoundly retarded epileptic child. *Journal of the Multihandicapped Person, 2*, 179–190.

Lent, J. R., & Spradlin, J. (1966). Cottage demonstration project. *Project News, 2*(7), 18–19.

Lovaas, O. I., Schreibman, L., Koegel, R. L., & Rehm, R. (1971). Selective responding by autistic children to multiple sensory input. *Journal of Abnormal Psychology, 77*, 211–222.

Lovaas, O. I., & Simmons, J. Q. (1969). Manipulation of self-destruction in three retarded children. *Journal of Applied Behavior Analysis, 2*, 143–157.

Luiselli, J. (1987). Behavior analysis of pharmacological and contingency management interventions for self-injury. *Journal of Behavior Therapy and Experimental Psychiatry, 17*, 275–284.

Lutzker, J. R. (1974). Social reinforcement control of exhibitionism in a profoundly retarded adult. *Mental Retardation, 5*, 46–47.

Lutzker, J. R. (1978). Reducing self-injurious behaviour in three classrooms by facial screening. *American Journal of Mental Deficiency, 83*, 510–513.

Lutzker, J. R. (1990). "Damn it, Burris, I'm not a product of Walden Two," or Who's controlling the controllers. In A. Repp & N. Singh (Eds.), *Severe behavior problems in developmental disabilities: Issues in nonaversive therapy* (pp. 495–501). Sycamore, IL: Sycamore Press.

Lutzker, J. R. (1991, August 16–20). Theoretical framework for an ecobehavioral approach. In J. R. Lutzker (Chair), *Project Ecosystems. Ecobehavioral prevention of child abuse in developmental disabilities.* Symposium presented at the 99th annual convention of the American Psychological Association, San Francisco, CA.

Lutzker, J. R., Campbell, R. V., Harrold, M., & Kiesel, K. (1992). Project Ecosystems: An ecobehavioral approach to families with children with developmental disabilities. *Journal of Developmental and Physical Disabilities, 4*, 1–14.

Lutzker, J. R., Campbell, R. V., Newman, M. R., & Harrold, M. (1989). Ecobehavioral interventions for abusive, neglectful, and high-risk families. In G. H. S. Singer & L. K. Irvin (Eds.), *Support for caregiving families* (pp. 313–326). Baltimore: Paul H. Brooks.

Lutzker, J. R., & Martin, J. A. (1981). *Behavior change.* Monterey, CA: Brooks/Cole.

Lutzker, J. R., Megson, D. A., Webb, M. E., & Dachman, R. S. (1985). Validating and training adult–child interaction skills to professionals and to parents indicated for child abuse and neglect. *Journal of Child and Adolescent Psychotherapy, 2*, 91–104.

Miller, R. M., & LeBlanc, J. M. (1973). *Experimental analysis of the effect of detailed and minimal instructions upon the acquisition of preacademic skills.* Paper presented at the 81st annual convention of the American Psychological Association, Montreal.

Matson, J. L., Sevin, J. A., Fridley, D., & Love, S. R. (1990). Increasing spontaneous language in three autistic children. *Journal of Applied Behavior Analysis, 23*, 227–233.

Moran, D. R., & Whitman, T. L. (1991). Developing generalized teaching skills in mothers of autistic children. *Child and Family Behavior Therapy, 13*, 13–37.

O'Brien, S., Repp, A. C., Williams, G. E., & Christophersen, E. R. (1991). Pediatric feeding disorders. *Behavior Modification, 15*, 394–418.

Parsons, M. B., & Reid, D. H. (1990). Assessing food preferences among persons with profound mental retardation: Providing opportunities to make choices. *Journal of Applied Behavior Analysis, 23*, 183–195.

Plummer, S., Baer, D. M., & LeBlanc, J. M. (1977). Functional considerations in the use of procedural timeout and an effective alternative. *Journal of Applied Behavior Analysis, 10*, 689–706.

Polvinale, R. A., & Lutzker, J. R. (1980). Elimination of assaultive and inappropriate sexual behavior by reinforcement and social restitution. *Mental Retardation, 18*, 27–30.

Repp, A. C., Deitz, S. M., & Speir, N. C. (1974). Reducing stereotypic responding of retarded persons through the differential reinforcement of other behaviors. *American Journal of Mental Deficiency, 79*, 279–284.

Sajwaj, T., Libet, J., & Agras, S. W. (1974). Lemon-juice therapy: the control of life threatening rumination in a six-month-old infant. *Journal of Applied Behavior Analysis, 7*, 552–563.

Sarber, R. E., Halasz, M. M., Messmer, M. C., Bickett, A. D., & Lutzker, J. R. (1983). Teaching menu planning and grocery shopping skills to a mentally retarded mother. *Mental Retardation, 21*, 101–106.

Scheerenberger, R. C. (1971). Mental retardation: Definition, classification, and prevalence. In J. H. Rothstein (Ed.), *Mental retardation: Readings and resources* (pp. 4–23). New York: Holt, Rinehart & Winston.

Singer, G. H. S., & Irvin, L. K. (Eds.). (1989). *Support for caregiving families.* Baltimore: Paul H. Brookes.

Singh, N. H. (1980). The effects of facial screening on infant self-injury. *Journal of Behavior Therapy & Experimental Psychiatry, 11*, 131–134.

Singh, N. H., & Aman, M. G. (1981). Effects of thioridazine dosage on the behavior of severely mentally retarded persons. *American Journal of Mental Deficiency, 85*, 580–587.

Tanner, B. A., & Zeiler, M. (1975). Punishment of self-injurious behavior using aromatic ammonia as the aversive stimulus. *Journal of Applied Behavior Analysis, 8*, 53–57.

Turnbull, A. P., & Turnbull, H. R. (1990). *Families, professionals and exceptionality: A special partnership.* Columbus, OH: Merrill.

Webster, D. R., & Azrin, N. H. (1973). Required relaxation: A method of inhibiting agitative disruptive behavior of retardates. *Behaviour Research and Therapy, 11*, 67–78.

Williams, G. E., & Cuvo, A. J. (1986). Training apartment upkeep skills to rehabilitation clients: A comparison of task analysis strategies. *Journal of Applied Behavior Analysis, 19*, 39–52.

Wolery, M., Kirk, K., & Gast, G. L. (1985). Stereotypic behavior as a reinforcer: Effects and side effects. *Journal of Autism and Developmental Disorders, 15*, 149–161.

Wolf, M. M., Risley, T., & Mees, H. (1964). Application of operant conditioning procedures to the behavior problems of an autistic child. *Behaviour Research and Therapy, 1*, 305–312.

Zegiob, L. E., Alford, A. S., & House, A. (1978). Response suppressive and generalization effects of facial screening on multiple self-injurious behaviors in a retarded boy. *Behavior Therapy, 9*, 688.

Zencius, A. H., Davis, P. K., & Cuvo, A. C. (1990). A personalized system of instruction for teaching checking account skills to adults with mild disabilities. *Journal of Applied Behavior Analysis, 23*, 245–252.

Zimmerman, E. H., & Zimmerman, J. (1962). The alteration of behavior in a special classroom situation. *Journal of Experimental Analysis of Behavior, 5*, 59–60.

5

Autism

Tristram Smith

Introduction

Of all the diagnostic categories in DSM-III-R (American Psychiatric Association [APA], 1987), Autistic Disorder may be associated with the most severe impairment in functioning. It begins at birth or within the first 2 or 3 years of life, and problems persist into adulthood in over 95% of untreated cases (Lotter, 1978; Rumsey, Rapoport, & Sceery, 1985; Rutter, 1970). About half of autistic individuals are unable to speak in words (Eisenberg, 1956; Rutter, 1970). Most of the rest do not speak communicatively. Instead, they simply echo what others say or repeat phrases over and over again (Kanner, 1943). When autistic individuals do have communicative speech, it is usually less advanced than that of their peers, and its content may be limited to stating demands or delivering monologues on topics that the speaker is preoccupied with, such as the weather (Rutter, 1970). Typically, autistic individuals make their needs known by taking others by the hand and pulling them over to what they want. They may lack other nonverbal forms of communication such as pointing, waving goodbye, nodding their head to mean "yes," shaking their head to mean "no," or motioning others to come toward them (Attwood, Frith, & Hermelin, 1988; Mundy, Sigman, Ungerer, & Sherman, 1986).

Autistic individuals often have as much trouble comprehending what is spoken to them as they do expressing themselves. Indeed, they may be so unresponsive when their name is called or a request is made of them that their families suspect they are deaf. Paradoxically, however, the same autistic individuals who fail to respond to words may be hypersensitive to other sounds. For example, they may cover their ears and look pained when an airplane flies far overhead (Ornitz & Ritvo, 1976).

Autistic individuals often appear to be in their own world, oblivious to the existence of others (Kanner, 1943). They may climb over others as if they were furniture. They may arch their backs and struggle to avoid affection offered by family members. They often evade eye contact. Unless closely supervised, they are

Tristram Smith • Department of Psychology, University of California, Los Angeles, Los Angeles, California 90024-1563.

Handbook of Effective Psychotherapy, edited by Thomas R. Giles. Plenum Press, New York, 1993.

apt to wander away from caregivers in public and show no concern about having done so. They may display little distress when separated from their parents and little joy when reunited (Sigman & Ungerer, 1984). In a group of peers, they are likely to be off by themselves, acting as if their peers were not present (Kanner, 1943). They seldom imitate actions performed by others (Dawson & Adams, 1984).

Autistic children seldom play with toys (Wulff, 1985). When they do play, they hardly ever engage in imaginative activities such as feeding dolls, inventing scenarios with action figures, or pretending that an object is something different from what is actually is (e.g., using a broom as a riding horse). Instead of playing, autistic children engage in repetitive, stereotyped activities that provide auditory, visual, or other sensory stimulation (Lovaas, Newsom, & Hickman, 1987). Common examples of stereotyped, self-stimulatory behaviors are flapping the hands from the wrists in front of the eyes, rocking the body back and forth, spinning in circles, gazing intently at spinning objects for extended periods of time, picking up and dropping objects over and over again, and lining objects into neat rows. Autistic individuals may also become unusually preoccupied with certain narrow topics, such as the alphabet, calendars, or automobile models. In addition, they may develop rituals, such as insisting that the family carry out household chores in a certain order or take a certain route on the way home. Further, they may become upset by minor changes such as a new picture on the wall. When their self-stimulatory behaviors or routines are disrupted, or when they do not get their way in other situations, many autistic individuals throw severe tantrums (Kanner, 1951). Frequently, these tantrums include assaulting others or injuring themselves by banging their head against the wall, biting or punching themselves, or poking at their eyes or kidneys. In some cases, the aggression is so severe that it poses a significant danger to autistic individuals or those around them (Rutter, Greenfeld, & Lockyer, 1967).

Most autistic individuals develop motor skills such as walking and sitting at a normal age, and they often show good gross and fine motor coordination throughout their lives. In addition, a sizable minority (perhaps 10%) have isolated abilities that are far beyond what might be expected from their functioning in other areas (Rimland & Fein, 1988; Treffert, 1988). Often, their special abilities take the form of memorizing large amounts of factual information or performing visual tasks such as completing complex puzzles. When young, many autistic individuals are physically attractive, with facial expressions that appear highly intelligent (Kanner, 1943). Nevertheless, about 75% perform in the mentally retarded range on standardized measures of intelligence (Freeman, Ritvo, Needleman, & Yokota, 1985). Moreover, they show little interest in and aptitude for acquiring self-help skills such as dressing, toileting, and avoiding common dangers (hot stoves, heights, oncoming traffic, etc.). Hence, their level of adaptive functioning is consistent with their performance on intelligence tests (Rutter, 1983). The vast majority require custodial care throughout their lives (Lotter, 1978; Rumsey *et al.*, 1985; Wing, 1989).

Autism is three to four times more common in boys than girls (APA, 1987), and it occurs in about 1 of every 2,500 people in the general population. There are also "autistic-like" individuals, who show many characteristics of the syndrome but who do not meet DSM-III-R (APA, 1987) criteria for the diagnosis. The number of autistic-like individuals is unknown but may be approximately equal to the number of autistic individuals.

Until the 1960s, most professionals believed that autism was caused by extremely hostile parents who forced their children to withdraw from the world (Bettelheim, 1967). This view has turned out to be false: Many investigations have shown that parents of autistic children are no different from parents of children with no history of behavioral disturbance, except that, not surprisingly, they are much more worried about their children's current behavior and future prospects (Cantwell & Baker, 1984). Furthermore, autistic children are much more severely disturbed than children who are known to have suffered extreme forms of abuse or neglect (Rutter, 1978). Thus, the etiology of autism is almost certainly organic. However, the precise cause or causes have yet to be identified (Rutter & Schopler, 1987).

The severity and chronicity of autistic individuals' problems create a compelling need to identify an effective treatment. At the same time, their youth, intelligent appearance, and strong families raise hopes that such a treatment will be discovered. Consequently, autism has attracted a great deal of attention. From a scientific standpoint, this attention has had both positive and negative effects. On the negative side, it has been all too easy to foist highly questionable treatments on harried parents and a credulous public eager for a "miracle cure." Even bizarre and illogical treatments, such as encouraging physical contact with dolphins, have received favorable media coverage that has been believed by many. More interventions have been devised for autism than any other behavioral disturbance, with the possible exception of schizophrenia.

On the positive side, autistic individuals have received extensive study. Indeed, autism has been described as the best studied of all childhood disorders (Rutter & Schopler, 1987), and many of the studies have concerned treatment. The severity and chronicity of autistic individuals' problems not only invites research but simplifies the investigators' task in some important ways. First, autistic individuals hardly ever stop being autistic without treatment. Second, most existing treatments, as we shall see, do not appear to be of any benefit in improving their functioning. Therefore, it is less important than with other clinical populations to be concerned with spontaneous remission and nonspecific treatment effects. Finding that treatment is superior to no treatment is often sufficient to validate an intervention.

Most existing interventions take place in psychotherapeutic or educational settings. These interventions may be grouped into four categories: relationship therapies, sensory-motor therapies, behavioral treatment, and special education. In addition, because autism is presumably organic in origin, researchers have made extensive efforts to develop effective psychopharmacological interventions. The remainder of this chapter will focus on psychotherapeutic and educational interventions, with a brief overview of psychopharmacology. For consistency, the chapter will refer to "therapists" and "clients" throughout, although there are some sections in which the terms "teachers" and "students" may seem more appropriate.

Psychotherapeutic and Educational Interventions: Rationale and Evidence for Efficacy

Relationship Therapies

From the 1940s, when autism was first hypothesized to be a distinct disorder (Kanner, 1943), to the 1960s, most autistic individuals were institutionalized and received little or no treatment (Lotter, 1978). When they did receive treatment, it was likely to be psychoanalysis. Bettelheim (1967) provided the most detailed and influential description of psychoanalytic treatment. According to Bettelheim and other psychoanalysts, mothers of autistic children are extremely cold individuals who treat their children like specimens in a science laboratory (Kanner, 1949) and harbor "murderous impulses" (Bettelheim, 1967, p. 70) toward them. In most cases, they act out these murderous impulses, killing their children or allowing them to die from neglect (Bettelheim, 1967, p. 421). The children who manage to survive develop autism as a defense against their horrible situation: They withdraw from the world as much as possible into a solitary (autistic) state.

As described by Bettelheim, psychoanalytic treatment begins by separating the autistic client from the mother. At minimum the separation consists of numerous psychotherapy sessions alone with the client. Preferably it involves a lengthy stay in a residential program. The client is given as much freedom as possible in an atmosphere of warmth and love. Therapists place particular emphasis on displaying warmth and love at times when, according to psychoanalysts, clients are withdrawing further into an autistic state—for example, when they display stereotypical or aggressive behavior. Therapists also offer interpretations of the behaviors that the client exhibits. While the client is undergoing treatment, the mother may also enter psychotherapy in order to work on the unconscious conflicts which, in the psychoanalytic view, produced her child's autistic state (Despert, 1951).

Although several studies (described in the section "Interorientation Comparisons") have tested the effectiveness of psychoanalysis and other relationship therapies against that of alternate treatments, no study has evaluated psychoanalysis alone. Psychoanalysts have opposed conducting such studies. They believe that autistic children have already suffered from an overdose of science at the hands of their mothers. Furthermore, they consider the psychoanalytic process to be too complex to be adequately evaluated in a data-based investigation (Bettelheim, 1967, pp. 1–9). Other professionals have concluded that psychoanalysis is probably harmful (e.g., Schopler, 1971). Parents may be devastated when blamed (erroneously, as noted in the introduction) for their child's condition. Other aspects of the treatment may also have deleterious effects (as shown in studies reviewed in the sections "Nonspecific Treatment Effects" and "Parameters of Treatment Outcome"). First, the treatment excludes parents, though parental participation appears to be an important component of successful intervention. Second, clients receive the most love and warmth when they display the most severe problems; in some situations, this has been shown to reinforce the problems and thereby make them even more severe. Finally, it allows clients to select their activities; studies have shown that clients benefit more from a structured environment.

The popularity of psychoanalysis has waned since the 1960s; but it remains very much in demand (Bettelheim, 1987), and it is still the dominant treatment in many parts of Europe. Furthermore, many of its concepts have been incorporated into other relationship therapies that have become popular. "Holding therapy" (Tinbergen & Tinbergen, 1983; Welch, 1987) views autism as a failure of the mother and child to "bond" and involves the mother forcibly holding the child close to her so as to cause "the autistic defense" to crumble (Welch, 1987, p. 48). Humanistic play therapy (Axline, 1965; DesLauriers & Carlson, 1969) emphasizes encouraging autistic children to play with toys in a setting where they receive unconditional positive regard. "Options" (Kaufman, 1976) provides individualized, loving attention for most of the child's waking hours in a residential setting.

"Gentle teaching" (McGee & Gonzalez, 1990) has the goal of showing autistic children that social interactions are rewarding, so that "bonding" occurs between the children and their therapists. This is accomplished by exhibiting "unconditional and authentic valuing" (McGee & Gonzalez, 1990). However, none of these therapies have been evaluated with autistic clients in controlled studies. Until proven otherwise, it may be assumed that the therapies are at best ineffective and at worst harmful because they share many of the weaknesses associated with psychoanalysis.

Sensory-Motor Therapies

One of the oldest and most popular notions about clients with delays, including those diagnosed with autism, is that they have difficulty processing sensory input from the environment and/or translating such input into effective action (Spitz, 1986). In this view, clients may be overaroused or underaroused by normal levels of stimulation they receive from the environment. Their nonoptimal arousal leads them to engage in self-stimulatory behaviors in order to modulate their arousal levels. It also prevents them from accurately perceiving and responding to environmental events.

Dating back to about 1800, a variety of different sensory-motor therapies have been proposed in an effort to alleviate these hypothesized deficits. At one time or another, many of the most influential figures in the history of special education have advocated such therapies: Itard, Seguin, Montessori, Frostig, Delacato, and others (Spitz, 1986). The most common sensory-motor therapy for autistic children is sensory integration (Ayres, 1972, 1979), which is based on the observation that autistic clients are unresponsive to sounds and other aspects of their environment. To increase their responsiveness, sensory integration stimulates their skin and vestibular system. This stimulation takes the form of activities such as swinging in a hammock suspended from the ceiling, spinning in circles on specially constructed chairs, brushing parts of clients' bodies, and engaging in physical exercises that require balance (Ayres, 1972).

In the only controlled study on the effects of sensory integration with autistic clients, Reilly, Nelson, and Bundy (1983) compared sensory integration to tabletop activities such as coloring and completing puzzles. Eighteen autistic children (mean age = 8.2 years) each participated in two 30-min sessions of sensorimotor integration and two of tabletop activities. The ordering of sessions was counterbalanced across subjects. The authors reported that, during tabletop activities, subjects spoke more appropriately than they did during sensorimotor integration. The authors did not assess other behaviors, nor did they examine whether changes occurred outside the treatment setting. These limitations, along with the extremely short duration of treatment, suggest that additional investigations of sensory integration are needed.

Another sensory-motor therapy, auditory integration training (Rimland & Edelson, 1991), is based on the observation that some autistic individuals are hypersensitive to certain sounds. Auditory integration training begins with an audiogram to determine the frequencies at which a client's hearing is overly acute. Once these frequencies have been identified, the client spends 10 hours listening to music played through a device that filters out sounds to which he or she is hypersensitive. Rimland and Edelson (in press) conducted the first controlled evaluation of auditory integration training. Eighteen autistic subjects, aged 4–22 years, were matched into pairs based on age, sex, history of ear infections, and severity of problems with hypersensitive hearing. One subject in each pair, selected at random, received auditory retraining. The other received a placebo treatment that consisted of listening to music that (unlike auditory integration training) had no sound frequencies filtered out. Subjects, their families, and therapists were not informed of the group assignments until the completion of the study. Despite the matching and randomization procedures, the experimental group prior to treatment displayed significantly more behavioral and auditory problems than the control group. Between pretreatment and posttreatment, the experimental group showed a greater decrease in these problems than the control group. The randomized, double-blind subject assignment is a laudable feature of this study, but the preexisting differences between groups make the results difficult to interpret. Another significant problem is that the measure of hypersensitive hearing (observations by trained clinicians) has not been shown to be reliable or valid. Rimland and Edelson (in press) considered their investigation to be a pilot study and have planned additional research.

Facilitated communication (Makarushka, 1991) views autistic children as having a motor deficit that prevents them from expressing themselves even though they are intellectually able to do so. To overcome this problem, a trained facilitator holds the client's forefinger, wrist, or arm to help the client type out messages on a keyboard. This treatment has attracted extensive publicity because of reports that it produces sudden increases in appropriate language. However, its proponents have opposed studies that evaluate its effectiveness. Objective evaluations of facilitated communication have been uniformly negative, revealing that, in all cases, the facilitator rather than the client was producing the messages that appeared on the keyboard (Rimland, 1992). Consequently, facilitated communication does not appear to be a valid treatment, although investigations are continuing.

Altogether, then, despite the widespread use of sensory-motor therapies, few controlled studies have examined their effects on autistic clients. A preliminary study on auditory integration training reported encouraging results (Rimland & Edelson, in press), but investigations of sensorimotor integration and facilitated communication did not (Reilly *et al.*, 1983; Rimland, 1992). More generally, Kavale and Mattson (1983) conducted a thorough meta-analysis of a variety of sensory-motor therapies across a variety of clinical populations (autistic, mentally retarded, language-delayed, learning-disabled, hyperactive, etc.) and across a variety of target behaviors. This meta-analysis produced no evidence of any benefits for sensory-motor therapies in any situation. Thus, whether or not sensory-motor therapies help clients remains to be demonstrated.

Behavioral Treatment

Behavioral treatment for autistic children (Lovaas & Smith, 1989) began in the 1960s. Behaviorists break down autism into separate behavioral problems and attempt to treat as many of these problems as possible. This approach differs from that of other professionals, who aim to identify a central problem, such as a failure to bond or a sensory-motor deficit, which becomes the main focus of treatment. Lovaas and Smith (1988) estimated that 500 behaviors would be separately targeted over the course of a behavioral treatment, including various language, social, emotional, academic, and self-care skills. Behavioral treatment has developed slowly and cumulatively, as interventions for different problems have been identified one at a time in data-based investigations. Thus, behavioral treatment has become increasingly complex over time, and advances continue to occur (Lovaas & Smith, 1989; Newsom & Rincover, 1989). Studies on behavioral treatment almost always use single-subject experimental designs. Experience with this kind of research has shown that the majority of effective interventions use principles derived from laboratory studies on learning, particularly in the area of operant conditioning. Hence, behaviorists view autism as a learning disorder. Although supervised by professionals (usually psychologists), behavioral treatment is most often provided by paraprofessionals and nonprofessionals such as students, parents, and employees without advanced degrees or licenses.

The literature contains hundreds of studies on behavioral treatment for autistic clients. Many additional studies have focused on behavioral treatment for other developmentally disabled populations, and these findings have often proved applicable to autistic clients. A complete review of this research is beyond the scope of this chapter. However, selected examples of research in two major areas—language and aggression—will serve as illustrations. Behavioral treatment has also been successful at, among other things, helping clients assist family members in the home (doing chores, cooperating with requests, etc.), teaching clients independent living skills (toileting, dressing, etc.), expanding clients' leisure activities (e.g., playing with toys), improving academic skills, providing job training, and enhancing cognitive skills (solving puzzles, detecting patterns, etc.). Additionally, behavioral treatment has had some success promoting interactions between autistic clients and "normal" or "average" peers, though this key area was neglected until the 1980s and remains very much in need of research. More complete overviews are provided by Koegel, Rincover, and Egel (1982), Lovaas (1977; Lovaas *et al.*, 1981; Lovaas & Smith, 1988, 1989), Newsom and Rincover (1989), and Schreibman (1988).

Language. Language training forms a central part of behavioral treatment for autistic clients. Studies have indicated that the most effective procedures for teaching communicative language simplify the instructional situation as much as possible so that the client can be successful. This simplification entails the use of procedures derived from laboratory research on operant conditioning and discrimination training, such as discrete trails, prompting, fading, shaping, and chaining (Lovaas, 1977). Prior to initiating language training, behavior therapists teach clients to comply with simple instructions and to imitate simple actions performed by the therapist (Lovaas, Freitas, Nelson, & Whalen, 1967). Then the therapist teaches clients to imitate simple sounds like "aah" and "mmm." Next comes instruction in imitating other sounds, combining these sounds into syllables, and forming words (Lovaas, Berberich, Perloff, & Schaeffer, 1966). Once clients are able to imitate words, they are instructed to use thee words to label common objects (Risley & Wolf, 1967). Subsequently, clients are instructed to combine these words to form simple sentences such as "I want . . ." and "This is a . . ." (Risley, Hart, & Doke, 1972). They are also instructed to use abstract concepts including yes/no (Hung, 1980), plurals (Baer, Guess, & Sherman, 1972), adjectives (Risley *et al.*, 1972), prepositions, pronouns, opposites such as big/little and hot/cold, and time relations such as first/last and before/after (Lovaas, 1977). If they master these concepts, they are taught to ask questions (Hung, 1977; Lovaas, 1977) and engage in simple conversations (Gaylord-Ross, Haring, Breen, & Pitts-Conway, 1984; Lovaas, 1977). Thus, experimentally validated procedures exist for helping clients progress from being mute to possessing many of the language skills displayed by typical preschool-age children.

Most of the reports on language training appeared in the 1960s and 1970s. Howlin (1981) reviewed these reports and found that, of the clients who were initially mute, 23% remained mute, 60% acquired one-word labels for objects, and only 17% acquired meaningful phrase speech. Almost half the clients who initially used single words acquired phrase speech. Finally, over 80% of clients who began treatment with some phrase speech acquired extensive meaningful phrase speech. As Howlin (1981) noted, the reliability of these figures is questionable. Most of the reports in the review contained methodological problems. Although single-subject experiments were numerous, so were uncontrolled case studies. Furthermore, even the single-subject experiments contained weaknesses. Many failed to obtain reliability data on behavior observations. Others failed to assess whether skills were maintained over time or generalized to situations outside the instructional setting. On the one hand, because of these problems, the data reported by Howlin may overestimate the effectiveness of behavioral approaches to teaching language. On the other hand, most of the reports in Howlin's review described attempts to teach specific skills rather than produce global improvements in language. Therefore, it is also possible that the data are underestimates.

Despite the foregoing difficulties in interpretation, several points are clear: Numerous investigations have documented that behavioral approaches help autistic clients acquire language. However, some clients benefit much more than others, and the extent to which gains maintain over time and generalize to new situations is in doubt.

Carr (1979) proposed using sign language with clients who are slow to develop vocal language. Many clients are better at visual tasks than auditory tasks. Therefore, sign language may be less frustrating and easier to acquire. Indeed, clients typically master sign language more rapidly than vocal speech (Barrera & Sulzer-Azaroff, 1983). In some cases, having had this success with language, clients go on to acquire vocal speech. However, in other cases, they continue to be dependent on sign language (Carr & Dores, 1981). Because sign language is so seldom used in everyday situations, switching to sign language is generally viewed as a last resort, but it is a viable option when attempts to teach vocal speech have been unsuccessful.

Another attempt to overcome the problems associated with standard behavioral language training is to make the teaching situation more natural. The inherent limitation of this strategy is that the more natural the teaching situation becomes, the more it resembles the situation in which clients initially failed to learn language. However, it may be that standard behavioral approaches are unnecessarily artificial in some respects. For example, perhaps therapists can place greater emphasis on allowing clients to select instructional materials and reinforcing clients by offering them the opportunity to handle these materials. Perhaps, in addition, therapists can increase motivation and minimize frustration by accepting partially correct responses even when clients have previously given superior ones (unlike shaping procedures, in which therapists hold out for better and better responses). Modifications such as these have served as the basis for two teaching approaches, the Natural Language Paradigm (NLP; Koegel, O'Dell, & Koegel, 1987) and incidental teaching (Hart & Risley, 1975). Advocates of both approaches believe that the approaches may produce more generalization than standard behavioral techniques because they make the treatment situation more like situations in everyday life. However, this contention has yet to receive an empirical test. Two studies have indicated that NLP increases the rate of language acquisition for some clients who had progressed at a slow rate with standard behavioral procedures (Koegel *et al.*, 1987; Laski, Charlop, & Schreibman, 1988). Additional studies have shown that incidental teaching can be used (1) to instruct clients to select an object when the therapist says its name (McGee, Krantz, Mason, & McClannahan, 1983) and (2) to help clients master prepositions (McGee, Krantz, & McClannahan, 1985). Thus, naturalistic teaching methods may supplement standard behavioral approaches for some clients.

Aggression. A functional analysis is the starting point for a behavioral intervention for aggression (Iwata, Vollmer, & Zarcone, 1990). In a functional analysis, the therapist observes the client's immediate environment for antecedents (events that immediately precede the aggression and hence may trigger it) and consequences (events that immediately follow the aggression and hence may serve to reinforce it). Some events commonly trigger aggression in autistic individuals, such as placing demands on them or denying them access to something they want. Other antecedents are idiosyncratic. For example, Lovaas, Freitag, Gold, and Kassorla (1965) demonstrated that a certain song triggered aggression in an autistic girl, while other songs did not. When the antecedent is easily avoided, as in the latter example, the aggression often can be eliminated simply by preventing the client from encountering the antecedent. However, in most cases it is unrealistic to remove the antecedent. For example, because most clients are very limited in their ability to function effectively without guidance, therapists and family members must occasionally place demands on them, even if the demands provoke self-injury.

When the antecedent cannot be removed, therapists examine the consequences of the aggression. Studies have identified three main kinds of consequences (Lovaas & Smith, in press): (1) positive reinforcement from others (e.g., attention or food), (2) negative reinforcement (e.g., escape from situations that are aversive to the client), and (3) self-stimulation (i.e., the aggression provides sensory feedback for the client). The preferred intervention for aggression serving any of these three functions is to teach alternative, adaptive behaviors that may replace the aggression. For example, when aggression produces positive or negative social reinforcement, it is often effective to teach clients to state what they want so that they do not need to resort to aggression to obtain it (Durand & Carr, 1991). When aggression produces self-stimulation, teaching appropriate leisure activities may be effective (Favell, McGimsey, & Schell, 1982). Usually, while these alternative behaviors are being taught, the therapist attempts to ignore the aggression when it occurs (in technical terms, the aggression is placed on extinction). Sometimes, however, teaching alternative behaviors is unsuccessful or proves to be too slow. For example, Lovaas and Simmons (1969) documented that, during extinction combined with teaching alternative behaviors, a client punched himself in the face with considerable force 10,000 times before his self-injury stopped. When the treatment moved to the next room, the client resumed punching himself at a high rate. Because of the near certainty that the client would maim himself if treatment continued at this pace, Lovaas and Simmons decided to consequate the punching with a mild dose of electric shock that had been determined to pose no risk of physical injury. The client stopped punching himself after only 12 administrations of the shock. Subsequent investigations have confirmed that shock rapidly suppresses self-injury (Carr & Lovaas, 1983).

Aversive interventions such as the use of shock constitute a very small part of behavioral treatment. Most clients do not receive such interventions at all. They come into consideration only when a crisis arises. Nevertheless, they have provoked considerable controversy (Axelrod & Apsche, 1983; Repp & Singh, 1990). One obvious concern is that they may produce negative side effects. However, numerous studies have shown that shock actually produces more positive side effects (particularly increases in social interactions) than negative side effects (Lichstein & Schreibman, 1976; Matson & Taras, 1989; Newsom, Favell, & Rincover, 1983) provided that it is administered properly. Research has shown that proper administration consists of targeting only one behavior at a time, administering the shock every time the behavior occurs, teaching alternative behaviors that may replace the targeted behaviors, monitoring the effects of the intervention closely (terminating the intervention if it does not result in an immediate cessation of the aggression), and making sure to obtain the approval and cooperation of everyone who has frequent contact with the child (Favell *et al.*, 1982; Lovaas & Favell, 1987).

Another valid concern is that aversive interventions could be misused or abused. Responding to this concern, many investigators have attempted to improve the effectiveness of procedures for teaching alternative behaviors (Carr & Durand, 1985). Other investigators have made extensive efforts to find alternatives that may be less risky than aversive interventions such as shock. Koegel and Covert (1972) found that a slap on the thigh or the buttocks may be effective. This punishment is similar to what most typical children would receive if their conduct put themselves or others in danger (Lichstein & Schreibman, 1976). However, this punishment may actually be more prone to abuse than electric shock because of the difficulty in monitoring the intensity with which the slap is given. Other investigators have attempted to identify aversive interventions that may be milder, such as time-out, saying "no" in a loud voice, holding the autistic individual's head down for a brief period of time, and spraying water mist (Axelrod & Apsche, 1983). However, it remains to be demonstrated whether autistic individuals in fact experience these interventions as less aversive. If so, it would then be important to determine whether the clients' interests are served by the increase in the length of treatment that may result from the use of a mildly aversive interventions (Newsom *et al.*, 1983; Smith, 1990b): Is a lengthy treatment that is mildly aversive preferable to a brief treatment that is strongly aversive? Perhaps the most promising approach to avoiding the use of aversive methods is to emphasize early intervention. The goal of early intervention is to begin treatment before clients become large enough to pose a significant danger to themselves or others. Treatment focuses on teaching clients to function as effectively as possible so that they will have little need to resort to aggression later on (Lovaas & Smith, in press). Despite these efforts, research has shown that situations continue to arise in which aversive interventions are the only approach known to be effective (Matson & Taras, 1989; Smith, 1990b).

In summary, behavioral investigators have demonstrated the effectiveness of a variety of procedures for reducing aggression. These interventions are successful in the large majority of cases (Matson & Taras, 1989) and usually (though not always) avoid the use of aversive procedures. An important limitation of this research should be noted: Many studies lack follow-up evaluations to determine whether treatment gains are maintained over time. When follow-ups are conducted, they rarely extend more than 18 months beyond the end of treatment. Thus, long-term effects have received insufficient investigation (Lovaas & Smith, in press).

Special Education

Since the passage of legislation in 1975 requiring that all handicapped children in the United States have the opportunity to receive a public school education, the most common intervention for autistic children has been placement in special education programs offered by public schools. Almost all autistic children participate in such programs. Project TEACCH, a statewide program in North Carolina founded by Eric Schopler (Schopler & Olley, 1982), has been the most influential special education agency. Schopler and his associates concur with the behavioral view that autism is best conceptualized as a learning disorder. They frequently draw upon behavioral procedures to teach self-help skills and manage disruptive behaviors. However, they depart from behavioral treatment in a major way by discouraging the use of other components of the treatment, particularly procedures for teaching language (Schopler, Reichler, & Lansing, 1980). They contend that such procedures are likely to result in poor generalization, and they assert that teaching methods derived from personal experience are more likely to produce satisfactory results. They have outlined the methods they have developed in a teaching manual (Schopler *et al.*, 1980), though they have not performed data-based studies to evaluate any of these methods. Project TEACCH clients spend most of the day in classrooms with children who have similar problems. However, they may be with "normal" or "average" children during recess, playtime, music, or other special activities (Wooten & Mesibov, 1986). Schopler and his associates place considerable emphasis on conducting an assessment incorporating normed instruments and clinical observations of the client. The purpose of the assessment is to identify developmentally appropriate targets for intervention, as well as instructional approaches that meet the individual needs of clients (Schopler & Reichler, 1979). Despite this emphasis on assessment and treatment planning, Schopler and his associates believe that establishing a warm relationship with clients and their families may be more important than choosing the right assessment or treatment procedures (Schopler, 1987). Thus, Project TEACCH is an eclectic mix of behavioral interventions, methods derived from personal experience, assessment practices common in educational settings, and concepts derived from relationship therapies.

Only one study (Schopler, Mesibov, & Baker, 1982) has evaluated the effectiveness of Project TEACCH classrooms. Subjects of this study were 657 past and present clients in Project TEACCH. Fifty-one percent had been diagnosed with autism; the remainder suffered from other unspecified communication handicaps. The clients ranged in age from 2 to 26 years old. One group had received only a diagnostic evaluation; a second group had received a diagnostic evaluation and parent training; a third group had had a diagnostic evaluation and placement in a classroom; and the fourth group had participated in a diagnostic evaluation, parent training, and a special education class. The authors supplied no information on the number of subjects in each group or the procedure for assigning subjects to groups. To evaluate the services that subjects received, parent questionnaires were sent to subjects' homes. Of these questionnaires, 348 (53%) were returned. The majority of respondents indicated that Project TEACCH had been very helpful. Those having the most contact with the agency gave the highest ratings. Staff members rated the effectiveness of Project TEACCH for a subset of 108 subjects. The procedure for selecting these subjects was not specified. The staff ratings also suggested that Project TEACCH had been successful. Finally, the autistic adolescents and adults in the sample were found to have an institutionalization rate of 7%, considerably lower than the rates of 39% to 74% recorded in studies of autistic clients in the 1960s. Unfortunately, this study contains a number of serious methodological difficulties: The subjects were extremely heterogeneous. The subject assignment procedures were not described. There is much missing data. It is not clear whether parent and staff ratings were anonymous; hence, respondents may have felt pressure to give favorable ratings. Finally, the hospitalization rate recorded by Schopler *et al.* is about what would be expected based on the sharp reduction in institutionalization between the time of the comparison studies and Schopler *et al.*'s report. Thus, this study provides no basis for determining the effectiveness of Project TEACCH (Smith, 1988). Sounder outcome studies are essential.

Special education classes outside Project TEACCH vary widely. However, it is likely that the typical class shares with Project TEACCH the eclectic mix of behavioral interventions, teaching methods derived from personal experience, reliance on detailed assessments, and emphasis on rapport with clients and families. Many school programs supplement classroom placement by referring clients for speech and language therapy 1–2 hours per week. There are many different speech and language therapies for autistic clients, none of which have been systematically investigated or proven effective (Snyder & Lindstedt, 1985). In the only controlled study of public school special education classes, Bartak and Rutter (1973; Rutter & Bartak, 1973) compared the effects of three different classes for autistic children (mean age = 8.5 years, range 3.5–15 years): Unit A (n = 8) provided relationship therapy; Unit B (n = 18) provided individualized intervention programs, with some clients engaging in structured academic activities and others spending most of their time in free play; Unit C (n = 24) emphasized teaching academic skills in a carefully planned, structured manner. Clients were assessed while in the classroom and during a follow-up approximately 4 years later. In the classroom, Unit C clients engaged in more constructive activities and fewer self-stimulatory behaviors than Unit B clients, who in turn surpassed Unit A clients on these measures. At follow-up, Unit C clients also showed superior educational attainment. Further, Unit C clients had a nonsignificant tendency to have more advanced speech. However, all clients remained severely delayed in these areas, I.Q. scores remained unchanged after treatment, and parental reports revealed no differences between units in clients' behavior at the home. Hence, Unit C outperformed the other two units, but its advantage was limited and may have been specific to the school setting. Moreover, at the beginning of the study, subjects in Unit C were functioning at a much higher level than subjects in the other units: Unit C had a mean I.Q. of 66, compared to 48 in Unit A and 52 in Unit B. This discrepancy, rather than the classroom environment, may account for the superior outcome of Unit C. Rutter and Bartak (1973) attempted to control for this possibility statistically, but no satisfactory procedure exists for doing so (Lord, 1967). In sum, Bartak and Rutter's study has many noteworthy features (comparison groups, detailed assessments, long-term follow-ups, etc.), and it is often cited as evidence that autistic children can benefit from structured classrooms such as the one in Unit C. However, it is more accurate to regard the results as inconclusive.

While no other controlled studies have evaluated special education programs for autistic clients in the public schools, Carlberg and Kavale (1980) have evaluated such programs for developmentally disabled children generally and found that clients tend to be slightly better off if they do not attend special education programs. Thus, although most autistic children receive special education, it remains to be seen whether these programs are helpful.

One alternative to public schools is the Higashi Program (Roland, McGee, Risley, & Rimland, 1988), which is based in Japan and also has a large school in Boston. The Higashi Program shares two features with behavioral treatment, though it was developed independently: (1) the use of prompt and prompt-fading procedures to teach new skills and (2) the reduction of behavior problems by extinction and positive practice (guiding the client through an adaptive behavior that may replace a disruptive behavior). However, other important behavioral procedures, such as discrete trials and shaping, are not emphasized, nor is language training. The curriculum focuses on academic skills, fine arts, and physical education. Rimland (1987a) sent questionnaires to 27 non-Japanese parents whose autistic children were enrolled in the Higashi Program in Japan. Nineteen parents responded. All reported that the program had been very helpful, surpassing other services their children had received. These results are open to question because the respondents formed a select group that may not have been representive of all the participants in the Higashi Program. Moreover, the improvements they reported may or may not be confirmed by independent assessments. Nevertheless, the results suggest that further evaluations are warranted.

Special education programs with a more thoroughgoing behavioral approach have also been set up. Behavioral classrooms typically use behavioral procedures to handle all of the problems that clients present. In addition, they incorporate several modifications that, according to some studies, help make the classroom situation beneficial. For example, Koegel and Rincover (1974) found that, prior to training, clients failed to pay attention in group settings. To correct this problem, the investigators taught skills such as raising hands and sitting quietly in a circle in a one-to-one situation. Then they instructed the classroom teacher to request and reinforce these behaviors when the child was in the class. Finally, they gradually and systematically increased the class size in which clients could function effectively. Russo and Koegel (1977) used this procedure to mainstream one autistic client into a regular class. Rincover and Koegel (1977) developed an alternative procedure for enabling clients to function in a class: instructing the teachers to work with each client one-to-one on a rotating basis. Strain (1983) found that autistic children benefit from having "normal" or "average" children in their class rather than being segregated with other autistic children. Some preliminary investigations (Fenske, Zalenski, Krantz, McClannahan, 1985; Harris, Handleman, Gordon, Kristoff, & Fuentes, 1991; Rincover, Taggart, Hyde, Cardella, &

Barany, 1985, as cited in Newsom & Rincover, 1989; Strain, Hoyson, & Jamieson, 1985) have reported that behavioral classrooms may allow children to go on to less restricted school placement and achieve average gains of about 20 points or more on standardized tests of intelligence or achievement. However, sounder and more complete investigations are required before these reports can be accepted.

Specific versus Nonspecific Treatment Effects

Schopler (1987) has written extensively about the need for treatment programs to garner the enthusiasm of autistic individuals, their families, the treatment staff, and the community at large. According to Schopler, "this nonspecific positive response . . . [is] likely to represent the program's heart and soul" (1987, p. 379). Although specific treatment techniques may be helpful, therapists' main task, in Schopler's view, is to maintain a warm, caring, supportive attitude.

Undoubtedly, it is essential to establish rapport with autistic individuals and their families, and it is certainly helpful to maintain good standing in the community. The question is whether nonspecific displays of warmth and attention meet these objectives and produce favorable outcomes. Two studies suggest they might. In the first, Wenar, Ruttenberg, Dratman, and Wolf (1967) compared three interventions for autistic children: a large custodial state institution (n = 8), a large state institution that provided psychoanalytic treatment (n = 15), and a small psychoanalytic day-care unit (n = 9). After a year in these settings, only children in the third setting showed significant improvement, as measured by a behavior observation instrument developed by the authors. The authors attributed this improvement to the individualized attention offered at the day-care unit.

In the second study, the same research group (Wenar & Ruttenberg, 1976) compared eight treatment centers that had enrolled a total of 46 autistic children. The authors classified each setting on three dimensions: (1) child-oriented versus authoritative, (2) residential versus day care, and (3) type of therapy (behavior modification, educational, psychoanalytic, or none). They reported that child-centered treatment settings, defined as those that were sensitive to the behaviors and needs of the children and that were "skillfully implemented by a dedicated and attentive staff" (p. 175), achieved the best outcome regardless of the type of setting or therapeutic orientation.

Both of these studies were weakened by small sample sizes that gave them little power to detect differences between treatments. They were further weakened by a failure to describe the different interventions in replicable detail. Additionally, subjects were not randomly assigned to treatment conditions. Hence, it is unclear whether the results reflect treatment effects or preexisting differences in subjects or both. Countering these studies, a large number of reports have suggested that specific treatment procedures are critical in achieving optimal outcomes.

Two studies indicated that adults must not only be attentive but must also provide structure. One of these studies (Bartak & Rutter, 1973) has already been reviewed and does not provide clear-cut results. The second study (Schopler, Brehm, Kinsbourne & Reichler, 1971) used an ABAB reversal design to compare the effects of structured versus unstructured teaching situations with four autistic children. These investigators found that the structured situation produced substantially more attention, displays of appropriate affect, social interactions, and nonpsychotic behavior than unstructured situations. This effect was particularly marked for the lower-functioning subjects in the study.

Lovaas and his associates (Lovaas *et al.*, 1965; Lovaas & Simmons, 1969) compared the effects of displaying warmth and affection when autistic individuals displayed aggression (as psychoanalysts advocate) to using behavioral interventions derived from a functional analysis. In two cases studied in ABAB reversal designs, the investigators found that displays of warmth and attention had to be discontinued because they produced a marked increase in aggression. In both cases, procedures derived from the functional analysis successfully eliminated the aggression.

A number of studies on specific treatment effects grew out of research on stimulus overselectivity (Lovaas, Koegel, & Schreibman, 1979), which is the tendency of autistic clients to focus on only parts of complex stimuli. For example, when presented with a buzzer and a light, they may attend only to the light. The presence of overselectivity has several treatment implications that have been supported by research: First, to maximize the likelihood that a client attends to the relevant portion of an instruction, it is best to keep the instructions as short and simple as possible (e.g., saying "sit" rather than "would you please sit down") (Koegel & Rincover, 1976). Second, when using a prompt such as physical guidance or modeling to help a client respond to an instruction, therapists should fade out the prompt as soon as possible to prevent the client from attending to the prompt rather than the therapists' instruction (Schreibman, 1975). Third, if possible, therapists should make prompts part of the instruction rather than separate from it (e.g., exaggerating the relevant words in the instruction rather than modeling the correct response) (Rincover, 1978; Schreibman, 1975). Finally, therapists should avoid giving inadvertent cues such as glancing at the correct response, always putting it in the same position, or giving instructions in a predictable sequence, because clients are likely to attend to these cues rather than to instructions (Koegel & Rincover, 1976).

A number of other studies have documented specific effects. For example, Koegel, Russo, and Rincover (1977) found that clients' performance in teaching situations deteriorated within minutes unless teachers used simplifications derived from research on operant conditioning (discrete trials, shaping, etc.; cf. Lovaas, 1977). Koegel, Dunlap, and Dyer (1980) found that the interval between the reinforcement of one response and the request for the next response should be limited to about 1 second in order to hold the client's attention. Koegel and Williams (1980) and Litt and Schreibman (1981) also found that, if possible, the reinforcement should be related to the response rather than arbitrarily selected (e.g., allowing the client to play with instructional materials rather than giving food). Several investigators have shown that training new responses should be interspersed with requests for other responses so as to maintain the client's motivation, help the child learn which response goes with which request, and promote retention of the correct response once training ends (Dunlap, 1984; Neef, Iwata, & Page, 1980; Smith, 1990a).

Many of the foregoing studies have not been replicated and may be open to question because they were performed by investigators who favor behavioral treatment. Nevertheless, the studies strongly indicate that careful adherence to behavioral approaches is necessary for achieving optimal results.

Interorientation Comparisons

Because behavioral treatment is the only intervention that has any significant experimental support, there has been little incentive to perform interorientation comparisons. Most of the interorientation comparisons have already been discussed: Bartak and Rutter (1973) compared three different models for classroom teaching and found that the one offering the most structure and teaching time was the most effective. Lovaas and his associates (Lovaas *et al.*, 1965; Lovaas & Simmons, 1969) compared psychoanalytic and behavioral approaches to the treatment of aggression with two subjects and found that behavioral approaches were more effective. Finally, Wenar and Ruttenberg (Wenar *et al.*, 1967; Wenar & Ruttenberg, 1976) reported that the provision of individualized attention was more important than the choice of treatment approach.

In addition, Ney, Palvesky, and Markely (1971) compared a group of 10 autistic children who received behavioral treatment to a group of equal size that received Jungian play therapy (not a common treatment for autistic clients, but one that has seen occasional use since the 1960s). These investigators found that the behavioral treatment group achieved significantly greater increases in mental age (as measured by standardized intelligence tests) and amount of speech than the play therapy group.

Most of these studies suggest that treatment for autistic clients should involve structured teaching of practical skills rather than relationship therapy or sensory-motor therapy. Contrary evidence comes from Wenar and Ruttenberg's studies, which indicate that the choice of treatment is relatively insignificant as long as clients receive individual attention. On balance, it seems reasonable to accept the view that structured teaching is important, because this view has more and better empirical support, particularly when the evidence presented in the preceding section is taken into account. No studies have directly compared different structured teaching approaches (behavioral treatment vs. typical special education classes, etc.). Consequently, although behavioral treatment appears to be the intervention of choice in studies on the validity of particular interventions and on the importance of specific factors, interorientation comparisons have yet to confirm (or refute) this perception.

Outcome Parameters

Factors That Influence Treatment Effectiveness

A consensus exists among researchers that certain variables are important in optimizing outcome (Simeonnson, Olley, & Rosenthal, 1987): early intervention, parental involvement, community focus, and intensity of treatment. Four reports have evaluated early intervention by comparing outcomes achieved by preschool-age children to those achieved by older clients. Three found that the preschoolers achieved superior outcomes (Fenske *et al.*, 1985; Rincover *et al.*, 1985; as cited in Newsom & Rincover, 1989; Wenar & Ruttenberg, 1976), but the fourth found the reverse (Howlin, 1981). One additional study indicated that, even in samples restricted to preschoolers, younger subjects attained better outcomes than older subjects (Strain, 1987). However, a second study of preschoolers found no correlation (Lovaas & Smith, 1988). None of these studies adequately controlled for the possibility that the younger and older subjects were dissimilar from the beginning. Hence, inequalities in outcome may reflect preexisting differences rather than differential treatment response. Nevertheless, the studies provide some evidence that early intervention increases the effectiveness of treatment.

Several studies have shown that autistic children achieve more favorable outcomes when their parents are involved in the treatment than when they are not (reviewed by Newsom & Rincover, 1989). For example, Lovaas, Koegel, Simmons, and Long (1973) found that autistic children who entered an institutional setting rather than returning home at the end of treatment relapsed. By contrast, autistic children who returned home to parents who had learned to implement behavioral techniques showed no relapse.

Some debate exists about how extensively the parents should be involved. Howlin and Rutter (1987) gave approximately 20 hours of parent training to mothers of autistic children and compared this group to parents who received no intervention. The authors reported that mothers who had received parent training managed disruptive behaviors and taught language skills more effectively than mothers in the control group. However, they were not able to provide increases in intellectual functioning (as measured by I.Q.) or spontaneous speech. Koegel, Schreibman, Britten, Burke, and O'Neill (1982) compared a 25–50-hour course of parent training to 1 year of behavioral treatment provided 4–5 hours a week in the home. Both groups showed improvements, but only the parent-training group demonstrated improvements during everyday situations at home. Other investigators have involved parents of autistic children much more extensively than these authors did. For example, Lovaas (1987) asked parents to work 10 hours a week with their autistic child under the apprenticeship of experienced therapists, with the goal that they would eventually equal the experienced therapists in their ability to implement behavioral treatment. An additional 30 hours a week were provided in which parents were encouraged to attend to other family members or take time to themselves. However, no data were collected on how proficient the parents became, and some professionals expressed concern that this intervention imposed a burden on the parents (Schopler, Short, & Mesibov, 1989), a point disputed by Lovaas and his associates (Lovaas, Smith, & McEachin, 1989). Thus, parental involvement appears to be important, but what form this involvement should take and what goals are realistic remain in dispute.

In addition to involving parents, many therapists recommend conducting treatment in the home and elsewhere in the community, as opposed to clinics, hospitals, and other professional settings. Such a community focus is intended to help clients use their new skills in everyday situations, not just during treatment sessions. Supporting this strategy, Rincover and Koegel (1975) and Cardella and Rincover (1985, cited in Newsom & Rincover, 1989) found that some clients experienced difficulties when the treatment situation differed from the situation in which they were expected to use their skills. However, Smith and Calouri (1989) failed to obtain such an effect. Hence, additional research may be needed to determine whether it is important to conduct treatment at home and in other everyday situations.

Little evidence exists on the appropriate level of treatment intensity. Lovaas and Smith (1989) suggested that autistic children may need to receive as much treatment as possible if they are to have any chance of catching up to "normal" or "average" children, who seem to learn during all their waking hours, while autistic children fail to do so. Accordingly, in a study that will be described in greater detail below, Lovaas (1987) provided a group of autistic children (n = 19) with about 40 hours of behavioral treatment a week for 2 or more years. This group was compared to a group that received 10 hours a week or less (n = 19) and a group that was never referred to his treatment program (n = 21). The group that received 40 hours a week showed substantial gains in I.Q. and school placements, whereas the other two groups showed no improvements on these measures and did not differ from each other. Anderson, Avery, DiPietro, Edwards, and Christian (1987) performed an uncontrolled study evaluating an intervention based in some respects on the Lovaas program, but providing only 20 hours a week of treatment. Subjects showed some increase in I.Q., but not nearly of the magnitude reported by Lovaas (1987). Thus, at least on the global measures employed in these studies, 10 hours a week of treatment may not differ from no treatment; 20 hours of treatment may produce only modest benefits; and as much as 40 hours a week may be needed to produce major improvements. This suggests that interventions may need to be very intensive.

Studies of Treatment Effectiveness

Only one research group, Lovaas and his associates (Lovaas, 1987; Lovaas & Smith, 1988; McEachin, Smith, & Lovaas, 1993), has published controlled evaluations of the effectiveness of a behavioral treatment program that includes all the foregoing components (early intervention, parental involvement, high intensity, and community focus). As already noted, Lovaas (1987) studied three groups of autistic children: (1) an intensive-treatment group (n = 19), (2) a minimal-treatment group (n = 19), and (3) a no-treatment group (n = 21). Subjects who were referred to the clinic were assigned to the intensive-treatment group or the minimal-treatment group based on therapist availability: If enough therapists were available they entered intensive treatment; otherwise, they entered minimal treatment. To be included in the study, subjects had to be under 40 months old at intake if they were mute, and under 46 months old if they spoke recognizable words. The age cutoff was extended for children with recognizable words because it was expected that the presence of some language would provide a head start, allowing treatment to be completed more quickly. Subjects also had to have a minimum ratio I.Q. of 37, as autism is difficult to distinguish from other diagnoses in children who have low I.Q.'s (Wing, 1981). The treatment groups did not differ at intake on 19 of 20 pretreatment variables; the twentieth variable, age at which treatment began, was not related to outcome and may have varied because of the lack of availability of therapists for the minimal-treatment group. Attrition was low: Only two subjects, both in the experimental group (not included in the final sample size of 19), dropped out during treatment, and one control subject dropped out between the first and second posttreatment evaluation.

In the first posttreatment evaluation, conducted when the subjects were 7 years old, the mean I.Q. of the intensive-treatment group had increased from 63 to 83, while the mean I.Q. of the minimal-treatment group declined from 57 to 52, and the mean I.Q. of the no-treatment group went from 59 to 58 (Lovaas & Smith, 1988). Of the 19 intensive-treatment subjects, 9 successfully passed first grade in regular (nonspecial education) classes without special intervention from the Lovaas clinic or the schools. These children also performed within normal range on standardized measures of intelligence. Hence, they were classified as normal in intellectual and educational functioning. Only 1 of 40 subjects in the two control groups achieved such a favorable outcome.

A second follow-up evaluation, conducted when the intensive-treatment subjects had reached an average age of 13 years, showed that eight of the nine children who had been classified as normal functioning had remained in regular classes. Further, when tested by examiners blind to their history of behavioral disturbance, these eight subjects performed in the normal range on tests of intelligence, adaptive behavior, and personality, as well as on ratings by the examiners. The ninth subject maintained an I.Q. score in the normal range, but showed significant adjustment difficulties in other respects. The intensive-treatment group as a whole had maintained its gains over the minimal-treatment group.

The results reported by Lovaas and his associates have come under close scrutiny. Schopler *et al.* (1989) suggested that at intake the subjects had unusually high I.Q. scores for a group of autistic children and hence may have had favorable prognoses. However, this does not appear to be the case. For example, the mean I.Q. of Lovaas's subjects is only 3 points higher than that in a sample reported by Schopler (Lord & Schopler, 1989). Furthermore, Lord and Schopler found that subjects with the highest I.Q.'s showed the least improvement. Perhaps the major weakness in the Lovaas study was the failure to use an arbitrary procedure for assigning subjects to groups. Although the groups appeared to be similar at intake, the subject assignment procedure left open the possibility that the assignment was somehow biased. By contrast, this research contained a number of methodological safeguards that enhance the believability of the results (McEachin *et al.*, 1992): control groups, extensive pretreatment and posttreatment evaluations conducted by independent examiners, and detailed descriptions of the treatment procedures (Lovaas *et al.*, 1981). Replications by independent investigators will be vital in determining whether behavioral treatment is as effective as suggested by the work of Lovaas and his associates.

Three other studies have also reported large gains in standardized test scores and/or educational placement (Fenske *et al.*, 1985; Harris *et al.*, 1991; Strain *et al.*, 1985). However, these studies all had small samples and/or few experimental controls. Other studies have examined small-scale interventions such as parent training of 20–50 hours in duration (Hemsley *et al.*, 1978; Howlin & Rutter, 1987; Koegel, Schreibman *et al.*, 1982; Kozloff, 1973) and home-based treatment of less intensity than in the Lovaas study (Anderson *et al.*, 1987; Schreibman & Koegel, 1975). These studies have shown that clients decrease disruptive behaviors and increase adaptive behaviors such as speech and self-help, but they stay the same on global measures such as I.Q. tests.

Lovaas *et al.* (1973) evaluated an early version of behavioral treatment. Subjects were 20 autistic children, aged 3–10 years. All subjects received 40 hours of treatment per week for 12 to 14 months. There was no comparison group of untreated subjects. However, some degree of control was provided by the fact that some clients received treatment in an ABAB design (no treatment, treatment, no treatment, treatment) and participated in studies on the effectiveness of specific behavioral procedures. Some subjects were inpatients; others were outpatients. Some parents received training; others did not. The treatment focused primarily on language, but efforts were made to increase self-help and reduce disruptive behaviors. Social skills, such as playing with peers, were not taught. The subjects increased their adaptive behavior, as measured by the Vineland Social Maturity Scale, from 48 to 71. They also showed modest increases in I.Q. scores, although all but one remained in the mentally retarded range. In addition, they improved on behavior observations. However, many subjects relapsed after treatment, and none achieved normal levels of functioning. This study and the evaluations of short-term interventions in other investigations led many professionals to conclude that behavioral treatment could effect only small and/or temporary changes (Rutter, 1985). However, many improvements have been made since the time of the Lovaas *et al.* (1973) study. The more recent results of Lovaas and his associates, as well as the preliminary results obtained by other investigators, suggest that the picture may have brightened considerably.

Psychopharmacological Interventions

At the present time, psychopharmacological interventions have limited use with autistic clients. They generally do not produce overall improvements in clients' functioning but may help control disruptive behaviors. The medications whose effects are best documented are the major tranquilizers, particularly nonsedating ones such as haloperidol (Haldol), which often produce rapid reductions in aggression (Locascio *et al.*, 1991). However, because of the frequency and severity of potential side effects, they are rarely prescribed to preadolescent clients.

A number of small studies indicate that fluoxetine (Prozac), an antidepressant, and naltrexone, an opiate, may suppress or reduce self-injury and excessive activity levels (Campbell *et al.*, 1990; Leboyer *et al.*, 1992). However, more extensive clinical trials are needed to validate the utility of these interventions. Interestingly, several double-blind, controlled investigations have found that megadoses of Vitamin B-6 (thiamine) help 40–50% of autistic clients (Rimland, 1987b). Megavitamin therapies generally have a poor reputation in the medical community but appear worth pursuing with autistic clients in view of the evidence supporting their efficacy. Many other medications have been studied, but none have been clearly demonstrated to be helpful (Campbell, 1989).

Conclusions and Implications

Research has indicated that behavioral treatment is the intervention of choice for autistic clients (DeMyer, Hingtgen, & Jackson, 1981; Rutter, 1985; Simeonnson *et al.*, 1987). In addition, psychopharmacological interventions, especially haloperidol, may help control disruptive behaviors in some cases. For the most part, behavioral treatment has achieved its preeminence by default, not by surpassing alternative interventions in direct comparisons: Hundreds of studies attest to the effectiveness of behavioral treatment, while none of the many other interventions in existence has any clear experimental support. In fact, some of these interventions may be harmful. Relationship therapies such as psychoanalysis seem to be particularly inappropriate. Unfortunately, special education programs offered by the public schools, which are by far the largest service providers for autistic children, have not received an adequate evaluation and may not be beneficial.

Almost all studies on behavioral treatment have used single-subject designs. These studies have been conducted by investigators interested in operant conditioning and its applications. Historically, such investigators have had a very strong preference for single-subject designs over group comparisons (Johnston, 1988). Their preference has served the field well in identifying specific interventions that modify individual behaviors exhibited by autistic clients. However, it has been considerably less useful in determining what happens when the interventions are combined into a comprehensive treatment package. Investigators have learned little about what proportion of clients are helped; the extent to which they stop displaying behaviors that would warrant a diagnosis of autism; the size of gains they make on I.Q. tests and other global measures of functioning; the improvements clients may make in their ability to cope with everyday situations, how long these improvements last, and so forth.

The main studies on the overall effectiveness of behavioral treatment have come from Lovaas and his associates (Lovaas, 1987; Lovaas & Smith, 1988; McEachin *et al.*, 1993). These investigators studied a treatment protocol that was intended to be as effective as possible, given the current state of knowledge. They emphasized early intervention (beginning in the preschool years), involvement of parents and other significant people in the children's everyday environment, many hours of treatment (40 hours a week for 2 or more-years), and implementation of the treatment in clients' communities rather than clinical settings. They found that nearly half their clients became indistinguishable from "normal" peers on a broad array of psychological tests. Other investigators, studying smaller interventions or now-obsolete versions of behavioral treatment, have reported only small or temporary improvements. The work of Lovaas and his associates needs to be replicated, and in the interim there will be uncertainty as to whether to accept the hopeful reports from these investigators or the more pessimistic view put forth by other studies.

An important question is what ramifications these studies have for professionals who work with autistic clients. In general, the author believes that, if research has identified a treatment of choice, it should be standard practice to implement that treatment or refer to another professional or agency that will. Research is fallible and from time to time will yield results that are wrong or misleading. Nevertheless, it is the best available way to identify effective interventions.

From this perspective, it is clear that therapists have an obligation to ensure that autistic clients receive behavioral treatment. Occasionally, exceptions may arise: Clients' caretakers may choose an alternative intervention even after being informed about behavioral treatment; clients may have already received an adequate trial of behavioral treatment that proved unsuccessful; and in the future (though not at present) it may be possible to identify clients who are poor candidates for behavioral treatment and might be better served by an alternative intervention. Additionally, caretakers often wish to enroll clients in alternative interventions as an adjunct to behavioral treatment. It is usually good practice to give them freedom to do so and to evaluate the interventions themselves, as long as the interventions do not appear to pose a risk to clients, take too much time away from behavioral treatment, or impose an excessive financial burden or other hardship.

Unfortunately, competent behavioral treatment is hard to find. Few professionals have received training in the use of behavioral procedures in one-to-one situations. Many are unfamiliar with essential concepts such as discrete trials and discrimination training. The Association for Behavior Analysis (located in Kalamazoo, MI) provides some information on training programs. Sadly, however, clients' families, rather than professionals, have had to give most of the impetus for the dissemination of behavioral treatment that has occurred. It may not be an exaggeration to say that behavioral treatment would have died out if families had not formed advocacy groups such as the Autism Society of America and supported this intervention. Families have also played a major role in pushing for the adoption of the improvements that have been made in behavioral treatment over time, and they have even corrected technical mistakes made by professionals who have criticized outcome research. Leading authorities, meanwhile, have often been extremely hostile, dismissing behavioral treatment altogether and chastising its proponents (e.g., Bettelheim, 1967; Schopler, 1988). For clients' sake, one may hope that in the future professionals will require less prodding to implement behavioral treatment and will be more attracted to the opportunity it offers to make a major difference in the lives of some extremely dysfunctional clients.

ACKNOWLEDGMENTS. The author thanks Annette Groen and Ivar Lovaas for their help in preparing this chapter.

References

American Psychiatric Association. (1987). *Diagnostic and statistical manual of mental disorders* (3rd ed.-revised). Washington, DC: American Psychiatric Association.

Anderson, S. R., Avery, D. L., DiPietro, E. K., Edwards, G. L., & Christian, W. P. (1987). Intensive home-based early intervention with autistic children. *Education and Treatment of Children, 10*, 352–266.

Attwood, A., Frith, U., & Hermelin, B. (1988). The understanding and use of interpersonal gestures by autistic and Down's Syndrome children. *Journal of Autism and Developmental Disorders, 18*, 241–257.

Axelrod, S., & Apsche, J. (Eds.). (1983). *The effects of punishment on human behavior*. New York: Academic Press.

Axline, V. M. (1965). *Dibs: In search of self: Personality development in play therapy*. Boston: Houghton Mifflin.

Ayres, A. J. (1972). *Sensory integration and learning disorders*. Los Angeles: Western Psychological Services.

Ayres, A. J. (1979). *Sensory integration and the child*. Los Angeles: Western Psychological Services.

Baer, D. M., Guess, D., & Sherman, J. (1972). *Adventures in simplistic grammar*. In R. L. Schiefelbusch (Ed.), Language of the mentally retarded (pp. 93–105). Baltimore: University Park Press.

Barrera, R. D., & Sulzer-Azaroff, B. (1983). An alternating treatment comparison of oral and total communication training programs with echolalic autistic children. *Journal of Applied Behavior Analysis, 16*, 379–394.

Bartak, L., & Rutter, M. (1973). Special educational treatment of autistic children: A comparative study. I. Design of study and characteristics of units. *Journal of Child Psychology and Psychiatry, 14*, 161–179.

Bettelheim, B. (1967). *The empty fortress*. New York: Free Press.

Bettelheim, B. (1987). The therapeutic milieu. In J. K. Zeig (Ed.), *The evolution of psychotherapy* (pp. 223–231). New York: Brunner/Mazel.

Campbell, M. (1989). Pharmacotherapy in autism: An overview. In C. Gillberg (Ed.), *Diagnosis and treatment of autism* (pp. 203–217). New York: Plenum.

Campbell, M., Anderson, L. T., Small, A. M., Locascio, J. J., Lynch, N. S., & Choroco, M. C. (1990). Naltrexone in autistic children; A double-blind and placebo-controlled study. *Psychopharmacology Bulletin, 26*, 130–135.

Cantwell, D. B., & Baker, L. (1984). Research concerning families of children with autism. In E. Schopler & G. B. Mesibov (Eds.), *The effects of autism on the family* (pp. 41–63). New York: Plenum.

Carlberg, C., & Kavale, K. (1980). The efficacy of special versus regular class placement for exceptional children: A meta-analysis. *Journal of Special Education, 14*, 295–309.

Carr, E. G. (1979). Teaching autistic children to use sign language: Some research issues. *Journal of Autism and Developmental Disorders, 9*, 345–359.

Carr, E. G., & Dores, P. A. (1981). Patterns of language acquisition following simultaneous communication with autistic children. *Analysis and Intervention in Developmental Disabilities, 1*, 347–361.

Carr, E. G., & Durand, V. M. (1985). Reducing behavior problems through functional communication training. *Journal of Applied Behavior Analysis, 18*, 111–126.

Carr, E. G., & Lovaas, O. I. (1983). Contingent electric shock as a treatment for severe behavior problems. In S. Axelrod & J. Apsche (Eds.), *The effects of punishment on human behavior* (pp. 221–246). New York: Academic Press.

Dawson, G., & Adams, A. (1984). Imitation and social responsiveness in autistic children. *Journal of Autism and Developmental Disabilities, 12*, 209–226.

DeMyer, M. R., Hingtgen, J. N., & Jackson, R. K. (1981). Infantile autism reviewed: A decade of research. *Schizophrenia Bulletin, 7*, 388–451.

DesLauriers, A. M., & Carlson, C. F. (1969). *Your child is asleep: Early infantile autism.* Homewood, IL: Dorsey Press.

Despert, J. (1951). Some considerations relating to the genesis of autistic behavior in children. *American Journal of Orthopsychiatry, 21*, 335–350.

Dunlap, G. (1984). The influence of task variation and maintenance tasks on the learning and affect of autistic children. *Journal of Experimental Child Psychology, 37*, 41–46.

Durand, V. M., & Carr, E. G. (1991). Functional communication training to reduce challenging behavior: Maintenance and application in new settings. *Journal of Applied Behavior Analysis, 24*, 251–264.

Eisenberg, L. (1956). The autistic child in adolescence. *American Journal of Psychiatry, 112*, 607–612.

Favell, J. E., Azrin, N. H., Baumeister, A. A., Carr, E. G., Dorsey, M. A., Forehand, R., Foxx, R. M., Lovaas, O. I., Rincover, A., Risley, T. R., Romanczyk, R. G., Russo, D. C., Schroeder, S. R., & Solmck, J. V. (1982). The treatment of self-injurious behavior. *Behavior Therapy, 13*, 529–554.

Favell, J. E., McGimsey, J. F., & Schell, R. M. (1982). Treatment of self-injury by providing alternative sensory activities. *Analysis and Intervention in Developmental Disabilities, 2*, 83–104.

Fenske, E. C., Zalenski, S., Krantz, P. J., & McClannahan, L. E. (1985). Age at intervention and treatment outcome for autistic children in a comprehensive intervention program. *Analysis and Intervention in Developmental Disabilities, 5*, 49–58.

Freeman, B. J., Ritvo, E. R., Needleman, R., & Yokota, A. (1985). The stability of cognitive and linguistic parameters in autism: A five-year prospective study. *Journal of the American Academy of Child Psychiatry, 24*, 459–464.

Gaylord-Ross, R. J., Haring, T. G., Breen, C., Pitts-Conway, V. (1984). The training and generalization of social interaction skills with autistic youth. *Journal of Applied Behavior Analysis, 17*, 229–247.

Harris, S., Handleman, J., Gordon, R., Kristoff, B., & Fuentes, F. (1991). Changes in cognitive and language functioning of preschool children with autism. *Journal of Autism and Developmental Disorders, 21*, 281–290.

Hart, B., & Risley, T. R. (1975). Incidental teaching of language in the preschool. *Journal of Applied Behavior Analysis, 8*, 411–420.

Hemsley, R., Howlin, P., Berger, M., Hersov, L., Holbrook, D., Rutter, M., Yule, W. (1978). Treating autistic children in a family context. In M. Rutter & E. Schopler (Eds.), *Autism: A reappraisal of concepts and treatment.* New York: Plenum.

Howlin, P. A. (1981). The effectiveness of operant language training with autistic children. *Journal of Autism and Developmental Disorders, 11*, 89–105.

Howlin, P. A., & Rutter, M. (1987). *Treatment of autistic children.* New York: Wiley.

Hung, D. W. (1977). Generalization of "curiosity" questioning behavior in autistic children. *Journal of Behavior Therapy and Experimental Psychiatry, 8*, 237–245.

Hung, D. W. (1980). Training and generalization of yes and no as mands in two autistic children. *Journal of Autism and Developmental Disorders, 10*, 139–152.

Iwata, B., Vollmer, T. R., & Zarcone, J. R. (1990). The experimental (functional) analysis of behavior disorders: Methodology, applications, and limitations. In A. C. Repp & N. N. Singh (Eds.), *Perspectives on the use of nonaversive and aversive interventions for persons with developmental disabilities* (pp. 301–330). Sycamore, IL: Sycamore Publishing.

Johnston, J. M. (1988). Strategic and tactical limits of comparison studies. *The Behavior Analyst, 11*, 1–9.

Kanner, L. (1943). Autistic disturbances of affective contact. *The Nervous Child, 2*, 217–250.

Kanner, L. (1949). Problems of nosology and psychodynamics in early infantile autism. *American Journal of Orthopsychiatry, 19,* 416–426.

Kanner, L. (1951). The conception of wholes and parts in early infantile autism. *American Journal of Psychiatry, 108,* 23–26.

Kaufman, B. N. (1976). *Son-rise.* New York: Harper & Row.

Kavale, K. A., & Mattson, P. D. (1983). "One jumped off the balance beam": Meta-analysis of perceptual-motor training. *Journal of Learning Disabilities, 16,* 165–173.

Koegel, R. L., & Covert, A. (1972). The relationship of self-stimulation to learning in autistic children. *Journal of Applied Behavior Analysis, 5,* 381–388.

Koegel, R. L., Dunlap, G., & Dyer, K. (1980). Intertrial interval duration and learning in autistic children. *Journal of Applied Behavior Analysis, 13,* 91–99.

Koegel, R. L., O'Dell, M. C., & Koegel, L. K. (1987). A natural language teaching paradigm for nonverbal autistic children. *Journal of Autism and Developmental Disorders, 17,* 187–200.

Koegel, R. L., & Rincover, A. (1974). Treatment of psychotic children in a classroom environment: I. Learning in a large group. *Journal of Applied Behavior Analysis, 7,* 45–59.

Koegel, R. L., & Rincover, A. (1976). Some detrimental effects of using extra stimuli to guide responding in autistic and normal children. *Journal of Abnormal Child Psychology, 4,* 59–71.

Koegel, R. L., Rincover, A., & Egel, A. L. (Eds.). (1982). *Educating and understanding autistic children.* San Diego: College-Hill Press.

Koegel, R. L., Russo, D. C., & Rincover, A. (1977). Assessing and training teachers in the generalized use of behavior modification with autistic children. *Journal of Applied Behavior Analysis, 10,* 197–205.

Koegel, R. L., Schreibman, L., Britten, K. R., Burke, J. C., & O'Neill, R. E. (1982). A comparison of parent training to direct child treatment. In R. L. Koegel, A. Rincover, & A. L. Egel (Eds.), *Educating and understanding autistic children* (pp. 260–279). San Diego: College-Hill Press.

Koegel, R. L., & Williams, J. A. (1980). Direct versus indirect response-reinforcer relationships in teaching autistic children. *Journal of Abnormal Child Psychology, 8,* 537–547.

Kozloff, M. A. (1973). *Reaching the autistic child: A parent training program.* Cambridge, MA: Brookline Books.

Laski, K. E., Charlop, M. H., & Schreibman, L. (1988). Training parents to use the natural language paradigm to increase their autistic children's speech. *Journal of Applied Behavior Analysis, 21,* 391–400.

Leboyer, M., Bouvard, M. P., Launay, J., Tabuteau, F., Waller, D., Dugas, M., Kerdelhue, B., Lensing, P., & Panksepp, J. (1992). A double-blind study of naltrexone in infantile autism. *Journal of Autism and Developmental Disorders, 22,* 311–313.

Lichstein, K. L., & Schreibman, L. (1976). Employing electric shock with autistic children: A review of the side effects. *Journal of Autism and Childhood Schizophrenia, 6,* 163–173.

Litt, M. D., & Schreibman, L. (1981). Stimulus-specific reinforcement in the acquisition of receptive labels by autistic children. *Analysis and Intervention in Developmental Disorders, 1,* 171–186.

Locascio, J. J., Malone, R. P., Small, A. M., Kafantaris, V., Ernst, M., Lynch, W. S., Overall, J. E., & Campbell, M. (1991). Factors related to haloperidol response and dyskinesias in autistic children. *Psychopharmacology Bulletin, 27,* 119–126.

Lord, C., & Schopler, E. (1989). The role of age at assessment, developmental level, and test in the stability of intelligence scores in young autistic children. *Journal of Autism and Developmental Disorders, 19,* 483–499.

Lord, F. M. (1967). A paradox in the interpretation of group comparisons. *Psychological Bulletin, 68,* 304–305.

Lotter, V. (1978). Follow-up studies. In M. Rutter & E. Schopler (Eds.), *Autism: A reappraisal of concepts and treatment* (pp. 475–495). London: Plenum.

Lovaas, O. I. (1977). *The autistic child: Language development through behavior modification.* New York: Irvington.

Lovaas, O. I. (1987). Behavioral treatment and normal educational and intellectual functioning in young autistic children. *Journal of Consulting and Clinical Psychology, 55,* 3–9.

Lovaas, O. I., Ackerman, A. B., Alexander, D., Firestone, P., Perkins, J., & Young, D. (1981). *Teaching developmentally disabled children: The ME book.* Austin, TX: Pro-Ed.

Lovaas, O. I., Berberich, J. P., Perloff, B. F., & Schaeffer, B. (1966). Acquisition of imitative speech by schizophrenic children. *Science, 151,* 705–707.

Lovaas, O. I., & Favell, J. E. (1987). Protection for clients undergoing aversive/restrictive interventions. *Education and Treatment of Children, 10,* 311–325.

Lovaas, O. I., Freitag, G., Gold, V. J., & Kassorla, I. C. (1965). Experimental studies in childhood schizophrenia: Analysis of self-destructive behavior. *Journal of Experimental Child Psychology, 2*, 67–84.

Lovaas, O. I., Freitas, L., Nelson, K., & Whalen, C. (1967). The establishment of imitation and its use for the development of complex behaviour in schizophrenic children. *Behaviour Research and Therapy, 5*, 171–181.

Lovaas, O. I., Koegel, R. L., & Schreibman, L. (1979). Stimulus overselectivity in autism: A review of research. *Psychological Bulletin, 86*, 1236–1254.

Lovaas, O. I., Koegel, R. L., Simmons, J. Q., and Long, J. S. (1973). Some generalization and follow-up measures on autistic children in behavior therapy. *Journal of Applied Behavior Analysis, 6*, 131–165.

Lovaas, O. I., Newsom C., & Hickman, C. (1987). Self-stimulatory behavior and perceptual reinforcement. *Journal of Applied Behavior Analysis, 20*, 45–68.

Lovaas, O. I., & Simmons, J. Q. (1969). Manipulation of self-destruction in three retarded children. *Journal of Applied Behavior Analysis, 2*, 143–157.

Lovaas, O. I., & Smith, T. (1988). Intensive behavioral treatment for young autistic children. In B. B. Lahey and A. E. Kazdin (Eds.), *Advances in clinical child psychology* (Vol. 11, pp. 285–324). New York: Plenum.

Lovaas, O. I., & Smith, T. (1989). A comprehensive behavioral theory of autistic children: Paradigm for research and treatment. *Journal of Behavior Therapy and Experimental Psychiatry, 20*, 17–29.

Lovaas, O. I., & Smith, T. (in press). Intensive and long-term treatments for clients with destructive behaviors. In T. Thompson & D. Gray (Eds.), *Treatment of destructive behavior in developmental disabilities* (Vol. II). Newbury Park, CA: Sage.

Lovaas, O. I., Smith, T., & McEachin, J. J. (1989). Clarifying comments on the Young Autism Study. *Journal of Consulting and Clinical Psychology, 57*, 165–167.

Makarushka, M. (1991, October 6). The words they can't say. *New York Times Magazine*, pp. 32–36, 70.

Matson, J. L., & Taras, M. E. (1989). A 20-year review of punishment and alternative methods to treat problem behaviors in developmentally delayed persons. *Research in Developmental Disabilities, 10*, 85–104.

McEachin, J. J., Smith, T., & Lovaas, O. I. (1993). Long-term outcome for children with autism who received early intensive behavioral treatment. *American Journal of Mental Retardation, 97*, 359–372.

McGee, G. G., Krantz, P. J., Mason, D., & McClannahan, L. E. (1983). A modified incidental-teaching procedure for autistic youth: Acquisition and generalization of receptive object labels. *Journal of Applied Behavior Analysis, 16*, 329–388.

McGee, G. G., Krantz, P. J., & McClannahan, L. E. (1985). The facilitative effects of incidental teaching on preposition use by autistic children. *Journal of Applied Behavior Analysis, 18*, 17–31.

McGee, J. J., & Gonzalez, L. (1990). Gentle teaching and the practice of human interdependence: A preliminary group study of 15 persons with severe behavioral disorders and their caregivers. In A. C. Repp & N. N. Singh (Eds.), *Perspectives on the use of nonaversive and aversive interventions for people with developmental disabilities* (pp. 215–230). Sycamore, IL: Sycamore Publishing.

Mundy, P., Sigman, M., Ungerer, J., & Sherman, T. (1986). Defining the social deficits of autism: The contribution of nonverbal communication measures. *Journal of Child Psychology and Psychiatry and Allied Disciplines, 27*, 657–669.

Neef, N. A., Iwata, B. A., & Page, T. J. (1980). The effects of interspersal training versus high density reinforcement on spelling acquisition and retention. *Journal of Applied Behavior Analysis, 13*, 153–158.

Newsom, C., Favell, J. E., & Rincover, A. (1983). The side effects of punishment. In S. Axelrod & J. Apsche (Eds.), *The effects of punishment on human behavior* (pp. 285–316). New York: Academic Press.

Newsom, C., & Rincover, A. (1989). Autism. In E. J. Mash & R. A. Barklay (Eds.), *Treatment of childhood disorders* (pp. 286–346). New York: Guilford Press.

Ney, P. G., Palvesky, A. E., & Markely, J. (1971). Relative effectiveness of operant conditioning and play therapy in childhood schizophrenia. *Journal of Autism and Childhood Schizophrenia, 1*, 337–349.

Ornitz, E. M., & Ritvo, E. R. (1976). The syndrome of autism: A critical review. *American Journal of Psychiatry, 133*, 609–621.

Reilly, C., Nelson, D. L., & Bundy, A. C. (1983). Sensorimotor versus fine motor activities in eliciting vocalizations in autistic children. *The Occupational Therapy Journal of Research, 3*, 199–211.

Repp, A. C., & Singh, N. N. (1990). *Perspectives on the use of nonaversive and aversive interventions for persons with developmental disabilities*. Sycamore, IL: Sycamore Publishing.

Rimland, B. (1987a). *Evaluation of the Tokyo Higashi Program for autistic children by parents of the international division students*. Unpublished manuscript.

Rimland, B. (1987b). Megavitamin B6 and magnesium in the treatment of autistic children and adults. In E. Schopler & G. B. Mesibov (Eds.), *Neurobiological issues in autism* (pp. 390–405). New York: Plenum.

Rimland, B. (1992, No. 4). Facilitated communication: What's going on? [Editor's Notebook]. *Autism Research Review International*, pp. 2–3.

Rimland, B., & Edelson, S. M. (1991). Improving the functioning of autistic persons: *A comparison of the Berard auditory training approach with the Tomatis audio-psycho-phonology approach* (Technical Report No. 111). San Diego: Autism Research Institute.

Rimland, B., & Edelson, S. M. (in press). Auditory integration training in autism: A pilot study. *Journal of Autism and Developmental Disorders*.

Rimland, B., & Fein, D. (1988). Special talents of autistic savants. In L. K. Obler & D. Fein (Eds.), *The exceptional brain* (pp. 474–492). New York: Guilford Press.

Rincover, A. (1978). Variables affecting stimulus fading and discriminative responding in psychotic children. *Journal of Abnormal Psychology, 87*, 541–553.

Rincover, A., & Koegel, R. L. (1975). Setting generality and stimulus control in autistic children. *Journal of Applied Behavior Analysis, 8*, 235–246.

Rincover, A., & Koegel, R. L. (1977). Classroom treatment of autistic children: II. Individualized instruction in a group. *Journal of Abnormal Child Psychology, 5*, 125–136.

Risley, T., Hart, B., & Doke, L. (1972). Operant language development: The outline of a therapeutic technology. In R. L. Schiefelbusch (Ed.), *Language of the mentally retarded* (pp. 107–123). Baltimore: University Park Press.

Risley, T., & Wolf, M. (1967). Establishing functional speech in autistic children. *Behaviour Research and Therapy, 5*, 73–88.

Roland, C. C., McGee, G. G., Risley, T. R., & Rimland, B. (1988). *Description of the Tokyo Higashi Program for autistic children* (ICBR Publication No. 77). San Diego: Autism Research Institute.

Rumsey, J., Rapoport, J., & Sceery, W. (1985). Autistic children as adults: Psychiatric, social and behavioral outcomes. *Journal of the American Academy of Child and Psychiatry, 24*, 465–473.

Russo, D. C., & Koegel, R. L. (1977). A method for integrating an autistic child into a normal public-school classroom. *Journal of Applied Behavior Analysis, 10*, 579–590.

Rutter, M. (1970). Autistic children: Infancy to adulthood. *Seminars in Psychiatry, 2*, 435–450.

Rutter, M. (1978). Diagnosis and definition. In M. Rutter and E. Schopler (Eds.), *Autism: A reappraisal of concepts and treatment* (pp. 1–25). New York: Plenum.

Rutter, M. (1983). Cognitive deficits in the pathogenesis of autism. *Journal of Child Psychology and Psychiatry, 24*, 513–531.

Rutter, M. (1985). The treatment of autistic children. *Journal of Child Psychology and Psychiatry, 26*, 193–214.

Rutter, M., & Bartak, L. (1973). Special educational treatment of autistic children: A comparative study. II. Follow-up findings and implications for services. *Journal of Child Psychology and Psychiatry, 14*, 241–270.

Rutter, M., Greenfeld, D., & Lockyer, L. (1967). A five to fifteen year follow-up of infantile psychosis. *British Journal of Psychiatry, 113*, 1183–1199.

Rutter, M., & Schopler, E. (1987). Autism and pervasive developmental disorders: Concepts and diagnostic issues. *Journal of Autism and Developmental Disorders, 17*, 159–186.

Schopler, E. (1971). Parents of psychotic children as scapegoats. *Journal of Contemporary Psychotherapy, 4*, 17–22.

Schopler, E. (1987). Specific and nonspecific factors in the effectiveness of a treatment system. *American Psychologist, 42*, 376–383.

Schopler, E. (1988). Concerns about misinterpretation and uncritical acceptance of exaggerated claims. *American Psychologist, 43*, 658.

Schopler, E., Brehm, S., Kinsbourne, M., & Reichler, R. J. (1971). Effect of treatment structure on development in autistic children. *Archives of General Psychiatry, 24*, 415–421.

Schopler, E., Mesibov, G. B., & Baker, A. (1982). Evaluation of treatment for autistic children and their parents. *Journal of the American Academy of Child Psychiatry, 21*, 262–267.

Schopler, E., & Olley, J. G. (1982). Comprehensive educational services for autistic children: The TEACCH model. In C. R. Reynolds & T. B. Gutkin (Eds.), *Handbook of school psychology* (pp. 626–643). New York: Wiley.

Schopler, E., & Reichler, R. J. (1979). *Individualized assessment and treatment for autistic and developmentally disabled children. Vol. 1. Psychoeducational profile (PEP)*. Austin, TX: Pro-Ed.

Schopler, E., Reichler, R. J., & Lansing, M. (1980). *Individualized assessment and treatment for autistic and developmentally disabled children. Vol. 2. Teaching strategies for parents and professionals*. Austin, TX: Pro-Ed.

Schopler, E., Short, A., & Mesibov, G. (1989). Relation of behavioral treatment to "normal functioning": Comment on Lovaas. *Journal of Consulting and Clinical Psychology, 57*, 162–164.

Schreibman, L. (1975). Effects of within-stimulus and extra-stimulus prompting on discrimination learning in autistic children. *Journal of Applied Behavior Analysis, 8*, 91–112.

Schreibman, L. (1988). *Autism*. Beverly Hills, CA: Sage.

Schreibman, L., & Koegel, R. L. (1975, March). Autism: A defeatable horror. *Psychology Today*, pp. 61–67.

Sigman, M., & Ungerer, J. A. (1984). Attachment behaviors in autistic children. *Journal of Autism and Developmental Disorders, 14*, 231–244.

Simeonnson, R. J., Olley, J. G., & Rosenthal, S. L. (1987). Early intervention for children with autism. In M. J. Guralnick & F. C. Bennett (Eds.), *The effectiveness of early intervention for at-risk and handicapped children* (pp. 275–296). Orlando, FL: Academic Press.

Smith, T. (1988). Concerns about nonspecific factors in the treatment of developmental disabilities. *American Psychologist, 43*, 657–658.

Smith, T. (1990a). Increasing memory to promote generalization of treatment gains in autistic children (Doctoral dissertation, University of California, Los Angeles, 1990). *Dissertation Abstracts International, 52*, 1005B.

Smith, T. (1990b). When and when not to consider the use of contingent aversives with autistic children. In N. Singh & A. Repp (Eds.), *Current practices in the use of non-aversive and aversive interventions with developmentally disabled persons* (pp. 287–297). Sycamore, IL: Sycamore Publishing.

Smith, T., & Calouri, K. A. (1989). [Context effects on the generalization of new responses acquired by autistic children]. Unpublished raw data.

Snyder, L. S., & Lindstedt, D. E. (1985). Models of child language development. In E. Schopler & G. B. Mesibov (Eds.), *Communication problems in autism* (pp. 17–35). New York: Plenum.

Spitz, H. H. (1986). *The raising of intelligence*. New Jersey: Lawrence Erlbaum.

Strain, P. S. (1983). Generalization of autistic children's social behavior change: Effects of developmentally integrated and segregated settings. *Analysis and Intervention in Developmental Disabilities, 3*, 23–34.

Strain, P. S. (1987, May). Early intervention for autistic children: The earlier the better. In G. Olley (Chair), *Comprehensive preschool services for autistic children*. Symposium conducted at the meeting of the Association for Behavior Analysis, Nashville, TN.

Strain, P. S., Hoyson, M. H., & Jamieson, B. J. (1985). Normally developing preschoolers as intervention agents for autistic-like children: Effects on class deportment and social interactions. *Journal of the Division for Early Childhood, 9*, 105–115.

Tinbergen, W., & Tinbergen, E. A. (1983). *Autistic children: New hope for a cure*. London: Allen and Unwin.

Treffert, D. A. (1988). The idiot savant: A review of the syndrome. *American Journal of Psychiatry, 145*, 563–571.

Welch, M. G. (1987). Toward prevention of developmental disorders. *Pennsylvania Medicine, 90*, 47–52.

Wenar C., & Ruttenberg, B. A. (1976). The use of BRIAC to evaluate therapeutic effectiveness. *Journal of Autism and Childhood Schizophrenia, 6*, 175–191.

Wenar, C., Ruttenberg, B. A., Dratman, M. L., & Wolf, E. G. (1967). Changing autistic behavior: The effectiveness of three milieus. *Archives of General Psychiatry, 17*, 26–35.

Wing, L. (1981). Language, social, and cognitive impairments in autism and severe mental retardation. *Journal of Autism and Developmental Disorders, 9*, 11–29.

Wing, L. (1989). Autistic adults. In C. Gillberg (Ed.), *Diagnosis and treatment of autism* (pp. 419–432). New York: Plenum.

Wooten, M., & Mesibov, G. B. (1986). Social skills training for elementary school autistic children with normal peers. In E. Schopler & G. B. Mesibov (Eds.), *Social behavior and autism* (pp. 305–319). New York: Plenum.

Wulff, S. B. (1985). The symbolic and object play of children with autism: A review. *Journal of Autism and Developmental Disorders, 15*, 139–148.

6

Treatment of Nocturnal Enuresis

Stuart L. Kaplan and Joan Busner

Epidemiology of Enuresis

Definition

Although functional enuresis is one of the more objectively measurable disorders clinicians treat, there is considerable disagreement about its definition.

Definitions of enuresis in the literature have varied mainly with regard to required age of patient and frequency of wetting episodes. There has also been disagreement regarding the time period required for labeling the enuresis as primary, that is, never having been preceded by the child's achieving a sustained period of dryness, or secondary, that is, acquired following an earlier sustained period of dryness.

The DSM-III-R (American Psychiatric Association [APA], 1987), currently sets the minimum age requirement for obtaining a diagnosis of enuresis at 5 years, with minimum wetting frequency requirements of two events per month for 5- to 6-year-olds, and one event per month for older children. The current DSM-III-R cutoff for making the primary and secondary distinction is a 1-year period of dryness. Unlike most definitions in the literature, including that of the earlier DSM-III, the DSM-III-R definition explicitly includes intentional, volitional wetting.

Enuresis is either nocturnal ("bed-wetting"), diurnal, or both.

In clinical practice, based on our own experience, and on an informal survey of the sample descriptions of approximately 100 published treatment outcome studies, the enuretic child presenting to practitioners is typically a nocturnal

Stuart L. Kaplan and **Joan Busner** • Rockland Children's Psychiatric Center, Orangeburg, New York 10962 and College of Physicians and Surgeons of Columbia University, New York, New York 10027.

Handbook of Effective Psychotherapy, edited by Thomas R. Giles. Plenum Press, New York, 1993.

enuretic who wets at least several times a week, if not nightly, and, by both the child's and parents' report, wets involuntarily.

Prevalence

Largely due to differences in definitions of enuresis, the available prevalence statistics differ widely by study (DeJonge, 1973). Rutter, Yule, and Graham (1973), in their classic epidemiological studies of the British Isle of Wight, found the prevalence of enuresis occurring at least weekly to be approximately 7% for 7-year-old boys and 3% for 7-year-old girls, 3% for 9- to 10-year-old boys and 2% for 9- to 10-year-old girls, and, by age 14, only 1% for boys and .5% for girls.

Overall, enuretics are twice as likely to be boys than girls (Crawford, 1989); three times as likely to wet only at night than to wet in the day (Mikkelson, 1991); and three times as likely to have always had the problem (i.e., have primary rather than secondary enuresis) (Rushton, 1989).

Although there is wide agreement that enuresis decreases with age, there is some disagreement regarding the prevalence decrease that accompanies each year's increase in age. The reported per year decreases in prevalence range from approximately 6% (Shaffer, 1985, 1988), to approximately 15% (Dejonge, 1973; Rushton, 1989). Extrapolations from these numbers can be used to provide rough estimates of the probability of a given youngster's achieving continence within a given time without treatment. For example, Scharf, Pravda, Jennings, Kauffman, and Ringel (1987), using the 15% per year prevalence decrease, note that a child who is enuretic at age 6 would still have a 70% chance of being enuretic by age 8. Using Shaffer's 6% estimate, 76% of enuretic 6-year-olds, untreated, would still be wetting at age 10.

Thus, according to most estimates, an untreated enuretic child will, in all likelihood, continue wetting for several years or more. Therefore, the advice given to parents as reason to avoid seeking treatment—"don't worry, he'll outgrow it"—though in the long term almost undoubtedly true, is misleading with regard to the likely time frame of such an occurrence. Nevertheless, the fact that enuresis does decrease, spontaneously, with age, is important as a baseline for evaluating the efficacy of long-term treatments.

Historical Bases for Current Treatment Approaches

Treatments for bed-wetting, which have appeared in published literature dating back to as early as 1500 B.C., have ranged from drinking wine in which had soaked the testicles of a hare (in Norgaard, Rittig, & Djurhuus, 1989), to severe beatings and rubbing of the face in the wet bedclothes (Scharf *et al.*, 1987). Predating the bell-and-pad device by several hundred years was the use by Nigerian witch doctors of a toad tied to the penis of the bed wetter; the "alarm" that rang upon contact with urine was the toad—who croaked! (as described in Mountjoy, Ruben, & Bradford, 1984).

In current times, the evolution of the major approaches to the treatment of enuresis can be traced to several theoretical schools.

Psychoanalytic Approach

From the psychoanalytic school comes the view that enuresis represents the outward symptom of an underlying unconscious conflict; bed-wetting has been understood as symbolizing masturbation, hostility toward the mother, exhibitionism, and, in girls, penis envy (see Doleys, 1979; Kupfersmid, 1989).

The treatment of bed-wetting that evolved from this view is long-term psychotherapy designed to cure the symptom by uncovering and working through unconscious conflicts.

Learning Theory

From learning theory comes the view of enuresis as a failure in learning to attend to the internal stimuli that immediately precede bladder emptying or to discriminate between appropriate and inappropriate sites for urination (Wagner, 1987).

The major treatment that evolved from learning theory is the bell-and-pad device (Mowrer & Mowrer, 1938). The bell-and-pad device (also known as a urine alarm) consists of an in-bed (or, more recently, on-body) sensor that, when it contacts urine, triggers an alarm, which awakens the child. According to the classical learning perspective, after repeated pairings of the alarm (unconditioned stimulus) with the act of urination (neutral stimulus), the bladder sensations that immediately precede the release of urine become a conditioned stimulus for the conditioned response of waking (Lovibond, 1963; Turner, Young, & Rachman, 1970).

Interestingly, operant learning theory can also be used to explain bell-and-pad treatment: for example, the eventual reduction in wetting that results from the application of the alarm can be explained using a punishment model, with the alarm as the punisher serving to decrease the likelihood of the wetting. Also, the reduction in wetting can be understood in terms of an avoidance model, with the child waking (or tightening the muscles that allow urine to be released) to avoid the onset of the alarm.

Although there have been some efforts at determining whether the bell and pad works by classical or operant conditioning, these studies have yielded inconclusive results (Lovibond, 1963), and many hold the view that both types of learning probably take place in bell-and-pad treatment (Hansen, 1979).

Treatments that have evolved from the operant learning perspective are, by and large, designed to enhance the operant aspects of standard bell-and-pad treatment; these include the addition of specific positive reinforcers, punishers, and other operant techniques to the bell and pad. Exemplars are the Dry Bed method (Azrin, Sneed, & Foxx, 1974) and the Tangible Rewards with Fading program (Kaplan, Breit, Gauthier, & Busner, 1989). Some programs call for operant training without the bell and pad (e.g., retention control training; Kimmel & Kimmel, 1970).

Biological Approach

A third major approach, not necessarily incompatible with the above two, is to view enuresis as a condition amenable to treatment by drugs. A slightly different biological approach is to view enuresis as the result of a subtle physical abnormality correctable by stretching of the bladder, surgery, or drugs.

Review of Treatments

In evaluating the relative efficacy of treatments for enuresis, it is important to consider the documented placebo, or intervention, effects known to occur (Lynch, Grunert, Vasudevan, & Severson, 1984). To some degree, a small percentage of cases of enuresis will respond to minimal, nonspecific interventions such as reassurance, having the child record the number of wet and dry nights, or, in what has been termed the "gadget effect," providing the child with an unconnected alarm, or even applying to the child's head an (unconnected) polygraph electrode (Alford, Zegiob & Bristow, 1982; Novick, 1966); such minimal interventions may reduce wetting in approximately 10% of enuretic children who present for treatment (Novick, 1966; Shaffer, Costello, & Hill, 1968). Studies that do not employ plausible controls for nonspecific effects must be interpreted with this information in mind.

Standard Bell and Pad Treatment

Treatment with the bell and pad has been extensively studied for decades (Forsythe & Butler, 1989). Doleys (1977), in an excellent review of the behavioral treatment of enuresis, selected from the bell-and-pad literature 12 studies (with a total subject number of 628) that contained credible comparison groups, a minimum of 15 subjects per group, quantitative data, and replicable procedures; using each study's individual criterion for the child's having achieved dryness (most often 14 consecutive dry nights), the average bell-and-pad initial dryness efficacy rate was 75%, with rates ranging between 62% and 90%. Of those studies reporting follow-up data, the average percentage of successfully treated children who then relapsed within 6 months (specific relapse criteria not reported) was 41%, of whom 68% were then successfully retreated.

Forsythe and Butler (1989) reviewed 26 studies, with a total subject number of 1,525. Although the review was limited to those works that specified initial dryness criteria and that consisted of a minimum of 15 subjects, there was no comparison group inclusion criterion. Using each study's own dryness criterion, (again, most often 14 consecutive dry nights), the average bell-and-pad efficacy rate was 68%, with rates ranging from 15% to 100%. Because of the difficulty in defining relapse across studies, there was no tally of relapses for the 26 studies; the authors do note that relapse rates reported in studies since 1980 have ranged from 29% within 6 months to 66% within 12 months.

Physical Modifications to the Bell and Pad

In attempts to maximize the effectiveness of the bell and pad, many studies have systematically varied physical characteristics of the bell and pad and then measured the effects on dryness achievement and relapse rate. These studies are reviewed below.

Continuous versus Intermittent Alarm Schedule. Several studies have compared alarms that ring on a continuous schedule, that is, every time the child wets (standard bell and pad), with alarms that ring on an intermittent schedule, that is, only some of the times the child wets. According to learning principles, conditioning under an intermittent rather than a continuous schedule takes longer to acquire but is more resistant to extinction (Reynolds, 1975). Applied to enuresis treatment, a child treated with an alarm that rings only some of the times the child wets should take longer to become dry but should relapse less than a child treated with an alarm that rings every time the child wets.

Turner *et al.* (1970) compared continuous with intermittent alarm schedules in a random assignment treatment study that included a 3-year follow-up. The intermittent schedule was 50%, meaning that the alarm rang an average of 50% of the times the child wet. This was accomplished by asking parents to unobtrusively switch off a standard bell-and-pad alarm according to a calendar supplied by the experimenters.

Of note, almost half of the 81 patients dropped out of treatment, with parents usually citing difficulty following the alarm schedule as the reason. Of the remaining subjects, the results indicated equivalent dryness efficacy for the two groups (84% overall), with the intermittent group showing an increase of approximately 4 weeks in time taken to achieve dryness (6.5 weeks versus 10.2 weeks—statistical significance not reported). The study provided tentative evidence for a lower relapse rate in the intermittent group than in the continuous group; although the respective relapse rates at 3-year follow-up for the continuous and intermittent groups were 65% versus 27%, respectively, this large difference was not statistically significant.

Finley, Besserman, Bennett, Clapp, and Finley (1973) also compared continuous with intermittent alarm schedules, but they used a specially designed programmable alarm constructed for the study, and a 70% rather than 50% intermittent schedule. In addition, they included a control group which received an identical alarm that rang only in the parents' room and only after a 20-min delay. After 6 weeks' treatment, none of the placebo, 80% of the intermittent alarm, and 90% of the continuous alarm subjects had reached a dryness criterion of seven consecutive nights. Dryness rates of the two active groups did not statistically differ, nor did the weekly reduction in wetting. At 3-month follow-up, however, 44% of the continuous alarm subjects, compared to 12.5% of the intermittent alarm subjects, had relapsed, which was significant statistically.

Additional study by Finley and his colleagues both supports the apparent advantage of intermittent over continuous alarm schedules and provides evidence that, in general, a 70% schedule is preferable to other schedules varying from 30% to 90% (Finley, Rainwater, & Johnson, 1982).

Unfortunately, there is no commercially available programmable alarm. It remains an open question whether a parent-assisted procedure could be devised that would be easy to administer and acceptable to parents.

On-Body versus In-Bed. Alarms that are worn on the body rather than placed in the bed represent a recent modification of the traditional bell-and-pad device. These devices typically consist of a small alarm unit strapped to the child's shoulder or wrist, and an attached wire leading to a urine sensor snapped to the child's underwear. The on-body devices are generally less bulky and cumbersome than the traditional bed-and-pad devices; also, because the urine sensor is placed in the child's underwear rather than the bed, there is theoretically a greater chance of the child awakening prior to soaking the bed.

On the one hand, because the alarm should ring sooner given the closer proximity of the sensor to the child's body, the on-body alarm might be expected to train the child faster. On the other hand, because the bell and pad requires the child to more fully awaken so as to get up from the bed to shut off the alarm unit (which is intentionally kept at some distance from the bed), the traditional bell and pad might be expected to train the child faster (Fordham & Meadow, 1989). Studies that have compared the two types of alarms show them to have equivalent dryness efficacy (Butler, Forsythe, & Robertson, 1990; Fordham & Meadow, 1989) and relapse rates (Butler *et al.*, 1990), although one study suggests a slight advantage for the body-worn alarm in speed of achieving dryness (Butler *et al.*, 1990). Based on available information, individual preference of child and parent should probably dictate the type of alarm used.

Behavior Modification Packages with Bell and Pad

Several treatment packages are available that add various behavior modification techniques to the bell and pad in efforts to improve dryness efficacy and reduce relapse rates. We review here those studies that have compared such packages to standard bell-and-pad treatment.

Dry-Bed Method. Probably the most widely studied package is the Azrin *et al.* (1974) Dry Bed method. This method, in addition to the bell and pad, makes use of bladder stretching and retention control training (giving fluids and asking the child to postpone urination), behavioral rehearsal of correct toileting, punishment via changing wet sheets and verbal expressions of disapproval for wetting, and social rewards in the form of expressions of approval for dryness.

The Dry Bed method begins with an "Intensive Training" night: 1 hour before bedtime the child engages in "Positive Practice," in which, for 20 repetitions, the child must lie on the bed, count to 50, walk to the toilet and attempt to urinate, and go back to bed. At bedtime, this first night, the child is encouraged to drink fluids, and the child sets the bell-and-pad device. If the alarm has not rung, the child is awakened by the parents every hour and told to walk to the bathroom. At the door of the bathroom the child is asked whether he or she can refrain from urinating for one more hour. If so, the child is returned to bed and given additional fluids to drink. This continues hourly throughout the first night. If the alarm rings during the night (i.e., the child wets), the child is reprimanded, he or she must remove wet clothes and bedding, obtain dry clothes and bedding, and change and remake the bed. Prior to returning to sleep, the child must then perform the Positive Practice routine (20 repetitions of lying in bed, counting to 50, walking to the bathroom and attempting to urinate in the toilet).

After the first training night, the routine is the same when the alarm rings with regard to the 20 repetitions of Positive Practice and the bed changing, but the routine is relaxed somewhat in that the child is awakened only once by the parents in the absence of the alarm ringing, instead of hourly, and the child is not given fluids during the night (Azrin *et al.*, 1974). This procedure continues until the child achieves seven consecutive dry nights.

Using this method, with experimenters serving as in-home trainers for the first night, Azrin *et al.* (1974) reported 100% dryness achievement within 3 weeks of training (with wetting all but ceased by only two weeks' training) for 26 enuretic children who had previously wet nightly. This was compared with 0% dryness achievement of 13 matched controls who received standard bell-and-pad treatment for two weeks' time.

Although 30% of the children who received Dry Bed training relapsed (defined as two wet nights in a 1-week period) within the 6 months following treatment, all were successfully retreated.

Bollard and Nettelbeck (1981), in a comprehensive multigroup design, replicated the 100% rate of dryness acquisition using in-home trainers, and further demonstrated a 100% rate using parents rather than professionals for the Intensive Training night; these rates were significantly higher than those of a wait-list control group asked only to record-keep (10% dryness acquisition rate), a group given the bell-and-pad alone (80% dryness acquisition rate), and a group given the (parent-administered) Dry Bed method without the bell and pad (25% dryness acquisition rate). Relapse rates of the five groups at 1-year follow-up did not significantly differ and averaged approximately 25%.

That the bell-and-pad component is necessary to achieve Dry Bed initial dryness acquisition superiority has been replicated by others (Keating, Butz, Burke, & Heimberg, 1983; Nettelbeck & Langeluddecke, 1979), as has the finding that parents and professional trainers are equally efficacious (Bollard & Woodroffe, 1977).

A dismantling study that attempted to reduce the difficulty of administering the Dry Bed method by removing some of its elements found the (parent-administered) Dry Bed method to fail to significantly surpass standard bell-and-pad treatment when any of the following components were removed: retention control, waking the child, and Positive Practice combined with bed and clothing changing. Only when those three components were included together were the dryness efficacies significantly different from that of the bell and pad alone (Bollard & Nettelbeck, 1982).

Doleys, Ciminero, Tollison, Williams, and Wells (1977) were unable to replicate the 100% efficacy rate of the Dry Bed method, instead reporting a 64% dryness acquisition rate after 6 weeks of treatment. The relapse rate, according to a later paper (Doleys, 1979), was only 14% (time period not given).

Breit, Kaplan, Gauthier, and Weinhold (1984), using parents as trainers, were also unable to replicate the extremely high efficacy rates of Azrin *et al.* (1974), instead reporting an 80% dryness acquisition rate with 50% relapsing within 6 months. In a subsequent comparison with a group treated with standard bell-and-pad treatment, the authors failed to find a significant advantage to the Dry Bed method and noted its substantial "cost" in terms of the complexity of procedures the family must perform (Kaplan *et al.*, 1989; cf. Fincham & Spettell, 1984).

Tangible Rewards with Fading. A package developed as an alternative to the Dry Bed method is the Tangible Rewards with Fading method developed by Kaplan *et al.* (1989). The method adds to the bell and pad tangible rewards and social approval for dryness and penalties and social disapproval for wetting; like the Dry Bed method, the package calls for the child to change wet pajamas and bedding should wetting occur.

When compared with standard bell-and-pad and parent-administered Dry Bed treatment groups, in a consecutive series study, the method resulted in an initial dryness acquisition rate of 85%, which did not significantly differ from the 80% Dry Bed or 67% standard bell-and-pad rates (Kaplan *et al.*, 1989). In an effort at reducing relapses, the authors included in the Tangible Rewards with Fading method a parent-administered system that gradually removed the tangible rewards and penalties contingent on the child maintaining dryness; the 6-month relapse rate, defined as two wets in any 7-day period, was 37%, in contrast to 50% and 67% for the Dry bed and standard bell-and-pad groups, respectively. The differences were not statistically significant.

Retention Control Training. There have been several reports of lower functional bladder capacity in enuretic than in nonenuretic children; enuretic children may void when their bladders contain less urine than those of nonenuretic children (Starfield, 1967; Troup & Hodgson, 1971).

These reports have led to the development of interventions, known collectively as retention control training (Kimmel & Kimmel, 1970), designed to increase functional bladder capacity. The techniques consist of forcing fluids and encouraging postponement of urination. This training is sometimes conducted throughout the day (e.g., Kimmel & Kimmel, 1970) and sometimes at night, either alone, or in conjunction with the bell and pad (e.g., Dry Bed training, Azrin *et al.*, 1974).

In direct comparisons of the bell and pad with retention control training, the bell and pad has been shown to be superior (Fielding, 1980).

When retention control training is used as an adjunct to the bell and pad, there are mixed results. Taylor and Turner (1975) added "overlearning," defined as bedtime fluid forcing following the attainment of seven dry nights, to bell-and-pad treatment, and compared this procedure to standard bell-and-pad treatment with regard to relapse rates. At approximately 1-year follow-up, the relapse rate of the group treated with overlearning was only 23%, which was significantly lower than the 70% rate of the group treated with standard bell and pad.

As discussed earlier, Bollard and Nettelbeck (1982), in their dismantling study of the Dry Bed method, did not find a significant advantage to adding retention control to the bell and pad, although relapse rates were not assessed.

One study suggests that the addition of retention control training to the bell and pad may be helpful in terms of initial dryness acquisition for children with small functional bladder capacities, but that it may actually increase wetting in children with normal or large functional bladder capacities (Geffken, Johnson, & Walker, 1986).

Most authors have not found retention control training to change functional bladder capacity, even when it results in successful enuresis treatment (Doleys *et al.*, 1977; Fielding, 1980), and the role played by the training is less than clear.

Findings, thus, are mixed. Retention control training alone is less efficacious than bell-and-pad training alone; the evidence is mixed as to whether retention control training is a useful adjunct to the bell and pad. For children who do not have smaller than normal functional bladder capacities, there may be a danger to adding retention control training.

Insight-Oriented Psychotherapy

No insight-oriented psychotherapy study has been conducted that has contained a relevant attention control group. An attention-controlled study is not warranted, however, because the studies that have included no-treatment control groups (DeLeon & Mandell, 1966; Werry & Cohrssen, 1965) have failed to demonstrate any benefit to insight-oriented psychotherapy in the treatment of enuresis over and beyond that of no treatment.

Pharmacotherapy

Drugs are frequently used in the treatment of enuresis and have been the subject of frequent study. Although dozens of drugs have been studied, we will limit this section to a review of the two agents most widely used.

Imipramine. The use of the antidepressant imipramine in the treatment of enuresis is one of the most studied areas in childhood psychopharmacology, although the drug's mechanism of action remains a subject of speculation (Ambrosini, 1984). Its effectiveness is not related to its anticholinergic effect (Korczyn & Kish, 1979), nor is it believed to be related to its antidepressant effect. Unlike its antidepressant effect, its response as an antienuretic is rapid in onset, occurring in the first week of treatment, and the effect occurs at relatively low doses—1 to 2 mg/kg; as an antidepressant, the agent requires 3 to 6 weeks of treatment and high doses—3.5 to 5 mg/kg.

There is considerable variation from study to study in reported efficacy of imipramine. In general, most studies support the finding that imipramine is superior to placebo in reducing the frequency of bed-wetting during the time the imipramine is administered, with wetting reduction rates ranging from 40% to 70% (Ambrosini, 1984). After the medicine is discontinued, some or all of the bed-wetting almost invariably returns (Blackwell & Currah, 1973). Patients who respond do so within the first week of treatment (Korczyn & Kish, 1979).

The heterogeneity of the findings defies easy generalization. To provide some information about the efficacy of imipramine, two of the more widely known studies will be briefly summarized with regard to treatment outcome.

In a comprehensive multigroup design that included measurement of plasma drug level and sleep EEGs, Rapoport *et al.* (1980) compared imipramine, desipramine, methscopolamine, and placebo as antienuretics. We will summarize only the imipramine findings. During a 10-day placebo-controlled trial, imipramine resulted in significantly more dry nights than placebo. Of the 40 subjects studied, 23 (58%) were dry five or more nights. The authors identitied three subgroups of responders in an additional month of treatment during which dose was altered: those who initially responded well and continued to respond well at the same dose (47% of subjects); those who initially did not respond and never responded, even with dose increases (17% of subjects); and a group of "transient responders," who initially responded, then began to wet, then responded anew to an increased dose, then again began to wet (36%).

Shaffer *et al.* (1968), in a comprehensive placebo-controlled trial, compared high and low doses of imipramine that were calculated on the basis of the patients' surface area; the doses in the high and low conditions reached maximums of 75 mg and 50 mg, respectively. Imipramine was significantly more effective than placebo, and dose was unrelated to outcome. Relapse rates were high. Of the 56 patients who took imipramine, 20 (36%) reached a 14-day dryness criterion while taking the medicine. After the medicine was withdrawn, 17 (85%) of this group immediately relapsed, with an additional child relapsing 9 weeks later. Only 2 of the 20 responders remained dry.

It should be noted that imipramine use is not without risks. In the dose range usually prescribed for the treatment of enuresis, 1–2 mg/kg, imipramine is a relatively safe medication compared to other medications prescribed for other medical and psychiatric conditions. But, as with any other medication, there are risks that must be weighed in the assessment of the risks/benefits ratio associated with the use of imipramine for the treatment of enuresis.

Imipramine often produces side effects such as dry mouth, constipation, and, less frequently, blurred vision, increases in pulse rate, and increases or decreases in blood pressure.

More serious risks exist. Imipramine is lethal on overdose, and there are reports of children overdosing and dying presumably in attempts to effect better cures of their bed-wetting (Bennett, 1982).

Further, there has been a recent report of three deaths of children prescribed desipramine ("Sudden Death in Children," 1990); desipramine, a metabolite of imipramine, is present in the body of any child taking imipramine. One of the deaths was an 8-year-old boy who had taken 50 mg of desipramine a day for only 6 months. The report has been discussed in the child psychiatric literature (Biederman, 1991; Popper & Elliott, 1990).

DDAVP. A more recent pharmacological intervention for enuresis is the intranasally administered synthetic antidiuretic hormone desmopressin (usually known as DDAVP for its chemical name, desamino-D-arginine vasopressin). The drug, the treatment of choice for diabetes insipidus, was first subject to clinical trials for enuresis in the 1970s, and has now been studied in at least a dozen placebo-controlled, double-blind trials (Klauber, 1989).

DDAVP has a well-documented record of efficacy in reducing wetting. Klauber (1989) presents wetting reduction results from 12 placebo-controlled studies that encompassed 516 patients. Across studies, there was an average of 37% fewer wet nights during DDAVP treatment, with rates ranging between 10% and 65%. Dryness acquisition rates were presented for only two of the studies: using five or more dry nights per week as the criterion, the rates were 41% and 30%.

Unfortunately, relapse rates are high. Janknegt and Smans (1990), in a placebo-controlled, 12-week trial of DDAVP, found 14 (64%) of 22 patients to show a 25% or greater reduction in wetting (rate of dryness acquisition not reported); of these patients, however, 13 (93%) relapsed as soon as the DDAVP was discontinued.

Similarly, Terho (1991) found significantly more dry nights during DDAVP than placebo administration in a 12-week crossover study of 52 children, with 29% of the children achieving a 5-day dryness criterion, but he also found 90% of the sample to resume near pretreatment levels of wetting upon discontinuation of the drug.

Thus, like imipramine, DDAVP is effective in a substantial proportion of patients but is associated with almost invariable relapse upon treatment cessation.

The drug's antienuretic mechanism of action is controversial. There is some evidence that enuretic children have abnormalities in nighttime urine concentrating ability, suggesting deficiency in nighttime production of antidiuretic hormone (Norgaard *et al.*, 1989). Other studies have failed to demonstrate abnormalities in nighttime urine concentration, casting doubt on deficiency of antidiuretic hormone as a mechanism for enuresis as well as on the mode of action of DDAVP in the treatment of enuresis (Aladjem *et al.*, 1982; Schmitt, 1990).

DDAVP is believed to be an extremely safe drug, with virtually no known adverse effects in short- or long-term use (Harris, 1989); however, it is expensive—approximately $90 per month, as compared with $5 a month for imipramine (Schmitt, 1990).

Interorientation Treatment Comparisons

Insight-Oriented Psychotherapy versus Bell and Pad

Two studies have directly compared the bell and pad with verbal psychotherapy. DeLeon and Mandell (1966) found an 18% dryness acquisition rate after 90 days (and an average of 12 treatment sessions) for 13 enuretic children treated weekly by a mental health practitioner (psychiatrist or psychologist) at a mental health clinic, using an unspecified treatment orientation; this rate was significantly different from an 86.3% dryness acquisition rate obtained after 90 days' treatment with the bell and pad, but not significantly different from an 11% rate obtained in a wait-list control group.

Werry and Cohrssen (1965) found 20% of children treated for 4 months with 6–8 sessions of "psychodynamically oriented" psychotherapy to be "greatly improved or cured," compared to 60% of children treated for 4 months with the bell and pad, and 10% placed in a wait-list control for 4 months. The therapy and wait-list efficacy rates did not significantly differ; both significantly differed from the bell and pad.

Imipramine versus Bell and Pad

Several studies have compared imipramine to the bell and pad. Wagner, Johnson, Walker, Carter, and Wittner (1982), in a three-group comparison of imipramine, bell-and-pad, and wait-list control treatments, found no significant difference between imipramine (33%) and control (8%) dryness acquisition rates after 14 weeks' treatment; both rates were significantly poorer than the bell-and-pad dryness rate of 83%. Further, in a week-by-week analysis of the data, there was no evidence that the imipramine worked more quickly than the bell and pad.

Fournier, Garfinkle, Bond, Beauchesne, and Shapiro (1987), in a comprehensive eight-group design, found no significant difference between imipramine and the bell and pad either after 6 weeks' treatment or at a 3-month follow-up. Also, there was no advantage to combining the two treatments over and above that of using either treatment alone.

Kolvin *et al.* (1972) compared placebo, imipramine, and bell and pad on wetting reduction relative to baseline. After 2 months' treatment, the imipramine and the bell and pad did not appreciably differ from each other in percentage improvement (approximately 63%); both appeared to differ from placebo (53%) (statistics not reported). The imipramine tended to work faster, judged by greater improvement in the first month than was found with the bell and pad. At 2-month follow-up, the dryness improvement over baseline had dropped to only 43% for the imipramine group, though it remained unchanged for the other two groups (no statistics reported).

Netley, Khanna, McKendry, and Lovering (1984) compared rates of dryness 2 months following 8-week trials of imipramine and the bell and pad. The authors defined dryness acquisition as complete absence of wetting for the 2 months following treatment; this definition is unusual in that it extends into the posttreatment relapse assessment period of most other studies. Using this definition, 28% of subjects who received imipramine were dry for the 2 months following treatment, compared to 58% of subjects who received the bell-and-pad device (only marginally significant, statistically).

Findings across studies thus show imipramine to be less efficacious than the bell and pad in overall dryness acquisition and relapse prevention; there is some evidence that its onset of wetting reduction is faster.

DDAVP versus Bell and Pad

There is only one controlled study that compares DDAVP with the bell and pad. Wille (1986) randomly assigned 24 children to 3 months' DDAVP treatment and 22 children to 3 months' bell-and-pad treatment. There was a significant advantage to DDAVP in the initial week of treatment, after which there were no significant differences until the eleventh week, when the bell and pad was superior. By the end of treatment, the bell-and-pad group had significantly less wet nights than the DDAVP group; both groups were significantly improved relative to baseline (actual numbers not given). By a 6-month follow-up, the bell-and-pad group showed a marked advantage, with 82% judged to be improved relative to baseline, compared with only 42% of the DDAVP group.

Thus, like imipramine, DDAVP may have a more rapid onset but a higher relapse rate than the bell and pad. The only attempt at combining the two treatments used a 2-week crossover design, in which the combination was compared with placebo and bell-and-pad conditions (Sukhai, Mol, & Harris, 1989). Although there were less wets in the DDAVP plus bell-and-pad condition than in the placebo plus bell-and-pad condition, the study design did not allow for the assessment of long-term effectiveness or relapse.

Treatments Not Tested against Relevant Controls

Current literature abounds with reports of a wide variety of enuresis treatments, among them acupuncture (Baozhu & Xiyou, 1985; Roje-Starcevic, 1990), hypnosis (Edwards & Van der Spuy, 1985; Olness, 1975), and chiropractic manipulation (Gemmell & Jacobson, 1989). However, these treatments have not yet been subjected to empirical study using relevant controls for nonspecific effects. The extant studies consist of open trials, case reports, and comparisons with no treatment controls. We defer discussion of these treatments in this chapter.

Conclusions and Discussion

There are three major enuresis treatment outcome parameters: acquisition of dryness, speed of acquiring dryness, and relapse rate. Perhaps the most relevant determinant of outcome is whether the child becomes dry. As extensively reviewed above, the bell and pad is the treatment consistently associated with the highest rates of dryness acquisition. The treatment with the fastest onset of wetting reduction is pharmacotherapy. High rates of relapse are unfortunately common to all of the treatments. The treatment associated with the highest rate of relapse is pharmacotherapy; the treatment with the lowest rate is bell and pad. As discussed, there is some evidence that bell-and-pad relapse rates can be reduced by the use of intermittent alarms, retention control training, or operant techniques such as gradual fading of reinforcers.

The weight of reviewed evidence clearly favors the bell and pad either alone or in combination with other behavioral interventions. It is an ironic commentary on the sociology of knowledge that less than 5% of American primary care practitioners prescribe the bell and pad for their enuretic patients (Rushton, 1989), and, despite the absence of any evidence supporting the efficacy of the approach, 73% of 196 therapist members of the American Association for Marriage and Family Therapy, when surveyed, chose individual psychotherapy or family therapy over behavioral conditioning as the treatment of choice for bed-wetting (Wagner & Hicks-Jimenez, 1986).

References

Aladjem, M., Wohl, R., Boichis, H., Orda, S., Lotan, D., & Freedman, S. (1982). Desmopressin in nocturnal enuresis. *Archives of Disease in Childhood, 57*, 137–140.

Alford, G. S., Zegiob, L., & Bristow, A. R. (1982). Use of instructions and apparatus-enhanced suggestion in treating a case of headaches, nightmares and nocturnal enuresis. *Psychotherapy: Theory, Research & Practice, 19*, 110–115.

Ambrosini, P. J. (1984). A pharmacological paradigm for urinary incontinence and enuresis. *Journal of Clinical Psychopharmacology, 4*, 247–252.

American Psychiatric Association. (1987). *Diagnostic and Statistical Manual of Mental Disorders* (3rd ed.-revised). Washington, DC: American Psychiatric Association.

Azrin, N. H., Sneed, T. J., & Fox, R. M. (1974). Dry-bed training: Rapid elimination of childhood enuresis. *Behaviour Research and Therapy, 12*, 147–156.

Baozhu, S., & Xiyou, W. (1985). Short-term effect in 135 cases of enuresis treated by wrist–ankle needling. *Journal of Traditional Chinese Medicine, 5*(1), 27–28.

Bennett, H. J. (1982). Imipramine and enuresis: Never forget its dangers [letter]. *Pediatrics, 69*, 831–832.

Biederman, J. (1991). Sudden death in children treated with a tricyclic antidepressant. *Journal of the American Academy of Child and Adolescent Psychiatry, 30*, 495–498.

Blackwell, B., & Currah, J. (1973). The psychopharmacology of nocturnal enuresis. In I. Kolvin, R. MacKeith, & S. R. Meadow (Eds.), *Bladder control and enuresis* (pp. 231–257). London: Heinemann.

Bollard, J., & Nettelbeck, T. (1981). A comparison of dry-bed training and standard urine-alarm conditioning treatment of childhood bedwetting. *Behaviour Research and Therapy, 19*, 215–226.

Bollard, J., & Nettelbeck, T. (1982). A component analysis of dry-bed training for treatment for bedwetting. *Behaviour Research and Therapy, 20*, 383–390.

Bollard, R. J., & Woodroffe, P. (1977). The effect of parent-administered dry-bed training on nocturnal enuresis in children. *Behaviour Research and Therapy, 15*, 159–165.

Breit, M., Kaplan, S. L., Gauthier, B., & Weinhold, C. (1984). The dry-bed method for the treatment of enuresis: A failure to duplicate previous reports. *Child & Family Behavior Therapy, 6*(3), 17–23.

Butler, R. J., Forsythe, W. I., & Robertson, J. (1990). The body-worn alarm in the treatment of childhood enuresis. *British Journal of Clinical Practice, 44*, 237–241.

Crawford, J. D. (1989). Treatment of nocturnal enuresis, introductory comments. *Journal of Pediatrics, 114*, 687–690.

DeJonge, G. A. (1973). Epidemiology of enuresis: A survey of the literature. In I. Kolvin, R. MacKeith, & S. R. Meadow (Eds.), *Bladder control and enuresis* (pp. 39–46). London: Heinemann.

DeLeon, G., & Mandell, W. (1966). A comparison of conditioning and psychotherapy in the treatment of functional enuresis. *Journal of Clinical Psychology, 22*, 326–330.

Doleys, D. M. (1977). Behavioral treatments for nocturnal enuresis in children: A review of the recent literature. *Psychological Bulletin, 84*, 30–54.

Doleys, D. M. (1979). Assessment and treatment of childhood enuresis. In A. J. Finch & P. C. Kendall (Eds.), *Clinical treatment & research in child psychopathology* (pp. 207–233). New York: Medical & Scientific Books.

Doleys, D. M., Ciminero, A. R., Tollison, J. W., Williams, C. L., & Wells, K. C. (1977). Dry-bed training and retention control training: A comparison. *Behavior Therapy, 8*, 541–548.

Edwards, S. D., & Van Der Spuy, H. I. J. (1985). Hypnotherapy as a treatment for enuresis. *Journal of Child Psychology, 26*(1), 161–170.

Fielding, D. (1980). The response of day and night wetting children and children who wet only at night to retention control training and the enuresis alarm. *Behaviour Research and Therapy, 18*, 305–317.

Fincham, F. D., & Spettell, C. (1984). The acceptability of dry bed training and urine alarm training as treatments of nocturnal enuresis. *Behavior Therapy, 15*, 388–394.

Finley, W. W., Besserman, R. L., Bennett, L. F., Clapp, R. K., & Finley, P. M. (1973). The effect of continuous, intermittent, and "placebo" reinforcement on the effectiveness of the conditioning treatment for enuresis nocturna. *Behaviour Research and Therapy, 11*, 289–297.

Finley, W. W., Rainwater, A. J., & Johnson, G. (1982). Effect of varying alarm schedules on acquisition and relapse parameters in the conditioning treatment of enuresis. *Behaviour Research and Therapy, 20*, 69–80.

Fordham, K. E., & Meadow, S. R. (1989). Controlled trial of standard pad and bell alarm against mini alarm for nocturnal enuresis. *Archives of Disease in Childhood, 64*, 651–656.

Forsythe, W. I., & Butler, R. J. (1989). Fifty years of enuretic alarms. *Archives of Disease in Childhood, 64*, 879–885.

Fournier, J. P., Garfinkel, B. D., Bond, A., Beauchesne, H., & Shapiro, S. K. (1987). Pharmacological and behavioral management of enuresis. *Journal of the American Academy of Child and Adolescent Psychiatry, 26*, 849–853.

Geffken, G., Johnson, S. B., & Walker, D. (1986). Behavioral interventions for childhood nocturnal enuresis: The differential effect of bladder capacity on treatment progress and outcome. *Health Psychology, 5*, 261–272.

Gemmell, H. A., & Jacobson, B. H. (1989). Chiropractic management of enuresis: Time-series descriptive design. *Journal of Manipulative and Physiological Therapeutics, 12*, 386–389.

Hansen, G. D. (1979). Enuresis control through fading, escape, and avoidance training. *Journal of Applied Behavior Analysis, 12*, 303–307.

Harris, A. S. (1989). Clinical experience with desmopressin: Efficacy and safety in central diabetes insipidus and other conditions. *Journal of Pediatrics, 114*, 711–718.

Janknegt, A., & Smans, A. J. (1990). Treatment with desmopressin in severe nocturnal enuresis in childhood. *Journal of Urology, 66*, 535–537.

Kaplan, S. L., Breit, M., Gauthier, B., & Busner, J. (1989). A comparison of three nocturnal enuresis treatment methods. *Journal of the American Academy of Child and Adolescent Psychiatry, 28*, 282–286.

Keating, J. C., Butz, R. A., Burke, E., & Heimberg, R. G. (1983). Dry bed training without a urine alarm: Lack of effect of setting and therapist contact with child. *Journal of Behavior Therapy and Experimental Psychiatry, 14*, 109–115.

Kimmel, H. D., & Kimmel, E. (1970). An instrumental conditioning method for the treatment of enuresis. *Journal of Behavior Therapy and Experimental Psychiatry, 1*, 121–123.

Klauber, G. T. (1989). Clinical efficacy and safety of desmopressin in the treatment of nocturnal enuresis. *Journal of Pediatrics, 114*, 719–722.

Kolvin, I., Taunch, J., Currah, J., Garside, R. F., Nolan, J., & Shaw, W. B. (1972). Enuresis: a descriptive analysis and a controlled trial. *Developmental Medicine and Child Neurology, 14*, 715–726.

Korczyn, A. D., & Kish, I. (1979). The mechanism of imipramine in enuresis nocturna. *Clinical and Experimental Pharmacology and Physiology*, *6*, 31–35.

Kupfersmid, J. (1989, fall). Treatment of nocturnal enuresis: A status report. *The Psychiatric Forum*, pp. 37–46.

Lovibond, S. H. (1963). The mechanism of conditioning treatment of enuresis. *Behaviour Research and Therapy*, *1*, 17–21.

Lynch, N. T., Grunert, B. K., Vasudevan, V., & Severson, R. A. (1984). Enuresis: Comparison of two treatments. *Archives of Physical Medicine Rehabilitation*, *65*, 98–100.

Mikkelsen, E. J. (1991). Modern approaches to enuresis and encopresis. In Melvin Lewis (Ed.), *Child and adolescent psychiatry, a comprehensive textbook* (pp. 583–591). Baltimore: Williams and Wilkins.

Mountjoy, P. T., Ruben, D. H., & Bradford, T. S. (1984). Recent technological advancements in the treatment of enuresis. *Behavior Modification*, *8*, 291–315.

Mowrer, O. H., & Mowrer, W. M. (1938). Enuresis: A method for its study and treatment. *American Journal of Orthopsychiatry*, *8*, 436–459.

Netley, C., Khanna, F., McKendry, J. B. J., & Lovering, J. S. (1984). Effects of different methods of treatment of primary enuresis on psychologic functioning in children. *Canadian Medical Association Journal*, *131*, 577–579.

Nettelbeck, T., & Langeluddecke, P. (1979). Dry-bed training without an enuresis machine. *Behaviour Research and Therapy*, *17*, 403–404.

Norgaard, J. P., Rittig, S., & Djurhuus, J. C. (1989). Nocturnal enuresis: An approach to treatment based on pathogenesis. *Journal of Pediatrics*, *114*, 705–710.

Novick, J. (1966). Symptomatic treatment of acquired and persistent enuresis. *Journal of Abnormal Psychology*, *71*, 363–368.

Olness, K. (1975). The use of self-hypnosis in the treatment of childhood nocturnal enuresis. *Clinical Pediatrics*, 273–279.

Popper, C. W. & Elliott, G. R. (1990). Sudden death and tricyclic antidepressants: Clinical considerations for children. *Journal of Child and Adolescent Psychopharmacology*, *1*, 125–132.

Rapoport, J. L., Mikkelsen, E. J., Zavadil, A., Nee, L., Gruenau, C., Mendelson, W., Gillin, J. L. (1980). Childhood enuresis: II. Psychopathology, tricyclic concentration in plasma, and antienuretic effects. *Archives of General Psychiatry*, *37*, 1146–1152.

Reynolds, G. S. (1975). *A primer of operant conditioning*. Glenview, IL: Scott, Foresman.

Roje-Starcevic, M. (1990). The treatment of nocturnal enuresis by acupuncture. *Neurologija*, *39*, 179–184.

Rushton, H. G. (1989). Nocturnal enuresis: Epidemiology, evaluation, and currently available treatment options. *Journal of Pediatrics*, *114*, 691–696.

Rutter, M., Yule, W., & Graham, P. (1973). Enuresis and behavioural deviance: Some epidemiological considerations. In I. Kolvin, R. MacKeith, & S. R. Meadow (Eds.), *Bladder control and enuresis* (pp. 137–147). London: Heinemann.

Scharf, M. B., Pravda, M. F., Jennings, S. W., Kauffman, R., & Ringel, J. (1987). Childhood enuresis. A comprehensive treatment program. *Psychiatric Clinics of North America*, *10*, 655–666.

Schmitt, B. D. (1990). Nocturnal enuresis: Finding the treatment that fits the child. *Contemporary Pediatrics*, *7*, 70–97.

Shaffer, D. (1985). Nocturnal enuresis: Its investigation and treatment. In D. Shaffer, A. A. Ehrhardt, & L. L. Greenhill (Eds.), *The clinical guide to child psychiatry* (pp. 29–47). New York: Free Press.

Shaffer, D. (1988). The clinical management of bedwetting in children. In C. J. Kestenbaum & D. T. Williams (Eds.), *Handbook of clinical assessment of children and adolescents* (pp. 689–710). New York: New York University Press.

Shaffer, D., Costello, A. J., & Hill, J. D. (1968). Control of enuresis with imipramine. *Archives of Diseases in Childhood*, *43*, 665–671.

Starfield, B. (1967). Functional bladder capacity in enuretic and nonenuretic children. *Journal of Pediatrics*, *70*, 777–781.

Sudden death in children treated with a tricyclic antidepressant. (1990, June). *Medical Letter on Drugs and Therapeutics*, p. 53.

Sukhai, R. N., Mol, J., & Harris, A. S. (1989). Combined therapy of enuresis alarm and desmopressin in the treatment of nocturnal enuresis. *European Journal of Pediatrics*, *148*, 465–467.

Taylor, P. D., & Turner, R. K. (1975). A clinical trial of continuous, intermittent and overlearning "bell and pad" treatments for nocturnal enuresis. *Behaviour Research and Therapy*, *13*, 281–293.

Terho, P. (1991). Desmopressin in nocturnal enuresis. *Journal of Urology*, *145*, 818–820.

Troup, C. W., & Hodgson, N. B. (1971). Nocturnal functional bladder capacity in enuretic children. *Journal of Urology, 105*, 129–132.

Turner, R. K., Young, G. C., & Rachman, S. (1970). Treatment of nocturnal enuresis by conditioning techniques. *Behaviour Research and Therapy, 8*, 367–381.

Wagner, W. G. (1987). The behavioral treatment of childhood nocturnal enuresis. *Journal of Counseling and Development, 65*, 262–265.

Wagner, W. G., & Hicks-Jimenez, K. (1986). Clinicians' knowledge and attitudes regarding the treatment of childhood nocturnal enuresis. *The Behavior Therapist, 9*(4), 77–78.

Wagner, W., Johnson, S., Walker, D., Carter, R., & Wittner, J. (1982). A controlled comparison of two treatments for nocturnal enuresis. *Journal of Pediatrics, 101*, 302–307.

Werry, J. S., & Cohrssen, J. (1965). Enuresis—an etiologic and therapeutic study. *Journal of Pediatrics, 67*, 423–431.

Wille, S. (1986). Comparison of desmopressin and enuresis alarm for nocturnal enuresis. *Archives of Disease in Childhood, 61*, 30–33.

7

Effective Psychological Treatment of Panic Disorder

Guylaine Côté and David H. Barlow

This chapter focuses on the psychological treatment of panic attacks and panic disorder as defined by DSM-III-R diagnostic criteria (American Psychiatric Association [APA], 1987). In this chapter, current available psychological treatments of panic disorder and evidence for their efficacy are reviewed. A brief discussion of developments in conceptualization and in the treatment of panic disorder as well as recent epidemiological data are presented before describing specific treatment procedures and their efficacies. Directions for future research are suggested in the conclusion.

Introduction

While panic attacks have been described in the literature for many years (e.g., Cohen & White, 1950; Da Costa, 1871; Freud, 1895/1961; Oppenheim, 1918), it is only a relatively recent development that panic attacks have been recognized as a unique form of anxiety. The importance attached to the concept of panic attacks and the creation of the diagnostic category of panic disorder is largely a result of research carried out by Donald Klein and his colleagues over the past 20 years. With the publication of the third edition of the *Diagnostic and Statistical Manual of Mental Disorders* (APA, 1980), anxiety neurosis was divided into panic disorder and generalized anxiety disorder. The two diagnostic categories of panic disorder and agoraphobia with panic attacks were created, and the presence of spontaneous panic attacks became a major criterion in the differential diagnosis of anxiety disorders. Since this time, there has been considerable evidence that panic attacks constitute an aspect of anxiety qualitatively distinct from chronic, generalized anxiety or agoraphobic avoidance (Barlow, 1988; Rapee, 1985). Following publication of DSM-III, there was an enormous increase in research on panic. The

Guylaine Côté and **David H. Barlow** • Center for Stress and Anxiety Disorders, State University of New York-Albany, Albany, New York 12203.

Handbook of Effective Psychotherapy, edited by Thomas R. Giles. Plenum Press, New York, 1993.

diagnostic criteria relating to agoraphobia and panic disorder were updated in the DSM-III-R, and more emphasis was placed on the presence of unexpected or "spontaneous" panic attacks by creating a separate category for panic disorder with different degrees of agoraphobia.

Recent epidemiological studies indicate that panic disorder, using the DSM-III definition, occurs in adults with a lifetime prevalence of about 2% and a 6-month rate of 1.2%. In reviewing epidemiological studies, Wittchen and Essau (1991) reported a remarkable consistency in the lifetime prevalence of panic found by researchers using similar methodology in different locations and in different cultural and racial groups. According to these authors, lifetime prevalence estimates would increase to about 4% under the definition of panic disorder based on the new DSM-III-R classification. Community studies suggest that the ratio for panic disorder is nearly equal for males and females (Wittchen & Essau, 1991).

There is good clinical and epidemiological evidence that panic disorder begins from the midteens through the mid-50s but most frequently during the late 20s and early 30s (Anderson, Noyes, & Crowe, 1984; Thyer, Parrish, Curtis, Nesse, & Cameron, 1985; Wittchen, 1988). Risk factors and various precipitating factors have not proven to be consistently and powerfully related to the development of panic disorder (Wittchen & Essau, 1991). A large percentage (72%) report the presence of identifiable stressors around the time of the first panic attack (Craske, Miller, Rotunda, & Barlow, 1990), but other evidence suggests that the incidence of stress may not be different from normals. Rather stressful events are more "impactful" in those who go on to develop panic disorder (Rapee, Litwin, & Barlow, 1990). In any case, panic disorder is a chronic and persistent condition. The course of symptoms is either stable and chronic or chronic with episodic exacerbations (Breier, Charney, & Heninger, 1986; Wittchen, 1988).

Panic disorder is often associated with other mental health problems. Among the various forms of anxiety disorders, panic disorder has one of the highest comorbidity rates with other anxiety disorders, including generalized anxiety disorder, social phobia, and simple phobia (Moras, Di Nardo, Brown, & Barlow, 1992; Sanderson, Di Nardo, Rapee, & Barlow, 1990; Weissman & Merikangas, 1986; Wittchen, 1988). There has also been clear evidence showing a high prevalence of major depression and an excessive prevalence of alcohol or drug abuse or dependence among patients with panic disorder (Wittchen & Essau, 1991). Also, in addition to hypochondriasis and somatic complaints, actual medical sequelae of panic disorder include increased risk of hypertension, peptic ulcer disease, and circulatory system dysfunctions (Katon, 1984; Katon *et al.*, 1986, 1987; King, Margraf, Ehlers, & Maddock, 1986). Studies of health care utilization indicate that individuals with panic disorder are heavy users of health services, actually using mental health services more often than individuals with other serious mental health problems, including schizophrenia, major affective disorder, somatization disorder, alcohol abuse or dependence, and drug abuse or dependence (Boyd, 1986). The severity and long-term debilitating effects of panic disorder and the heavy utilization of health services underline the importance of developing effective, economical, and ethical treatments.

Traditionally, the treatment of choice for panic attacks has been medication. Many valuable drug treatments for panic attacks have been investigated. However, the possible role of psychological factors in the understanding of panic was neglected, and psychological treatments for panic were largely overlooked. Indeed, until recently, no research had been conducted on the use of psychological procedures in the specific alleviation of panic attacks. One possible reason for this may be that drug studies were the major stimulus for the creation of the diagnostic category of panic disorder and formed the foundation for the biological explanation of panic.

Two broad psychological approaches provide theoretical perspectives that have led to treatment approaches for panic disorder: the psychodynamic approach and the cognitive-behavioral approach.

Psychodynamic Approach

Core elements of the current psychoanalytic understanding of panic continue to be based on Freud's thinking about anxiety (Shear, 1991). The analytical approach is based on the development of insight by association. By recalling events and thoughts that precede the panic attack, associations are made with repressed impulses that allow catharsis to occur and anxiety episodes to diminish (Dittrich *et al.*, 1983). This follows from the analytical view that anxiety signals the potential eruption of threatening impulses into conscious awareness and, in effect, helps to keep the impulses repressed by directing attention toward the symptomology of anxiety (Nemiah, 1981). Panic is an acute form of signal anxiety (see, Shear, 1991, for a more complete explanation of the psychodynamic thinking about anxiety and panic). Psychodynamic theories of anxiety have received scant attention. There is no formal body of prospective clinical research data pertaining to the psychodynamic treatment of panic disorder (Shear, 1991).

Cognitive-Behavioral Approach

Recent investigations have isolated psychological factors (hyperventilation, catastrophic misinterpretation, limited sense of control, interoceptive conditioning) as having potentially causative and/or maintaining roles in panic attacks (Beck, Laude, & Bohnert, 1974; Hibbert, 1984; Lum, 1981; Rapee, 1986; Rapee, Mattick, & Murrell, 1986; Salkovskis, Warwick, Clark, & Wessels, 1986; Sanderson, Rapee, & Barlow, 1989; van den Hout, 1988). This increased interest in psychological factors has culminated in the development of cognitive-behavioral theories and models of panic attacks (Barlow, 1988; Beck, 1988; Clark, 1986; Ley, 1985; van den Hout & Griez, 1983). While these theories differ with respect to the amount of emphasis placed on the psychological and physiological aspects of the disorder, all accent the importance of the psychological response to a set of physiological sensations, and they conceptualize panic attacks as a fear reaction to a specific set of somatic sensations (Rapee & Barlow, 1988).

The first systematic attempts to research the effectiveness of cognitive-behavioral treatment for panic attacks utilized multicomponent packages containing a combination of cognitive, relaxation, breathing, and specialized exposure techniques. While continuing to include a combination of procedures, more recent treatment studies highlight specific components that appear to target mechanisms that seem to play a crucial role in the etiology and maintenance of panic disorder as more advanced conceptualizations of panic disorder emerge. The three major panic treatment components that have been emphasized in the psychological treatment of panic attacks are breathing retraining, cognitive reattribution, and interoceptive exposure.

Breathing Retraining. It is believed that hyperventilation may produce the various somatic sensations that occur during panic attacks for a certain proportion of patients (Rapee, 1985). In the conception of panic attacks that emphasizes hyperventilation, panic attacks are viewed as stress-induced respiratory changes that provoke fear because they are perceived as frightening or because they augment fear already elicited by other stimuli. The increased apprehension produces further hyperventilation and a vicious cycle results (Clark *et al.*, 1985). Treatment implications point to the potential benefit of breathing retraining as a means of increasing respiratory control and reestablishing normal breathing patterns.

Cognitive Reattribution. According to the cognitive model of panic, panic attacks result from misinterpretation of bodily sensations which are evaluated as frightening, dangerous, or lethal. Catastrophic appraisal results in powerful and rapid escalations in anxiety, triggering further arousal, and eventual panic (Beck, 1988). Cognitive treatment involves formulating more realistic interpretations of sensations by providing corrective information about features of panic and specific identification and critical evaluation of cognitive factors that lead to misinterpretations.

Interoceptive Exposure. Another development in the understanding of the nature of panic disorder posits that extreme sensitivity to and fear of interoceptive cues in panic may result from interoceptive conditioning. The conceptualization of panic attacks as "conditioned" or learned alarm reactions to salient bodily cues (Barlow, 1988) forms the theoretical basis for the implementation of interoceptive exposure. Interoceptive exposure techniques are intended to disrupt associations between somatic sensations and panic attacks. The treatment entails repeated exposure to the physical sensations by the use of procedures that induce panic-related symptoms reliably, such as physical exercise, inhalations of carbon dioxide, and hyperventilation.

It is recognized that none of these hypothesized mechanisms of action may be "causal" in anxiety and panic reduction procedures. Rather, all may contribute to effectiveness through increasing perceptions of control (Barlow, 1988).

Single-Subject Designs

Psychodynamic Treatment

Several case reports document the successful use of hypnotherapy, psychoanalytic dream analysis, and other forms of psychodynamic therapy for the treatment of patients with panic attacks (Fewtrell, 1984; Malan, 1976; Mann, 1973; McDougall, 1985; Sandler, 1988; Sifneos, 1972; Silber, 1984; Van Pelt, 1975; Woods, 1972). However, these case studies do not enable the demonstration of the specific treatment components responsible for success due to a lack of experimental control. There is no research that demonstrates the specific treatment effect of psychodynamic therapy for panic disorder using a single-subject experimental design.

Cognitive-Behavioral Treatment

Two large-scale investigations, using time series designs, provide evidence for the effectiveness of the combination of breathing training and cognitive reattribution. Clark *et al.* (1985) reported on 18 panic patients who were selected because they perceived a similarity between the effects of hyperventilation and naturally occurring panic attacks. These patients received two weekly sessions of respiratory control training, including the application of corrective breathing techniques and cognitive reinterpretation after brief hyperventilation. Compared to a stable baseline period, panic attacks lessened from an average of ten to an average of five per week in patients whose panic was associated with specific situations, and from an average of five to two per week in patients with apparent spontaneous panic. Patients received an average number of 10 additional sessions involving cognitive-behavioral treatment and *in vivo* exposure, during which the frequency of panic continued to diminish and stabilized at zero. A 2-year follow-up assessment indicated that panic and generalized anxiety ratings had maintained. However, the study does not allow examination of the long-term effects of breathing control techniques, given the nature of the additional treatment sessions.

In a replication and extension of Clark *et al.* (1985), Salkovskis, Jones, and Clark (1986) reported similar findings in a series of nine unselected panicking patients. The treatment consisted of four weekly sessions of forced hyperventilation, corrective information, and breathing retraining, after which *in vivo* exposure was provided if necessary. Panic frequency lessened, on average, from seven to three attacks per week after respiratory control training and maintained at that level during *in vivo* exposure. Furthermore, there was some evidence that outcome was positively correlated with the extent to which patients perceived a similarity between the effects of voluntary overbreathing and naturally occurring attacks.

As noted by Clark (1988), while neither study included a wait-list control group, stable baselines were established before treatment, and significant improvements from baseline occurred in a treatment period shorter than the baseline. Thus, the efficacy of a breathing control training plus cognitive intervention treatment was demonstrated in the two studies. However, as suggested by Clark (1988), the amount of improvement obtained from the treatment might be positively associated with the extent to which patients perceive similarities between sensations due to hyperventilation and their naturally occurring panic attacks.

A recent study used an experimental single-case methodology to evaluate the effectiveness of a multicomponent cognitive-behavioral treatment for panic attacks (Laberge, Gauthier, Côté, Plamondon, & Cormier, in press). Two multiple-baseline-across-subjects designs with follow-up and direct replication were used, one to test eight patients with a primary diagnosis of panic disorder and an additional diagnosis of major depression, and the second to test seven patients with a primary diagnosis of panic disorder without an additional diagnosis of major depression. After a stabilized baseline, a program of information on panic attacks presented as psychotherapy was instituted to assess the effects of nonspecific factors. After a second stabilized baseline, cognitive-behavior therapy was introduced. In the information-based treatment phase, patients received detailed information on the nature of anxiety and panic attacks, but no instructions on cognitive restructuring, symptoms reduction techniques, or interoceptive exposure were provided. The cognitive-behavior therapy consisted of a combination of symptom reduction techniques, such as breathing training and relaxation in addition to cognitive-restructuring techniques, and interoceptive exposure. Cognitive-behavior therapy was significantly superior to the information-based treatment in reducing panic attack frequency for both nondepressed and depressed panic patients. At the end of the cognitive-behavior treatment, all subjects were panic-free and 87% of them remained panic-free at 6-month follow-up, with no significant differences between depressed and nondepressed patients. Furthermore, the significant improvement in panic symptomatology cannot be explained by a sudden change in the dosage or type of medication since medication intake was constant during baseline and cognitive-behavior therapy. Together, these methodological controls led the authors to suggest that cognitive-behavior therapy acted as a specific therapeutic agent in this study. According to this study, the simple provision of accurate information regarding the source and the nature of the physiological sensations associated with panic attacks is not sufficient to eliminate the attacks.

In summary, research with single-subject designs provides evidence on the efficacy of combined cognitive-behavioral treatment programs in panic disorder. Evaluations of specific treatment components, such as cognitive restructuring, breathing retraining, and interoceptive exposure, not used in combination, and using a single-case experimental methodology, are presently nonexistent.

Treatment Comparisons with Nonspecific Effects

Psychodynamic Treatment

Controlled research evaluating the efficacy of psychoanalytic interventions for the treatment of panic is unavailable. Indeed, these treatment approaches have never been compared to a waiting-list or credible placebo control or to an established alternative psychotherapeutic intervention.

Cognitive-Behavioral Treatment

Multicomponent Treatment. In the first controlled study evaluating multicomponent cognitive-behavioral treatment for panic disorder (Barlow *et al.*, 1984), 11 patients with panic disorder were assigned to treatment or a waiting-list control group. None of the DSM-III panic-disordered patients had more than minimal agoraphobic avoidance. Treatment consisted of 18 weekly sessions in which patients were treated with a combination of progressive muscle relaxation training, muscle tension biofeedback, and cognitive restructuring specifically designed to address panic disorder. Compared with controls, treated subjects improved significantly on clinical ratings, psychophysiological, and self-report anxiety measures, including daily self-monitoring measures of background anxiety and episodes of high anxiety and panic. The improvements were maintained 3 months after treatment completion. However, results from this study indicated that the decreases in muscle tension were not correlated with any outcome measure, which suggests that progressive muscle relaxation and biofeedback were not effective through their intended mechanisms. This also makes evident the need for nonspecific treatment comparisons.

Relaxation. Applied relaxation training (ART) has been used successfully in behavioral treatments of anxiety and phobic disorders. However, only two controlled outcome studies examining the efficacy of ART as a treatment for panic disorder have been published as of this writing. Applied relaxation involves training in progressive muscle relaxation until patients are skilled in the use of cue-control procedures which they apply when practicing items from a hierarchy of anxiety-provoking tasks. Öst (1988) compared ART to progressive muscle relaxation in the treatment of 16 panic-disordered patients who underwent individual therapy for 14 sessions. While both interventions were beneficial with respect to clinical ratings, self-reports of generalized anxiety and depression, and self-monitoring of panic attacks, the ART condition was superior on most of the measures at posttreatment and on all measures at follow-up, approximately 19 months after treatment completion. One hundred percent of the ART group were panic-free after treatment and at follow-up in comparison to 71% of the progressive muscle relaxation group at posttreatment and 57% at follow-up. Furthermore, all of the ART group were classified as having high end-state status at follow-up in comparison to 25% of the progressive muscle relaxation group. It is important to note that exposure to interoceptive cues, which are highly salient to panic disorder responding, were included in the ART group. Therefore, it is difficult to completely attribute the results primarily to ART.

Barlow and colleagues (1989) recently reported the results of a long-term clinical outcome study testing variations of behavioral treatments for panic disorder with mild or no agoraphobic avoidance. In that study, ART was compared with a treatment condition combining exposure to somatic sensations associated with panic attacks, cognitive therapy directed at catastrophic thoughts associated with panic attacks, and breathing retraining (referred to as Panic Control Treatment [PCT]). In a third condition, these two treatments were combined. All three conditions were compared with a waiting-list control. At termination, the percentage of patients in the relaxation group (60%) who completed treatment and reported no panic attacks did not differ significantly from the waiting-list group (36%). Thus, the relaxation intervention was not found to be effective in eliminating panic. Moreover, a significantly greater number of subjects dropped out of the relaxation condition (33%). Therefore, when dropouts are included in the final analysis, with the assumption that panic episodes continue, the percentage of patients who were panic-free falls to 40% in the relaxation condition. Relaxation, however, tended to effect greater reductions in generalized anxiety. These results suggest that ART as administered in this treatment protocol, is a less specific treatment for panic attacks than the other treatment conditions.

In a recent report on the long-term follow-up results of this clinical outcome study, Craske, Brown, and Barlow (1991) observed that 81% of the group who received PCT were free of panic attacks 2 years after termination of treatment in contrast to 43% for the combination treatment group and 36% for the relaxation treatment group when dropouts were included in the analyses and were assumed to be continuing to panic. The authors speculated that a dilution effect, or perhaps a detrimental effect of the addition of relaxation procedures, accounted for the lower success rate of the combination treatment group. Furthermore, the relaxation group showed significant deterioration on measures of general anxiety, somatic symptoms, and depression as well as clinical ratings of severity, while subjects in the interoceptive and cognitive treatment groups evidenced maintenance or continued improvement.

In summary, these findings suggest that progressive muscle relaxation taught for application to a hierarchy of anxiety-producing tasks has limited effectiveness in the control of panic attacks in the short term, and any success as a result of treatment may be more prone to relapse over the long term. These results contrast with Öst's (1988) report of the efficacy of ART. The inclusion of interoceptive exposure tasks in the anxiety hierarchies in Öst's relaxation treatment may explain this discrepancy.

Breathing Retraining. Breathing control training is used to treat panic based on evidence that hyperventilation can play a role in at least some panic attacks (Ley, 1988; Lum, 1981; Salkovskis, Warwick, Clark, & Wessels, 1986). However, in controlled outcome studies, breathing control has been combined with other treatment interventions, thereby providing no evidence on the efficacy of breathing control training alone.

Cognitive Restructuring. Evidence appears to be accumulating that cognitive factors are associated with the experience of panic, suggesting that cognitive restructuring may be of value in the treatment of panic attacks (Beck *et al.*, 1974; Bonn, Harrison, & Rees, 1973; Hibbert, 1984; Rapee, 1985, 1986; Sanderson, Rapee, & Barlow, 1987). Cognitive treatment intended for panic attacks began with Beck's (1988) extension of his cognitive model of depression to anxiety and panic, in which he focuses on the role of catastrophic interpretations of sensations related to panic attacks, particularly those associated with loss of control or death. At this time, the only evidence of the efficacy of cognitive interventions from controlled trials appears to be from studies in which cognitive therapy is conducted in conjunction with behavioral techniques, but the effective mechanism of change is assumed to lie in the cognitive realm. Sokol-Kessler and Beck (1987, cited in Beck, 1988) reported on a controlled outcome study involving 29 panic-disordered patients in which a 12-week cognitive therapy program including interoceptive exposure and *in vivo* exposure was compared with a control treatment consisting of 8 weeks of self-monitoring and brief weekly supportive therapy. The cognitive therapy program was associated with significantly greater reduction in frequency of panic attacks per week, compared to supportive therapy when pretest mean panic scores were covaried out. Mean panic responses lessened from 5.06 per week at intake to zero at termination for the cognitive therapy program group, while no significant gains were obtained for the control group. Although the inclusion of a controlled comparison permits the conclusion that the treatment effect was greater than that achieved from time alone, the inclusion of specific behavioral treatment procedures precludes discussion of the effectiveness of cognitive procedures alone.

Interoceptive Exposure. The purpose of interoceptive exposure is to disrupt conditioned associations between somatic sensations and panic attacks by repetitive exposure to the somatic sensations. The theoretical principles underlying interoceptive exposure is one of fear extinction, given the conceptualization of panic attacks as conditioned responses to sensations that have been associated with panic attacks (Barlow, 1988).

The available evidence on the efficacy of interoceptive exposure alone in the treatment of panic is scant, although interoceptive exposure has been combined with other interventions in controlled studies. As described earlier, Barlow *et al.* (1989) examined the efficacy of combination treatments that emphasized interoceptive exposure, comparing them to relaxation alone. The combined interventions were (1) interoceptive exposure and cognitive restructuring (PCT) and (2) interoceptive exposure, cognitive restructuring, and ART. Interoceptive exposure entailed repeated exposures using induction techniques such as forced hyperventilation, spinning, and cardiovascular effort. Treatments consisted of 15 weekly sessions. At termination, the percentage of patients reporting no panic attacks differed significantly across groups. In the two treatment conditions containing exposure to somatic sensations plus cognitive therapy, either alone or in combination with relaxation, over 85% of clients were free of panic attacks during a 2-week period after treatment in comparison to 60% in the relaxation condition and 35% in the waiting-list control group. Only those groups receiving exposure plus cognitive therapy were significantly improved compared to the waiting-list control subjects on this measure. However, as the investigators point out, the study does not provide evidence on the efficacy of interoceptive exposure alone.

Griez and van den Hout (1986) reported the first controlled study of interoceptive exposure alone. They used inhalations of 35% CO_2/65% O_2 as a way of repeatedly exposing patients to the bodily sensations which accompany panic attacks. Inhalation of 35% CO_2/65% O_2 is a highly effective technique for inducing the bodily sensations of panic (van den Hout & Griez, 1984). Using a crossover design, Griez and van den Hout (1986) evaluated the short-term effectiveness of six sessions of repeated, graded CO_2 inhalation over 2 weeks, which was compared with a 2-week regimen of propranolol, chosen because of its ability to suppress sensations induced by CO_2 inhalations. The inhalation therapy was associated with significant reductions in two primary measures of panic: panic attack frequency and fear of autonomic sensations. Propranolol failed to produce significant effects on either of these measures. However, the difference between the two treatments, based on raw difference scores, only reached significance on the measure of fear of sensations. Although the inhalation therapy was associated with substantial drops in panic frequency, most patients were not panic-free at the end of the 2 weeks. Further improvements might have been observed if the therapy had been extended.

While these data indicate that interoceptive exposure may be a valuable treatment technique in the alleviation of panic attacks, more extensive and controlled evaluations of this specific component used alone are still needed to fully measure its effectiveness.

Summary

Controlled research regarding the efficacy of psychoanalytic approaches for the treatment of panic is unavailable. Multicomponent cognitive-behavioral treatments for panic seem to be more effective than the passage of time alone and are consistently associated with reduction, and often, elimination of panic attacks. Moreover, combination treatments that focus on fear of internal sensations evidenced greater efficacy than interventions that rely on relaxation. At the present time, conclusions on the efficacy of separate cognitive and behavioral interventions are limited because these interventions have been combined in panic treatment controlled studies. The only specific intervention for which evidence was found for its efficacy when used alone in the treatment of panic is interoceptive exposure (Griez & van den Hout, 1986). However, conclusions on the maintenance of its effects are precluded by the use of a crossover experimental design.

Interorientation Comparisons

At the present time, there is no evidence supporting the effectiveness of traditional psychotherapy for treating panic disorder (National Institutes of Health [NIH], 1991). Cognitive-behavioral treatment programs including a combination of cognitive restructuring and interoceptive exposure procedures have been shown to be far more effective than supportive psychotherapy (Sokol-Kessler & Beck, 1987, cited in Beck, 1988). Although it is not possible to say whether the apparent effectiveness of the cognitive-behavioral treatments is due to their specific emphasis on fear of internal sensations, treatment focusing on interoceptive exposure and cognitive restructuring of misinterpretations of bodily sensations is associated with a higher efficacy than treatment relying on relaxation (Clark *et al.*, 1990; Craske *et al.*, 1991).

Outcome Parameters

Most studies evaluating cognitive-behavioral treatments for panic disorder have used panic-free status as an indicator of treatment success at termination of treatment as well as at follow-up phases. Short-term clinical outcome from controlled studies indicate that the panic-free status in the cognitive-behavioral procedures reviewed varies between 80% to 100%. Treatments including a combination of interoceptive and cognitive-restructuring procedures are associated with a higher percentage of patients free of panic at termination of treatment, while treatments focusing on relaxation techniques are associated with a lower percentage of panic-free patients (Barlow *et al.*, 1989). Relatively few studies have systematically examined the long-term clinical outcome from psychological treatment of panic disorder, and the only long-term outcome available is from cognitive-behavioral treatment approaches. Moreover, most of the follow-up findings from the cognitive-behavioral treatments of panic disorder are based on uncontrolled studies (Clark *et al.*, 1985; Salkovskis, Jones, & Clark, 1986; Sokol & Beck, 1987, cited in Beck, 1988). Only two controlled investigations of the follow-up effects of cognitive-behavioral treatments for panic disorder have been done, and both used panic-free status to indicate success rates. In one of these studies, in which the relative efficacy of applied relaxation training and progressive muscle relaxation was compared (Öst, 1988), 100% of the applied relaxation group achieved panic-free status at a 19-month follow-up assessment in contrast to 57% of the progressive muscle relaxation group. The second controlled study reporting long-term clinical outcome of psychological treatment of panic disorder (Craske *et al.*, 1991) brings evidence to suggest maintenance and continued improvement in subjects receiving exposure and cognitive treatment procedures. Fully 81% of the exposure and cognitive-restructuring treatment group (including dropouts) were reportedly free of panic at a 24-month assessment in contrast to 43% of the group that received exposure and cognitive treatment in combination with relaxation and 36% of the relaxation group. However, as it has been suggested (Barlow, 1988) panic-free status, as the central outcome measure, may be an overly optimistic indicator of therapeutic success since panic-disordered patients, who are free of panic, often continue to evidence significant symptomatology (e.g., general anxiety, avoidance) that keeps them impaired. For example, Craske *et al.* (1991) observed that, while the majority of subjects who received interoceptive and cognitive-restructuring procedures were panic-free at 24-month follow-up, only 50% met high end-state status criteria. These criteria include a combination of measures on major phenomenological components of panic disorder—namely, panic-free status, subjective anxiety, avoidance behavior, and functional impairment—that might indicate that the patient is essentially cured. Used as outcome measures, these criteria are important because they highlight the possible differential effects of interventions directed at panic on other aspects of functioning.

Attrition rate is also an important criteria of treatment effectiveness. While a few studies on the psychological treatment of panic disorder did not report the number of dropouts (e.g., Sokol-Kessler & Beck, 1987, cited in Beck, 1988), the typical attrition rate of cognitive-behavioral treatments of panic disorder averages somewhere between 10% and 20%. In one study, relaxation procedures were found to produce a differential attrition compared to other psychological treatments (Barlow *et al.*, 1989). The dropout rate in the relaxation group (33%) was higher than rates typically observed in most psychological treatments and approach dropout rates reported from drug studies (Barlow, 1988). This finding may be related to the fact that in the early stages of treatment, relaxation may induce anxiety (Heide & Borkovec, 1984) or panic (Adler, Craske, & Barlow, 1987). However, the conclusions that can be drawn from the dropout findings about differential efficacy of the treatments in Barlow *et al.*'s study (1989) are limited since outcome assessment data at the time of dropout were not reported, and thus it cannot be concluded that dropouts were treatment failures. Nevertheless, the different dropout rates for the treatments are suggestive of differential efficacy and, thus, highlight the importance of reporting dropout data in treatment comparison studies.

Psychological treatment directed at the control of panic attacks is still a relatively new area. While the overall efficacy of cognitive-behavioral treatments for panic disorder have been demonstrated, exploration of the various parameters in an attempt to improve the efficacy of psychological interventions is yet to be conducted.

Psychopharmacology

Several classes of drugs have been studied and/or proposed as possible treatment for panic disorder: antidepressant medications, including both tricyclic and monoamine oxidase (MAO) inhibitors; benzodiazepines, including drugs such as diazepam and alprazolam; beta-blockers, best represented by propranolol; and clonidine, an antihypertensive medication (see Fyer, Sandberg, and Klein, 1991, for a literature review on the pharmacological treatment of panic disorder).

Although several studies have examined the comparative and combined efficacy of therapeutic exposure and pharmacotherapy in the treatment of panic disorder with varying degrees of agoraphobic avoidance (e.g., Mavissakalian & Michelson, 1986; Telch, Agras, Taylor, Roth, & Gallen, 1985), few studies to date have compared cognitive-behavioral panic control treatments to pharmacological treatments for panic disorder without agoraphobia.

Recently, Klosko, Barlow, Tassinari, and Cerny (1990) reported the results of a study comparing the efficacy of their panic control treatment (consisting of cognitive restructuring, breathing retraining, relaxation, and exposure to somatic cues) to alprazolam, placebo, and a waiting-list control in 57 patients with panic disorder. At posttreatment, 87% of the patients undergoing panic control treatment were free of panic attacks compared to 50% for alprazolam, 36% for placebo, and 33% for waiting-list control. Although the panic control treatment was not statistically superior to alprazolam, it was significantly better than the waiting-list and the placebo. Nevertheless, the panic control group demonstrated a broader pattern of positive therapeutic change than the alprazolam group. Unfortunately, follow-up data were not available.

Clark *et al.* (1990) compared the efficacy of cognitive therapy for panic to imipramine, applied relaxation, and a waiting-list condition in 64 patients with panic disorder with and without agoraphobia. The three treatments were delivered across 12 sessions in conjunction with self-exposure assignments. All three active treatments appeared to be effective when compared with the waiting-list group. However, at posttreatment, cognitive therapy was significantly more effective on several measures than either imipramine or applied relaxation, which did not differ from each other. At a 3-month follow-up assessment, cognitive therapy remained more effective than applied relaxation on several measures. However, by this time, the subjects in the imipramine group, who had not yet begun tapering of imipramine, tended to catch up with those treated with cognitive therapy. Clark *et al.* (1990) are currently collecting 12- and 24-month follow-up data on these subjects. Given the lack of long-term follow-up data on the functioning of treated panic-disordered patients, these results will be particularly informative.

Another important coming stage of research is evaluating the comparative and combined efficacy of newly developed cognitive-behavioral treatments of panic and extant pharmacological approaches. Recently, a large-scale collaborative study sponsored by the National Institute of Mental Health has been initiated to address this need. Central to this study is the collaboration of four research sites (SUNY-Albany, Pittsburgh, Hillside/Columbia, and Yale) representing both psychological and pharmacological orientations. The following five conditions are being evaluated: imipramine, pill placebo, the panic control treatment recently developed at Albany, and a combination of this latter treatment with either imipramine or placebo. A total of 480 panic-disordered patients with no or mild agoraphobic avoidance will be enrolled over the 5-year course of the study. This large sample size will allow sufficient statistical power to detect subtle yet potentially important effects that may predict outcome, such as subject variables or interactions between subject variables and treatment conditions. Moreover, the examination of differences between sites will provide important information regarding the generalizability of treatment procedures. In addition, this design will allow the exploration of comparative mechanisms of action of psychological and pharmacological treatment.

Although there is little direct evidence from controlled studies supporting the effects of medication on panic disorder without substantial agoraphobic avoidance, medication nevertheless has long been recognized as the generally accepted form of treatment for panic-disordered patients. Pharmacological treatments are easy to deliver, can act quickly, and demand little effort from the patient, apart from compliance. Many of the disadvantages of pharmacological treatment are related to the side effects of drugs, the dropout rate, the possibility of long-term dependence, and the problems of discontinuation of treatment. The side effects that often occur for some patients may be troublesome, debilitating, or even dangerous. The dropout rates are high, particularly for tricyclics such as imipramine because of anticholinergic side effects during the first few weeks of treatment. Currently available research suggests that when treatment is discontinued the rate of relapse is quite high, particularly with the benzodiazepines and the MAO inhibitors. In patients withdrawn from benzodiazepine, relapse approaches 100% (Barlow, 1988). There is little systematic evidence on the rate of relapse over the months and years following discontinuation of tricyclic antidepressants such as imipramine. Panic disorder is frequently seen in women of childbearing age, and while research on the safety of pharmacological treatment during pregnancy and lactation is limited, medication use in this population seems particularly problematic and undesirable (Kerns, 1986; Robinson, Stewart, & Flak, 1986). Other disadvantages of pharmacological treatment are the reluctance of some patients to take medication and risks of chemical dependency in patients with alcohol and drug problems.

Given the contention, most often based on the theories of state-dependent learning or attributions, to the effect that pharmacological interventions may impede progress when anxiety is treated through psychological procedures, Côté, Gauthier, and Laberge (1992) compared the differential efficacy of cognitive-behavioral therapy (including breathing retraining, cognitive therapy, and exposure to internal and external cues) in panic-disordered patients divided into two groups on the basis of presence/absence of concurrent medication use (antidepressant, antianxiety). All medicated patients were taking benzodiazepines either alone or with an antidepressant. After the 17-week trial of cognitive-behavior therapy, no significant differences were found in the frequency and apprehension of panic attacks between medicated patients and nonmedicated patients, and both groups significantly improved on these measures, indicating that concurrent medication use had no impact on outcome. Moreover, 85% of medicated patients and 88% of nonmedicated patients were panic-free. At a 12-month follow-up, all the nonmedicated patients were free of panic attacks compared to 92% of medicated patients. These results suggested that patients who relied on medication to deal with their panic attacks and those who did not responded equally well to newly developed cognitive-behavioral treatments for panic disorder. Newman, Beck, Beck, and Tran (1990) obtained similar results when comparing the benefit of cognitive therapy obtained by panic-disordered patients with or without medication.

Conclusion

Several key issues have emerged in this review of the psychological treatment of panic disorder. Psychological approaches that have addressed the treatment of panic disorder are the psychodynamic approach and the cognitive-behavioral approach. Psychoanalytic treatment for panic disorder has not been demonstrated to be effective. Indeed, evidence supporting the effectiveness of this treatment on panic attacks is restricted to uncontrolled case reports and therefore remains inconclusive. Cognitive-behavioral treatments have been shown to be very effective for the control of panic attacks in the short term and, more importantly, up to 2 years following treatment completion.

Effective cognitive-behavioral treatments for panic have been compared with alternative psychological treatment such as applied relaxation and supportive psychotherapy and have been found to provide superior results. At the present time, it is not possible to say whether the apparent effectiveness of the cognitive-behavioral treatments is due to their specific emphasis on fear of interoceptive sensations. Nevertheless, it is encouraging to note that cognitive-behavioral treatments have been found to be effective with panic-disordered patients because these patients, for a long time, formed a group for whom there was no generally accepted psychological treatment. Cognitive-behavioral treatments have been recognized to be the only psychological treatments shown to be effective for panic disorder (NIH, 1991). In the absence of any controlled data on efficacy of treatment of other widely used approaches, such as psychodynamic psychotherapy, and given the risks of maintaining individuals in nonvalidated treatments of panic disorder, cognitive-behavioral treatment should be the treatment of choice.

Although the developments reviewed in this chapter represent remarkable advancement, existing research suggests that important issues need to be addressed in future treatment studies of panic disorder. Follow-up status is crucial to the evaluation of these psychological treatment procedures. Conclusions about the maintenance of effects are only available for combined cognitive-behavioral treatment, and the results from controlled studies are very promising. Therapeutic effects from short-term cognitive-behavioral treatments tend to be maintained for up to 2 years following treatment completion, particularly for interoceptive exposure combined with cognitive-restructuring treatment procedures. However, more substantial follow-up data are needed.

While cognitive-behavioral treatment is effective for panic disorder, it is not known which treatment component is responsible for the success of treatment. To date, past panic treatment studies, advocating one particular approach, have included a combination of at least one of the other components, and it is not clear which procedures are most responsible for producing the therapeutic effects. The concern of researchers and clinicians is the identification of the simplest combination of procedures for maximal effectiveness. Consequently, an important step in future research would be to dismantle the multicomponent cognitive-behavioral treatments of panic disorder in an attempt to identify the essential components. Such research could have a major impact on our understanding of the psychological mechanisms underlying these treatment effects and, consequently, would be very helpful to developing the most effective treatments. In light of the paucity of data isolating the essential components of panic control treatments, two attempts have recently been initiated to address this need. First, a large clinical trial, sponsored by the National Institute of Mental Health, has been conducted for the past few years at the Center for Stress and Anxiety Disorders at the State University of New York at Albany to isolate the essential components of panic control treatment (Barlow, Brown, Craske, Rapee, & Anthony, 1991). The four treatment conditions in this study are cognitive restructuring only, cognitive restructuring plus breathing retraining, cognitive restructuring plus interoceptive exposure, and cognitive restructuring plus breathing retraining plus interoceptive exposure. Second, a controlled trial comparing cognitive therapy alone, interoceptive exposure therapy alone, their combination, and a waiting-list control is currently underway at Philipps-University, Marburg, West Germany (Margraf, Dornier, & Schneider, 1991). The results from these two studies, still in progress, will be particularly valuable.

The question of which patients are going to benefit from these cognitive-behavioral treatments is also important. Although existing studies indicate that cognitive-behavioral treatments focusing on the fear of interoceptive cues are highly efficacious for patients with a principal diagnosis of panic disorder with no or mild agoraphobia, the generalizability of their effectiveness remains to be assessed. Indeed, little is known about the efficacy of the treatments when panic disorder is accompanied by the presence of mood states like depression, moderate or severe agoraphobia, comorbid DSM-III-R Axis I disorders and Axis II personality disorders, and the presence of medical conditions such as asthma or heart disease that have symptoms similar to panic sensations. Recent clinical assessment studies have indicated high comorbidity rates between panic disorder and other major anxiety and mood disorders (Barlow, Di Nardo, Vermilyea, Vermilyea, & Blanchard, 1986; Breier, Charney, & Heninger, 1984; Di Nardo & Barlow, 1990; Moras *et al.*, 1991). At the present time, only one study supports the clinical efficacy of cognitive-behavioral procedures for treating panic-disordered patients with secondary major depression (Laberge *et al.*, in press). Further research is needed to assess the efficacy of cognitive-behavioral treatments with panic-disordered patients who have other co-occurring syndromes and/or medical conditions. It is possible that the relevance of each specific cognitive-behavioral treatment component will differ depending on various patient characteristics, and that the choice of a specific treatment or combination of treatments will be dependent upon a thorough initial evaluation. It is also possible that alternative psychotherapeutic procedures might be important in the treatment of panic disorder that is accompanied by other Axis I and Axis II disorders. Sokol and Beck (1986, cited in Beck, 1988) found that the implementation of cognitive-behavioral procedures for panic was noticeably less effective for panic-disordered patients with various personality disorders.

A major problem for the proponents of psychological treatment is the limited accessibility of effective cognitive-behavioral treatments for the average individual with panic disorder. It is possible that the existence of manuals and workbooks that can be handed directly to the patient working under minimal clinical supervision (e.g., Barlow & Craske, 1989; Côté, Gauthier, & Laberge, 1988) might make these interventions more available. Determining the best methods of disseminating these treatments will be important. At the present time, only one controlled study has evaluated a cognitive-behavioral treatment program for panic disorder with mild or no agoraphobic avoidance utilizing minimal therapist contact designed to make this treatment more accessible (Côté *et al.*, 1990). Results of this study demonstrated that the treatment providing minimal contact with the therapist was as effective as the therapist-directed treatment in eliminating panic attacks, with the results being maintained or furthered at a 6-month follow-up. Additional evaluation of the effectiveness of self-administered treatment via manuals combined with minimal therapist contact is an important priority for increasing the accessibility of these new, effective cognitive-behavioral treatments for panic disorder.

To improve the accessibility of effective cognitive-behavioral treatment for panic disorder, training programs for the combined treatments for panic attacks that are being used in major research centers are now available. Training in the treatment used in Beck's studies (Beck, 1988) can be obtained at Beck's Center for Cognitive Therapy in Philadelphia, Pennsylvania. Clark and Salkovskis described their treatment in a book chapter (Clark, 1989). Barlow and colleagues have written two treatment manuals describing the combined cognitive-behavioral treatment (Panic Control Treatment) currently used for panic disorder at the Phobia and Anxiety Disorders Clinic at Albany, New York. One is for practitioners (Barlow & Cerny, 1988), and the other—a therapist-guided, self-help manual—is appropriate for patient use (Barlow & Craske, 1989). The latter manual comes with a therapist's guide (Craske & Barlow, 1990).

References

Adler, C. M., Craske, M. G., & Barlow, D. H. (1987). Relaxation-induced panic (RIP): When resting isn't peaceful. *Integrative Psychiatry, 5,* 94–112.

American Psychiatric Association. (1980). *Diagnostic and statistical manual of mental disorders (3rd ed.).* Washington, DC: Author.

American Psychiatric Association. (1987). *Diagnostic and statistical manual of mental disorders (3rd ed.-revised).* Washington, DC: Author.

Anderson, D. J., Noyes, R., & Crowe, R. R. (1984). A comparison of panic disorder and generalized anxiety disorder. *American Journal of Psychiatry, 141,* 572–575.

Barlow, D. H. (1988). *Anxiety and its disorders.* New York: Guilford Press.

Barlow, D. H., Brown, T. A., Craske, M. G., Rapee, R. M., & Antony, M. (1991, November). *Treatment of panic disorder: Follow-up and mechanisms of action.* Paper presented at the meeting of the Association for Advancement of Behavior Therapy, New York.

Barlow, D. H., & Cerny, J. A. (1988). *Psychological treatment of panic.* New York: Guilford Press.

Barlow, D. H., Cohen, A. S., Waddell, M. T., Vermilyea, B. B., Klosko, J. S., Blanchard, E. B., & Di Nardo, P. A. (1984). Panic and generalized anxiety disorders: Nature and treatment. *Behavior Therapy, 15,* 431–449.

Barlow, D. H., & Craske, M. G. (1989). *Mastery of your anxiety and panic.* Albany, NY: Graywind Publications.

Barlow, D. H., Craske, M. G., Cerny, J. A., & Klosko, J. S. (1989). Behavioral treatment of panic disorder. *Behavior Therapy, 20,* 261–282.

Barlow, D. H., Di Nardo, P. A., Vermilyea, B. B., Vermilyea, J., & Blanchard, E. B. (1986). Co-morbidity and depression among the anxiety disorders: Issues in diagnosis and classification. *Journal of Nervous and Mental Disease, 174,* 63–72.

Beck, A. T. (1988). Cognitive approaches to panic disorder: Theory and therapy. In S. Rachman & J. D. Maser (Eds.), *Panic: Psychological perspectives* (pp. 91–109). Hillsdale, NJ: Lawrence Erlbaum.

Beck, A. T., Laude, R., & Bohnert, M. (1974). Ideational components of anxiety neurosis. *Archives of General Psychiatry, 31,* 319–325.

Breier, A., Charney, D. S., & Heninger, G. R. (1984). Major depression in patients with agoraphobia and panic disorder. *Archives of General Psychiatry, 41,* 1129–1135.

Breier, A., Charney, D. S., & Heninger, G. R. (1986). Agoraphobia with panic attacks: Development, diagnostic stability, and course of illness. *Archives of General Psychiatry, 43,* 1029–1036.

Bonn, J. A., Harrison, J., & Rees, L. (1973). Lactate infusion in the treatment of "free-floating" anxiety. *Canadian Psychiatric Association Journal, 18,* 41–45.

Boyd, J. H. (1986). Use of mental health services for the treatment of panic disorder. *American Journal of Psychiatry, 143,* 1569–1574.

Clark, D. M. (1986). A cognitive approach to panic. *Behaviour Research and Therapy, 24,* 461–470.

Clark, D. M. (1988). A cognitive model of panic attacks. In S. Rachman & J. D. Maser (Eds.), *Panic: Psychological perspectives* (pp. 71–89). Hillsdale, NJ: Lawrence Erlbaum.

Clark, D. M. (1989). Anxiety states: Panic and generalized anxiety. In K. Hauton, P. M. Salkovskis, J. Kirk, & D. M. Clark (Eds.), *Cognitive behaviour therapy for psychiatry problems: A practical guide* (pp. 52–96). Oxford: Oxford University Press.

Clark, D. M., Gelder, M. G., Salkovskis, P. M., Hackmann, A., Middleton, H., & Anastasiades, P. (1990, May). *Cognitive therapy for panic: Comparative efficacy*. Paper presented at the meeting of the American Psychiatry Association, New York.

Clark, D. M., Salkovskis, P. M., & Chakley, A. J. (1985). Respiratory control as a treatment for panic attacks. *Journal of Behavioral Therapy and Experimental Psychiatry, 16*, 23–30.

Cohen, M. E., & White, P. D. (1950). Life situations, emotions and neurocirculatory asthenia (anxiety neurosis, neurasthenia, effort syndrome). In H. G. Wolff (Ed.), *Life stress and bodily disease*. Baltimore: Williams & Wilkins.

Côté, G. Gauthier, J., & Laberge, B. (1988). *Vaincre la panique et l'agoraphobie*. Unpublished manuscript.

Côté, G., Gauthier, J., & Laberge, B. (1992, November). *The impact of medication use on the efficacy of cognitive-behavior therapy for panic disorder*. Paper presented at the meeting of the Association for the Advancement of Behavior Therapy, Boston, MA.

Côté, G., Gauthier, J. G., Laberge, B., Fillion, L., Cormier, H., & Plamondon, J. (1990, November). *Clinic-based vs. home-based treatment with minimal therapist contact for panic disorder*. Paper presented at the meeting of the Association for Advancement of Behavior Therapy, San Francisco.

Craske, M. G., & Barlow, D. H. (1990). *Master your anxiety and panic: Therapist's guide*. Albany, NY: Graywind Publishing.

Craske, M. G., Brown, T. A., & Barlow, D. H. (1991). Behavioral treatment of panic: A two-year follow-up. *Behavior Therapy, 22*, 289–304.

Craske, M. G., Miller, P. P., Rotunda, R., & Barlow, D. H. (1990). A descriptive report of features of initial unexpected panic attacks in minimal and extensive avoiders. *Behaviour Research and Therapy, 28*, 395–400.

Da Costa, J. M. (1871). On irritable heart: A clinical study of a form of functional cardiac disorder and its consequences. *American Journal of the Medical Sciences, 61*, 17–52.

Di Nardo, P. A., & Barlow, D. H. (1990). Syndrome and symptom co-occurrence in the anxiety disorders. In J. D. Maser & C. R. Cloninger (Eds.), *Comorbidity of mood and anxiety disorders* (pp. 205–230). Washington, DC: American Psychiatry Press.

Dittrich, J., Houts, A. C., & Lichstein, K. L. (1983). Panic disorder: Assessment and treatment. *Clinical Psychology Review, 3*, 215–225.

Fewtrell, W. D. (1984). Psychological approaches to panic attack—Some recent developments. *British Journal of Experimental and Clinical Hypnosis, 1*, 21–24.

Freud, S. (1961). On the grounds for detaching a particular syndrome from neurasthenia under the description of anxiety neurosis. In J. Strachey (Ed.), *The standard edition of the complete psychological works of Sigmund Freud* (Vol. 3, pp. 85–116). London: Hogarth Press. (Original work published 1895).

Fyer, A. J., Sandberg, D., Klein, D. F. (1991). The pharmacologic treatment of panic disorder and agoraphobia. In J. R. Walker, G. R. Norton, & C. A. Ross (Eds.), *Panic disorder and agoraphobia: A comprehensive guide for the practitioner* (pp. 211–251). Pacific Grove, CA: Brooks/Cole.

Griez, E., & van den Hout, M. A. (1986). CO_2 inhalation in the treatment of panic attacks. *Behaviour Research and Therapy, 24*, 145–150.

Heide, F., & Borkovec, T. (1984). Relaxation-induced anxiety: Mechanisms and theoretical implications. *Behaviour Research and Therapy, 24*, 1–12.

Hibbert, G. A. (1984). Ideational components of anxiety: Their origin and content. *British Journal of Psychiatry, 144*, 618–624.

Katon, W. (1984). Panic disorder and somatization: A review of 55 cases. *The American Journal of Medicine, 77*, 101–106.

Katon, W., Vitaliano, P. P., Russo, J., Cormier, L. (1986). Panic disorder: Epidemiology and primary care. *Journal of Family Practice, 23*, 233–239.

Katon, W., Vitaliano, P. P., Russo, J., Jones, M., & Anderson, K. (1987). Panic disorder: Spectrum of severity and somatization. *Journal of Nervous and Mental Disease, 175*, 12–19.

Kerns, L. L. (1986). Treatment of mental disorders in pregnancy: A review of psychotropic drug risks and benefits. *Journal of Nervous and Mental Disease, 174*, 652–659.

King, R., Margraf, J., Ehlers, A., & Maddock, R. (1986). Panic disorder—Overlap with symptoms of somatization disorder. In I. Hand & H. U. Wittchen (Eds.), *Panic and phobias* (Vol. 1, pp. 72–77). Heidelberg: Springer.

Klosko, J. S., Barlow, D. H., Tassinari, R. B., & Cerny, J. A. (1990). A comparison of alprazolam and behavior therapy in the treatment of panic disorder. *Journal of Consulting and Clinical Psychology, 58*, 77–84.

Laberge, B., Gauthier, J., Côté, G., Plamondon, J., & Cormier, H. (in press). Cognitive-behavior therapy of panic disorder with secondary major depression: A preliminary investigation. *Journal of Consulting and Clinical Psychology.*

Ley, R. (1985). Blood, breath, and fears: A hyperventilation theory of panic attacks and agoraphobia. *Clinical Psychology Review, 5*, 271–285.

Ley, R. (1988). Hyperventilation and lactate infusion in the production of panic attacks. *Clinical Psychology Review, 8*, 1.

Lum, L. C. (1981). Hyperventilation and anxiety states. *Journal of the Royal Society of Medicine, 74*, 1–4.

Malan, D. (1976). *The frontier of brief psychotherapy.* New York: Plenum.

Mann, J. (1973). *Time-limited psychotherapy.* Cambridge, MA: Harvard University Press.

Margraf, J., Dornier, C., & Schneider, S. (1991, November). *Outcome and active ingredients of cognitive-behavioral treatments for panic disorder.* Paper presented at the meeting of the Association for Advancement of Behavior Therapy, New York.

Mavissakalian, M., & Michelson, L. (1986). Agoraphobia: Relative and combined effectiveness of therapist-assisted *in vivo* exposure and imipramine. *Journal of Clinical Psychiatry, 47*, 117–122.

McDougall, J. (1985). *Theaters of the mind.* New York: Basic Books.

Moras, K., Di Nardo, P. A., Brown, T. A., & Barlow, D. H. (1992). *Comorbidity and depression among the DSM-III-R anxiety disorders.* Manuscript submitted for publication.

National Institutes of Health. (1991, September). *Treatment of panic disorder: Consensus development conference statement,* Washington, D.C.

Nemiah, J. C. (1981). The psychoanalytic view of anxiety. In D. F. Klein & J. Rabkin (Eds.), *Anxiety: New research and changing concepts* (pp. 291–300). New York: Raven Press.

Newman, C. F., Beck, J. S., Beck, A. T., & Tran, G. Q. (1990, November). *Efficacy of cognitive therapy in reducing panic attacks and medication.* Paper presented at the meeting of the Association for Advancement of Behavior Therapy, San Francisco.

Oppenheim, B. S. (1918). Report on neurocirculatory asthenia and its management. *Military Surgeon, 42*, 711–744.

Öst, L. G. (1988). Applied relaxation in the treatment of panic disorder. *Behaviour Research and Therapy, 26*, 13–22.

Rapee, R. (1985). Distinctions between panic disorder and generalized anxiety disorder: Clinical presentation. *Australian and New Zealand Journal of Psychiatry, 19*, 227–232.

Rapee, R. (1986). Differential response to hyperventilation in panic disorder and generalized anxiety disorder. *Journal of Abnormal Psychology, 95*, 24–28.

Rapee, R., & Barlow, D. H. (1988). The assessment of panic disorder. In P. McReynolds, J. C. Rosen, & G. Chelune (Eds.), *Advances in psychological assessment* (Vol. 7, pp. 203–228). New York: Plenum.

Rapee, R. M., Litwin, E. M., & Barlow, D. H. (1990). Impact of life events on subjects with panic disorder and on comparison subjects. *American Journal of Psychiatry, 147*, 640–644.

Rapee, R., Mattick, R., & Murrell, E. (1986). Cognitive mediation in the affective component of spontaneous panic attacks. *Journal of Behavior Therapy and Experimental Psychiatry, 17*, 245–253.

Robinson, G., Stewart, D., & Flak, E. (1986). The rational use of psychotropic drugs in pregnancy and postpartum. *Canadian Journal of Psychiatry, 31*, 183–190.

Salkovskis, P. M., Jones, D. R. O., & Clark, D. M. (1986). Respiratory control in the treatment of panic attacks: Replication and extension with concurrent measurement of behavior and pCO_2. *British Journal of Psychiatry, 148*, 526–532.

Salkovskis, P. M., Warwick, H. M. C., Clark, D. M., & Wessels, D. J. (1986). A demonstration of acute hyperventilation during naturally occurring panic attacks. *Behaviour Research and Therapy, 24*, 91–94.

Sanderson, W. C., Di Nardo, P. A., Rapee, R. M., & Barlow, D. H. (1990). Syndrome co-morbidity in patients diagnosed with a DSM-III-revised anxiety disorder. *Journal of Abnormal Psychology, 99*, 308–312.

Sanderson, W. C., Rapee, R. M., & Barlow, D. H. (1989). The influence of an illusion of control on panic attacks induced via inhalation of 5.5% CO_2 enriched air. *Archives of General Psychiatry, 46*, 157–164.

Sandler, A. (1988). Aspects of the analysis of a neurotic patient. *British Journal of Psychoanalysis, 69*, 317–326.

Shear, M. K. (1991). The psychodynamic approach in the treatment of panic disorder. In J. R. Walker, G. R. Norton, & C. A. Ross (Eds.), *Panic disorder and agoraphobia: A comprehensive guide for the practitioner* (pp. 335–351). Pacific Grove, CA: Brooks/Cole.

Sifneos, P. E. (1972). *Short-term psychotherapy and emotional crisis.* Cambridge, MA: Harvard University Press.

Silber, A. (1984). Temporary disorganization facilitating recall and mastery: An analysis of symptom. *Psychoanalytic Quarterly, 53,* 498–501.

Telch, M. J., Agras, W. S., Taylor, C. B., Roth, W. T., & Gallen, C. C. (1985). Combined pharmacological and behavioural treatment for agoraphobia. *Behaviour Research and Therapy, 23,* 325–335.

Thyer, B. A., Parrish, R. T., Curtis, G. C., Nesse, R. M., & Cameron, O. G. (1985). Age of onset of DSM-III anxiety disorders. *Comprehensive Psychiatry, 26,* 113–122.

van den Hout, M. A. (1988). Panic, perception, and pCO_2. In I. Hand, & H. H. Wittcher (Eds.), *Panic and phobias* (Vol. 2, pp. 117–128). Heidelberg: Springer.

van den Hout, M. A., & Griez, E. (1983). Some remarks on the nosology of anxiety states and panic disorders. *Acta Psychiatrica Belgica, 83,* 33–42.

van den Hout, M. A., & Griez, E. (1984). Panic symptoms after inhalation of carbon dioxide. *British Journal of Psychiatry, 144,* 503–507.

Van Pelt, S. J. (1975). Hypnosis and panic. *Journal of the American Institute of Hypnosis, 16,* 39–46.

Weissman, M. M., & Merikangas, K. R. (1986). The epidemiology of anxiety and panic disorders: An update. *Journal of Clinical Psychiatry, 47,* 11–17.

Wittchen, H. U. (1988). Natural course and spontaneous remissions of untreated anxiety disorders: Results of the Munich Follow-Up Study (MFS). In I. Hand & H. U. Wittchen (Eds.), *Panic and phobia* (Vol. 2, pp. 3–17). Heidelberg: Springer.

Wittchen, H. U., & Essau, C. A. (1991). The epidemiology of panic attacks, panic disorder, and agoraphobia. In J. R. Walker, G. R. Norton, & C. A. Ross (Eds.), *Panic disorder and agoraphobia: A comprehensive guide for the practitioner* (pp. 103–149). Pacific Grove, CA: Brooks/Cole.

Woods, M. M. (1972). Violence: Psychotherapy of pseudohomosexual panic. *Archives of General Psychiatry, 27,* 255–258.

8

Treatment of Agoraphobia

Lawrence E. Shapiro, C. Alec Pollard, and Cheryl N. Carmin

Introduction

Agoraphobia, a potentially chronic and debilitating psychiatric syndrome, is seen more often in clinical settings than any other phobia (Marks, 1969) and is believed to affect approximately 2% to 6% of the general population (Myers *et al.*, 1987). The relative prevalence and clinical significance of agoraphobia underscores the importance of identifying effective treatments. However, consumers and practitioners may find it difficult to evaluate existing treatment options. Representatives of many psychotherapeutic approaches claim to be able to treat this disorder successfully, and reviewers of the general psychotherapy literature have often concluded that all approaches are equally beneficial (Luborsky, Singer, & Luborsky, 1975; Smith & Glass, 1977).

The purpose of the present chapter is to evaluate that portion of the outcome literature that specifically addresses the treatment of agoraphobia and to offer some conclusions regarding the efficacy of available treatments.[1] First, however, some background regarding the definition and diagnosis of agoraphobia is provided, followed by brief descriptions of each of the major psychotherapeutic approaches to this syndrome.

Definition and Diagnosis

The term *agoraphobia* was coined by Westphal, a German psychiatrist, in the late 1800s (Westphal, 1888). Use of the Greek word *agora* reflected Westphal's view

[1]The reader is advised that the literature in this chapter explores only that research specifically related to the treatment of agoraphobia. Although some research addressing the treatment of panic disorder includes agoraphobic patients, investigations of panic disorder were not included unless data were provided on the agoraphobic subsample. For information regarding the treatment of panic disorder, the reader is referred to Chapter 7, this volume, by Côté and Barlow.

Lawrence E. Shapiro, C. Alec Pollard, and **Cheryl N. Carmin** • St. Louis University Medical Center, Division of Behavioral Medicine, St. Louis, Missouri 63104.

Handbook of Effective Psychotherapy, edited by Thomas R. Giles. Plenum Press, New York, 1993.

of the disorder as a fear of the "marketplace" or "place of assembly." One year earlier, however, Benedikt (1870) used the term *platzschwindel* (place dizziness) to describe the same condition. In fact, agoraphobia has appeared in the literature under various names, including *platzangst*, or place fear (Cordes, 1871), anxiety hysteria (Freud, 1919), locomotor anxiety (Abraham, 1953), street fear (Miller, 1953), phobic-anxiety-depersonalization syndrome (Roth, 1959), phobic anxious states (Klein, 1964), and nonspecific insecurity fears (Snaith, 1968). The variety of names assigned to agoraphobia over the years reflects differences in emphases upon specific symptoms of the disorder, differences still found in disputes among contemporary authorities (e.g., Klein & Klein, 1989 versus Marks, 1987). Perhaps even more striking, however, is the consistency with which the disorder has typically been described. In particular, two aspects of agoraphobic fear have been repeatedly mentioned as defining features.

One feature is the fear of environmental situations in which escape or access to safety might be hampered. Among phobias, agoraphobia is distinguished by the variety of stimuli typically feared. Examples of situations commonly avoided or dreaded by agoraphobics are public transportation, traveling long distances from home, being alone, crowded settings, and elevators or other physically constraining environments (Chambless, Caputo, Bright, & Gallagher, 1984; Marks, 1970). In addition to avoiding situations perceived as dangerous, agoraphobics tend to actively seek situations in which they feel safe, such as being home or in the company of a trusted companion (Rachman, 1984).

A second feature of agoraphobia is the experience of disturbing physical sensations and the excessive somatic concerns that accompany them. From Benedikt's (1870) emphasis upon dizziness to contemporary concepts of symptom attacks (American Psychiatric Association, 1987), agoraphobia has frequently been portrayed as involving more than just a fear of environmental situations (Benedikt, 1870; Freud, 1936; Goldstein & Chambless, 1978; Klein, 1964; Sheehan & Sheehan, 1982; Weekes, 1976; Wolpe, 1990). It has been suggested that agoraphobic fear is influenced by internal as well as external stimuli. This recurrent observation has clearly influenced contemporary conceptual models in which agoraphobia is described as a fear of the symptoms of panic attacks (Goldstein & Chambless, 1978; Hallam, 1978; Klein, 1964; Weekes, 1976). In fact, from this perspective, phobic avoidance is viewed as a by-product of the fear of panic. Agoraphobics avoid situations in which they fear that the disturbing symptoms of a panic attack will lead to some catastrophic consequence like loss of control, death, insanity, or humiliation (Pollard & Frank, 1990).

Currently, agoraphobia is defined in DSM-III-R (American Psychiatric Association, 1987) as a "fear of being in places or situations from which escape might be difficult or embarrassing or in which help might not be available in the event of a panic attack" (p. 238) or another ". . . symptom that could be incapacitating or embarrassing" (p. 241). This contemporary definition incorporates both the environmental and the interoceptive (internal, physiological) stimuli generally believed to constitute the object of agoraphobic fear. Also, two diagnostic options are available, depending on the nature of the symptom attack feared. The first option, "Panic Disorder with Agoraphobia," is assigned when the disorder is associated with panic attacks. A second option, "Agoraphobia without History of Panic Disorder," is diagnosed in cases in which agoraphobic patterns are associated with a fear of symptom attacks other than panic. Examples of these symptom attacks include vomiting, cardiac distress, loss of bladder or bowel control, migraine headache, depersonalization, and dizziness (Pollard & Kenney, 1992).

Before discussing treatment, one additional note on the nature of agoraphobia is warranted. Despite the fact that examples of agoraphobia involving symptom attacks other than panic were described as long as a century ago (Benedikt, 1870; Freud, 1924), the diagnostic category of "Agoraphobia without History of Panic Disorder" has only recently received attention in the literature (Pollard & Kenney, 1992). Data from clinical settings (Pollard, Bronson, & Kenney, 1989) and samples of the general population (Weismann, Leaf, Blazer, Boyd, & Florio, 1986) indicate that a portion of agoraphobics experience symptom attacks that cannot be categorized as panic. Nonetheless, because the bulk of the literature on agoraphobia refers to cases involving panic attacks, conclusions outlined in the present chapter may not be pertinent to Agoraphobia without History of Panic Disorder. An adequate appraisal of the relevance of this chapter to the latter form of agoraphobia must await additional research.

Treatment Approaches

Treatments for agoraphobia have been developed from a variety of different psychological orientations. It is not within the scope of this chapter to provide detailed accounts of every treatment option, but a basic understanding of the way in which the major schools of psychotherapy approach agoraphobia is necessary to evaluate the literature. Therefore, brief overviews of psychodynamic, existential/humanistic, and cognitive-behavioral psychotherapies are presented.

An understanding of psychodynamic approaches to the treatment of agoraphobia begins with the ideas of Sigmund Freud. Freud (1924) viewed all phobias as attempts to deal with anxiety; that is, anxiety, generated by unacceptable sexual or aggressive id impulses, is displaced onto a more socially appropriate or acceptable external object. He also proposed that phobic objects had unconscious symbolic meaning. For example, an agoraphobic in conflict over sexual impulses might become anxious in public situations where the temptation to express sexual impulses is greatest (Deutsch, 1929). Freud's views of agoraphobia have been expanded or modified by therapists representing several different psychodynamic perspectives, including traditional psychoanalysis (Deutsch, 1929), object relations theory (Frances & Dunn, 1975), self-psychology (Diamond, 1985), ego psychology (Weiss, 1964), and short-term dynamic psychotherapy (Sifneos, 1972). Though specific procedures and concepts vary, psychodynamic psychotherapies are characterized by the use of primarily verbal interaction (e.g., interpretation, free association) to help patients gain insight into the nature of underlying psychological conflicts or historical traumas believed to be responsible for agoraphobic symptoms.

A second major school of psychotherapy, the existential/humanistic, has had little to say specifically about agoraphobia. However, it should not be assumed that clinicians from this school of psychotherapy never see individuals with an agoraphobic symptom presentation. The conceptual and philosophical models that guide existential and humanistic psychotherapists tend to address more global challenges of human existence and typically do not discuss patients in terms of specific nosological categories like agoraphobia. Therapeutic issues related to anxiety in general, however, have been discussed extensively (Bugental, 1978; May, 1980; Rogers, 1951). From existential and humanistic perspectives, clinical anxiety represents the perception of a fundamental threat to the individual; for example, a threat to the self-concept (Rogers, 1951) or to basic values held essential for existence (May, 1950). Existential and humanistic psychotherapists tend to differ in their basic view of human nature, but both adhere to clinical models which emphasize the necessity of creating a facilitative therapeutic relationship within which clients can experience, learn from, and integrate anxiety. The therapist's behavior is typically nondirective, and the focus of therapy is primarily on the client's subjective experience in the therapy session.

A third approach to the treatment of agoraphobia has come from cognitive and behavioral psychotherapies. Based upon the prevailing conditioned-learning models, early behavioral treatments for agoraphobia, like systematic desensitization and *in vivo* exposure (Marks, 1969; Weekes, 1976; Wolpe, 1990), were designed to decondition or extinguish anxiety responses and phobic behavior in agoraphobic situations. Whether through imagination or in real life, whether performed gradually or rapidly, "exposure" procedures confront patients with some form of the phobic object. Another group of interventions is designed to address deficits in anxiety management (Suinn, 1971), marital communication (Arnow, Taylor, Agras, & Telch, 1985), assertion (Emmelkamp, van der Hout, & de Vries, 1983), or self-statements (Emmelkamp, Kuipers, & Eggeraat, 1978), based on hypothesized relationships between these deficits and agoraphobic symptoms. Recently, a multicomponent cognitive-behavioral treatment designed specifically for panic disorder has been applied to agoraphobia (Beck & Emory, 1985; Clark, 1986; Klosko, Barlow, Tassinari, & Cerny, 1990). In addition to *in vivo* exposure, this treatment typically includes education, training in panic and anxiety management skills, cognitive restructuring of maladaptive beliefs, and interoceptive exposure (to the physical sensations associated with panic). All cognitive and behavioral treatments attempt to help patients change current maladaptive response patterns. The focus is upon modifying factors believed to be maintaining the agoraphobic symptoms. These treatments are further distinguished by the active and directive role played by therapists and procedures that emphasize patients' applying lessons or techniques learned in therapy to situations outside the treatment setting.

It is the goal of this chapter to examine research on these various techniques and orientations to answer some basic questions: What treatments have been found to be most effective with agoraphobia? Among them, which ones have been compared with placebo or another treatment condition? Under what conditions and for which symptoms has each treatment been effective? What are the apparent limitations and advantages of each treatment? Are the treatments cost-effective? What components of treatment are essential?

To help answer these questions, several aspects of the outcome literature on agoraphobia will be discussed. First, research involving single-case studies, treatment comparisons with nonspecific effects, and interorientation comparisons will be examined. Second, in the section on outcome parameters, overarching issues relevant to the evaluation of extant research will be addressed. Third, implications of pharmacotherapy research for assessing the merits and limitations of psychological treatments will be outlined. Finally, general conclusions will be summarized.

Single-Case Study Designs

Most single-case reports of the treatment of agoraphobia are anecdotal and tend to report significant clinical change, regardless of the intervention. Case reports have described agoraphobic patients successfully treated with hypnosis (London, 1981; Milne, 1988; Tilton, 1983; Wood, 1986; Yager, 1988), client-centered therapy (Tensch & Bohme, 1991), Jacobsonian-type relaxation (Jansson, Jerremalm, & Ost, 1986), marital therapy (Chernan & Friedman, 1990), psychoanalysis (Vangaard, 1987), and multimodal/eclectic approaches (Beckfield, 1987; Biran, 1987; Jackson, & Elton, 1985; Schwartz & Val, 1984). However, these reports do not include baseline levels of symptomatology, standardized measures, or comparisons with other treatment conditions. Thus, conclusions regarding the effectiveness of these interventions are difficult to make.

Two single-case studies, however, represent advances over the aforementioned reports. Frame, Turner, Jacob, and Szekeley (1984) evaluated the utility of graded self-exposure therapy using a single-subject design including baseline (35 days), treatment (60 days), posttest, and follow-up (18 months) scores on standard objective and subjective measures. They found clinically significant improvement from baseline to posttest on all measures, although there was evidence of deterioration at 18-month follow-up. Since the authors did not report their criteria for "clinically significant improvement," it is not clear if the subject maintained her level of improvement. However, no measures returned to baseline levels, suggesting that at least some clinically relevant gains were maintained. Frame *et al.*'s conclusions supported the use of self-directed exposure, but cautioned that the subject in this study was only moderately impaired and highly motivated to change.

Another single-case study (Zarate, Craske, & Barlow, 1990) included baseline data and standardized measures but also compared more than one treatment condition. Using a within-subjects design, Zarate *et al.* compared two forms of *in vivo* exposure (self-shaping and therapist-assisted) to a panic control treatment (PCT) consisting of education, challenging maladaptive cognitions, breathing retraining, and controlled exposure to somatic or interoceptive symptoms. Assessments were made at baseline, after each treatment, at posttreatment, and at 2-year follow-up. The PCT component appeared to be more effective than either of the exposure treatments in decreasing both anxiety and avoidance. While this study represents a substantial advance over prior case reports, conclusions must be tempered by its remaining limitations. Most notably, the fact that exposure therapy involved fewer sessions than, and was administered prior to, PCT may have blunted the apparent effects of exposure and inflated those of PCT. Limitations of this study notwithstanding, the idea that interventions which focus primarily on the cognitive and interoceptive features of panic may be useful for the treatment of agoraphobia is intriguing and merits further study.

Treatment Comparisons with Nonspecific Effects

As discussed in the section on single-case studies, specificity of a treatment effect cannot be established simply by demonstrating beneficial results. A treatment's unique and essential effects must be directly compared to those of other treatment conditions. Unfortunately, there are no studies comparing different psychodynamic therapies to one another or to placebo, nor have such comparisons been made regarding the humanistic/existential psychotherapies. Studies reviewed in this section are limited primarily to those examining cognitive-behavioral interventions. Among these interventions, exposure-based therapies are the most thoroughly studied. Three types of investigations have been conducted: (1) comparisons of *in vivo* exposure versus some other cognitive-behavioral intervention, (2) comparisons of different ways to administer *in vivo* exposure, and (3) comparisons of *in vivo* exposure with and without another treatment.

Comparisons of In Vivo *Exposure to Other Treatments*

***In Vivo* versus Imaginal Exposure.** The literature comparing the effects of *in vivo* versus imaginal exposure is limited. *In vivo* exposure has produced more significant improvement than imaginal exposure on behavioral and subjective measures of phobic avoidance, and the concurrent use of imaginal exposure does not appear to enhance the effects of *in vivo* exposure (Emmelkamp & Wessels, 1975). However, subjects receiving *in vivo* treatment have demonstrated less phobic avoidance when pretreated with imaginal exposure than subjects receiving *in vivo* exposure alone (Mathews, Johnston, Shaw, & Gelder, 1974). This finding suggests that imaginal exposure may have a "priming" effect that could enhance the effectiveness of subsequent *in vivo* exposure.

***In Vivo* Exposure versus Relaxation Training.** There is some evidence that relaxation training may play a role in the treatment of agoraphobia, but results have been inconsistent. In one study comparing *in vivo* exposure to applied relaxation (Jansson *et al.*, 1986), both treatments improved subjective and behavioral measures of agoraphobic symptoms at posttest and 15-month follow-up. Although the relaxation group deteriorated after 7 months, it had recovered by the 15-month follow-up assessment. The effects of exposure may be more stable, but these findings suggest that relaxation techniques produce comparable long-term results.

In another study (Alstrom, Nordlund, Persson, Harding, & Ljungqvist (1983), relaxation training was found to be more successful in decreasing symptoms associated with agoraphobia than either self-exposure or therapist-assisted exposure in women "suitable for insight-oriented therapy." Alstrom *et al.* (1983) also found that prolonged, therapist-assisted exposures were least helpful in decreasing symptoms. Dropouts occurred only in the prolonged exposure group.

In contrast, McNamee, O'Sullivan, Lelliot & Marks (1989) found that a group of housebound agoraphobics given self-exposure instructions over the phone and by mail improved significantly more than a group of housebound agoraphobics given relaxation tapes. Differences between the two groups were maintained at 12 weeks posttreatment and at 32 weeks follow-up. Interestingly, even though the exposure group improved more than the relaxation group, the former experienced greater dropout.

Comparisons of Different Ways to Administer In Vivo *Exposure*

Massed versus Gradual Exposure. Both massed and gradual administrations of exposure have been effective at posttreatment. Massed exposure produces higher dropout rates when compared to graded exposure (Emmelkamp & Wessels, 1975), but reduces avoidance more rapidly for those patients who complete treatment (Foa, Jameson, Turner, & Payne, 1980). Relapse rates for subjects participating in prolonged, massed exposure tend to exceed those of gradual, self-paced exposure (Jansson & Ost, 1982; Trull, Neitzel, & Main, 1988), though this finding has not been universal (Chambless, 1990).

Group versus Individual Exposure. Despite the personal attention received in individual therapy, Gray and McPherson (1982) found group treatment at least as effective as individual treatment, and Trull *et al.* (1988) found a larger effect size for group treatment. Better outcomes were associated with group treatment at anxiety disorder or outpatient clinics, but individual treatment had superior results at university psychiatry settings (Trull *et al.*, 1988). Although the reasons for these findings are not clear, differences in training and/or experience of the therapist could have been a contributing factor.

Self-Directed versus Therapist-Assisted Exposure. Several studies suggest that self-directed and therapist-assisted methods of administering exposure are of equal benefit (Carr, Ghosh, & Marks, 1988; Ghosh & Marks, 1987; Jannoun, Munby, Catalan, & Gelder, 1980; Mathews, Teasdale, Munby, Johnston, & Shaw, 1977). In addition to being less expensive, self-directed exposure has been found to instill a sense of mastery over treatment and symptoms (Ghosh & Marks, 1987) and encourages patients to decrease dependency on their therapist (Mathews *et al.*, 1977). In particular, Mathews *et al.* (1977) noted that treatment gains tended to diminish if dependency on the therapist developed, suggesting that, for some individuals, self-directed exposure may provide more stable improvement. However, it is likely that a subsample of agoraphobics requires the assistance of a therapist.

Comparisons of In Vivo *Exposure with and without Another Treatment*

Given that *in vivo* exposure is not consistently effective, some investigators have explored whether certain interventions are able to augment the effects of exposure treatment. Marital or couples therapy, cognitive therapy, and paradoxical intention are the only treatments that have been systematically evaluated as adjuncts to *in vivo* exposure.

Exposure versus Exposure Plus Couples Therapy. The effects of the marital relationship on agoraphobic symptoms has been demonstrated by a number of investigators (Craske, Burton, & Barlow, 1989; Emmelkamp, 1980; Milton & Haffner, 1979). These studies suggest that marital communication is important for treatment success and maintenance, but they do not directly compare exposure with and without marital therapy. Data that are available, however, suggest that including spouses in treatment enhances the effects of exposure-based therapy.

Barlow, O'Brien, and Last (1984) found that agoraphobic women demonstrated greater improvement on behavioral and subjective measures of phobic avoidance when spouses were included in treatment than when spouses did not participate. Both groups had improved at posttreatment, but subjects in the spouse-assisted group demonstrated significantly greater improvement. Interestingly, there was no difference in the amount of *in vivo* practice between spouse-assisted and non-spouse-assisted groups. Cerny, Barlow, Craske, and Himadi (1987) found similar results. A group that received *in vivo* exposure with spouse involvement had higher end-state functioning and greater marital satisfaction for up to 2 years posttreatment than a group that received *in vivo* exposure without spouse involvement.

Improving couples' communication skills has also been found to enhance the effects of graded, *in vivo* exposure, when compared to relaxation training for couples (Arnow *et al.*, 1985). Arnow *et al.* found that all subjects in the study improved on subjective and behavioral measures of agoraphobic avoidance after 4 weeks of spouse-assisted *in vivo* exposure. However, the group with couples that received communication training subsequent to the exposure component of treatment demonstrated significantly greater improvement than the group with couples receiving postexposure relaxation training. These differences were maintained at 8-months follow-up.

Only one study (Cobb, Mathews, Childs-Clarke, & Blowers, 1984) failed to find greater clinical improvement in agoraphobics whose spouses were involved in treatment than in those whose spouses were uninvolved. However, uninvolved spouses did have limited contact with the therapist, which could have influenced these findings.

Exposure versus Exposure Plus Cognitive Interventions. There is conflicting evidence regarding the efficacy of cognitive interventions as an adjunct to exposure. Cognitive interventions do not appear to be effective as the sole means of modifying agoraphobia (Emmelkamp *et al.*, 1978; Emmelkamp & Mersch, 1982). For example, Williams and Rappoport (1983) found that improvements in phobic avoidance were no different between agoraphobics with driving phobias receiving *in vivo* driving exposure alone versus those receiving the same exposure plus cognitive interventions, (i.e., distraction, coping statements, and positive self-statements). Subjects reported that cognitive interventions were helpful 79% of the time, but these interventions did not appear to add to the efficacy of the driving exposure.

Emmelkamp, Brilman, Kuiper, and Mersch (1986) found similar results comparing the effects of self-instructional training, rational emotive therapy (RET), and therapist-assisted *in vivo* exposure. Self-instruction included relabeling, homework assignments of identifying and countering negative thoughts, and practicing these interventions in imagination. RET followed a standard A-B-C format, with A being the activating event, B being the belief about the event, and C being the emotional or behavioral consequence. This component also included readings on RET and active challenging of subjects' beliefs by the therapist. Only the therapist-assisted group received exposures. The authors found that *in vivo* exposure was consistently superior to cognitive interventions, as assessed by performance on a behavioral approach test and an assessment battery including measures of phobic anxiety and avoidance. When *in vivo* exposure was added to the two cognitive interventions, all subjects improved significantly. The authors concluded that cognitive interventions do not enhance the effects of *in vivo* exposure. However, the design of the study does not control adequately for order of treatment.

One study has found that cognitive interventions enhance the effects of *in vivo* exposure (Marchione, Michelson, Greenwald, & Dancu, 1987). Comparing graded, therapist-assisted *in vivo* exposure alone and the same exposure protocol combined either with 1 hour a week of Beckian cognitive therapy or with 1 hour a week of relaxation training, subjects in the two combined treatment groups completed a behavioral approach test at posttreatment with significantly less anxiety than subjects receiving graded exposure alone. In addition, the combined treatment groups improved more on measures of physiological arousal, and only the cognitive therapy group increased the number of positive self-statements during exposure. End-state functioning was highly improved for 100% of the subjects in the two combined therapy groups, while only 25% of the exposure-alone group was highly improved, based on composite measures of phobic anxiety and avoidance, self-ratings of severity, and therapists' global assessment of severity.

It is clear that the role of cognitive interventions in the treatment of agoraphobia requires further study. One consideration for future research designs is that the impact of cognitive interventions may be delayed compared to behavioral interventions like exposure (Emmelkamp & Mersch, 1982). Also, cognitive therapy is a term that refers to several different interventions and approaches that may not be applied uniformly across studies. Therefore, it is difficult to draw general conclusions regarding the utility of "cognitive therapy."

Exposure versus Exposure Plus Paradoxical Intention. Paradoxical intention has been described by some authors as a "cognitive" intervention (e.g., Michelson, Mavissakalian, & Marchione, 1985) and by others as a "behavioral" intervention (Ascher, 1981). For the purpose of this chapter, paradoxical intention is examined separately from cognitive therapy.

Asking subjects to focus on and attempt to increase symptoms of anxiety is the way in which the principle of paradoxical intention has been applied to agoraphobia (Ascher, 1981). Paradoxical intention was designed to enhance the effects of *in vivo* exposure by helping patients reduce self-induced anxiety in phobic situations (Michelson & Ascher, 1984).

Ascher (1981) found that subjects given instructions in paradoxical intention prior to starting *in vivo* exposure improved more rapidly on a behavioral approach test than subjects who started with *in vivo* exposure and received instructions for paradoxical intention later. One problem with this study is that informal criteria were used to diagnose agoraphobia. However, similar results have been found by Mavissakalian, Michelson, Greenwald, Kornblith, & Greenwald (1983) and by Ascher, Schotte, & Grayson (1986) using subjects meeting DSM-III criteria for agoraphobia. Ascher *et al.* (1986) also found that paradoxical intention itself can be enhanced by the addition of cognitive restructuring and paradoxical intention in imagination.

The ability of paradoxical intention to enhance the effects of exposure has not been a universal finding, however. Michelson *et al.* (1985, 1988) found no significant posttreatment differences on behavioral, physiological, and subjective measures of anxiety and phobic avoidance between agoraphobic groups receiving either therapist-assisted *in vivo* exposure alone, self-exposure in combination with paradoxical intention, or self-exposure in combination with relaxation training. Although the exposure-alone and relaxation training groups appeared to change more rapidly than the paradoxical intention group, it should be noted that there was no condition in which paradoxical intention was paired with therapist-assisted exposure which would have been a more appropriate control group to compare with therapist-assisted exposure alone.

Interorientation Comparisons

Another way to assess a treatment is to compare its effects with those of treatments derived from other theoretical models. In this section, we review outcome studies that have included direct comparisons between psychological treatments from two or more different schools of psychotherapy. Thus far, interorientation comparisons involving agoraphobia have been limited to studies examining the relative efficacy of psychodynamic and cognitive-behavioral approaches. There are no published studies comparing existential/humanistic psychotherapies with either a psychodynamic or a cognitive-behavioral psychotherapy.

Four studies have directly compared psychodynamic and cognitive-behavioral treatments for agoraphobia (Alstrom *et al.*, 1984; Gelder, Marks, Wolff, & Clark, 1967; Hoffart & Martinsen, 1990; and Klein, Zitrin, Woerner, & Ross, 1983). However, because all of the subjects in these studies appear to have received exposure of some kind, conclusions about the independent effects of treatments cannot be made. It is possible, however, to begin to evaluate the relative additive effects of psychodynamic psychotherapy versus cognitive-behavioral interventions other than *in vivo* exposure. Thus far, results have been inconsistent.

Two studies found no differences between psychodynamic and behavioral procedures. Gelder *et al.* (1967) compared individual psychodynamic psychotherapy, analytically oriented group therapy, and individual, graded self-exposure combined with imaginal desensitization. At posttreatment, the desensitization group had experienced a more rapid improvement than the other two groups. However, by follow-up, differences between groups were no longer significant because of eventual improvements in the two nonbehavioral groups.

Klein *et al.* (1983) also found little difference in effectiveness between behavior therapy (imaginal desensitization, self-directed *in vivo* exposure, and assertion training) plus either imipramine or placebo, and psychodynamically oriented supportive psychotherapy plus either imipramine or placebo. All groups improved equally on self-report, therapist report, and independent observer evaluations. However, the supportive psychotherapy group also received instructions to confront their fears, though this was not considered part of the experimental protocol. They did not report follow-up data, so it is unknown if the treatments continued to be equally effective.

One study (Alstrom *et al.*, 1984) found psychodynamic psychotherapy superior to behavior therapy. Agoraphobic women "not suitable for insight-oriented therapy" improved more when self-exposure, education, and anxiolytic medication was combined with insight-oriented therapy than when combined with either therapist-assisted, massed, *in vivo* exposure or relaxation training. These results must be interpreted with caution because the authors did not define a number of important variables, including what constituted nonsuitability for insight-oriented therapy, measures used to assess symptoms, or what constituted "recovery."

A fourth study (Hoffart & Martinsen, 1990) found behavior therapy more effective than psychodynamic psychotherapy. Inpatient agoraphobics concurrently treated with psychodynamically oriented group therapy, occupational and milieu therapy, and individual psychotherapy improved more when formal training in self-exposure was added to their treatment plan. They found that 58% of subjects trained in self-exposure improved on measures of avoidance compared to 41% of subjects simply advised to confront their fears. By follow-up, the importance of training in self-exposure was more evident. They found that 51% of the self-exposure group had maintained improvement on measures of avoidance, while only 26% of the psychotherapy-only group had.

Three of the four studies comparing psychodynamic and cognitive-behavioral treatments reported dropout rates. Two studies found that subjects who received behavior therapy were more likely to drop out (Alstrom *et al.*, 1984; Gelder *et al.*, 1967), while one study found that subjects given psychotherapy only dropped out at a greater rate than subjects who were also given exposure therapy (Hoffart & Martinsen, 1990). Additionally, Hoffart and Martinsen (1990) reported that nearly 30% of the group receiving only psychotherapy failed to return follow-up data at 1-year posttreatment, compared to full compliance by the exposure group.

Outcome Parameters

Results of single-case studies, treatment comparisons with nonspecific effects, and interorientation comparisons must be interpreted in light of a number of factors. The data currently available leave many unanswered questions regarding the impact of potentially crucial variables on treatment outcome. In this section, we discuss three types of deficiencies in the research literature that should be considered before drawing conclusions about the efficacy of treatments available for agoraphobia: (1) failures to report critical information, (2) methodological limitations, and (3) inattention to alternative indices of outcome.

Failures to Report Critical Information

This section focuses on information missing from treatment outcome reports that could be important in forming judgments regarding treatment efficacy. For example, many studies fail to indicate the experience level of the treatment staff (e.g., Emmelkamp *et al.*, 1978; Liddell *et al.*, 1986). This oversight is important given that level of training may be related to the effectiveness with which treatment for agoraphobia is applied (Aronson, 1987). One meta-analysis of agoraphobia treatment studies revealed a more positive outcome associated with more experienced therapists (Trull *et al.*, 1988).

Studies also often neglect to fully describe treatment interventions (e.g., Alstrom *et al.*, 1983, 1984). In a study by Franklin (1989), for example, the design excludes a specific exposure component, yet all conditions appear to involve self-directed exposure. Authors may fail to provide the details of a particular treatment intervention (e.g., Emmelkamp, 1974; Emmelkamp & Mersch, 1982; Emmelkamp & Wessels, 1975; Everaerd, Rijken, & Emmelkamp, 1973) or neglect to describe any of the interventions used (e.g., Aronson, 1987; Liddell *et al.*, 1986). Inadequate descriptions of treatment leave the reader at a disadvantage and make it difficult for researchers and clinicians to replicate interventions.

Another frequent reporting failure is the absence of sufficient information about medication. When patients receive concomitant drug treatments, details concerning the types or dosages of the drugs presented are often not reported (e.g., Burns, Thorpe, & Cavallaro, 1986; Franklin, 1989; Liddell *et al.*, 1986; Mavissakalian, 1986; Zitrin, Klein, & Woerner, 1980). Assessing outcome is always more complicated when two forms of treatment are confounded. However, the demonstrated effectiveness of pharmacotherapy makes the omission of this type of information particularly problematic when attempting to evaluate the efficacy of psychological interventions for agoraphobia.

Methodological Limitations

Problems Related to Diagnosis. Another difficulty in evaluating treatments for agoraphobia is the use of different diagnostic criteria in various studies. In some cases, DSM-III (American Psychiatric Association, 1983) criteria are used (e.g., Ascher *et al.*, 1986). More recent studies use DSM-III-R nosology (American Psychiatric Association, 1987) (e.g., Zarate *et al.*, 1990). In other studies (e.g., Ascher, 1981), diagnostic criteria are based on clinical judgment. As a result, different diagnostic criteria are likely to result in different sample characteristics, which of course complicates the process of evaluating and comparing various studies.

One significant way in which samples may vary is comorbidity. Between 40%and 65% of a sample of agoraphobics has been found to have a personality disorder (Brooks, Baltazar, & Munjack, 1989). Gray and McPherson (1982) observed that early studies used severely agoraphobic subjects and did not exclude subjects diagnosed with major depression. Greater levels of psychopathology have been found to be related to increased avoidance (Rapee & Murrell, 1988), and comorbidity is likely to influence the duration of an anxiety disorder (Aronson, 1987).

Problems in Subject Selection. Research subjects are never selected randomly from the larger population of agoraphobics. Uniformity across patients who participate in research and those who do not cannot be assumed (Chambless, 1985, 1990). This issue is particularly germane to the agoraphobia literature. For example, distance from the clinic, the nature of the patient's fears, and availability of a "safe" person may all influence whether an agoraphobic individual agrees to, or remains in, treatment. The extent to which treatments applied to patients who volunteer for research are applicable to other agoraphobics is unclear.

Inconsistencies in Therapist Behavior. Another important source of influence on treatment outcome may involve informal or subtle aspects of the therapist's behavior. Behavioral approach tests have been found to improve from an average of 28.7% to 68% of end goal when therapists gradually decreased their use of empathy and included instruction and education. In contrast, an approach which relied more on negotiation and reminding patients of negative consequences resulted in poorer outcomes (Gustavson, Jensson, Jerremalm, & Öst, 1985). In addition, a significant association has been found between improvement on behavioral approach tests and therapists whose behavior was perceived as self-confident, caring, and involved (Williams & Chambless, 1990). These aspects of the therapist's behavior have seldom been systematically addressed in agoraphobia research and may contribute to differences in outcome between groups or between studies.

Lack of External Validity. Evaluation of treatment outcome studies must also consider the extent to which treatments are externally valid, that is, how well they represent the way in which treatment is or can be practiced in most clinical settings. For example, although necessary for research purposes, the isolation of cognitive and behavioral components of a treatment intervention (e.g., Emmelkamp *et al.*, 1978; Emmelkamp & Mersch, 1982; Klosko *et al.*, 1990; Michelson *et al.*, 1985; Zarate *et al.*, 1990) may not reflect how treatment is actually conducted by clinicians.

Along these same lines, protocol-driven or standardized therapies may be effective, but they do not represent the way in which therapy is conducted in the clinician's office. Additionally, agoraphobics are not necessarily in treatment for the 8 to 12 weeks that research protocols often specify. Clinicians typically design therapy to meet the needs of the individual patient rather than follow a standardized protocol. It is therefore difficult to assess the external validity of treatment outcome studies until attempts are made to document the application of experimental treatments in clinical settings.

Limitations of Frequently Used Outcome Measures. Another problem concerns how change is assessed and whether what is measured is clinically meaningful for agoraphobic individuals. One complication arises when scores from several self-report instruments are combined to yield an agoraphobia end-state functioning score. The magnitude of these scores can be inflated due to uncontrolled multicollinearity. Measurement problems also arise when researchers investigating agoraphobia treatment create instruments specific to the needs of their own study (e.g., Alstrom *et al.*, 1984). Use of such idiosyncratic instruments makes comparisons across studies difficult, and the frequent absence of psychometric data further limits confidence in the accuracy of whatever outcome measures are used.

Finally, few studies use reports of significant others or independent quality-of-life indicators as a means of determining outcome. As a result, use of multimethod batteries for assessing change in agoraphobic symptoms has been recommended (Ogles, Lambert, Weight, & Payne, 1990), a reasonable suggestion given the degree to which anxiety and avoidance affect the quality of an agoraphobic's life. Likewise, use of multiple behavioral approach tests would help assess if treatment gains have generalized to commonly encountered phobic situations.

Inattention to Alternative Indices of Outcome

Traditionally, the utility of treatments has been determined by evaluating the posttreatment status of patients' symptoms. However, more recently, the importance of other indices of outcome has been recognized. In this section, we discuss outcome indicators that are less frequently addressed in the literature—acceptance and completion rates, maintenance of treatment gains, and consumer satisfaction.

Acceptance and Completion of Treatment. Two of the standards by which treatment outcome has recently begun to be evaluated are treatment completion, or dropout rate, and treatment acceptance. Unfortunately, neither of these standards is uniformly handled by researchers.

Learning more about differences between subjects who dropout and those who remain in treatment could influence how future treatments for agoraphobia are designed. For instance, Chambless (1990) found no significant differences in dropout rates for subjects participating in massed versus spaced exposure groups. She did caution, however, that a number of potential subjects refused to participate because of possible assignment to the massed-exposure condition. Additionally, Aronson (1987) found that dropout rates were higher for patients referred by their physician compared to rates for those who were self-referred.

Subjects are an important source of information for the reasons behind treatment failures and dropouts, yet only one study (Gournay, 1991) systematically queried subjects to determine possible differences between treatment successes and failures. Treatment failure was defined by objective criteria on both behavioral measures and questionnaires, and included individuals who had not responded to treatment, relapsed, dropped out of treatment, or refused treatment. By this definition, 44% of the patients failed treatment. The most common reasons for treatment dropout were feeling the therapist did not understand, being frightened of therapy, finding out that the treatment approach was not what was expected, and believing that one had to overcome ones fears without the help of others. The most common reasons for treatment failure were too much anxiety, symptom improvement, feeling the therapist did not understand, receipt of further help, and a worsening of symptoms. The only significant difference between those who successfully completed treatment and those who failed was that the former reported higher levels of marital satisfaction.

Maintenance of Initial Gains. Just as it is important to evaluate outcome when treatment is terminated, it is equally important to assess whether treatment gains are stable or change over time. In general, benefits from treatment of agoraphobia have been maintained at follow-up (Chambless, 1985; Jacobson, Wilson, & Tupper, 1988). However, specific treatments may vary in the length of time necessary for gains to be consolidated. For example, between-group differences apparent at posttreatment have lost significance by follow-up assessment (e.g., Emmelkamp & Mersch, 1982). The effects of certain interventions, such as cognitive therapy, may take longer to be effective, and gains may be apparent only at longer-term follow-up (Emmelkamp & Mersch, 1982). It is also possible that one intervention primes a patient in such a way that the efficacy of interventions which follow are enhanced (e.g., Franklin, 1989; Mathews *et al.*, 1974). It is easy to see how different conclusions regarding efficacy are possible depending upon whether outcome is evaluated at posttreatment or at follow-up.

The definition of relapse is another issue relevant to assessing maintenance of gains. A fairly consistent finding across studies is that agoraphobic patients improve as a result of treatment but are neither symptom-free nor "cured" (Burns *et al.*, 1986; Chambless, 1985; Franklin, 1989; Jacobson *et al.*, 1988; Klosko *et al.*, 1990). As residual symptoms remain, it is not surprising to find that subjects often receive additional treatment during the follow-up period (e.g., Burns *et al.*, 1986; McPherson, Brougham, & McLaren, 1980). In some cases, receiving additional treatment has been interpreted as a relapse. However, as Chambless (1985) has observed, those seeking additional treatment may want to reduce agoraphobic symptoms further or work on another problem altogether. Likewise, one cannot assume that subjects have not relapsed just because they have not pursued further treatment. For agoraphobics in particular, logistical or financial constraints may interfere with the pursuit of treatment (Chambless, 1985). Relapse can also be defined by the persistence of symptoms subsequent to treatment, but patients sometimes note that they are confident they can cope with their residual anxiety (Liddell *et al.*, 1986) and consequently may not feel impaired. Because there is no simple way to define and measure relapse, various methods may need to be used if the long-term outcome of treatment is to be fully understood.

Consumer Satisfaction. Consumer satisfaction is another neglected index of outcome. Satisfaction with treatment may influence whether patients apply the skills they learn in therapy or may affect their willingness to seek further help in the future. The agoraphobia literature has not, thus far, evaluated consumer satisfaction with any form of psychological treatment.

Psychopharmacology

In addition to the psychological treatments reviewed in this chapter, a number of drugs have been used to treat agoraphobia. It is not within the scope of this chapter to provide a comprehensive review of the pharmacotherapy of agoraphobia. Rather, our discussion is limited to those aspects of the pharmacotherapy literature relevant to evaluating the relative benefits and limitations of psychological treatments.

In controlled trials, medications like alprazolam (Ballenger *et al.*, 1988; Charney *et al.*, 1986; Dunner, Ishiki, Avery, Wilson, &Hyde, 1986; Fyer *et al.*, 1987; Pecknold, Swinson, Kuch, & Lewis, 1988), clonazepam (Tesar & Rosenbaum, 1986), phenelzine (Sheehan, Ballenger, & Jacobsen, 1980), and imipramine (Ballenger *et al.*, 1988; Evans, Kenardy, Schneider, & Hoey, 1986; Marks *et al.*, 1983; Matuzas, Uhlenhuth, Glass, Javaid, & Davis, 1986; Mavissakalian & Michelson, 1986; Zitrin *et al.*, 1980; Zitrin, Klein, Woerner, & Ross, 1983) have been found to be more effective than placebo in reducing one or more of the primary symptoms of agoraphobia. Presently, the effects of these different drugs appear to be equivalent (Ballenger *et al.*, 1988; Charney *et al.*, 1986; Herman, Rosenbaum, & Brotman, 1987; Rizley, Kahn, McNair, & Frankenthaler, 1986; Sheehan *et al.*, 1980).

One important area of research concerns how the outcome of psychological treatment compares to that of pharmacotherapy. The number of studies directly comparing drug and psychological treatments is limited, but some preliminary conclusions can be drawn by examining outcome data such as dropout rates, success rates, and relapse rates across studies. In a recent review of both controlled and uncontrolled studies of the treatment of agoraphobia, Clum (1989) found that 18% of individuals receiving behavior therapy dropped out before completing treatment. This rate was not significantly different than the 14% dropout rate reported for patients receiving high-potency benzodiazepines (e.g., alprazolam, clonazepam), and it was significantly lower than the 34% and 41% rates reported for patients taking either tricyclic antidepressants or monoamine oxidase inhibitors, respectively. Because data were pooled from various studies with different methodologies, Clum's comparisons between types of treatment are vulnerable to many uncontrolled sources of error. However, similar findings have been reported by the few investigators who have directly compared dropout rates from psychological and pharmacological treatments in the same study (Klosko *et al.*, 1990; Zitrin *et al.*, 1983). Again, these limited data suggest that behavioral therapies and benzodiazepines have lower dropout rates than do the antidepressants.

For patients who complete therapy, psychological and pharmacological treatments appear to be roughly equivalent in reducing the symptoms of agoraphobia by posttreatment assessment. Clum's (1989) review, for instance, found that the percentage of agoraphobics classified as "significantly improved" after treatment was between 60% and 65% both for behavioral as well as drug treatments and for drugs such as alprazolam and imipramine. Outcomes have also been roughly equivalent the few times behavioral and drug treatment approaches have been applied independently and compared within the same investigation (Klosko *et al.*, 1990; Telch *et al.*, 1985).

Even if psychological and pharmacological interventions have comparable effects upon global assessments of clinical improvement, they might have differential effects upon specific symptoms of agoraphobia. Drug treatments like imipramine or alprazolam were originally believed to impact agoraphobia specifically by suppressing panic attacks (Klein, 1964; Sheehan & Sheehan, 1982). Alternatively, behavioral strategies like *in vivo* exposure were proposed to have a more immediate effect upon phobic avoidance (Klein, Ross, & Cohen, 1987; Mavissakalian, 1984). However, outcome data have not unequivocally supported assumptions regarding treatment specificity. Drug treatments have reduced phobic avoidance (Mavissakalian, Michelson, & Dealy, 1983; Ballenger *et al.*, 1988), and *in vivo* exposure has resulted in the elimination of panic attacks (Marks *et al.*, 1983; Mavissakalian & Michelson, 1986). Psychological and drug treatments may impact different symptoms of agoraphobia, but further research is needed to establish the nature and extent of these differential effects.

Some differences do emerge from data on the long-term effects of treatment. Existing data suggest that clinical benefits derived from medication are not maintained as well as those derived from psychological treatment, particularly when medication is terminated. Clum (1989) found a relapse rate of 18% for behavior therapies versus 27% for high-potency benzodiazepines and 23–34% for tricyclic antidepressants, but some of these drug treatments were used in combination with psychological treatments. There are currently no follow-up data available beyond 1-year posttreatment for patients treated with medication alone. When medication has been discontinued and no psychological treatment provided, relapse rates have ranged from 30% to 100% (Mavissakalian & Michelson, 1986; Sheehan, 1986; Solyom *et al.*, 1973).

Given that neither psychological nor drug treatment is consistently effective, it is not surprising that many authorities (Balestrieri, Ruggori, & Bellatuono, 1989; Lydiard & Ballenger, 1987; Mavissakalian, 1990) recommend integrating the two forms of therapy. However, it has been argued that medication might retard the efficacy of behavior therapy, either by interfering with the habituation of anxiety or by diminishing self-confidence because patients would attribute their recovery to the drug instead of themselves (Gray, 1987; Telch, 1988). There are several studies documenting the efficacy of combining pharmacotherapy with a psychological therapy in the treatment of agoraphobia (Cox *et al.*, 1988; Nagy, Krystal, Woods, & Charney, 1989; Sheehan *et al.*, 1980), but there are very little data available to indicate whether a combined approach is significantly more effective than either treatment alone.

One exception has been the combined use of imipramine and *in vivo* exposure. A small number of studies (Mavissakalian & Michelson, 1986; Telch *et al.*, 1985; Zitrin *et al.*, 1980, 1983) suggest that the effects of *in vivo* exposure on agoraphobic avoidance are enhanced by the concomitant use of imipramine. Only one study (Marks *et al.*, 1983) did not obtain this result. However, another finding suggests that adding imipramine to behavior therapy may increase the relapse rate (Zitrin *et al.*, 1980). Assessing the impact of adding exposure to imipramine is hampered by, among other things, the frequent coadministration of the two treatments. The one study (Telch *et al.*, 1985) which did administer the two treatments separately found that exposure enhanced imipramine's effects. There is preliminary evidence that the addition of behavior therapy to drug therapy might increase the number of patients that can withdraw from medication safely and effectively (Cottraux, Mollard, Duinat, & Riviere, 1986), but more studies are needed.

One final point should be made concerning outcome data on the pharmacotherapy of agoraphobia. Most drug studies have confounded some form of psychological treatment, typically *in vivo* exposure, with pharmacotherapy. This has led some reviewers (Cox, Swinson, & Endler, 1991; Marks & O'Sullivan, 1988; Telch, Tearman, & Taylor, 1983) to question whether sufficient evidence exists to justify conclusions about the independent effects of drug therapies upon agoraphobia. While medications like alprazolam and imipramine do seem to have some impact on agoraphobic symptoms, elucidation of the extent of that impact must await research designed to assess independent as well as combined effects of pharmacological and psychological treatments.

Conclusions

Agoraphobia is now recognized as a clinically significant psychiatric disorder that affects a substantial portion of the general population. A review of uncontrolled case reports alone would suggest that agoraphobia can be treated successfully with a variety of different psychological interventions and psychotherapeutic approaches. However, although limitations of the existing research literature preclude designating any single intervention as necessary and sufficient, the evidence does indicate that successful treatment of agoraphobia is the result of more than nonspecific factors. Some conclusions can be offered.

An impressive collection of outcome studies provide compelling evidence that having agoraphobics confront the situations they fear is sometimes sufficient, frequently necessary, and usually beneficial. Approximately 60–70% of patients treated with *in vivo* exposure experience moderate or greater reductions in symptoms. This finding is relatively consistent across studies, irrespective of whether the exposure is administered individually or in a group format, or whether it is largely self-directed or therapist-assisted.

Given that 30–40% of agoraphobic patients receive limited or no benefit from *in vivo* exposure, it can also be concluded that exposure to feared stimuli is sometimes insufficient or not beneficial. It is therefore imperative that careful attention be given to determining the most effective ways to administer exposure, developing interventions that enhance the effects of exposure, and discovering effective alternative treatments for patients who do not respond to exposure-based therapies.

Regarding the administration of exposure, there appears to be a variety of ways to confront phobic situations that have therapeutic value. However, graded or gradual exposure may result in lower dropout and relapse rates than rapid or massed exposure. There is some evidence that the effects of exposure can be enhanced by the use of adjunctive treatments. For example, selective inclusion of spouses or significant others in therapy can be helpful. In addition, providing patients with cognitive or behavioral strategies for managing anxiety and panic may potentiate the effects of exposure. It has been proposed that newly developed cognitive-behavioral treatments designed specifically to reduce panic attacks may be useful adjuncts or alternatives to *in vivo* exposure, but data to support this position are preliminary.

The difficulty of evaluating the efficacy of psychological treatments other than *in vivo* exposure is that outcome studies have rarely tested these treatments except in combination with some form of *in vivo* exposure. Therefore, the existing literature does not allow an adequate assessment of the independent effects of non-exposure-based psychotherapies. Results of studies that do evaluate the relative additive effects of psychodynamic versus cognitive-behavioral psychotherapies have been inconsistent and, in aggregate, suggest that neither approach is superior, either to the other or to *in vivo* exposure alone. There are currently no controlled studies upon which to base an evaluation of existential, humanistic, or systems-based psychotherapies as treatments for agoraphobia, with or without exposure therapy.

When compared to pharmacotherapy, cognitive-behavioral interventions have generally had equivalent effects at posttreatment assessment. Compared to medication, psychological treatments tend to take longer to be effective and require more effort on the part of the patient, but have better long-term outcome and fewer physical side effects. At least for *in vivo* exposure therapy, dropout rates are comparable to those found for the benzodiazepines, but lower than those reported for the antidepressants. The benefits and liabilities of combining psychological and pharmacological treatments have rarely been examined systematically, but some evidence suggests that a combination of *in vivo* exposure and imipramine is more effective than either treatment alone.

As with most areas of psychotherapy research, study of the treatment of agoraphobia needs a great deal more attention. Controlled investigations are needed which use standardized and multiple measures of outcome and which address one or more specific research questions or issues. One important goal for future research is to attempt to discover ways to improve the efficacy of *in vivo* exposure by increasing the proportion of individuals that respond favorably or by increasing the extent of recovery experienced by each individual. For example, cognitive-behavioral treatments that have been effective in reducing panic attacks may prove to be useful adjuncts, or even alternatives, to *in vivo* exposure. The same may be said for psychodynamic, existential/humanistic, or other forms of psychotherapy which emphasize different aspects of psychological adjustment than those addressed directly by *in vivo* exposure. Accordingly, more attention should be devoted to evaluating interventions from schools of psychotherapy other than those derived from cognitive and behavioral models. It will be particularly important to assess treatment effects that are independent of, as well as those that are additive to, the effects of exposure. Likewise, the interactions between and comparative benefits of psychological and pharmacological treatments deserve further investigation.

It has been 25 years since Gordon Paul (1967) first provided the exemplar psychotherapy research question: "What treatment, by whom, is most effective for this individual with that specific problem, under which set of circumstances?" (p. 111). We are a long way from fully answering this question as it relates to agoraphobia. Nonetheless, there is now sufficient evidence to suggest that *in vivo* exposure applied in a variety of different ways and under a number of different circumstances is beneficial for most people with agoraphobia. In fact, there is reason to question the ethics of continuing to treat agoraphobic individuals without at least informing them of the option of exposure-based procedures. There is also enough evidence to at least consider including significant others in treatment and teaching patients strategies (e.g., relaxation, paradoxical intention) for managing the symptoms of anxiety and avoidance. Recognition of the value of these interventions represents the first step toward a comprehensive understanding of the psychological treatment of agoraphobia. The rapidly growing literature on this topic promises a better understanding in the near future.

References

Abraham, K. (1953). A constitutional basis of locomotor anxiety. In *Selected papers* (pp. 235–243). New York: Basic Books. (Original work published 1913).

Alstrom, J. E., Nordlund, C. L., Persson, G., Harding, M., & Ljungqvist, C. (1983). Effects of four treatment methods on agoraphobic women not suitable for insight-oriented psychotherapy. *Acta Psychiatrica Scandinavica, 70*, 1–17.

Alstrom, J. E., Nordlund, C. L., Persson, G., & Ljungqvist, C. (1984). Effects of three non-insight-oriented treatment methods on agoraphobic women suitable for insight-oriented psychotherapy. *Acta Psychiatrica Scandinavica, 70*, 18–27.

American Psychiatric Association. (1983). *Psychiatry update* (Vol. 111). Washington DC: Author.

American Psychiatric Association. (1987). *Diagnostic and statistical manual of mental disorders* (3rd ed.-revised). Washington, DC: Author.

Arnow, B. A., Taylor, C., Agras, W. S., & Telch, M. J. (1985). Enhancing agoraphobic treatment outcome by changing couples' communication patterns. *Behavior Therapy, 16*, 425–467.

Aronson, T. A. (1987). A follow-up of two panic disorder-agoraphobic study populations: The role of recruitment biases. *The Journal of Nervous & Mental Disease, 175*, 595–598.

Ascher, L. M. (1981). Employing paradoxical intention in the treatment of agoraphobia. *Behaviour Research and Therapy, 19*, 533–542.

Ascher, L. M., Schotte, D. E., & Grayson, J. B. (1986). Enhancing effectiveness of paradoxical intention in treating travel restriction in agoraphobia. *Behavior Therapy, 17*, 124–130.

Balestrieri, M., Ruggeri, M., & Bellatuono, C. (1989). Drug treatment of panic disorder—A critical review of a controlled clinical trial. *Psychiatric Development, 4*, 337–350.

Ballenger, J. C., Burrows, G. D., DuPont, R. L., Jr., Lesser, L. M., Noyes, R., Jr., Pecknold, J. C., Rifkin, A., & Swinson, R. P. (1988). Alprazolam in panic disorder and agoraphobia: Results from a multicenter trial. 1. Efficacy of short-term treatment. *Archives of General Psychiatry, 45*, 413–423.

Barlow, D. H., O'Brien, G. T., & Last, C. G. (1984). Couples treatment for agoraphobia. *Behavior Therapy, 15*, 41–58.

Beck, A. T., & Emory, G. (1985). *Anxiety disorders and phobias: A cognitive perspective*. New York: Basic Books.

Beckfield, G. F. (1987). Importance of altering global response style in the treatment of agoraphobia. *Psychotherapy, 24*, 752–758.

Benedikt, M. (1870). Uber Platschwindel. *Allegemeine Wiener Medizinsche Zeitung, 15*, 488.

Biran, M. W. (1987). Two-stage therapy for agoraphobia. *American Journal of Psychotherapy, 41*, 127–136.

Brooks, R. B., Baltazar, P. L., & Munjack, D. J. (1989). Co-occurrence of personality disorders with panic disorder, social phobia, and generalized anxiety disorder: A review of the literature. *Journal of Anxiety Disorders, 3*, 259–285.

Bugental, J. F. T. (1978). *Psychotherapy and process: The fundamentals of an existential-humanistic approach*. Reading, MA: Addison-Wesley.

Burns, L. E., Thorpe, G. E., & Cavallaro, L. A. (1986). Agoraphobia 8 years after behavioral treatment: A follow-up study with interview, self-report, and behavioral data. *Behavior Therapy, 17*, 580–591.

Carr, A. C., Ghosh, A., & Marks, I. M. (1988). Computer-supervised exposure treatment for phobias. *Canadian Journal of Psychiatry, 33*, 112–117.

Cerny, J. A., Barlow, D. H., Craske, M. G., & Himadi, W. G. (1987). Couples treatment of agoraphobia: A two-year follow-up. *Behavior Therapy, 18*, 401–415.

Chambless, D. L. (1985, November). *Follow-up research on agoraphobia*. Paper presented at the annual convention of the Association for the Advancement of Behavior Therapy, Houston, TX.

Chambless, D. L. (1990). Spacing of exposure sessions in treatment of agoraphobia and simple phobia. *Behavior Therapy, 21*, 217–229.

Chambless, D. L., Caputo, G. C., Bright, P., & Gallagher, R. (1984). Assessment of fear in agoraphobics: The body sensations questionnaire and the agoraphobic cognitions questionnaire. *Journal of Consulting and Clinical Psychology, 52*, 1090–1097.

Chambless, D. L., Goldstein, A. J., Gallagher, R., & Bright, P. (1986). Integrating behavior therapy and psychotherapy in treatment of agoraphobia. *Psychotherapy: Theory, Research, and Practice, 23*, 150–159.

Charney, D. S., Woods, S. W., Goodman, W. K., Rifkin, B., Kinch, M., Aiken, B., Quandrino, L. M., & Heninger, G. R. (1986). Drug treatment of panic disorder: The comparative efficacy of imipramine, alprazolam, and trazodone. *Journal of Clinical Psychiatry, 47*, 580–586.

Chernan, L., & Friedman, F. (1990, November). *Collateral spouse treatment to enhance the efficacy of individual behavior therapy with the agoraphobic*. Paper presented at the meeting of the Association for the Advancement of Behavior Therapy, San Francisco, CA.

Clark, D. M. (1986). A cognitive approach to panic. *Behaviour Research and Therapy, 24*, 461–470.

Clum, G. A. (1989). Psychological interventions vs. drugs in the treatment of panic. *Behavior Therapy, 20*, 429–457.

Cobb, J. P., Mathews, A. M., Childs-Clarke, A., & Blowers, C. M. (1984). The spouse as cotherapist in the treatment of agoraphobia. *British Journal of Psychiatry, 144*, 282–287.

Cordes, E. (1871). Die Platzangst (agoraphobie): Symptom einer erschopfungsparese. *Archiv fur Psychiatrie und Nervendrankheiten, 3*, 521–524.

Cottraux, J., Mollard, E., Duinat, A., & Riviere, B. (1986, November). *Psychotropic medication suppression or reduction after behavior therapy in 81 agoraphobics with panic attacks*. Paper presented at the American Association for the Advancement of Behavior Therapy, Chicago.

Cox, B. J., Ballenger, J. C., Laraia, M., Hobbs, W. R., Peterson, G. A., & Hucek, A. (1988). Different rates of improvement of different symptoms in combined pharmacological and behavioral treatment of agoraphobia. *Journal of Behavior Therapy and Experimental Psychiatry, 19*, 119–126.

Cox, B. J., Swinson, R. P., & Endler, N. S. (1991). A review of the psychopharmacology of panic disorder: Individual differences and non-specific factors. *Canadian Journal of Psychiatry, 36*, 130–138.

Craske, M. G., Burton, T., & Barlow, D. H. (1989). Relationships among measures of communication, marital satisfaction and exposure during couples treatment of agoraphobia. *Behaviour Research and Therapy, 27*, 131–140.

Deutsch, H. (1929). The genesis of agoraphobia. *International Journal of Psychoanalysis, 10*, 51–69.

Diamond, D. (1985). Panic attacks, hypochondriasis, and agoraphobia: A self-psychology formulation. *American Journal of Psychotherapy, 39*, 114–125.

Dunner, D. L., Ishiki, D., Avery, D. H., Wilson, L. G., & Hyde, T. S. (1986). Effect of alprazolam and diazepam on anxiety and panic attacks in panic disorder: A controlled study. *Journal of Clinical Psychiatry, 138*, 458–460.

Emmelkamp, P. M. G. (1974). Self-observation versus flooding in the treatment of agoraphobia. *Behaviour Research and Therapy, 12*, 229–237.

Emmelkamp, P. M. G. (1980). Agoraphobics' interpersonal problems. *Archives of General Psychiatry, 37*, 1303–1306.

Emmelkamp, P. M. G., Brilman, E., Kuipers, H., & Mersch, P. (1986). Treatment of agoraphobia; Self-instructional training, rational-emotive therapy, and exposure *in vivo*. *Behavior Modification, 10*, 37–53.

Emmelkamp, P. M. G., Kuipers, A. C. M., & Eggeraat, J. B. (1978). Cognitive modification versus prolonged exposure *in vivo*: A comparison with agoraphobics as subjects. *Behaviour Research and Therapy, 16*, 33–41.

Emmelkamp, P. M. G., & Mersch, P. P. (1982). Cognition and exposure *in vivo* in the treatment of agoraphobia: Short-term and delayed effects. *Cognitive Therapy & Research, 6*, 77–88.

Emmelkamp, P. M. G., & Wessels, H. (1975). Flooding in imagination vs. flooding *in vivo*: A comparison with agoraphobics. *Behaviour Research and Therapy, 13*, 7–15.

Emmelkamp, P. M. G., van der Hout, A., & De Vries, K. (1983). Assertive training for agoraphobia. *Behaviour Research and Therapy, 21*, 63–68.

Evans, L., Kenardy, J., Schneider, P., & Hoey, H. (1986). Effect of a selective serotonin uptake inhibitor in agoraphobia with panic attacks: A double-blind comparison of zimelidine, imipramine, and placebo. *Acta Psychiatrica Scandinavia, 73*, 49–53.

Everaerd, W. T., Rijken, A. M., & Emmelkamp, P. N. G. (1973). A comparison of "flooding" and "successive approximation" in the treatment of agoraphobia. *Behaviour Research and Therapy, 11*, 105–117.

Foa, E. B., Jamesen, J. S., Turner, R. M., & Payne, L. L. (1980). Massed vs. spaced exposure sessions in the treatment of agoraphobia. *Behaviour Research and Therapy, 18*, 333–338.

Frame, C. O., Turner, S. M., Jacob, R. G., Szekely, B. (1984). Self-exposure treatment of agoraphobia. *Behavior Modification, 8*, 115–122.

Francis, A., & Dunn, P. (1975). The attachment-autonomy conflict in agoraphobia. *International Journal of Psycho-Analysis, 56*, 435–440.

Franklin, J. A. (1989). A 6-year follow-up of the effectiveness of respiratory retraining, in-situ isometric relaxation, and cognitive modification in the treatment of agoraphobia. *Behavior Modification, 13*, 139–167.

Freud, S. (1919). Turnings in the world of psychoanalytic therapy. In *Collected papers* (Vol. 2). (J. Riviera, Trans.) London: Hogarth Press and Institute of Psychoanalysis.

Freud, S. (1924). *The justification for detaching from neurasthenia a particular syndrome: The anxiety neurosis* (J. Riviera, Trans.). In Collected Papers (Vol. 1). Vienna: International Psychoanalytic Press. (Original manuscript written 1894).

Freud, S. (1936). *The problem of anxiety*. Albany, NY: Psychoanalytic Quarterly Press.

Fyer, A., Liebowitz, M., Gorman, J., Compeas, R., Levin, A., Davies, S., Goetz, D., & Klein, D. (1987). Discontinuation of alprazolam treatment in panic patients. *American Journal of Psychiatry, 144*, 303–308.

Gelder, M. G., Marks, I. M., Wolff, H. H., & Clark, M. (1967). Desensitization and psychotherapy in the treatment of phobic states: A controlled inquiry. *British Journal of Psychiatry, 113*, 53–73.

Ghosh, A., & Marks, I. M. (1987). Self-treatment of agoraphobia by exposure. *Behavior Therapy, 18*, 3–16.

Goldstein, A. J., & Chambless, D. L. (1978). A reanalysis of agoraphobia. *Behavior Therapy, 9*, 47–59.

Gournay, K. J. M. (1991). The failure of exposure treatment in agoraphobia: Implications for the practice of nurse therapists and community psychiatric nurses. *Journal of Advanced Nursing, 16*, 1099–1109.

Gray, J. (1987). Interactions between drugs and behavior therapy. In H. J. Eysenck & I. Martins (Eds.), *Theoretical foundations of behavior therapy* (pp. 433–447). New York: Plenum.

Gray, M. A., & McPherson, I. G. (1982). Agoraphobia: A critical review of methodology in behavioral treatment research. *Current Psychological Reviews, 2*, 19–46.

Gustavson, B., Jensson, L., Jerremalm, A., & Öst, L. G. (1985). Therapist behavior during exposure treatment of agoraphobia. *Behavior Modification, 9*, 491–504.

Hallam, R. S. (1978). Agoraphobia: A critical review of the concept. *British Journal of Psychiatry, 133*, 314–319.

Herman, J. B., Rosenbaum, J. F., & Brotman, A. W. (1987). The alprazolam to clonazepam switch for the treatment of panic disorder. *Journal of Clinical Psychopharmacology, 7*, 175–178.

Hoffart, A., & Martinsen, E. W. (1990). Exposure-based integrated vs. pure psychodynamic treatment of agoraphobic inpatients. *Psychotherapy, 27*, 210–218.

Jackson, H. J., & Elton, C. (1985). A multimodal approach to the treatment of agoraphobia: Four case studies. *Canadian Journal of Psychiatry, 30*, 539–543.

Jacobson, N. S., Wilson, L., & Tupper, C. (1988). The clinical significance of treatment gains resulting from exposure-based interventions for agoraphobia: A reanalysis of outcome data. *Behavior Therapy, 19*, 539–554.

Jannoun, L., Munby, M., Catalan, J., & Gelder, M. (1980). A home-based treatment program for agoraphobia: Replication and controlled evaluation. *Behavior Therapy, 11*, 294–305.

Jansson, L., Jerremalm, A., & Öst, L. G. (1986). Follow-up of agoraphobic patients treated with exposure *in vivo* or applied relaxation. *British Journal of Psychiatry, 149*, 486–490.

Jansson, L., & Öst, L. (1982). Behavioral treatment for agoraphobia: An evaluative review. *Clinical Psychology Review, 2*, 311–336.

Klein, D. F. (1964). Delineation of two drug-responsive anxiety syndromes. *Psychopharmacologia, 5*, 397–408.

Klein, D. F., & Klein, H. M. (1989). The nosology, genetics, and theory of spontaneous panic and phobia. In P. J. Tyrer (Ed.), *The psychopharmacology of anxiety* (pp. 163–195). New York: Oxford University Press.

Klein, D. F., Ross, D. C., & Cohen, P. (1987). Panic and avoidance in agoraphobia: Application of path analysis to treatment studies. *Archives of General Psychiatry, 44*, 377–385.

Klein, D. F., Zitrin, C. M., Woerner, N. G., & Ross, D. C. (1983). Treatment of phobias: II. Behavior therapy and supportive psychotherapy: Are there any specific ingredients? *Archives of General Psychiatry, 40*, 139–145.

Klosko, J. S., Barlow, D., Tassinari, R., & Cerny, J. (1990). A comparison of alprazolam and behavior therapy in the treatment of panic disorder. *Journal of Consulting and Clinical Psychology, 58*, 77–84.

Liddell, A., Mackay, W., Dawe, G., Galutira, B., Hearn, S., & Walsh-Doran, M. (1986). Compliance as a factor in outcome with agoraphobic clients. *Behaviour Research and Therapy, 24*, 217–220.

London, R. W. (1981). Agoraphobia: Hypnosis treatment with cognitive, affective and behavioral change. *The Australian Journal of Clinical Hypnotherapy and Hypnosis, 2*, 71–89.

Luborsky, L., Singer, B., & Luborsky, L. (1975). Comparative studies of psychotherapies. *Archives of General Psychiatry, 32*, 995–1008.

Lydiard, R. B., & Ballenger, J. C. (1987). Antidepressants in panic disorder and agoraphobia. *Journal of Affective Disorders, 13*, 153–168.

Marchione, K. E., Michelson, L., Greenwald, M., & Dancu, C. (1987). Cognitive behavioral treatment of agoraphobia. *Behaviour Research and Therapy, 25*, 319–328.

Marks, I. M. (1969). *Fears and phobias*. London: Academic Press.

Marks, I. M. (1970). Agoraphobic syndrome (phobic anxiety state). *Archives of General Psychiatry, 23*, 538–553.

Marks, I. M. (1987). *Fears, phobias, and rituals: Panic, anxiety, and their disorders*. Oxford: Oxford University Press.

Marks, I. M., Gray, S., Cohen, D., Hill, R., Dawson, D., Ramm, E., & Stern, R. S. (1983). Imipramine and brief therapist-aided exposure in agoraphobics having self-exposure homework. *Archives of General Psychiatry, 40*, 153–162.

Marks, I. M., & O'Sullivan, G. (1988). Drugs and psychological treatments for agoraphobia/panic and obsessive–compulsive disorders: A review. *British Journal of Psychiatry, 153*, 650–658.

Mathews, A. M., Johnston, D. W., Shaw, P. M., & Gelder, M. G. (1974). Process variables and the prediction of outcome in behavior therapy. *British Journal of Psychiatry, 125*, 256–264.

Mathews, A., Teasdale, J., Munby, M., Johnston, D., & Shaw, P. (1977). A home-based treatment program for agoraphobia. *Behavior Therapy, 18*, 915–924.

Matuzas, W., Uhlenhuth, E. H., Glass, R. M., Javaid, J., & Davis, J. M. (1986, December). *Alprazolam and imipramine in panic disorder—A life table analysis*. Paper presented at the 25th Annual Meeting of the American College of Neuropsychopharmacology, Washington, DC.

Mavissakalian, M. (1984). Agoraphobia: Behavioral therapy and pharmacotherapy. In B. D. Beitman and G. L. Keiman (Eds.), *Combining psychotherapy and drug therapy in clinical practice*. New York: Spectrum Publications, pp. 187–211.

Mavissakalian, M. (1986). Clinically significant improvement in agoraphobia research. *Behaviour Research and Therapy, 24*, 369–370.

Mavissakalian, M. (1987). The placebo effect in agoraphobia. *The Journal of Nervous and Mental Disease, 175*, 95–99.

Mavissakalian, M. (1990). Sequential combination of imipramine and self-directed exposure in the treatment of panic disorder with agoraphobia. *Journal of Clinical Psychiatry, 51*, 184–188.

Mavissakalian, M., & Michelson, L. (1986). Agoraphobia: Relative and combined efforts of therapist-assisted *in vivo* exposure and imipramine. *Journal of Clinical Psychiatry, 47*, 117–122.

Mavissakalian, M., Michelson, L., & Dealy, R. S. (1983). Pharmacological treatment of agoraphobia: Imipramine versus imipramine with programmed practice. *British Journal of Psychiatry, 143*, 348–355.

Mavissakalian, M., Michelson, L., Greenwald, D., Kornblith, S., Greenwald, M. (1983). Cognitive-behavioral treatment of agoraphobia: Paradoxical intention versus self-statement training. *Behaviour Research and Therapy, 21*, 75–86.

May, R. (1980). Value conflicts and anxiety. In I. L. Kutash, L. B. Schlesinger, & Associates (Eds.), *Handbook on stress and anxiety* (pp. 241–248). San Francisco: Jossey-Bass.

McNamee, G., O'Sullivan, G., Lelliott, P., & Marks, J. (1989). Telephone-guided treatment for housebound agoraphobics with panic disorder: Exposure vs. relaxation. *Behavior Therapy, 20*, 491–497.

McPherson, F. M., Brougham, L., & McLaren, S. (1980). Maintenance of improvement in agoraphobia patients treated by behavioral methods—A four year follow-up. *Behaviour Research and Therapy, 18*, 150–152.

Michelson, L., & Ascher, L. M. (1984). Paradoxical intention in the treatment of agoraphobia and other anxiety disorders. *Journal of Behavior Therapy and Experimental Psychiatry, 15*, 215–220.

Michelson, L., & Mavissakalian, M. (1983). Temporal stability of self-report measures in agoraphobia research. *Behavior Research and Therapy, 21*, 695–698.

Michelson, L., Mavissakalian, M., & Marchione, K. (1985). Cognitive and behavioral treatments of agoraphobia: Clinical, behavioral, and psychophysiological outcomes. *Journal of Consulting and Clinical Psychology, 53*, 913–925.

Michelson, L., Mavissakalian, M., & Marchione, K. (1988). Cognitive, behavioral, and psychophysiological treatments of agoraphobia: A comparative outcome investigation. *Behavior Therapy, 19*, 97–120.

Miller, M. L. (1953). On street fear. *International Journal of Psychoanalysis, 34*, 232–252.

Milne, G. (1988). Hypnosis in the treatment of single phobia and complex agoraphobia: A series of case studies. *Australian Journal of Clinical and Experimental Hypnosis, 16*, 53–65.

Milton, F., & Hafner, J. (1979). The outcome of behavior therapy for agoraphobia in relationship to marital adjustment. *Archives of General Psychiatry, 36*, 807–811.

Myers, J. K., Weissman, M. M., Tischler, G. L., Holzer, C. E., III, Orvaschel, H., Anthony, J. C., Boyd, J. H., Burke, J. D., Jr., Kramer, M., & Stolzman, R. (1984). Six-month prevalence of psychiatric disorders in three communities. *Archives of General Psychiatry, 41*, 959–967.

Nagy, L., Krystal, J., Woods, S., & Charney, D. (1989). Clinical and medication outcome after short-term alprazolam and behavioral group treatment in panic disorder. *Archives of General Psychiatry, 46*, 993–999.

Ogles, B. M., Lambert, M. G., Weight, D. G., & Payne, I. R. (1990). Agoraphobia outcome measurement: A review and meta-analysis. *Journal of Consulting and Clinical Psychology, 2*, 317–325.

Paul, G. L. (1967). Strategy of outcome research in psychotherapy. *Journal of Consulting and Clinical Psychology, 31*, 109–118.

Pecknold, J. C., Swinson, R. P., Kuch, K., & Lewis, C. P. (1988). Alprazolam in panic disorder and agoraphobia: Results from a multicenter trial. III. Discontinuation effects. *Archives of General Psychiatry, 45*, 429–439.

Pollard, C. A., Bronson, S. S., & Kenney, M. R. (1989). Prevalence of agoraphobia without panic in clinical settings. *American Journal of Psychiatry, 146*, 559.

Pollard, C. A., & Frank, M. (1990). Catastrophic cognitions and physical sensations of panic attacks associated with agoraphobia. *Phobia Practice and Research Journal, 3*, 3–18.

Pollard, C. A., & Henderson, J. G. (1987). Prevalence of agoraphobia: Some confirmatory data. *Psychological Reports, 60*, 1305.

Pollard, C. A., & Kenney, M. R. (1992). *Agoraphobia without panic: A review and commentary*. Unpublished manuscript.

Rachman, S. J. (1984). Agoraphobia: A safety-signal perspective. *Behaviour Research and Therapy, 22*, 59–70.

Rapee, R. M., & Murrell, E. (1988). Predictors of agoraphobic avoidance. *Journal of Anxiety Disorders, 2*, 203–217.

Rizley, R., Kahn, R. J., McNair, D. M., & Frankenthaler, L. M. (1986). A comparison of alprazolam and imipramine in the treatment of agoraphobia and panic disorder. *Psychopharmacology Bulletin, 22*, 167–172.

Rogers, C. R. (1951). *Client-centered therapy*. Boston: Houghton Mifflin.

Roth, M. (1959). The phobic anxiety—Depersonalization syndrome. *Proceedings of the Royal Society of Medicine, 52*, 587–595.

Schwartz, L. S., & Val, E. R. (1984). Agoraphobia: A multimodal treatment approach. *American Journal of Psychotherapy, 28*, 35–46.

Sheehan, D. V. (1986). *The anxiety disease* (rev. ed.). New York: Bantam.

Sheehan, D. V., Ballenger, J., & Jacobsen, G. (1980). Treatment of endogenous anxiety with phobic hysterical and hypochondriacal symptoms. *Archives of General Psychiatry, 37*, 51–59.

Sheehan, D. V., & Sheehan, K. H. (1982). The classification of phobic disorders. *International Journal of Psychiatry in Medicine, 12*, 243–266.

Sifneos, P. E. (1972). *Short-term psychotherapy and emotional crisis*. Cambridge: Harvard University Press.

Smith, M. L., & Glass, G. U. (1977). Meta-analysis of psychotherapy outcome studies. *American Psychologist, 32*, 752–760.

Snaith, R. P. (1968). A clinical investigation of phobias. *British Journal of Psychiatry, 114*, 673–698.

Solyom, L., Meseltine, G. F. D., McClure, D. J., Solyom, C., Ledwidge, B., & Steinberg, G. (1973). Behavior therapy versus drug therapy in the treatment of phobic neurosis. *Canadian Psychiatric Association Journal, 18*, 25–37.

Suinn, R. M. (1971). Anxiety management training. *Behavior Therapy, 2*, 498–510.

Telch, M. J. (1988). Combined pharmacologic and psychological treatments for panic sufferers. In S. Rachman and J. D. Maser (Eds.), *Panic: Psychological perspectives*. Hillsdale, NJ: Erlbaum.

Telch, M. J., Agras, W. S., Taylor, C. B., Roth, W. T., & Gallen, C. (1985). Combined pharmacologic and behavioral treatment for agoraphobia. *Behaviour Research and Therapy, 23*, 325–335.

Telch, M. J., Tearnan, B. H., & Taylor, C. (1983). Antidepressant medication in the treatment of agoraphobia: A critical review. *Behavior Research and Therapy, 21*, 505–527.

Tensch, L., & Bohme, H. (1991). What is the result of an inpatient treatment program with client-centered psychotherapy emphasis in patients with agoraphobia and/or panic? Results of a 1-year follow-up. *Psychotherapie, Psychosomatik, Medizinische Psychologie, 41*, 68–76.

Tesar, G. E., & Rosenbaum, J. F. (1986). Successful use of clonazepam in patients with treatment-resistant panic disorder. *The Journal of Nervous and Mental Disease, 174*(8), 477–482.

Tilton, P. (1983). Pseudo-orientation in time in the treatment of agoraphobia. *American Journal of Clinical Hypnosis, 25*, 267–269.

Trull, T. J., Nietzel, M. T., & Main, A. (1988). The use of meta-analysis to assess the clinical significance of behavior therapy for agoraphobia. *Behavior Therapy, 19*, 527–538.

Vangaard, T. (1987). *Panic: The course of a psychoanalysis*. New York: W. W. Norton & Co.

Weekes, C. (1976). *Simple effective treatment for agoraphobia*. New York: Hawthorne.

Weiss, E. (1964). *Agoraphobia in the light of ego psychology*. New York: Grune & Stratton.

Weissmann, M. M., Leaf, P. J., Blazer, D. G., Boyd, J. H., & Florio, L. (1986). The relationship between panic disorder and agoraphobia: An epidemiologic perspective. *Psychopharmacology Bulletin, 22*, 787–791.

Westphal, C. (1888). *Agoraphobia, a nemopathic phenomenon*. (T. J. Knapp & M. T. Schumacker, Trans.) Lahnan, ME: University Press of America. (Original work published 1871).

Williams, K. E., & Chambless, D. L. (1990). The relationship between therapist characteristics and outcome of *in vivo* exposure treatment for agoraphobia. *Behavior Therapy, 21*, 111–116.

Williams, S. L., & Rappoport, A. (1983). Cognitive treatment in the natural environment for agoraphobics. *Behavior Therapy, 14*, 299–313.

Wolpe, J. (1990). *The practice of behavior therapy* (4th ed.) New York: Pergamon Press.

Wood, A. B. (1986). Hypnosis and audiotapes as a treatment for agoraphobia. *The Australian Journal of Clinical Hypnotherapy and Hypnosis, 7*, 100–104.

Yager, E. T. (1988). Treating agoraphobia with hypnosis, subliminal therapy and paradoxical intention. *Medical Hypnoanalysis Journal, 3*, 156–160.

Zarate, R., Craske, M. G., & Barlow, D. H. (1990). Situational exposure treatment versus panic control treatment for agoraphobia: A case study. *Journal of Behavior Therapy and Experimental Psychiatry, 21*, 211–224.

Zitrin, C. M., Klein, D. F., & Woerner, M. G. (1980). Treatment of agoraphobia with group exposure *in vivo* and imipramine. *Archives of General Psychiatry, 37*, 63–72.

Zitrin, C. M., Klein, D. F., Woerner, M. G., & Ross, D. C. (1983). Treatment of phobias: I. Comparison of imipramine hydrochloride and placebo. *Archives of General Psychiatry, 40*, 125–138.

9

Treatment Efficacy in Posttraumatic Stress Disorder

Dudley David Blake, Francis R. Abueg, Steven H. Woodward, and Terence M. Keane

Introduction

Life, some contend, is punctuated by accidental as well as developmental crises (Caplan, 1964). Developmental crises are disruptive but reasonably predictable life changes experienced as milestones in growth and cognitive development. Accidental crises, by contrast, almost always occur at unpredictable times, are disruptive, and involve some primary loss, such as the death of loved ones, loss of job, or debilitating illness. With both types of crises, however, how well an individual manages the crisis influences future functioning. If a crisis is resolved successfully, the individual may become more confident, more skilled, and better able to handle future crises. If not, an individual may become less confident and able in managing future crises (Caplan, 1964).

At one extreme on the continuum of accidental crises are traumatic events that people can experience once or more during their lifetime. These accidental crises or traumas tend to be more extreme in terms of unpredictability, speed of onset, and extent of loss incurred. These traumas also tend to produce more extreme psychological consequences, which are often evident in pervasive and long-term impairment. Impairments are generally seen in one or more symptom groupings: recurrent, intrusive reexperiencing of the trauma, emotional numbing and affective constriction, and physiological hyperarousal (American Psychiatric Association, 1987).

Trauma, from the Greek word, *traumat(o)*, meaning ". . . a wound, hence in Psychiatry a mental shock" (Partridge, 1983), lies at the literal and conceptual core of Post-traumatic Stress Disorder (PTSD). Trauma can be conceived as an experi-

David Dudley Blake, Francis R. Abueg, and **Steven H. Woodward** • Clinical Laboratory and Education Division, National Center for PTSD, Palo Alto VAMC, Palo Alto, California 94304. **Terence M. Keane** • Behavioral Science Division, National Center for PTSD, Boston VAMC, Boston, Massachusetts 02130.

Handbook of Effective Psychotherapy, edited by Thomas R. Giles. Plenum Press, New York, 1993.

ence which is out of the range of usual human experience that would evoke significant psychological distress in nearly everyone (American Psychiatric Association, 1987). Conceiving of trauma in this way retains the perspective that PTSD is a function of both event and person factors (Keane, 1985). PTSD results from the interplay between extreme events and an individual's ability to tolerate those events.

As we approach the dawning of a new century, it is clear that trauma has emerged as a field of human inquiry. Clinicians, researchers, educators, and laypersons are increasingly conscious of trauma and its consequences. A survey of the published works found in *Psychological Abstracts* between 1970 and 1990 attests to the steady increase in interest in trauma (Figure 9.1; Blake, Albano, & Keane, 1992). As is apparent, the professional literature on trauma has burgeoned over past 20 years. This increase is likely due to the official acceptance of posttraumatic stress disorder as a diagnostic entity (American Psychiatric Association, 1980, 1987) and to the increased research with war veterans, prisoners during wartime, and victims of rape. As is apparent from the figure, treatment research has also grown and, in fact, comprises an increasingly larger proportion of the trauma literature (Blake *et al.*, 1992).

A variety of treatments have been employed with individuals diagnosed with PTSD. Empirical data supporting the efficacy of various pharmacological agents with PTSD have been reported (e.g., Friedman, 1988; Krystal *et al.*, 1989). Various forms of psychotherapy have also been advocated and show promise for PTSD treatment (e.g., Blank, 1985; Cryer & Beutler, 1980; Egendorf, 1975; Fairbank & Brown, 1987; Figley, 1988; Lyons & Keane, 1989). Each of these approaches to

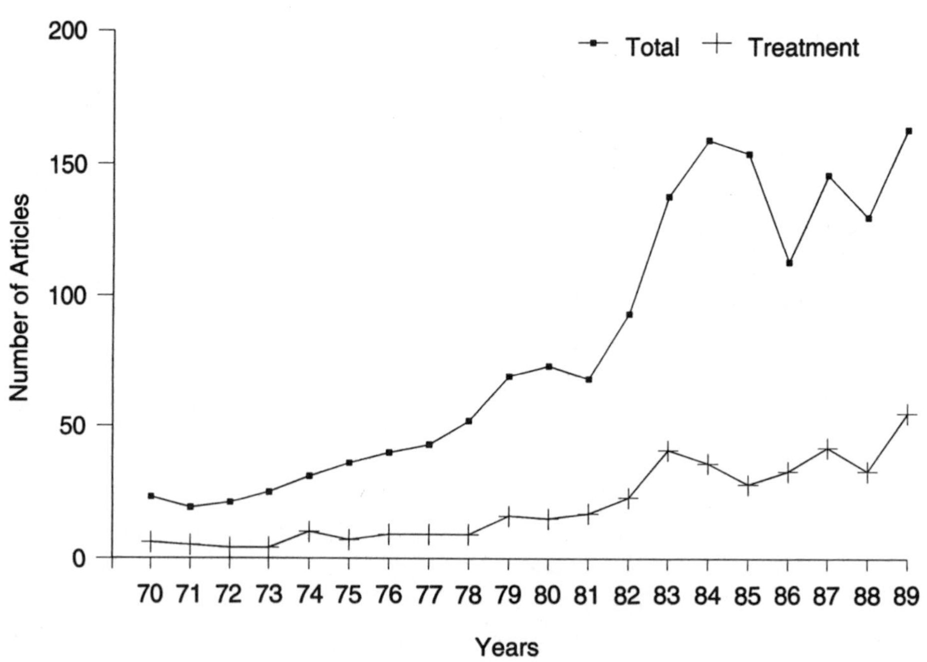

Figure 9.1. Yearly count of trauma publications found in *Psychological Abstracts* from 1970 through 1989.

PTSD treatment has received varying degrees of support in the professional literature, but little empirical data have been produced to demonstrate or compare their efficacies.

In the following sections the published empirical work involving the treatment of individuals with PTSD is reviewed. First, the history of PTSD as a diagnostic and conceptual entity is reviewed, followed by sections describing PTSD prevalence, demographics, development, course, and severity. Next, the theoretical bases behind each PTSD treatment orientation are described. Published work involving these treatments for particular trauma groups is reviewed with a critical eye toward treatment benefits. A section is then provided to discuss an emerging area of interest in PTSD research: eye movement desensitization. Finally, the comparative efficacies of extant PTSD treatments are summarized and suggestions for future directions are outlined.

History

With little question, the occurrence of prolonged, adverse reactions to trauma in both animals and humans predates recorded history. Laboratory-induced "experimental neurosis" also doubtlessly has real-life parallels for all living organisms. It is likely that reactions of this type are adaptive and serve as reminders to avoid repeated exposure to life-threatening circumstances. Persistent reminders of the trauma may help animals and humans to avoid attacks from predators and exposure to natural calamities.

Formal recognition of adverse reactions to trauma has a relatively recent history, which can be traced along specific trauma types. For example, in regard to natural disasters, the physician Samuel Pepys described reactions to the great London fire of 1666 (Daly, 1983) without recognizing these reactions as a syndrome. With regard to war trauma, DaCosta provided clear descriptions of war stress reactions during and following the American Civil War, which he coined "irritable heart" (later termed "DaCosta syndrome"; Scrignar, 1988). Clear accounts of this clinical phenomenon, although known by various names, were provided after World War I ("soldier's heart and effort syndrome"; Lewis, 1919) and World War II ("battle fatigue"; Grinker & Spiegel, 1945). Individuals who experienced traumatic persecution in German concentration camps during World War II also have received recognition, and their clinical presentation has been labeled the "survivor syndrome" (Koranyi, 1969; Niederland, 1981). Trauma reactions following vehicular accidents have also been described and labeled ("post-accident anxiety syndrome"; Modlin, 1967), as have reactions to sexual assault ("rape trauma syndrome"; Burgess, 1974; Burgess & Holmstrom, 1983).

The most explicit recognition of adverse trauma effects can be found in the psychiatric diagnostic nomenclature. In the *Diagnostic and Statistical Manual for Mental Disorders* (DSM; American Psychiatric Association, 1952), the term, "gross stress reaction" was used to describe the adverse reactions people can have to a broad range of traumatic events. In 1968, the second edition of the diagnostic manual, DSM-II (American Psychiatric Association, 1968), discontinued this term, and it nearest equivalent became "transient situational disturbances." With DSM-III (American Psychiatric Association, 1980), the concept of a discrete trauma reaction was revivified and has since been given the classification "post traumatic stress disorder."

Prevalence

A recent prevalence estimate holds that 1% to 1.5% of the general population in America have diagnosable, current PTSD (Helzer, Robins, & McEvoy, 1988). While some argue that, due to the use of conservative measures, this estimate may seriously underestimate PTSD prevalence (e.g., Keane & Penk, 1988), this figure suggests that 4½ million people in America currently meet criteria for PTSD. With regard to selected high-risk populations, it has been estimated that 15.2% or 479,000 male Vietnam veterans meet the current criteria for PTSD, and another 11.1% or 350,000 show partial PTSD (Kulka *et al.*, 1990). It has also been reported that nearly a quarter of the women (23.3%) in a community sample had been raped during their lifetime, and it is estimated that over half of all rape victims (57.1%) eventually develop PTSD (Kilpatrick, Saunders, Veronen, Best, & Von, 1987). While the consequences of PTSD are not yet known, injury and property loss from natural accidents and disaster are estimated to affect 2 million people in America each year (Rossi, Wright, Weber-Burdin, & Perina, 1983, cited in Solomon, 1989). Few or no estimates are available for percentage or number of individuals who have been traumatized from other events such as vehicular accidents, terrorist activities, violent crime, or child abduction (stranger or parental). However, if the available estimates are accurate, PTSD represents a significant problem in America, and quite likely in the rest of the world. As the scope of PTSD as a problem is increasingly recognized, so is the need for effective treatments.

Demographics

As a general rule, trauma is democratic and cuts across all demographic and cultural groups. Anyone, at any time and place, may be exposed to a traumatic event, be it war, violent crime, devastating accidents, or disaster. However, certain population subgroups may be at greater risk for exposure to traumatic events. For example, women are much more likely than men to be victims of sexual abuse and assault. Young men in the late 1960s, who reported troubles in school and had lower educational status, could not get deferments from the military, placing them at greater risk for military service. Vietnam veterans with these characteristics were also more likely to have later adjustment problems (Worthington, 1978).

Exposure to trauma itself may be a risk factor for subsequent trauma. For example, veterans traumatized by war have a greater likelihood of engaging in risky and self-destructive behaviors (e.g., alcohol and drug abuse, high-risk vocations, and criminal behavior), which in turn exposes them to the possibility of further trauma. Similarly, women who have been sexually assaulted may be at somewhat greater risk for sexual revictimization (Miller *et al.*, 1978). Victims of violent crime have a greater likelihood of repeated victimization than nonvictims (Ziegenhagen, 1976).

Development

By definition PTSD is a unique disorder in that its development can be traced to an environmental precipitant. DSM-III-R criteria for PTSD stipulate that this precipitant must involve a

> . . . psychologically distressing event that is outside the range of usual human experience (i.e., outside the range of such common experiences as simple

> bereavement, chronic illness, business losses, and marital conflict). The stressor producing this syndrome would be markedly distressing to almost anyone. (American Psychiatric Association, 1987, p. 247)

The most robust factor found in the development of PTSD is the trauma itself. Exposure to combat is the single best predictor of PTSD in Vietnam veterans (Foy, Carroll, Donahoe, 1987; Foy, Sipprelle, Rueger, & Carroll, 1984). In victims of rape, degree of life threat, physical injury, and rape completion (hence greater exposure) have been found to be the greatest predictors of PTSD status (Kilpatrick *et al.*, 1989).

Generally, signs and symptoms of the disorder occur almost immediately after the trauma and, for a diagnosis to be made, must persist for at least 1 month. Most persons exposed to trauma return to pretrauma or near-pretrauma functioning (some may in fact become higher functioning following a successful negotiation of a traumatic event). Symptoms of PTSD may persist over long periods of time, evolving from an acute to a chronic form.

Course

While PTSD was once generally regarded as having both continuous and delayed onset forms (American Psychiatric Association, 1980; see also Figley, 1978; Horowitz & Solomon, 1975; Klein, 1974), more recent understanding is that the avoidance symptoms of PTSD may begin immediately, while the reexperiencing symptoms may be presented later. The reexperiencing symptoms emerge later when the individual is retraumatized, exposed to significant life stressors, abuses substances, or experiences a natural event in the aging process. This revised understanding about the course of PTSD is consistent with the psychodynamic model of PTSD (Horowitz, 1986; see description later in this chapter). However, it is not clear whether the reexperiencing symptoms are actually present immediately after the trauma but are ignored and tolerated. More systematic study is required to adequately address this issue.

Severity

In the diagnosis of PTSD (American Psychiatric Association, 1980, 1987) there is no means for rating severity of the disorder, such as a fifth-digit code used with many diagnostic classes. DSM-III-R's five-axial diagnostic system does, however, allow for ratings of the individual's global functioning over the past year and of the severity of psychosocial stressors, both of which provide indirect measures of symptom severity. Evaluation of PTSD can be made in other ways as well, such as by considering total number of symptoms and their distribution across the three main criterion subgroupings in the DSM-III-R (Reexperiencing, Numbing, and Hyperarousal), levels of social and occupational impairment, and presence of other features associated with the disorder, such as relationship problems and substance abuse.

PTSD Theories

From a broad perspective, theories about PTSD come in many shapes and sizes, from psychoanalytic to sociological to Gestaltist. However, most treatments for PTSD have generally been of three types, each with separate theoretical frameworks: psychodynamic, behavioral, and psychopharmacological. The theories underlying these orientations and the treatments proposed within each are presented and discussed below.

Psychodynamic Theories

Psychodynamic theories, posited by Cohen (1981), Emery and Emery (1985), Horowitz (1986), Lifton (1973), Parson (1984), and Haley (1978), largely involve disruptions of ego development, violations of ego integrity and defense structure, vulnerability produced from early life trauma, or combinations of each. Although there are other psychodynamic approaches to treatment (e.g., Blackburn, O'Connell, Richman, 1984; Crump, 1984; Scrignar, 1988), the most widely recognized treatment is short-term psychodynamic psychotherapy (Horowitz, 1986), which is described briefly in this section.

Horowitz (1986) describes the most detailed and widely accepted psychodynamic theory for PTSD, which involves an individual's failure to modulate emotional reactions to trauma, which in turn leads to a cycling of intrusion and denial or avoidance processes. In this theory, the traumatized individual has a compulsive tendency to repeat or relive some aspect of the traumatic experience. This repetition is accomplished through recurrent dreams, thoughts, images, and emotions related to the experience, and in behaviors which help reenact the trauma (e.g., compulsively talking about the experience, physiological hyperarousal, engaging in thrill-seeking behavior or self-destructive acts, etc.). At the same time, the individual seeks to ward off this painful repetition of the trauma and invokes psychological denial, emotional numbing, and cognitive and behavioral avoidance. Problems result when the traumatized individual shows excessive and rigid control over the intrusion, or fails to adequately suppress the intrusion. A balance between over- and undercontrol of this process enables the individual to cognitively and emotionally assimilate or accommodate the traumatic experience and move on. A simplified schematic of this process is shown in Figure 9.2.

In psychodynamic treatment, the form that therapy assumes must depend on how much control the individual exerts over the repetition/intrusion. Weaker controls are buttressed by support, structure, and rest. Excessive controls are reduced through abreactive and cathartic treatments which allow the individual to work through conflict, guilt, fear, and the like engendered by the trauma. The traumatized individual is helped to abandon rigid and excessive control mechanisms, alter maladaptive defense mechanisms, and regain effective modulation of emotions.

Behavioral Theories

Behavioral theories (e.g., Fairbank & Brown, 1987; Holmes & St. Lawrence, 1983; Keane, Zimering, & Caddell, 1985; Rychtarik, Silverman, Van Landingham, & Prue, 1984) as a rule rely on the two-factor theory of learning (Mowrer, 1960), which includes both instrumental (operant) and respondent (classical) conditioning mechanisms. In brief, a traumatic event occurs within a classical learning situation in which the event (or unconditioned stimulus, UCS) becomes associated with more neutrally valenced stimuli. These previously neutral stimuli (conditioned stimuli or CSs) begin to evoke responses which were once elicited only when

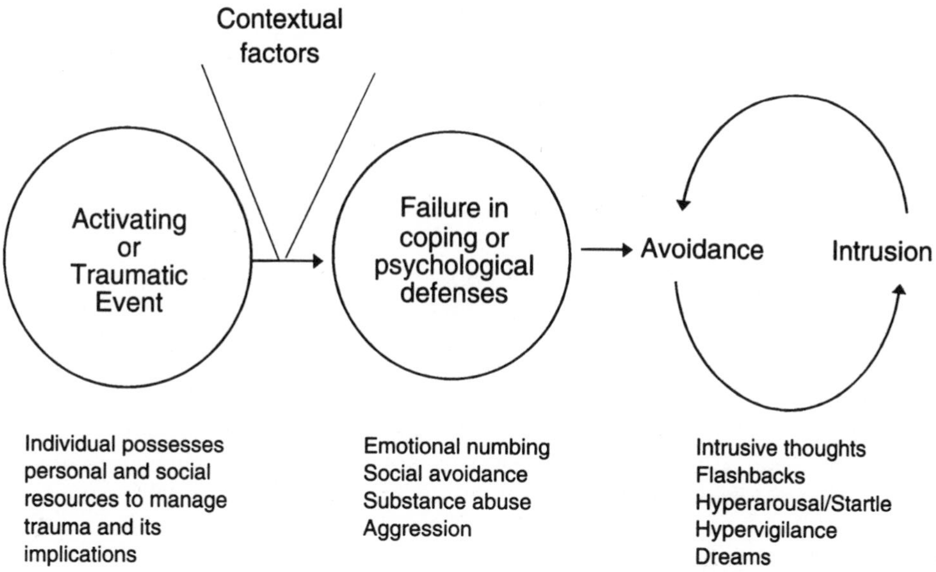

Contextual factors
Activating or Traumatic Event
Failure in coping or psychological defenses
Avoidance
Intrusion
Individual possesses personal and social resources to manage trauma and its implications
Emotional numbing
Social avoidance
Substance abuse
Aggression
Intrusive thoughts
Flashbacks
Hyperarousal/Startle
Hypervigilance
Dreams

Figure 9.2. Schematic diagram of a psychodynamic formulation for PTSD pathogenesis.

the UCS occurred. An example of this process is an earthquake which leads to autonomic arousal, feelings of fear, and maladaptive cognitions. These cues become conditioned responses (CRs), and are later produced in the presence of earthquake-associated sights, sounds, smells, such as in the case of ground rumbling when heavy vehicles drive by, the occurrence of approaching cracking and popping sounds, visions involving heat-produced shimmering, and so on. A schematic of this learning paradigm is presented in Figure 9.3. Instrumental, or

Unconditioned Stimuli (UCS)
(Traumatic Event)
Contiguously linked to the . . .
Conditioned Stimuli (CS)
(contextual variables accompanying trauma)
Unconditioned fear/pain response (UCR)
Conditioned fear/pain response (CR)
Environmental and internalized trauma cues
UCR/CR pain or fear response serves as a stimulus for instrumental behavior
Instrumental behavior
Avoidance response
Intrusive thoughts
Flashbacks
Hyperarousal/Startle
Hypervigilance
Dreams
Emotional numbing
Social avoidance
Substance abuse
Aggression

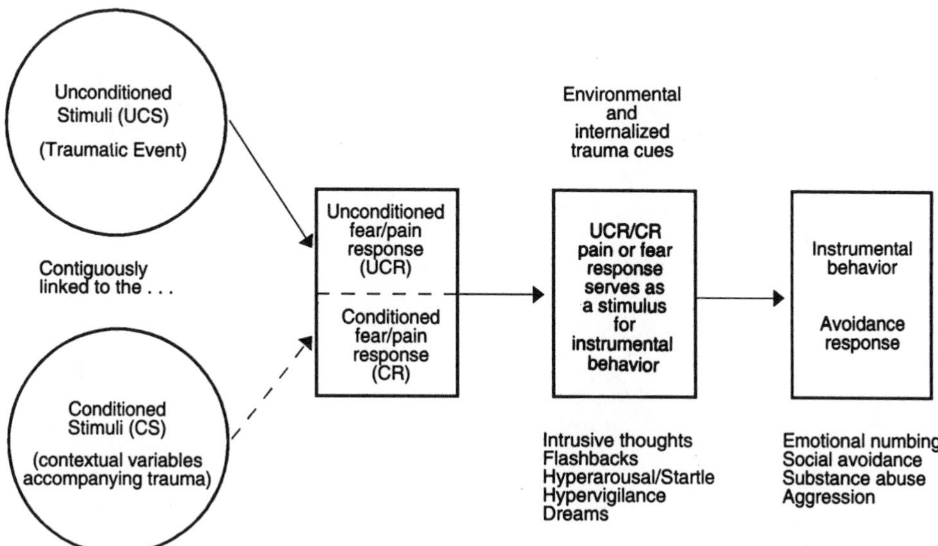

Figure 9.3. Schematic diagram of behavioral two-factor learning theory of PTSD.

operant, behavior is often engaged in to escape or avoid an elicitation of the UCRs. When this escape or avoidance is successful, the behavior is reinforced (and hence more likely to occur again in the future). This process, and the classical conditioning process preceding it, is shown in the right-hand section of Figure 9.3. Examples of this operantly reinforced behavior include avoidance of reminders of trauma, inappropriate expressions of anger (which helps to detract attention away from the CSs), and drug/alcohol abuse. Thus, the combined classical–operant two-factor model explains a great deal in terms of PTSD etiology and phenomenology.

Behavioral treatment for PTSD, which has taken several distinct forms, includes systematic desensitization, implosive therapy, relaxation training, biofeedback, cognitive-behavior therapy, and skills training. Each of these forms of treatment is described briefly below.

Systematic desensitization procedures are based on the principle of "reciprocal inhibition," posited by Wolpe (1958). In this principle, particular behaviors take precedence over, and thus "inhibit," the expression of others. The most prominent application of reciprocal inhibition is systematic desensitization, which typically involves three elements: (1) establishing a desired behavior (usually relaxation) that is incompatible with, or will inhibit, the undesired targeted behavior (usually a fear response), (2) making explicit a hierarchy of feared stimuli or images associated with the undesired behavior to which the individual can gradually receive full exposure to the entire range of (imagined) fear stimuli, and (3) during a desensitization session or sessions, exposing the individual to the feared stimuli in a gradually increasing manner, while he or she engages in the inhibitory behavior (e.g., relaxation), such that the undesired response (fear) is replaced in its association with the feared stimuli.

Implosive therapy is based on early work by Stampfl and Levis (1967), who derived their approach from the two-factor learning theory of Mowrer (1960; see Levis and Hare, 1977, and Keane, Fairbank, Caddell, Zimering, and Bender, 1985, for descriptions of this conceptualization and derivation). In implosive therapy, the therapist serves as a facilitator in a supportive treatment context, directing the individual to repeatedly and systematically imagine all aspects of the traumatic incident(s). The treated individual is guided to recall the event as if it were happening that very instant, and he or she is encouraged to employ as many senses (visual, auditory, gustatory, olfactory, tactile) as possible during the imagery (Lyons & Keane, 1989). In contrast to systematic desensitization, implosive therapy involves inducing the individual to actually experience the undesired, and conditioned (fear), responses that are associated with the fear-provoking stimuli. The fear responses are deliberately maintained until they are eliminated via the natural extinction process. Within and across these sessions, the individual eventually becomes less fearful since the unconditioned stimuli are not present during exposure trials. While implosive therapy involves the presentation of trauma-specific *and* hypothesized stimuli or cues, such as cognitions involving themes of guilt, loss of control, and rejection, a variant of this procedure, called *flooding*, entails having the individual imagine only trauma-specific stimuli.

Relaxation training is often used to help traumatized individuals gain control over hyperaroused physiology and to assist them in gaining mastery over important parts of life functioning (e.g., sleep, anger, unimpaired concentration and thinking). This training often takes the form of autogenic training or progressive muscle relaxation (Jacobsen, 1938), and it is sometimes accompanied by thermal or electromyographic (EMG) biofeedback. *Biofeedback* comprises a broad array of methods whose purpose is to help individuals gain control over their physiological processes. Control is attained by measuring an identified physiological response system (e.g., blood pressure, muscle tension, heart rate, respiration, etc.) and "feeding" that information back to the individual so that he or she can utilize skills to decrease or increase the rate, duration, or magnitude of that response. Relaxation and biofeedback may be particularly valuable for individuals with PTSD, given the physiological hyperarousal characteristic of this population.

Recently, *cognitive-behavioral* and *information-processing models* for explaining posttrauma symptomatology have appeared in the literature (Chemtob, Roitblat, Hamada, Carlson, & Twentyman, 1988; Foa, Steketee, & Olasov-Rothbaum, 1989; Jones & Barlow, 1990; Kreitler & Kreitler, 1988; Litz & Keane, 1989). Each of these theoretical formulations contains various common components that focus on cognitive processing, attention, perception, and memory integration. Cognitive therapy applications can be found in the work of Beck (1976; Beck & Emery, 1985), the rational emotive therapy of Ellis (Ellis & Grieger, 1986), the cognitive-behavior modification of Meichenbaum (1977); Meichenbaum & Turk, 1976), and the self-efficacy theory of Bandura (1977, 1986). Treatment typically involves changing cognitive patterns by modifying maladaptive cognitions, irrational beliefs, negative self-statements, or by increasing self-efficacy. It is important to recognize, however, that cognitive change occurs in other, noncognitive, treatments as well; for example, increased behavioral mastery is typically accompanied by increased self-efficacy.

Skills training in PTSD treatment generally involves anger management (McWhirter & Liebman, 1988) or stress inoculation training (Pearson, Poquette, & Wasden, 1983). Both approaches combine aspects of exposure-based treatments, the identification of high-risk situations, stimulus control procedures, cognitive restructuring, relaxation training, guided imagery, role playing, and behavioral rehearsal with specific methods for helping individuals better manage their stress or anger. Since exposure to trauma can fragment or inhibit learned behavior or patterns of behavior, individuals with PTSD may be particular beneficiaries of skills training (Keane, Fairbank *et al.*, 1985).

Biological Theories

To date, the literature on pharmacotherapy with PTSD is largely composed of uncontrolled pretest–posttest group studies. Biologically based theories of PTSD have been described in excellent detail elsewhere (e.g., Friedman, 1988; Kolb & Mutalipassi, 1982; Krystal *et al.*, 1989; van der Kolk, 1983, 1987; Wolfe, Alavi, & Mosnaim, 1987), so only brief descriptions will be provided here.

Van der Kolk, Greenberg, Boyd, and Krystal (1985) conceptualized posttraumatic stress as neurochemically mediated autonomic hyperarousal and hyperreactivity (involving nonadrenergic pathways) occurring in response to inescapable stress. This physiological state potentiates the release of endogenous opioids, and, over time, dependence on these opioids develops, much as in other addictions. Certain medications, like tricyclic antidepressants, appear to promote endogenous opioid release by potentiating seratonergic mechanisms, and they may be useful in PTSD for activating this process. Kolb and Mutalipassi (1982) conceptualized the symptoms of PTSD as conditioned emotional responses to environmental stimuli that are reminiscent of the traumatic event; this conditioned response is thought to be related to excessive central and peripheral adrenergic sympathetic activation. Benzodiazepines have often been the drug of choice for many anxiety disorders. The anxiolytic effects of these drugs appear to be due to their effect on the CNS GABAergic system, which directly influences the symptoms of autonomic arousal and anxious mood by exerting an inhibitory effect in the central nervous system. An alternative conceptualization of posttraumatic stress as a result of a neurobehavioral kindling process has provided a rationale for trials of the anticonvulsant carbamazepine.

Treatment Research

Numerous case studies and clinical case descriptions have appeared in the professional literature since 1945. Unfortunately, many of the studies have employed inadequately controlled methodologies which are particularly vulnerable to selection biases, history and maturation effects, and other threats to internal validity. By their tendency to rely on case-study designs, these studies are also likely to possess weak external validity. Nonetheless, these studies are important as initial demonstrations of novel and viable treatment tactics, and they are critical in the evolution of new areas of scientific inquiry. As a result of their importance, this section begins with a schematic presentation of the extensive uncontrolled PTSD treatment literature. Table 9.1 outlines these studies, with information presented on specific methodological aspects.

In addition to methodological shortcomings, these studies share other characteristics, including the use of standardized, physiological, or behavioral measures. These studies are also almost entirely examinations of a behavioral procedure or procedures. Nonbehavioral studies are conspicuously absent from this cluster of somewhat rudimentary clinical research efforts.

Controlled Single-Subject and Multiple-Baseline Studies

A handful of single-subject PTSD treatment studies have included adequate experimental controls for attributing observed effects to the specific treatment employed. These reports are presented in Table 9.2 and are described below.

Blanchard and Abel (1976) describe the heart rate biofeedback and imaginal exposure treatment of a 30-year-old female who had been raped 16 years previously. Since the rape, the patient had experienced "spells" which involved nausea, vomiting, choking sensations, tachycardia, and parasthesias. Using an ABAB design, the patient demonstrated mastery over her heart rate during audiotaped exposure to narrated rape scenes and was able to initiate and maintain contact with men in situations which previously would have provoked a spell. However, the investigators note that the treatment did not appear to affect her depressive symptomatology and appetite loss following marital conflicts.

Using a multiple-baseline across traumatic memories, Fairbank and Keane (1982) demonstrated that implosive therapy produced dramatic reductions in specific intrusive trauma memories of two Vietnam combat veterans. In addition, subjective distress and psychophysiological arousal (heart rate and skin conductance) related to trauma recall were reduced. Experimental control was elegantly demonstrated when changes were noted only in the memories being targeted across successive baselines.

In a series of multiple-baseline treatments, Saigh (1986, 1987a, 1987b) demonstrated the viability of flooding with traumatized children and adolescents who were innocent witnesses to fighting in Lebanon during the 1980s. In the first case, Saigh (1986) treated a 6½-year-old boy who had been exposed to a bomb blast and subsequently evidenced a variety of school and behavior problems, nightmares, distressing and intrusive recollections of the blast, avoidance behavior, and depression. In a multiple-baseline-across-traumatic-scenes design, the child showed clear reductions in trauma-specific fear, and after 10 sessions demonstrated improvement in all problems areas. These findings were replicated in a study involving three children, ages 11, 11, and 12 (Saigh, 1987a), and in a third study with an adolescent (Saigh, 1987b). In each of these studies, behavioral assessments were conducted which involved rating avoidance at the actual site where the traumas occurred. While failing to control for the effects from additional exposure from this source, Saigh built a compelling case for the utility of exposure-based methods with war-traumatized youths.

Utilizing a statistical method derived from classical test theory, Mueser, Yarnold, and Foy (1991) examined the efficacy of flooding in the treatment of four Vietnam combat veterans diagnosed with PTSD. Two of the veterans showed significant improvements in within-session heart rate, daily symptom ratings, depression, anxiety, and intrusive thoughts. One veteran showed no significant improvement, and the remaining veteran showed a worsening of symptom status. The latter veteran also declined to participate in the follow-up assessments.

Several conclusions can be stated about the studies reviewed above. First, experimental control was amply demonstrated in each study, providing strong support for the viability of each treatment employed. Second, the treatments employed seem to have had their greatest impact on the more obvious, anxiety-based symptoms, such as intrusive thoughts, nightmares, startle, and physiological arousal, while it is not certain whether symptoms involving anhedonic or social estrangement symptoms were affected. While the single-subject design is not without methodological problems, such as generalizing the observed effects to the larger trauma population, these studies do provide evidence that these primarily behavioral treatments do affect specific symptoms with selected traumatized individuals. Unfortunately, nonbehavioral studies are again absent from this group of empirical examinations of treatment efficacy.

Treatment Comparisons with Nonspecific Effects

A number of recent studies have examined the efficacy of PTSD treatments in comparison with no-treatment control conditions. These reports have provided support for the contention that psychologically based treatment is better than no treatment. A schematic summary of the PTSD treatment–no-treatment comparisons is presented in summary form in Table 9.3.

An EMG biofeedback-assisted systematic desensitization procedure was employed by Peniston (1986) in the treatment of eight Vietnam combat veterans with PTSD. As compared to a no-treatment control group, the treated subjects evidence marked reductions in EMG forehead tension and fewer disturbing nightmares and flashbacks at posttest. These effects were maintained throughout a 2-year follow-up

Table 9.1. Published Reports of Case Studies and Uncontrolled Group Treatments for PTSD

Article	Target poulation	Research method	*n*	Form of treatment	Number of sessions	Changes observed	Follow-up
Black & Keane (1982)	WW-II combat veteran	Case study	1	Implosive therapy	3	"Dramatic reduction in anxiety."	24 mo
Blonstein (1988)	41-year-old female car accident survivor	Case study	1	Imaginal exposure *In vivo* exposure with response prevention	22 wk 11 wk	Within- and between-session decreases in anxiety; decrease phobic avoidance.	no
Bowen & Lambert (1986)	Vietnam veterans, WW II POW, air crash witness	Pre–post	8 1 1	Systematic desensitization	several	Decreased psychophysiological arousal (HR & frontalis EMG) during exposure to combat stimuli; decreased subjective stress during exposure to combat stimuli.	no
Fairbank, DeGood, & Jenkins (1981)	32-year-old female car acident survivor	Case study	1	Relaxation training Behavioral rehearsal	3 weekly	Decreased self-reported startle and anxiety while driving.	6 mo
Fairbank, Gross, & Keane (1983)	Vietnam combat veteran	Case study	1	Imaginal Flooding	9	Decreased anxiety, depression, and intrusive recollections; decreased motoric arousal during exposure to trauma stimuli.	
Grigsby (1987)	Vietnam combat veteran	Case study	1	"Imploding psychodynamic themes"	10	Decreaed use of aprazolam; decreased intrusive thoughts.	?
Hickling, Sison, & Vanderploeg (1986)	Vietnam and WW II combat veterans	Pre–post	5 1	Relaxation training Frontalis EMG biofeedback	2–3 7–14	Decreased forntalis muscle tension within and across treatment sessions; decreased self-reported state anxiety, depression; decrease in MMPI scale scores; veteran reports of increased sense of control and accomplishment	no

Keane & Kaloupek (1982)	Vietnam combat veteran	Case study	1	Imaginal flooding	19	Increased sleep; decreased anxiety; decreased psychophysiological arousal (HR) to combat stimuli	12 mos
Kingsbury (1988)	Car and industrial accident survivors, assault victim, and needle phobic	Case study	4	Hypnosis	?	Decreased amnesic episodes, sleep disturbance, and trauma-specific fears (including panic attacks).	2 mo to "several years"
Kipper (1977)	Israeli combat veterans (Yom Kippur War)	Case study	4	Desensitization therapy	?	Increased exposure to steps higher on the hierarchy.	no
Kraft & Al-Issa (1965)	37-year-old male hit twice by car as a pedestrian	Case study	1	Systematic desensitization	22	Decreased irritability; improved sleep and sexual relations with wife; decreased anxiety related to traffic; decreased self-reported neuroticism and anxiety.	6 mo
Kuch (1987)	Car accident survivors	Descriptive report	12	Flooding Imaginal *In vivo* exposure	4–12 hr	"Marked" improvement in half the subjects; four more subjects improved by adding anxiolytic and cognitive treatment; two subjects showed no improvement; five of seven subjects experienced cessation or reduction in trauma-related pain.	6 mos to 9 yr
Kushner (1965)	17-year-old male car accident survivor	Case study	1	Systematic desensitization	6	Self-reported "ninety percent better"; decreased anxiety while driving; increased concentration at school; return to normal appetite; decreased irritability and sleep disturbance.	3 mo

(*continued*)

Table 9.1. Published Reports of Case Studies and Uncontrolled Group Treatments for PTSD (*continued*)

Article	Target poulation	Research method	*n*	Form of treatment	Number of sessions	Changes observed	Follow-up
McCaffrey & Fairbank (1985)	Transportation accident survivors (helicopter and automobile)	Case studies	2	Relaxation training Imaginal Flooding	6 9	Decreased self-rated anxiety; decreased trauma-related dreams; decreased subjective distress and psychophysiological arousal (heart rate and skin resistance) during exposure sessions.	3 mos
McCormack (1985)	Vietnam combat veteran	Case study	1	Cognitive behavior therapy	?	Decreased intrusive recollections; increased ability to communicate emotions to wife; increased control over anger outbursts; increased positive communiation with children; decreased frequency and duration of depression.	no
Mueser, Yarnold, & Foy (1991)	Vietnam combat veterans	Case studies	4	Imaginal Flooding	4–17	Significant improvement in two subjects; worsening of symptoms with one subject; improvements reflected in decreased self-reported daily symptoms, anxiety, and depression, and heart rate during imaginal exposure.	
Mueser & Butler (1987)	Vietnam, Korea, and WW II combat veterans (four with auditory hallucinations)	Pre–post	13	Imaginal Flooding	?	80%+ reduction of PTSD symtoms (3); 20–80% redution of PTSD symptoms (4); less than 20% reduction of PTSD symptoms (3); terminated treatment prematurely (3).	no

Pearson, Poquette, & Wasden (1983)	Female rape victim	Case study	1	Relaxation training Cognitive restructuring Systematic desensitization	?	Increased rational cognitions about phobic stimuli (males); increased effective coping skills.	6 mo
Olasov-Rothbaum & Foa (1983)	Female rape victim	Case study	1	Imaginal and *in vivo* exposure	9	Decreased anxiety, depression, and PTSD symptoms; regained use of voice (in context of trauma-induced elective mutism).	1 yr
Rychtarik, Silverman, Van Landingham, & Prue (1984)	Female incest victim	Case study	1	Implosive therapy	5	Decreased state anxiety; decrease skin conductance; decreased incest thoughts and dreams.	1 yr
Saul, Rome, & Leuser (1946)	WW II combat veterans	Descriptive	14	Systematic desensitization	12	Desensitization of startle reaction; decreased anxiety ("to some degree").	no
Schindler (1980)	Vietnam combat veteran	Case study	1	Systematic desensitization	5	Cessation of recurring nightmare of traumatic incident.	3 mo 7 mo
Venn (1988)	Car accident survivor	Case study	1	Hypnosis	4	Decreased tension, worry, intrusive thoughts, and night-driving fears.	24 mo
Wolff (1977)	Female rape victim	Case study	1	Systematic desensitization	5	Decreased anxiousness; decreased unecessary home "checking" behavior.	2 yr

Table 9.2. Published Reports of Controlled Single-Subject Studies Involving Treatment of PTSD

Article	Target poulation	Research method	n	Form of treatment	Number of sessions	Changes observed	Follow-up
Blanchard & Abel (1976)	Female rape victim	ABAB design	1	Heart rate biofeedback Imaginal exposure	54	Mastery of heart rate during exposure to audiotape-narrated rape scenarios; significant reduction in psychogenic "spells."	4 mo
Fairbank & Keane (1982)	Vietnam combat veteans	Multiple baseline	2	Imaginal Flooding	4 4	Decreased subjective distress and intrusive recollections; decreased arousal to trauma stimuli.	no
Saigh (1986)	Bomb blast and war-traumatized 6½-year-old child	Multiple baseline	1	Imaginal Flooding	9	Decreased subjective discomfort during flooding sessions; decreased self-reported depression and anxiety; improved teacher-rated school behavior; improved intelligence test performance.	6 mos
Saigh (1987a)	Postabduction and war-traumatized 14-year-old adolescent	Multiple baseline	1	Imaginal Flooding	6	Decreased subjective discomfort during flooding sessions; decreased self-reported depression and anxiety, and behavioral avoidance; improved intelligence test performance.	4 mos.
Saigh (1987b)	War-traumatized Lebanese children (11, 11, and 12 years old)	Multiple baseline	3	Imaginal Flooding	9–10	Decreased subjective discomfort during flooding sessions; decreased intrusive thoughts; decreased self-reported depression and anxiety, and behavioral avoidance; improved intelligence test performance.	6 mos

period (during which five of the no-treatment group and none of the treatment group reported hospitalizations for PTSD). Unfortunately, no data were provided on changes in the affective numbing/social avoidance or non-EMG hyperarousal aspects of PTSD.

In a more recent treatment outcome study, Keane, Fairbank, Caddell, and Zimering (1989) provided implosive therapy to 11 Vietnam veteran outpatients diagnosed with PTSD, and compared the results with 13 veterans who did not receive implosive therapy. Implosive therapy was found to be superior to no treatment (waiting-list control), as evidenced by changes in self-report measures of depression, anxiety, and fear, as well as decreases on selected MMPI scales (Hypochondriasis, Depression, and Hysteria). Furthermore, the treated veterans showed significant reductions in therapist-rated PTSD symptoms of reexperiencing of the trauma, startle, memory and concentration problems, guilt, and associated features (anxiety, depression, irritability, impulsivity, and legal problems). Not ameliorated were affective numbing, social avoidance, and self-reported social adjustment. These treatment gains were maintained at a 6-month follow-up. This study demonstrates the effectiveness of behavioral implosion for reducing the DSM-III-R PTSD symptoms associated with reexperiencing phenomena (Criterion B) and hyperarousal (Criterion D), but not affective numbing (Criterion C).

Frank *et al.* (1988) compared the efficacy of a cognitive therapy treatment to systematic desensitization in treating female rape victims. Both treatments were found to lead to improvements in psychometrically measured anxiety, depression, and fear, and these effects were found whether the subject sought treatment immediately after or several months following the assault (although Kilpatrick and Calhoun, 1988, provide a compelling argument that treatment provided immediately after the assault may not have been as efficacious as the investigators conclude). Posttreatment results of 34 subjects who received cognitive-behavior therapy where compared with those of 26 subjects who received systematic desensitization. Multivariate analyses revealed no statistically significant difference between the two treatments.

The studies reviewed in this section lend solid support for the view that psychologically based treatment is better than no treatment. As with the single-subject studies, the treatments appear to have greatest impact on the more observable aspects of the PTSD complex of symptoms. In addition, these empirical efforts were also limited to behavioral interventions, so it is unclear whether conventional psychological treatments can make the same claims about efficacy.

Interorientation Comparisons

Several outcome studies comparing psychological treatments for PTSD have appeared in the published literature over the past decade. The compared treatments have included transcendental meditation, stress inoculation, conventional and brief psychodynamic psychotherapy, and implosive therapy. The studies are described in this section and are summarized in Table 9.4.

In what appears to be the first comparative treatment study in PTSD, Brooks and Scarano (1985) randomly assigned help-seeking Vietnam combat veterans to either transcendental meditation (TM) or psychotherapy (eclectic) conditions. After 3 months of weekly sessions, the TM subjects showed improvement in eight dependent variables, which included PTSD symptoms, alcoholic consumption,

Table 9.3. Published Reports Involving Treatment Comparisons with Nonspecific Effects

Article	Target population	Research method	n	Form of treatment	Number of sessions	Changes observed	Follow-up
Keane, Fairbank, Caddell, & Zimering (1989)	Vietnam combat veterans	Controlled treatment outcome	11 13	Imaginal Flooding	14–16	Decreased self-reported anxiety, depression, and fear; decrease MMPI scales (1, 2, and 3); decrease in therapist-rated re-experiencing and hyperarousal symptoms	6 mos
Frank, Anderson, Stewart, Dancu, Hughes, & West (1988)	Female rape victims	Controlled treatment outcome	26 34	Systematic desensitization Cognitive therapy	14	Decreased anxiety, depression, and fear for both groups.	6 mos
Peniston (1986)	Vietnam combat veterans	Controlled treatment outcome	8 8	EMG biofeedback-assisted Systematic desensitization	48	Decreased forehead muscle tension, nightmares, and flashbacks; fewer hospital readmissions than controls.	2 yr

and family problems, while the psychotherapy subjects showed no significant change in any of these measures. Although the investigators provide scant detail about the psychotherapy condition (such as level of therapist training, content of sessions, etc.), these findings raise some doubt about the efficacy of generic psychotherapy as a treatment for PTSD. Transcendental meditation, by contrast, produced a substantial impact as measured by the selected variables.

In a more recent treatment outcome study, with acutely distressed rape victims (within 3 months of assault), Resick, Jordan, Girelli, Hutter, and Marhoefer-Dvorak (1988) examined the comparative efficacy of two behavioral treatments—assertion training and stress inoculation—and supportive psychotherapy plus information. These three treatments, provided in a brief therapy format (i.e., six sessions), all led to significant improvements on measures of anxiety and depression. Well over half of the participants (59%) improved by at least a half standard deviation on a standardized global symptom index, and nearly one-third (32%) improved by a full standard deviation. No treatment was found to be superior to any other. However, the investigators quite appropriately reported that their study possessed relatively low statistical power (between 10% and 15%), making it less likely to determine significant differences between the treatments. Furthermore, since recently victimized women were employed as subjects, any real difference between the treatments may have been obscured by naturally occurring gains that can be expected with this population (see Kilpatrick and Calhoun, 1988, for a discussion).

In what is perhaps the earliest controlled study of flooding and combat-related PTSD, Cooper and Clum (1989) compared seven Vietnam combat veterans who received a conventional individual and group PTSD treatment program with seven veterans who received this same treatment regimen supplemented with imaginal flooding (implosive therapy). Only the flooded veterans showed significant symptom reduction, in the form of decreased sleep disturbance, nightmares, and state anxiety, along with decreased discomfort during a combat-oriented behavioral avoidance task. The flooded group also maintained their reduced sleep disturbance and exhibited fewer psychoticlike symptoms when assessed at 3-month follow-up. Unfortunately, but significantly, the flooded group experienced a nearly 50% dropout rate.

Boudewyns and Hyer (1990) randomly assigned 38 PTSD inpatients to receive either 10–12 sessions of imaginal flooding or the same number of conventional one-to-one counseling sessions. While the veterans in neither group showed significant decreases in daily self-rated anxiety, the flooding group members did show decreased arousal—especially heart rate—when exposed to combat slides. In addition, flooding group members showed a significant improvement in a composite measure of anxiety/depression, vigor, alienation, and confidence in skills, at 3 months posttreatment. These findings suggest that, relative to conventional psychotherapy, implosive therapy is an efficacious treatment for combat-related PTSD.

In a study of the impact of direct therapeutic exposure with 58 Vietnam veteran PTSD program inpatients, Boudewyns *et al.* (1990) compared program graduates who were judged to be "successes" with those deemed as "failures." Subjects were randomly assigned to either a conventional inpatient treatment or a conventional treatment plus direct therapeutic exposure. The success or failure classification was based on the top and bottom quartiles as measured by adjustment scale residual gains scores (15 subjects in each group). No significant differences between these groups were found on pretreatment demographic, life history, and

Table 9.4. Published Reports Involving Interorientation Comparisons

Article	Target population	Research method	n	Form of treatment	Number of sessions	Changes observed	Follow-up
Boudewyns & Hyer (1990)	Vietnam combat veterans (inpatients)	Controlled treatment outcome	19 19	Imaginal Flooding	10–12	Decreased subjective anxiety and psychophysiological arousal (HR) when exposed to combat stimuli; improvements in self-reported anxiety/depression, depression, vigor, alienation, and confidence in skills.	3 mo
Boudewyns, Hyer, Woods, Harrison, & McCranie (1990)	Vietnam combat veterans (inpatients)	Controlled treatment outcome	26 32	Imaginal Flooding	10–12	More "successes" (38% and fewer failures (15.6%), based on social adjustment indices, than control group (11.5% and 37.5%, respectively).	3 mo
Brom, Kleber, & Defares (1989)	Trauma survivors (violent crime; traffic mishaps; spouse loss by murder/suicide, traffic accidents, or illness)	Comparative treatment outcome	31 29 29 23	Trauma desensitization Hypnotherapy Psychodynamic psychotherapy Wait-list control	14–19 (mean # sessions by group)	Significant improvements on psychometrically measured anxiety, trauma, and PTSD symptoms for all treatment groups; no significant differences among the treatments.	3 mo

Brooks & Scarano (1985)	Vietnam combat veterans (outpatients)	Comparative treatment outcome	10 8	Transcendental medication (TM) Psychotherapy	10–12	TM group showed decreases on measures of PTSD, emotional numbness, anxiety, depression, alcohol consumption, insomnia, and family problems; TM group showed increases in employment status.	3 mo
Cooper & Clum (1989)	Vietnam combat veterans	Comparative treatment outcome	8 8	Imaginal Flooding	6–14	Decreased subjective discomfort when exposed to combat stimuli; decreased nightmares; decreased self-reported state anxiety, nightmares, and sleep disturbance.	6 mo
Resick, Jordan, Girelli, Hutter, & Marhoefer-Dvorak (1988)	Rape victims	Comparative treatment outcome	12 13 12	Stress inoculation Assertion training Supportive therapy	6 (2 hr each)	All three conditions produced significant gains on global symptom index, phobic anxiety, and depression; no significant differences among the groups.	3 & 6 mo

psychometric variables. Analyses revealed a significantly greater number of treatment successes had received flooding therapy (10 of 15), whereas the failure group primarily comprised patients who had received only the conventional treatment (12 of 15).

Brom, Kleber, and Defares (1989) assessed the treatment efficacy of traumatic desensitization (treatment based on cognitive and two-factor learning theories), hypnotherapy, short-term psychodynamic psychotherapy, with a waiting-list control condition. One hundred and twelve persons diagnosed with PTSD who were within 5 years of their exposure to trauma (mostly victims of crime and vehicular accidents) were randomly assigned to one of these treatments. Psychological functioning, as measured by self-report psychometric instruments, showed improvements for all groups excepting the waiting-list control (about 60% improvement for treated subjects versus 26% improvement for the controls), and no significant differences between the treatment conditions. The investigators conclude: "The treatments do benefit some in comparison with a control group and using stringent methodological techniques, but they do not benefit everyone, the effects are not always substantial, and the differences between the therapies are small" (p. 610). While these findings parallel the conclusions reached by other investigators in psychotherapy outcome research, some aspects of the study suggest methodological shortcomings, for example, lack of adequate definition of the treatments being compared; failure to specify method for determining, and lack of detail about, symptom severity; reliance on psychometric measures as dependent measures; failure to standardize or statistically control number of sessions among the treatments, and so forth.

The treatment outcome studies reviewed above provide further data on the effectiveness of psychologically based treatment for PTSD. Four of the studies found a superiority for either transcendental meditation or imaginal flooding over conventional psychotherapy treatment of PTSD. Two studies reported significant benefits from behavioral and psychodynamic treatment but found no difference in outcome from the two treatment approaches.

Psychopharmacotherapy

Medications that have been utilized with trauma patients include mood stabilizers (antidepressants and lithium), beta-blockers, anticonvulsants, and minor tranquilizers. Nearly all of the studies examining pharmacotherapy in PTSD, unfortunately, are uncontrolled groups studies and as such are vulnerable to internal validity threats. Nevertheless, several medications have demonstrated effectiveness with at least some symptoms of PTSD.

Hogben and Cornfield (1981) reported that the monoamine oxidase inhibitor phenelzine was effective in the rapid remission of nightmares, flashbacks, startle response, panic, and anxiety in five traumatized patients. Milanes, Mack, Dennison, and Slater (1984) reported that phenelzine worked to reduce nightmares, hyperalertness, irritability, and anxiety in traumatized individuals. However, van der Kolk (1983) reported an increase in the vividness of traumatic memories in four of seven patients treated with phenelzine.

Kolb and Mutalipassi (1982) found the antihypertensive clonidine and the beta-adrenergic blocker propranolol to improve sleep and decrease hyperalertness in traumatized combat veterans. In a more recent study (Kolb, Burris & Griffiths,

1984), patients who were treated with either clonidine or propranolol reported a decrease in startle responses, explosiveness, and intrusive reexperiencing, while those on both drugs concurrently reported decreased nightmares. Follow-up at 6 months revealed continued symptom reduction for the majority of subjects (reduced explosiveness, decreased nightmares, improved sleep, decreased intrusive recollections, less startle, reduced hyperarousal).

Burstein (1984) found a reduction of reexperiencing and hyperarousal symptoms in 10 PTSD patients treated with imipramine, but no change in, or an exacerbation of, avoidant symptoms. Falcone, Ryan and Chamberlain (1985) compared the effects of amitriptyline, imipramine, desipramine, and doxepin with 17 combat veterans. Results suggest the most beneficial effects were evidenced with amitriptyline, which led to reductions of nightmares, flashbacks, and panic symptoms. Most recently, Davidson *et al.* (1990) compared the use of amitriptyline with placebo regimens in 46 PTSD-diagnosed combat veterans of World War II, Korea, and Vietnam. They found that the tricyclic (but not the placebo) produced significant reductions in depression and anxiety and in number and severity of PTSD symptoms. Lithium carbonate has also been used to treat the symptoms of loss of control and anger outbursts seen in trauma patients (van der Kolk, 1983). Of 22 patients treated with lithium, 14 reported gaining a subjective sense of control over their lives with a decrease in the hyperreactivity to stress and hyperarousal.

Lipper, Davidson, Grady, Edinger, and Cavenar (1986) found that the anticonvulsant carbamazepine produced significant improvement in traumatic dreams, flashbacks, and intrusive recollections of combat veterans. In a similar study, Wolfe, Alavi, and Mosnaim (1988) showed carbamazepine to be effective in reducing violent behavior and angry outbursts.

In summary, several medications have been found to have beneficial effects in the treatment of PTSD symptoms. These effects appear to be especially pronounced in the amelioration of the florid, anxiety-based symptoms, without remediating the less conspicuous symptoms such as emotional numbing, social estrangement, and anhedonia. This characteristic is not unlike that found with the imaginal flooding or implosive therapy treatments for PTSD, which appear most helpful in remediating the reexperiencing and hyperarousal aspects of PTSD. Due to their propensity for adverse side effects and misuse, however, it is particularly important to weigh the benefits of a given medication with its short- and long-term costs.

Eye Movement Desensitization

A controversial procedure for treating the negative affect associated with traumatic memories has been described recently in the professional literature (Shapiro, 1989a, 1989b, 1991; Wolpe & Abrams, 1991). The procedure, called eye movement desensitization (EMD), involves rapid therapist-directed, rhythmic or saccadic eye movements during the recollection of a painful traumatic memory. With head held still, the patient visually tracks the therapist's pen or finger as it is moved back and forth while the traumatic memory is recalled. Twenty-two individuals who had survived a variety of traumatizing experiences were reported to have dramatic anxiety reduction with the use of this procedure, with maintenance of gains at 1-month and 3-month follow-up (Shapiro, 1989b). Wolpe and Abrams (1991) presented comparable, anecdotal results with a rape victim. Just how this procedure produces these changes is unclear and awaits further research. Careful controlled research is also needed. One critical variable which must be controlled for in future investigations of EMD is patient expectancy and demand characteristics presented by the procedure. It is with keen interest that we await the results of controlled clinical trials on this novel and promising treatment.

Outcome Parameters

The reports reviewed suggest that current treatments affect primarily the more observable aspects of PTSD. Most studies, however, actually failed to examine other indices of functioning, such as emotional constriction, anhedonia, or social withdrawal. This failure to attend to "negative" PTSD symptoms (i.e., those which are less observable and anxiety based) is unfortunate. Information is lost that may be critically important in PTSD phenomenology and treatment. As an example, evidence is emerging that the sleep disturbances seen in PTSD are more than sources of subjective aggravation, but may contribute substantially to excess morbidity and mortality. To wit, a main cause of excess mortality in Vietnam veterans is motor vehicle accidents (Centers for Disease Control, 1987; Hearst, Newman, & Hulley, 1986). Though direct causal links between sleep loss and accidental death are hard to establish, both sleep apneic and insomniac groups have exhibited elevated numbers of vehicular accidents. Though sleep need varies tremendously between individuals, in many, impairments become marked as sleep is chronically restricted to a range of 4 hours per night or less (Naitoh, 1969). Do trauma victims lose this much sleep? In the case of chronic, severe combat-related PTSD, the answer seems to be yes. Furthermore, there appear to be subgroups at exceptional risk. Woodward (1991) has reported that frequent ("almost nightly") traumatic nightmare sufferers report significantly less time in bed and longer sleep latencies. These data, though preliminary, compel the PTSD clinician-researcher to assess sleep disturbance in each patient, not only from the standpoint of basic sleep hygiene but from that of risk reduction. Prominent in this assessment should be frequency of trauma-related and non-trauma-related nightmares, time spent in bed, sleep latency, and frequency of sleep disruptions. Also deserving attention is the fact that most medically related dyssomnias and parasomnias increase in prevalence in older persons: As PTSD patients age, severe sleep problems may be expected to emerge in these already sleep-compromised individuals. Ultimately, treatments should focus on basic sleep hygiene (cf. Hauri & Esther, 1990) and the translation of sleep-related treatments into the group therapy modalities dominant in many mental health settings (e.g., Brockway, 1987). Other PTSD features or associated features warranting attention include substance abuse, panic disorder, depression, marital and familial problems, and health status.

Although individuals exposed to different traumatic events may generally resemble one another in their behavioral presentation, they may differ in other important ways, for example, in levels of hyperarousal, degrees of survivor guilt, extent of dissociative symptoms, and so on. Two people diagnosed with PTSD but who differ in these ways can also be expected to respond differentially to treatment. For example, there is growing evidence that not all traumatized Vietnam veterans respond well to implosive therapy (e.g., Mueser & Butler, 1987; Pitman *et al.*, 1991). To determine which patients respond best to what treatments, future studies must include a careful examination of the full range of PTSD symptomatology, preferably by using a standardized diagnostic measure, such as the Structured Clinical Interview for DSM-III-R (SCID-R; Spitzer & Williams, 1989) or the Clinician Administered PTSD Scale (CAPS; Blake *et al.*, 1991).

Conclusions

In reviewing the results of both single-case and group studies, it is clear that the existing PTSD treatments, particularly behavioral and pharmacological, can significantly reduce PTSD signs and symptoms. The effects of these treatments are most likely to be seen in reduced psychophysiological arousal and startle, intrusive thoughts and nightmares, and irritability and anger. It is not clear whether these treatments also reduce numbing, alienation, and restricted affect (Keane, 1989;[1] Keane, Gerardi *et al.*, 1992). It may be that these treatments are effective primarily in suppressing the more easily observed PTSD symptoms and that adjunctive, alternative treatments may be necessary for adequately treating less evident aspects of PTSD. Alternatively, this apparent differential impact may be research artifact and reflect a widespread failure to adequately measure the less evident symptoms. In this case, one solution lies in conducting studies that report on a treatment's impact on the entire range of PTSD symptoms.

Several observations can be made about the extant PTSD treatment outcome literature. First, aside from pharmacotherapy trials, behavioral studies predominate in empirically based clinical research, and they do so absolutely in single-*n*, group pre–post, and simple, controlled studies. Little published data exist demonstrating the efficacy of psychodynamic psychotherapy with PTSD. The behavior therapy predominance in empirical research is not surprising in light of that orientation's foundation in the experimental and applied analyses of behavior. Behavior is also usually measured more easily than are internal, hypothesized constructs, and demonstrating prediction and control is a central interest in the science of behavior. Ironically, it is likely that most PTSD treatment being employed would not be considered behavioral (i.e., not involving direct therapeutic exposure, stress inoculation, etc.); the prevailing therapies are most likely eclectic, supportive, and developmental/psychodynamic in orientation (which may not be incompatible with behavior therapy). Because of their widespread use, the nonbehavioral treatments should be scrutinized more extensively; nonbehavioral clinician-researchers should engage in empirical research, not only to test the theory on which they have based their treatments, but to advance the assessment and treatment of PTSD.

In four of six interorientation comparison studies reported here, the behavioral treatments show a statistical and clinical superiority over conventional treatments (i.e., Boudewyns & Hyer, 1990; Boudewyns *et al.*, 1990; Brooks & Scarano, 1985; Cooper & Clum, 1989). In their description, the elements of these conventional therapies bore clear resemblance to that found in general supportive and

[1]Keane (1989) compared PTSD phenomenology to that of schizophrenia in the sense of being composed of these "positive" PTSD symptoms, while "negative" symptoms involved less conspicuous symptoms such as emotional constriction and feelings of guilt, anhedonia, and estrangement from others. The differential symptom impact seen in exposure-based and pharmacotherapy appears to follow this delineation.

psychodynamic therapy, which, in application to PTSD, is strikingly similar to short-term psychodynamic psychotherapy *a la* Horowitz. As such, the behavioral treatment appears to be a more efficacious treatment than the more traditional, psychodynamic treatment. This contention, however, is conjectural and awaits research involving direct comparisons between these two treatments. A fourth study, furthermore, failed to show any advantage of behavioral treatment over supportive therapy (Resick *et al.*, 1988). In the only study involving a direct comparison (Brom *et al.*, 1989), albeit with the methodological flaws cited above, the behavioral and psychodynamic treatments also produced equivalent outcomes. These studies give warning that more comparative research is necessary to assess their relative impact as well as their unique contributions for ameliorating PTSD symptomatology.

In concluding this chapter, it is worth recognizing several issues which have relevance to PTSD treatment and outcome research. First, PTSD phenomenology appears to vary according to the type of trauma experienced. The behavioral and psychological manifestations of PTSD in a war veteran may differ markedly from a rape victim, who in turn may differ from a survivor of a natural disaster. As a consequence, certain treatments may be more suited to one PTSD population than another. Implosive therapy has been considered to be an important treatment option for traumatized war veterans (e.g., Fairbank & Brown, 1987; Lyons & Keane, 1989) but has been criticized as a technique for victims of sexual assault (Kilpatrick & Best, 1984). Much of the research reviewed in this chapter was with traumatized combat veterans. Clearly, treatments involving other trauma populations warrant study as well.

Second, in part because the diagnostic category of PTSD was not formally codified until 1980 (American Psychiatric Association, 1980), published reports prior to that time did not report information about the full range of trauma-induced symptomatology; that is, exposure to trauma and subsequent help-seeking behavior justified study inclusion. Thus, it is difficult to ascertain whether the populations treated prior to 1980 are comparable to those treated more recently. Even the most recent studies have not included rigorous methods of determining PTSD status and severity (e.g., Blake *et al.*, 1991; Spitzer & Williams, 1989). These studies suffer serious threats to their external validity and clinical utility. In addition, since PTSD tends to have a high co-morbidity with other disorders (substance abuse, depression, panic disorder), assessment of those problem areas is also important.

A third issue pertains to the choice of dependent measure by researchers of PTSD treatment outcomes. The majority of studies, including those involving behavioral research, have relied solely upon self-report or paper-and-pencil psychometric measures to assess treatment effects. If the behavioral, cognitive, and physiological response domains are indeed critical for treatment and understanding of psychological functioning (e.g., Lang, 1977, 1979), this overreliance is disturbing. Future studies should supplement self-report and standardized psychometric measures with behavioral and psychophysiological measures.

Since PTSD is often a chronic disorder, with symptoms continuing for many years (Klonoff, McDougall, Clark, Kramer, & Horgan, 1976; Kluznik, Speed, Van Valkenburg, & Magraw, 1986), studies of its treatments therefore need to substantiate their durability over time. All of the reports reviewed in this chapter involved relatively short follow-up periods, reported largely in months rather than years.

Information regarding long-term maintenance of gains is critical for determining the relative efficacy of PTSD treatments. Future studies might also attend to less "mainstream" clinical populations and treatment interventions. Controlled treatments applied to specific PTSD populations, such as disaster- and crime-related PTSD, are needed. Careful study of PTSD treatments such as short-term dynamic psychotherapy and eye movement desensitization is also needed, as well as empirical scrutiny of lesser-known treatments such as anger management (McWhirter & Liebman, 1988), transcendental meditation (Brooks & Scarano, 1985) and hypnotherapy (Kingsbury, 1988; Spiegel, 1988; Venn, 1988).

A final, overarching problem with the current PTSD outcome research relates to its correspondence with existing treatments. While adhering to their respective theoretical bases, the treatments researched thus far may depart substantially from usual and customary clinical practice. The interventions exposed to empirical scrutiny may poorly reflect the dynamic and multidimensional nature of contemporary PTSD treatment. As necessary as it is to determine the efficacy of theoretically pure treatments, it also important to identify and examine the critical features of existing PTSD treatments as they are practiced by seasoned PTSD clinicians and in established outpatient and inpatient PTSD services. While it is important to acknowledge the publication descriptions of established PTSD services (Adams, 1982; Arnold, 1985; Berman, Price, & Gusman, 1982; Beysner, 1985; Starkey & Ashlock, 1984, 1986), information from front-line clinicians who have ongoing exposure to trauma survivors may yet provide the key to advancing effective treatment for this population.

References

Adams, M. F. (1982). PTSD: An inpatient treatment unit. *American Journal of Nursing, 82*, 1704–1705.

American Psychiatric Association. (1952). *Diagnostic and statistical manual of mental disorders*. Washington, DC: Author.

American Psychiatric Association. (1968). *Diagnostic and statistical manual of mental disorders* (2nd ed.). Washington, DC: Author.

American Psychiatric Association. (1980). *Diagnostic and statistical manual of mental disorders* (3rd ed.). Washington, DC: Author.

American Psychiatric Association. (1987). *Diagnostic and statistical manual of mental disorders* (3rd ed.-revised). Washington, DC: Author.

Arnold, A. L. (1985). Inpatient treatment of Vietnam veterans with post-traumatic stress disorder. In S. M. Sonnenberg, A. J. Blank, & J. A. Talbots (Eds.), *The trauma of war: Stress and recovery in Vietnam veterans* (pp. 239–261). Washington, DC: American Psychiatric Press.

Bandura, A. (1977). Self-efficacy: Toward a unifying theory of behavioral change. *Psychological Review, 84*, 191–215.

Bandura, A. (1986). *Social foundations of thought and action: A social cognitive theory*. Engelwood Cliffs, NJ: Prentice-Hall.

Beck, A. T. (1976). *Cognitive therapy and emotional disorders*. New York: International University Press.

Beck, A. T., & Emery, G. (1985). *Anxiety disorders and phobias: A cognitive perspective*. New York: Basic Books.

Berman, S., Price, S., & Gusman, F. (1982). An inpatient program for Vietnam combat veterans in a Veterans Administration hospital. *Hospital and Community Psychiatry, 33*, 919–922.

Beysner, J. K. (1985). Multimodal inpatient treatment of Vietnam veterans with post-traumatic stress disorder. *Psychotherapy in Private Practice, 3*, 43–47.

Black, J. L., & Keane, T. M. (1982). Implosive therapy in the treatment of combat related fears in a World War II veteran. *Journal of Behavior Therapy and Experimental Psychiatry, 13*, 163–165.

Blackburn, A. B., O'Connell, W. E., & Richman, B. W. (1984). Post-traumatic stress disorder, the Vietnam veteran, and Adlerian natural high therapy. *Journal of Adlerian Theory, Individual Psychology, 40*, 317–332.

Blake, D. D., Albano, A. M., & Keane, T. M. (1992). Twenty years of trauma: *Psychology Abstracts* 1970 through 1989. *Journal of Traumatic Stress, 5*, 477–484.

Blake, D. D., Weathers, F., Nagy, L. M., Kaloupek, D. G., Klauminzer, G., Charney, D. S., & Keane, T. M. (1991). A clinician rating scale for assessing current and lifetime PTSD: The CAPS-1. *The Behavior Therapist, 14*, 187–188.

Blanchard, E. B., & Abel, G. G. (1976). An experimental case study of the biofeedback treatment of a rape-induced psychophysiological cardiovascular disorder. *Behavior Therapy, 7*, 113–119.

Blank, A. S. (1985). Psychological treatment of war veterans: A challenge for mental health professionals. *Medical Hypnoanalysis, 6*, 91–96.

Blonstein, C. H. (1988). Treatment of automobile driving phobia through imaginal and *in vivo* exposure plus response prevention. *The Behavior Therapist, 11*, 70, 86.

Boudewyns, P. A., & Hyer, L. (1990). Physiological response to combat veterans and preliminary treatment outcome in Vietnam veteran PTSD patients treated with direct therapeutic exposure. *Behavior Therapy, 21*, 63–87.

Boudewyns, P. A., Hyer, L., Woods, M. G., Harrison, W. R., & McCranie, E. (1990). PTSD among Vietnam veterans: An early look at treatment outcome with direct therapeutic exposure. *Journal of Traumatic Stress, 3*, 359–368.

Bowen, G. R., & Lambert, J. A. (1986). Systematic desensitization therapy with post-traumatic stress disorder cases. In C. R. Figley (Ed.), *Trauma and its wake* (Vol. II, pp. 281–291). New York: Brunner/Mazel.

Brockway, S. S. (1987). Group treatment of combat nightmares in post-traumatic stress disorder. *Journal of Contemporary Psychotherapy, 17*, 270–284.

Brom, D., Kleber, R. J., & Defares, P. B. (1989). Brief psychotherapy for posttraumatic stress disorders. *Journal of Consulting and Clinical Psychology, 57*, 607–612.

Brooks, J. S., & Scarano, T. (1985). Transcendental meditation in the treatment of post-Vietnam adjustment. *Journal of Counseling and Adjustment, 64*, 212–215.

Burgess, A. W. (1974). Rape trauma syndrome. *Behavioral Sciences Law, 1*, 97–114.

Burgess, A. W., & Holmstrom, L. L. (1983). Rape trauma syndrome. *American Journal of Psychiatry, 131*, 981–986.

Burstein, A. (1984). Treatment of post-traumatic stress disorder with imipramine. *Psychosomatics, 25*, 681–687.

Caplan, G. *Principles of preventive psychiatry*. (1964). New York: Basic Books.

Centers for Disease Control Vietnam Experience Study (1987). Postservice mortality among Vietnam veterans. *Journal of the American Medical Association, 257*, 790–795.

Chemtob, C., Roitblat, H. L., Hamada, R. S., Carlson, J. G., & Twentyman, C. T. (1988). A cognitive action theory of post-traumatic stress disorder. *Journal of Anxiety Disorders, 2*, 253–275.

Cohen, J. A. (1981). Theories of narcissism and trauma. *American Journal of Psychotherapy, 35*, 93–100.

Cooper, N. A., & Clum, G. A. (1989). Imaginal flooding as a supplementary treatment for PTSD in combat veterans: A controlled study. *Behavior Therapy, 20*, 381–391.

Crump, L. E. (1984). Gestalt therapy in the treatment of Vietnam veterans experiencing PTSD symptomatology. *Journal of Contemporary Psychotherapy, 14*, 90–98.

Cryer, L., & Beutler, L. (1980). Group therapy: An alternative approach for rape victims. *Journal of Sex and Marital Therapy, 6*, 40–46.

DaCosta, J. M. (1871). On irritable heart: A clinical study of a form of functional cardiac disorder and its consequences. *American Journal of Medical Science, 61*, 17–52.

Daly, R. J. (1983). Samuel Pepys and post-traumatic stress disorder. *British Journal of Psychiatry, 143*, 64–68.

Davidson, J., Kudler, H., Smith, R., Mahorney, S. L., Lipper, S., Hammett, E., Saunders, W. B., & Cavenar, J. O., Jr. (1990). Treatment of posttraumatic stress disorder with amitriptyline and placebo. *Archives of General Psychiatry, 47*, 259–266.

Egendorf, A. (1975). Vietnam veteran rap groups and themes of postwar life. *Journal of Social Issues, 31*, 111–124.

Ellis, A., & Grieger, R. (1986). *Handbook of Rational Emotive Therapy (Vol. 2)*. New York: Springer.

Emery, P. E., & Emery, O. B. (1985). The defense process in posttraumatic stress disorders. *American Journal of Psychotherapy, 39*, 541–553.

Fairbank, J. A., & Brown, T. A. (1987). Current behavioral approaches to the treatment of posttraumatic stress disorder. *The Behavior Therapist, 10*, 57–64.

Fairbank, J. A., DeGood, D. E., & Jenkins, C. W. (1981). Behavioral treatment of a persistent posttraumatic startle response. *Journal of Behavior Therapy and Experimental Psychiatry, 12*, 321–324.

Fairbank, J. A., Gross, R. T., & Keane, T. M. (1983). Treatment of posttraumatic stress disorder: Evaluating outcome with a behavioral code. *Behavioral Modification, 7*, 557–568.

Fairbank, J. A., & Keane, T. M. (1982). Flooding for combat-related stress disorders: Assessment of anxiety reduction across traumatic memories. *Behavior Therapy, 13*, 499–510.

Falcone, S., Ryan, C., & Chamberlain, K. (1985). Tricyclics: Possible treatment for posttraumatic stress disorder. *Journal of Clinical Psychiatry, 46*, 385–389.

Figley, C. R. (1978). Symptoms of delayed combat stress among a college sample of Vietnam veterans. *Military Medicine, 143*, 107–110.

Figley, C. R. (1988). A five-phase treatment of post-traumatic stress disorder in families. *Journal of Traumatic Stress, 1*, 127–141.

Foa, E. B., Steketee, G., & Olasov-Rothbaum, B. (1989). Behavioral/cognitive conceptualizations of posttraumatic stress disorder. *Behavior Therapy, 20*, 155–176.

Foy, D. W., Carroll, E. M., & Donahoe, C. P. (1987). Etiological factors in the development of PTSD in clinical samples of Vietnam combat veterans. *Journal of Clinical Psychology, 43*, 17–27.

Foy, D. W., Sipprelle, R. C., Rueger, D. B., & Carroll, E. M. (1984). Etiology of PTSD in Vietnam veterans: Analysis of premilitary, military, and combat exposure influences. *Journal of Consulting and Clinical Psychology, 52*, 79–87.

Frank, E., Anderson, B., Stewart, B. D., Dancu, C., Hughes, C., & West, D. (1988). Efficacy of cognitive behavior therapy and systematic desensitization in the treatment of rape trauma. *Behavior Therapy, 19*, 403–420.

Friedman, M. J. (1988). Toward rational pharmacotherapy for posttraumatic stress disorder: An interim report. *American Journal of Psychiatry, 145*, 281–285.

Grigbsy, J. P. (1987). The use of imagery in the treatment of posttraumatic stress disorder. *Journal of Nervous and Mental Disease, 175*, 55–59.

Grinker, R., & Spiegel, J. P. (1945). *Men under stress.* Philadelphia: Blakiston.

Haley, S. A. (1978). Treatment implications of post-combat stress response syndrome for mental health professionals. In C. R. Figley (Ed.), *Stress disorders among Vietnam veterans* (pp. 254–267). New York: Brunner/Mazel.

Hauri, P. J., & Esther, M. S. (1990). Insomnia. *Mayo Clinic Proceedings, 65*, 869–882.

Hearst, N., Newman, T. B., & Hulley, S. B. (1986). Delayed effects of the military draft on mortality. A randomized natural experiment. *The New England Journal of Medicine, 314*, 620–624.

Helzer, J. E., Robins, L. N., & McEvoy, L. (1988). Post-traumatic stress disorder in the general population. *New England Journal of Medicine, 317*, 1630–1634.

Hickling, E. J., Sison, G. F. P., Jr., & Vanderploeg, R. D. (1986). Treatment of posttraumatic stress disorder with relaxation and biofeedback training. *Biofeedback and Self-Regulation, 11*, 125–134.

Hogben, G. L., & Cornfield, R. B. (1981). Treatment of traumatic war neurosis with phenelzine. *Archives of General Psychiatry, 38*, 440–445.

Holmes, M. R., & St. Lawrence, J. S. (1983). Treatment of rape-induced trauma: Proposed behavioral conceptualization and review of the literature. *Clinical Psychology Review, 3*, 417–433.

Horowitz, M. J. (1986). *Stress response syndromes* (2nd ed.). Northvale, NJ: Jason Aronson.

Horowitz, M. J., & Solomon, G. F. (1975). A prediction of delayed stress response syndromes in Vietnam veterans. *Journal of Social Issues, 31*, 67–80.

Jacobsen, E. (1938). *Progressive relaxation.* Chicago, IL: University of Chicago Press.

Jones, J. C., & Barlow, D. H. (1990). The etiology of post-traumatic stress disorder. *Clinical Psychology Review, 10*, 299–328.

Keane, T. M. (1985). Defining traumatic stress: Some comments on the current terminological confusion. *Behavior Therapy, 16*, 419–423.

Keane, T. M. (1989). Post-traumatic stress disorder: Current status and future directions. *Behavior Therapy, 20*, 149–153.

Keane, T. M., Albano, A. M., & Blake, D. D. (1992). Current trends in the treatment of post-traumatic stress symptoms. In M. Basoglu (Ed.), *Torture and its consequences* (pp. 363–401). London: Cambridge University Press.

Keane, T. M., Fairbank, J. A., Caddell, J. M., & Zimering, R. T. (1989). Implosive (flooding) therapy reduces symptoms of PTSD in Vietnam combat veterans. *Behavior Therapy, 20*, 245–260.

Keane, T. M., Fairbank, J. A., Caddell, J. M., Zimering, R. T., & Bender, M. E. (1985). A behavioral approach to the assessment and treatment of post-traumatic stress disorder in Vietnam veterans. In C. R. Figley (Ed.), *Trauma and its wake: The study and treatment of post-traumatic stress disorders* (pp. 257–294). New York: Brunner/Mazel.

Keane, T. M., Gerardi, R. J., Quinn, S. J., & Litz, B. T. (1992). Behavioral treatment of post-traumatic stress disorder. In S. Turner, K. Calhoun, & H. Adams (Eds.), *Handbook of Behavior Therapy* (2nd ed., pp. 87–97). New York: John Wiley & Sons.

Keane, T. M., & Kaloupek, D. G. (1982). Imaginal flooding in the treatment of a post-traumatic stress disorder. *Journal of Consulting & Clinical Psychology, 50*, 138–140.

Keane, T. M., & Penk, W. E. (1988). The prevalence of post-traumatic stress disorder [Letter to the editor]. *New England Journal of Medicine, 318*, 1690–1691.

Keane, T. M., Scott, O. N., Chavoya, G. A., Lamparski, D. M., & Fairbank, J. A. (1985). Social support in Vietnam veterans with post-traumatic stress disorder: A comparative analysis. *Journal of Consulting and Clinical Psychology, 53*, 95–102.

Keane, T. M., Zimering, R. T., & Caddell, J. M. (1985). A behavioral formulation of post-traumatic stress disorder in combat veterans. *The Behavior Therapist, 8*, 9–12.

Kilpatrick, D. G., & Best, C. L. (1984). Some cautionary remarks on treating sexual assault victims with implosion. *Behavior Therapy, 15*, 421–423.

Kilpatrick, D. G., & Calhoun, K. S. (1988). Early behavioral treatment for rape trauma: Efficacy or artifact? *Behavior Therapy, 19*, 421–427.

Kilpatrick, D. G., Saunders, B. E., Amick-McMullen, A., Best, C. L., Veronen, L. J., & Resnick, H. S. (1989). Victim and crime factors associated with the development of crime-related post-traumatic stress disorder. *Behavior Therapy, 20*, 199–214.

Kilpatrick, D. G., Saunders, B. E., Veronen, L. J., Best, C. L., & Von, J. M. (1987). Criminal victimization: Lifetime prevalence, reporting to police, and psychological impact. *Crime and Delinquency, 33*, 479–489.

Kingsbury, S. J. (1988). Hypnosis in the treatment of posttraumatic stress disorder: An isomorphic intervention. *American Journal of Clinical Hypnosis, 31*, 81–90.

Kipper, D. A. (1977). Behavior therapy for fears brought on by war experiences. *Journal of Consulting and Clinical Psychology, 45*, 216–221.

Kolb, L. C., Burris, B. C., & Griffiths, S. (1984). Propranalol and clonidine in the treatment of chronic post-traumatic stress disorders of war. In B. van der Kolk (Ed.), *Post-traumatic stress disorder: Psychological and biological sequelae* (pp. 97–105). Washington, DC: American Psychiatric Press.

Kolb, L. C., & Mutalipassi, L. R. (1982). The conditioned emotional response: A subclass of the chronic and delayed post-traumatic stress disorders. *Psychiatric Annals, 12*, 979–987.

Koranyi, E. K. (1969). A theoretical review of the survivor syndrome. *Diseases of the Nervous System, 30*, 115–118.

Klein, H. (1974). Delayed affects and after effects of severe traumatization. *Israel Annals of Psychiatry & Related Disciplines, 12*, 293–303.

Klonoff, H., McDougall, G., Clark, C., Kramer, P., & Horgan, J. (1976). The neuropsychological, psychiatric, and physical effects of prolonged and severe stress: 30 years later. *Journal of Nervous and Mental Disease, 163*, 246–252.

Kluznik, J. C., Speed, N., Van Valkenburg, C., & Magraw, R. (1986). Forty-year follow-up of United States prisoners of war. *American Journal of Psychiatry, 143*, 1443–1446.

Kraft, T., & Al-Issa, I. (1965). The application of learning theory to the treatment of traffic phobia. *British Journal of Psychiatry, 111*, 277–279.

Kreitler, S., & Kreitler, J. (1988). Trauma and anxiety: The cognitive approach. *Journal of Traumatic Stress, 1*, 35–56.

Krystal, J. H., Kosten, T. R., Perry, B. D., Southwick, S., Mason, J. W., & Giller, E. L., Jr. (1989). Neurobiological aspects of PTSD: Review of clinical and preclinical studies. *Behavior Therapy, 20*, 177–198.

Kuch, K. (1987). Treatment of PTSD following automobile accidents. *The Behavior Therapist, 10*, 224–242.

Kulka, R. A., Schlenger, W. E., Fairbank, J. A., Hough, R. L., Jordan, B. K., Marmar, C. R., & Weiss, D. S. (1990). *Trauma and the Vietnam War generation*. New York: Brunner/Mazel.

Kushner, M. (1965). Desensitization of a post-traumatic phobia. In L. P. Ullmann & L. Krasner (Eds.), *Case studies in behavior modification* (pp. 193–196). New York: Holt, Rinehart, & Winston.

Lang, P. J. (1977). Imagery in therapy: An information processing analysis of fear. *Behavior Therapy, 8*, 495–510.

Lang, P. J. (1979). A bioinformational theory of emotional imagery. *Psychophysiology, 16*, 495–510.

Levis, D. J., & Hare, N. A. (1977). A review of the theoretical rationale and empirical support for the extinction approach of implosive (flooding) therapy. In M. Hersen, R. M. Eisler, & P. M. Miller (Eds.), *Progress in behavior modification* (Vol. 4, pp. 299–374). New York: Academic Press.

Lewis, T. (1919). *The soldier's heart and the effort syndrome*. New York: Hoeber.

Lifton (1973). *Home from the war*. New York: Simon & Schuster.

Lipper, S., Davidson, J. R. T., Grady, T. A., Edinger, J., & Cavenar, J. O. (1986). Preliminary study of carbamazepine in post-traumatic stress disorder. *Psychosomatics, 27*, 849–854.

Litz, B. T., & Keane, T. M. (1989). Information processing in anxiety disorders: Application to the understanding of post-traumatic stress disorder. *Clinical Psychology Review, 9*, 243–257.

Lyons, J. A., & Keane, T. M. (1989). Implosive therapy for the treatment of combat-related PTSD. *Journal of Traumatic Stress, 2*, 137–152.

McCaffrey, R. J., & Fairbank, J. A. (1985). Behavioral assessment and treatment of accident-related posttraumatic stress disorder: Two case studies. *Behavior Therapy, 16*, 406–416.

McCormack, N. A. (1985). Cognitive therapy of posttraumatic stress disorder: A case report. *American Mental Health Counselors Association Journal, 7*, 151–155.

McWhirter, J. J., & Liebman, P. C. (1988). A description of anger-control therapy groups to help Vietnam veterans with PTSD. *Journal for Specialists in Group Work, 13*, 9–16.

Meichenbaum, D. (1977). *Cognitive-behavior modification: An integrative approach*. New York: Plenum.

Meichenbaum, D. H., & Turk, D. C. (1976). The cognitive behavioral management of anxiety, anger, and pain. In P. O. Davidson (Ed.), *The behavioral management of anxiety, depression and pain* (pp. 1–34). New York: Brunner/Mazel.

Milanes, F. J., Mack, C. N., Dennison, J., & Slater, V. L. (1984). Phenelzine treatment of post-Vietnam syndrome. *VA Practitioner, 1*, 40–49.

Miller, J., Moeller, D., Kaufman, A., DiVasto, P., Pathak, D., & Christy, J. (1978). Recidivism among sex assault victims. *American Journal of Psychiatry, 135*, 1103–1104.

Modlin, H. (1967). The post-accident anxiety syndrome: Psychosocial aspects. *American Journal of Psychiatry, 123*, 1008–1012.

Mowrer, O. H. (1960). *Learning theory and behavior*. New York: Wiley.

Mueser, K. T., & Butler, R. W. (1987). Auditory hallucinations in combat-related posttraumatic stress disorder. *American Journal of Psychiatry, 144*, 299–302.

Mueser, K. T., Yarnold, P. R., & Foy, D. W. (1991). Statistical analysis for single-case designs: Evaluating outcome of imaginal exposure treatment of chronic PTSD. *Behavior Modification, 15*, 134–155.

Naitoh, P. (1969). *Sleep loss and its effects on performance*. Report Number 68-3, Bureau of Medicine and Surgery, Department of the Navy (Research Task MF12. 524.004-9008).

Niederland, W. G. (1981). The survivor syndrome: Further observations and dimensions. *Journal of the American Psychoanalytic Association, 29*, 413–425.

Olasov-Rothbaum, B., & Foa, E. B. (1991). Exposure treatment of PTSD in concomitant with conversion mutism: A case study. *Behavior Therapy, 22*, 449–456.

Parson, E. R. (1984). The reparation of the self: Clinical and theoretical dimensions in the treatment of Vietnam combat veterans. *Journal of Contemporary Psychotherapy, 14*, 90–98.

Partridge, E. (1983). *Origins: A short etymological dictionary of modern English* (4th ed.). New York: Greenwich House.

Pearson, N. A., Poquette, B. N., & Wasden, R. E. (1983). Stress inoculation and the treatment of post-rape trauma. *The Behavior Therapist, 6*, 58–59.

Peniston, E. G. (1986). EMG biofeedback-assisted desensitization treatment for Vietnam combat veterans post-traumatic stress disorder. *Clinical Biofeedback and Health, 9*, 35–41.

Pitman, R. K., Altman, B., Greenwald, E., Longpre, R. E., Macklin, M. L., Poire, R. E., & Steketee, G. S. (1991). Psychiatric complications during flooding therapy for posttraumatic stress disorder. *Journal of Clinical Psychiatry, 52*, 17–20.

Resick, P. A., Jordan, C. G., Girelli, S. A., Hutter, C. K., & Marhoefer-Dvorak, S. (1988). A comparative outcome study of behavioral group therapy for sexual assault victims. *Behavior Therapy, 19*, 385–401.

Rossi, P. H., Wright, J. D., Weber-Burdin, E., & Perina, J. (1983). Victimization by natural hazards in the United States 1970–1980: Survey estimates. *International Journal of Mass Emergencies and Disaster, 1*, 467–482.

Rychtarik, R., Silverman, W., Van Landingham, W., & Prue, D. (1984). Treatment of an incest victim with implosive therapy: A case study. *Behavior Therapy, 15*, 410–420.

Saigh, P. A. (1986). *In vitro* flooding in the treatment of a 6-yr-old boy's posttraumatic stress disorder. *Behaviour Research and Therapy, 24*, 685–688.

Saigh, P. A. (1987a). *In vitro* flooding of childhood posttraumatic stress disorders: A systematic replication. *Professional School Psychology, 2*, 135–146.

Saigh, P. A. (1987b). *In vitro* flooding of an adolescent's post-traumatic stress disorder. *Journal of Clinical Child Psychology, 16*, 147–150.

Saul, L. J., Rome, H., & Leuser, E. (1946). Desensitization of combat fatigue patients. *American Journal of Psychiatry, 102*, 476–478.

Schindler, F. E. (1980). Treatment by systematic desensitization of a recurring nightmare of a real life trauma. *Journal of Behavior Therapy and Experimental Psychiatry, 11*, 53–54.

Scrignar, C. B. (1988). *Post-traumatic stress disorder: Diagnosis, treatment, and legal issues* (2nd ed.). New Orleans, LA: Bruno Press.

Shapiro, F. (1989a). Efficacy of eye movement desensitization procedure in the treatment of traumatic memories. *Journal of Traumatic Stress, 2*, 199–223.

Shapiro, F. (1989b). Eye movement desensitization: A new treatment for post-traumatic stress disorder. *Journal of Behavior Therapy and Experimental Psychiatry, 20*, 211–217.

Shapiro, F. (1991). Eye movement desensitization and reprocessing procedure: From EMD to EMD/R—a new treatment model for anxiety and related traumata. *Behavior Therapist, 14*, 133–135.

Solomon, S. (1989). Research issues in assessing disasters and their effects. In R. Gist & B. Lubin (Eds.), *Psychosocial aspects of disaster* (pp. 308–340). New York: Wiley.

Spiegel, D. (1988). Dissociation and hypnosis in post-traumatic stress disorder. *Journal of Traumatic Stress, 1*, 17–33.

Spitzer, R. L., & Williams, J. B. (1989). *Structured clinical interview for DSM-III-R, patient version*. New York: New York State Psychiatric Institute, Biometrics Research Department.

Stampfl, T. G., & Levis, D. J. (1967). Essentials of implosive therapy: A learning-theory-based psychodynamic behavioral therapy. *Journal of Abnormal Psychology, 72*, 157–163.

Starkey, T. W., & Ashlock, L. (1984). Inpatient treatment of PTSD: An interim report of the Miami model. *VA Practitioner, 1*, 41–44.

Starkey, T. W., & Ashlock, L. (1986). Inpatient treatment of PTSD: Final results of the late, great Miami model. *VA Practitioner, 3*, 41–44.

van der Kolk, B. (1987). The drug treatment of post-traumatic stress disorder. *Journal of Affective Disorders, 13*, 203–213.

van der Kolk, B. (1983). Psychopharmacological issues in post-traumatic stress disorder. *Hospital and Community Psychiatry, 34*, 683–691.

van der Kolk, B., Greenberg, M., Boyd, H., & Krystal, J. (1985). Inescapable shock, neurotransmitters, and addiction to trauma: Toward a psychobiology of post-traumatic stress. *Biological Psychiatry, 20*, 314–325.

Venn, J. (1988). Hypnotic intervention in accident victims during acute phase of posttraumatic adjustment. *American Journal of Clinical Hypnosis, 31*, 114–117.

Wolfe, M. E., Alavi, A., & Mosnaim, A. D. (1987). Pharmacological interventions in Vietnam veterans with post traumatic stress disorder. *Research Communications in Psychology, Psychiatry and Behavior, 12*, 169–176.

Wolfe, M. E., Alavi, A., & Mosnaim, A. D. (1988). Posttraumatic stress disorder in Vietnam veterans: Clinical and EEG findings; possible therapeutic effects of carbamazepine. *Biological Psychiatry, 23*, 642–644.

Wolff, R. (1977). Systematic desensitization and negative practice to alter the aftereffects of a rape attempt. *Journal of Behavior Therapy and Experimental Psychiatry, 8*, 423–425.

Wolpe, J. (1958). *Psychotherapy by reciprocal inhibition*. Stanford, CA: Stanford University Press.

Wolpe, J., & Abrams, J. (1991). Post-traumatic stress disorder overcome by eye movement desensitization: A case report. *Journal of Behavior Therapy and Experimental Psychiatry, 22*, 39–43.

Woodward, S. H. (1991). *Sleep disturbance and a health risk factor in PTSD*. Paper presented at the annual meeting of the American Psychological Association, San Francisco.

Worthington, E. R. (1978). Demographic and pre-service variables as predictors of post-military service adjustment. In C. R. Figley (Ed.), *Stress disorders among Vietnam veterans* (pp. 173–187). New York: Brunner/Mazel.

Ziegenhagen, E. A. (1976). The recidivist victim of violent crime. *Victimology, 1*, 538–550.

10

Social Phobia

Debra A. Hope, Craig S. Holt, and Richard G. Heimberg

Following its inclusion in the psychiatric nomenclature with the publication of DSM-III (American Psychiatric Association, 1980), social phobia has been recognized as a significant mental health problem. The 1987 revision of DSM-III (DSM-III-R; American Psychiatric Association, 1987) defined social phobia as "a persistent fear of one or more situations (the social phobic situations) in which the person is exposed to possible scrutiny by others and fears that he or she may do something or act in a way that will be humiliating or embarrassing" (p. 243). The social phobic situations include public speaking, eating, drinking, or writing in the presence of others, using public restrooms, and conversations with others. Although DSM-III suggested that fears were generally limited to one situation with little interference in functioning, research has revealed that most social phobics fear, and consequently avoid, two or more of these situations (Holt, Heimberg, Hope, & Liebowitz, 1992; Turner, Beidel, Dancu, & Keys, 1986), with a portion fearing most social contact with others. This latter portion has been identified as a *generalized* subtype in DSM-III-R (American Psychiatric Association, 1987).

Not surprisingly, social phobics' fear and avoidance impair their social and occupational functioning. In fact, 92% of Turner *et al.*'s sample believed their social phobia inhibited their career advancement, while nearly 85% and 70% reported disability in academic or general social functioning, respectively. Liebowitz, Gorman, Fyer, and Klein (1985) described similar impairment. Sanderson, DiNardo, Rapee, and Barlow (1990) reported that half of the social phobics in their sample (mean age = 33.8 years) had never married compared to 36% of individuals with panic disorder and agoraphobia and 18% of those with generalized anxiety disorder.

Nearly 60% of individuals with a primary diagnosis of social phobia met criteria for at least one additional Axis I disorder, including dysthymia (21%),

Debra A. Hope • Department of Psychology, University of Nebraska-Lincoln, Lincoln, Nebraska 68588-0308. **Craig S. Holt** • Iowa City VA Medical Center, Iowa City, Iowa 52246. **Richard G. Heimberg** • Center for Stress and Anxiety Disorders, University at Albany-State University of New York, Pine West Plaza #4, Albany, New York 12205.

Handbook of Effective Psychotherapy, edited by Thomas R. Giles. Plenum Press, New York, 1993.

simple phobia (25%), or panic disorder with agoraphobia (17%), in one sample of 24 social phobics (Sanderson *et al.*, 1990). Turner and colleagues (Turner, Beidel, Borden, Stanley, & Jacob, 1991) found a somewhat lower comorbidity rate, with 43% of 71 social phobics receiving an additional Axis I disorder, most commonly generalized anxiety disorder. Nearly one-fifth of the Sanderson *et al.* sample used benzodiazepines on a daily basis to control their social anxiety. Studies of alcoholics reveal a high prevalence of social phobia, with indications that many of these individuals may be drinking to reduce their social anxiety (Chambless, Cherney, Caputo, & Rheinstein, 1987; Mullaney & Trippett, 1979; Smail, Stockwell, Canter, & Hodgson, 1984).

One area of recent controversy has been the relationship between social phobia and avoidant personality disorder (APD), especially with the inclusion of the generalized subtype of social phobia in DSM-III-R. The percentage of social phobics who received an additional diagnosis of APD in four recent studies ranged from 22.1% to 70% (Herbert, Hope, & Bellack, 1992; Holt, Heimberg, & Hope, 1992; Schneier, Spitzer, Gibbon, Fyer, & Liebowitz, 1991; Turner, Beidel, & Townsley, 1992). Despite this great variability, all authors concluded that features of APD (if not fully meeting the diagnostic criteria) are common among social phobics, particularly among those with the generalized subtype. This line of research has led some to conclude that individuals with APD are simply the most severely impaired social phobics, with quantitative but not qualitative distinctions between social phobia and APD (Herbert *et al.*, 1992; but see also Holt, Heimberg, & Hope, 1992).

Epidemiological data place the prevalence of social phobia at about 2% of the general population (Myers *et al.*, 1984). It is equally common among men and women (Bourdon *et al.*, 1988).

Theories of Social Phobia

A review of the literature reveals that three comprehensive models of social phobia have gained at least a moderate level of acceptance. Each of these models will be described briefly below.

Self-Presentational Model of Social Anxiety

The self-presentational model of social anxiety, proposed by Schlenker and Leary (1982), states that social anxiety occurs when an individual desires to make a particular impression on others and doubts that he or she will be successful in doing so. Both conditions must be met; the individual must be sufficiently concerned about how he or she will appear to others *and* there must be apprehension about his or her ability to engage in adequate impression management. In later refinements of the model (summarized in Leary, 1988), Leary has identified situational and dispositional factors which may increase the motivation to engage in impression management and/or decrease one's self-efficacy in achieving the desired impression.

High need for approval is one of the factors which may increase an individual's desire to make a particular impression according to Leary (1988). In fact, the desire to avoid disapproval or fear of negative evaluation is a hallmark of social phobia, and change on this variable may be essential to treatment success (Hope, Heimberg, & Bruch, 1990; Mattick & Peters, 1988; Mattick, Peters, & Clarke, 1989).

In addition to factors which increase motivation to create a desired impression, Leary identified several factors which influence a person's confidence that he or she will meet impression management goals. These factors include real or perceived social skills deficits, low self-esteem, and low outcome expectations. Low self-esteem may contribute to social anxiety because such individuals likely presume that others will view them as poorly as they regard themselves. Real or perceived social skills deficits exemplify low efficacy expectations (the confidence that one can perform a given behavior) as defined by Bandura (1977). Additionally, socially anxious individuals may believe that even if they perform adequately, the desired impression will not be created. These low outcome expectancies (Bandura, 1977) may result from low self-esteem or a harsh view of social interactions. For example, Leary, Kowalski, and Campbell (1988) found that socially anxious individuals expected interaction partners to evaluate them negatively. However, they also expected interaction partners to evaluate other people negatively, even when only minimal contact was made.

The self-presentational model offers an excellent framework with which to predict whether a given individual will experience social anxiety in a given situation. Furthermore, later elaborations on the model have incorporated related concepts such as the role of social skills in social anxiety. The model proposes that clients are anxious for different reasons and identifies important areas to address in assessment. Is the client overly motivated to make a good impression or does he or she doubt his or her ability to perform adequately? Is the client's doubt grounded in behavioral deficits or in a distorted picture of themselves, other people, or social interactions? The answers to these questions are useful in selecting a treatment strategy, a point that will be addressed in more detail later.

Beck's Cognitive Theory of Social Anxiety

In their 1985 book, Beck and Emery elaborated a cognitive model of phobias and anxiety with specific applications to social phobia. The core of the cognitive model is the concept of *schema,* the basic cognitive structure which guides the processing of information. Schemata are conceptualized as rules which classify, prioritize, and interpret information. Schemata also facilitate the recall of relevant information from memory. They are grouped into *modes* which create an overall bias or cognitive set which the individual carries from one situation to another. According to Beck and Emery, anxiety-disordered individuals usually function in the *vulnerability* mode. In the vulnerability mode, the world is viewed as a dangerous place in which the individual must constantly be vigilant to potential threat. As a result of this hypervigilance, neutral or mildly positive cues are interpreted negatively. Positive or safety cues are discounted or ignored, as are memories or judgments of personal resources or successes.

For social phobics, the danger comes from social interactions, and social phobics are hypervigilant to social threat cues. Evidence suggests social phobics devote excessive attentional resources to the detection of social threat cues (Hope, Rapee, Heimberg, & Dombeck, 1990; Mattia, Heimberg, & Hope, 1991). These cues may then be exaggerated so that a barely noticeable stutter during a conversation is perceived as incoherence, and the refused request for a date predicts a lonely and isolated existence.

Psychobiological/Ethological Model

The stress-appraisal model developed by Trower and Turland (1984) in the early 1980s has recently been expanded to include an ethological perspective (Trower & Gilbert, 1989). Trower and Gilbert have proposed that social anxiety occurs as part of an intricate scheme to handle intraspecies threat, which evolved to facilitate the development of complex social groups. First, the earlier stress-appraisal model will be described briefly, then it will be incorporated into the broader ethological model.

Trower and Turland (1984; updated by Trower and Gilbert, 1989) proposed that two interdependent systems guide social functioning among humans. The *appraisal system* continuously evaluates information from the social environment and from within the person and compares the current state of affairs with a desired standard. If there is a discrepancy between the current situation and the desired situation, the *coping system* is automatically activated to reduce the discrepancy. As with Leary's self-presentational model described above, Trower and Turland's coping system evaluates outcome and efficacy expectancies in selecting a response (or nonresponse) to reduce the discrepancy. The emotional, cognitive, and physiological arousal characteristic of social anxiety is a result of the discrepancy between current and desired circumstances. However, unlike Leary, who postulates multiple pathways to social anxiety, Trower and colleagues trace the primary cause to inappropriate goals/standards in the appraisal system which are derived from evolutionarily prepared systems to handle intraspecies conflict.

The evolution of hierarchically organized social groups facilitated the sharing of territory among members of the same species. In the *defense system*, group cohesion is maintained by individuals' behaviors which demonstrate their role in the social hierarchy. Subordinates signal their submission to dominant members of the group in order to avoid hostile encounters and maintain their access to the group's resources. Thus subordinates must constantly remain alert and ready to engage in the appropriate submissive or appeasement-oriented behaviors to avoid falling in status or being ousted from the group. In the defense system, social anxiety among subordinates is essential to the continuation of the hierarchy.

Although social hierarchies play an important role even among humans, they need not depend upon submissive gestures by subordinates. In a more highly evolved strategy found in some chimpanzees and humans and known as the *safety system*, conflict among members of the group is prevented and group cohesion is increased by reassuring signals from dominant members to subordinates. This reduces the need for subordinates to maintain a defensive posture and allows them to engage in a broader range of behavior than under the defense system. Social anxiety need not play a role in the safety system as group members are bound together by mutuality rather than threats. However, social phobics do not appear to interpret social situations in this manner.

The appraisal system of social phobics, described in the original Trower and Turland model described above, utilizes the hierarchical defensive system rather than the cooperative safety system. The standard or desired state to which current experience is compared is derived from the defensive system. The initial desired state is to be in the dominant position. However, socially anxious individuals have low expectancies that they will be able to achieve this goal. Therefore, they become anxious and select another goal which will minimize their loss of access to the resources controlled by the dominant individual. The next goal or desired state is to attempt to maintain proximity to the dominant other by adopting a submissive posture and utilizing submissive behaviors. If the appraisal system determines the person is failing to meet the revised goal, the goal may be further revised to basic survival with escape or avoidance of the dominant other being the best alternatives. If this strategy also fails, the individual may give up any attempts to maintain status and become helpless, avoidant, and depressed.

In summary, Trower and Gilbert hypothesize that social phobics fail to recognize that their relationships with others can occur on a cooperative basis. By construing social relationships as hierarchical, they engage in a competition in which they have low expectancies of achieving their goals.

Review of Treatment Outcome Research

Single-Subject Designs

There are five published studies employing single-subject designs with social phobics. Four of the five examined cognitive-behavioral treatments.

Cognitive-Behavioral Treatments. Vermilyea, Barlow and O'Brien (1984) treated two social phobics and one simple phobic as part of an investigation of treatment integrity. Only the results for the social phobics will be discussed here. Both social phobics were women, one with public-speaking fears (Subject 1) and one with more generalized fears including eating in restaurants and attending meetings and church (Subject 3). Ratings on individualized fear and avoidance hierarchies served as the primary outcome measure. Following a 1-week baseline, subjects practiced replacing negative self-statements with positive, coping statements for 4 to 6 weeks. Subjects were specifically instructed not to seek out anxiety-provoking situations but to practice using the positive self-statements in any naturally occurring feared events. The second phase of treatment added graduated *in vivo* exposure to self-statement training. Exposure occurred within the treatment sessions as well as through homework assignments. The combined treatment phase lasted 8 weeks for Subject 1 and 6 weeks for Subject 3. An examination of the fear and avoidance hierarchy ratings completed during each treatment session revealed minimal change for either subject during self-statement training alone. However, during the combined treatment phase, substantial improvement was reported by Subject 3. Subject 1 made more modest gains. Examination of self-monitoring records revealed that Subject 3 tripled her baseline exposure rate to an average of 8.3 exposures per week compared to Subject 1, who reported only 1–2 exposures per week throughout baseline and treatment. These results suggest that a combined treatment of *in vivo* exposure and self-statement modification is effective for individuals with multiple social fears. Whether such a treatment would be effective for public-speaking phobics is unclear since the subject in this study failed to comply with the treatment guidelines. These data do not support the use of self-statement training alone, because subjects reported little change in fear and avoidance until exposure was added to the treatment protocol.

Stravynski (1983) treated a social phobic with psychogenic vomiting using *in vivo* exposure, social skills training, and cognitive modification in a multiple-baseline design across target situations. Because Stravynski conceptualized the vomiting as secondary to the subject's social anxiety, he did not target it directly. Rather he focused on controlling anxiety in four target situations related to socializing with the subject's girlfriend's family and going to movies and restaurants. Vomiting decreased immediately after treatment started and was completely eliminated by the sixth therapy session. Subjective anxiety fell below 100 (0–100 scale) only after each situation was specifically targeted and fluctuated dramatically from week to week. However, at the first follow-up, 6 weeks after the end of the 8-week treatment, subjective anxiety ratings were down to 20 for all four target situations. Gains were maintained at 1-year follow-up. At an informal 2-year follow-up, the subject reported occasional, but tolerable, social anxiety.

Three women with scriptophobia (fears about writing in the presence of others) were treated with *in vivo* exposure alone or following cognitive restructuring in a multiple-baseline design (Biran, Augusto, & Wilson, 1981). Primary dependent measures were subjective anxiety and behavioral approach to a hierarchy of feared situations. Subjects A and B received cognitive restructuring alone followed by exposure. Subject C received only exposure. All subjects reported dramatic increases in approach behavior and reductions in subjective fear with five sessions of exposure. Cognitive restructuring alone had little impact for the two subjects who received it. At 9-month follow-up gains on approach behavior remained, but subjective fear had increased for all three subjects. These data suggest exposure represents an effective treatment for avoidance of feared writing situations with little additional benefit from cognitive intervention which preceded the exposure.

Heimberg, Becker, Goldfinger, and Vermilyea (1985) treated seven social phobics—five with public-speaking fears and two with heterosocial fears—in a combined treatment of imaginal exposure, role-played exposure in the group therapy sessions, cognitive restructuring, and homework for *in vivo* exposure. Subjects were divided into two treatment groups with 6 and 10 weeks of baseline in a multiple-baseline design. At the end of the 14-week treatment, all subjects improved on a range of behavioral, physiological, and subjective measures. Gains were maintained at 6-month follow-up for six of seven subjects.

Non-Cognitive-Behavioral Treatment. One of the rare published studies of a non-cognitive-behavioral treatment for social anxiety-related problems involved a single subject treated in a multiple-baseline design across problem areas using brief (three sessions) Morita therapy (Ishiyama, 1986). Morita therapy is a Japanese therapy that uses confrontation and discussion to encourage clients to accept their anxiety and reconstrue it in a more positive light, using strategies such as "positive reinterpretation." For example, social anxiety is seen as a normal experience, not a personal weakness. Social anxiety reflects one's sensitivity to others and should be accepted and redirected to handling the situation, not avoided.

In this study, the subject presented with anxiety when speaking in public and when approaching strangers. Ishiyama did not report a formal diagnostic assessment, but it appears the subject would have met DSM-III-R criteria for social phobia. The dependent measures were three self-report scales designed for this study which measured anxiety acceptance, problem severity, and coping effectiveness. Treatment consisted of three sessions spaced over 5 weeks with data collected every week. Examination of the data revealed improvement on all three measures for the target problem at the introduction of the intervention, with stronger results for public-speaking anxiety. However, both problems showed significant gains on all three measures 28 weeks after the first baseline measure. Informal reports from significant others suggested behavioral changes were evident.

Comments and Discussion. A total of fourteen subjects, seven from one study, have been treated in single-subject designs. Eleven of the fourteen subjects were women. Six were treated primarily for public-speaking fears, three for scriptophobia, and five for general social interaction fears. However, the scriptophobics had more generalized fears that were not the focus of the treatment reported in the study. Although one subject was identified as a psychogenic vomiter, treatment focused on his fears in various social interactions. With one or two exceptions, treatment appeared to be successful.

These single-subject design studies raise several issues which make comparisons between studies difficult. Because these same concerns also characterize the larger-sample studies, they will be outlined briefly here but discussed in detail later. The most salient point in this literature is the lack of nonbehavioral studies. Only one nonbehavioral study was available. Studies vary widely on assessment measures, with the most common being some measure of subjective anxiety in feared situations and avoidance behavior. Similar treatment techniques are employed differently in different studies. For example, some cognitive interventions involve replacing negative self-statements with more positive ones (e.g., Vermilyea *et al.*, 1984), while others use logical reanalyses (e.g., Biran *et al.*, 1981; Heimberg *et al.*, 1985; Stravynsky, 1983). Some studies explicitly employ homework for exposure between sessions (Heimberg *et al.*, 1985; Stravynsky, 1983; Vermilyea *et al.*, 1984), while others leave it to the client's discretion (Biran *et al.*, 1981; Ishiyama, 1986), making it unclear whether homework played an important role in change or not. Finally, two of the studies (Heimberg *et al.*, 1985; Stravynsky, 1983) employed treatment packages consisting of a number of interventions. Although this strategy is suitable when first developing treatments, it makes it difficult to evaluate which part(s) of the package may be most important.

Comparison to Waiting-List or Attention Control Treatments

One of the most basic questions to address when evaluating a newly developed intervention is whether the new treatment works better than no intervention at all. This question is best addressed by comparison to a no-treatment condition. Most often researchers operationalize "no treatment" as being on a waiting list for some period of time with the promise of later treatment. Comparisons between the active treatment and no treatment address whether the therapy results in more remediation of symptoms than simply waiting for the benefit of whatever curative factors may be operating within the person or his or her environment. A more stringent test asks whether the new treatment works better than the nonspecific effects of treatment such as meeting with a therapist or having a rationale for the problem

(Frank, 1982). Studies designed to answer the latter question employ attention control or so called placebo treatments.

Cognitive-Behavioral Treatments. Numerous studies have compared several different cognitive-behavioral and behavioral interventions for social phobia to waiting-list or attention control conditions. These studies have investigated social skills training, relaxation, systematic desensitization, exposure, and various cognitive strategies.

Only two studies have compared social skills training and systematic desensitization to a no-treatment control condition. No study has utilized an attention control condition for either treatment. Marzillier, Lambert, and Kellett (1976) reported that subjects receiving skills training or systematic desensitization improved relative to baseline, but neither group did significantly better than subjects on the waiting list. Unfortunately, some procedural difficulties and excessive dropout in the systematic desensitization condition make findings for that treatment difficult to interpret. Kanter and Goldfried (1979) utilized a modified version of systematic desensitization called "self-control desensitization" and found it to be somewhat more effective than the waiting-list condition.

One study has compared relaxation therapy to an attention control condition, and a second has compared it to a waiting list. Jerremalm, Jansson, and Öst (1986) examined a modified form of relaxation, called "applied relaxation," which included practicing the relaxation skills in role plays of feared situations. Subjects receiving applied relaxation demonstrated improvement across a variety of measures and were more improved that waiting-list subjects. No follow-up data were reported. The second study, which utilized a more standard relaxation therapy, found minimal differences between a basal therapy condition (an attention control or minimal therapy condition which included education, self-exposure advice, support, and unspecified anxiolytic medication) and relaxation plus the basal therapy (Alstrom, Nordlund, Persson, Harding, & Ljungqvist, 1984). This lack of difference is not attributable to equal improvement above baseline for both conditions. Rather, neither relaxation nor basal therapy alone was effective. This poor showing for relaxation is particularly striking given that subjects receiving basal therapy alone were seen monthly (average number of sessions was 2.3), and subjects who also received relaxation were seen weekly (average number of sessions was 9.4). Interpretation of Alstrom and colleagues' findings is complicated by the fact that only social phobics who were deemed "unsuitable for insight-oriented therapy" were included in the study. The precise meaning of this selection criterion and its potential impact on treatment outcome are unclear.

Exposure to feared situations represents a standard intervention for the treatment of phobias and other anxiety disorders (Barlow & Beck, 1984). Not surprisingly, numerous researchers have investigated the efficacy of exposure, either alone or in combination with cognitive interventions, for social phobia. Studies which compared exposure alone to a waiting-list or attention control condition will be examined first.

Four studies have compared various types of exposure to waiting-list or attention control conditions. Three of the studies utilized primarily *in vivo* exposure, and the fourth used role-played exposure in the context of group treatment with homework for *in vivo* exposure. The study by Alstrom and colleagues (1984) described above also included a prolonged *in vivo* exposure condition (combined with the minimal treatment basal therapy) compared to basal therapy alone. Exposure was the most effective treatment in this study, with subjects showing improvement relative to the basal therapy alone across a variety of measures and generally maintaining gains at a 9-month follow-up assessment. Mattick *et al.* (1989) found that subjects who received 6 weeks of *in vivo* exposure improved more than waiting-list subjects at posttreatment. Although follow-up data were unavailable for waiting-list subjects, subjects treated with exposure showed some deterioration in the 3 months posttreatment. Butler and colleagues (Butler, Cullington, Munby, Amies, & Gelder, 1984) reported similar results for the efficacy of exposure versus a waiting-list control group at posttest despite declining treatment credibility ratings for the exposure condition. Using role-played exposure conducted in the context of group therapy combined with homework for *in vivo* exposure, Hope, Heimberg, and Bruch (1990) also reported that exposure therapy yielded greater symptom reduction than a waiting-list control at the end of 12 weeks of treatment.

Three studies have compared cognitive interventions to a waiting-list control condition (Jerremalm *et al.*, 1986; Kanter & Goldfried, 1979; Mattick *et al.*, 1989). All three found that cognitive treatment was more effective than waiting-list control groups on a variety of measures. Interpretation of these findings is complicated by the fact that only the Mattick *et al.* study did not include some type of exposure in addition to the cognitive therapy. Kanter and Goldfried had subjects practice cognitive skills during imaginal exposure, and Jerremalm *et al.* included homework for *in vivo* exposure. The implications of this point will be discussed in further detail below.

Some researchers have explicitly combined cognitive therapy and exposure, hypothesizing that the combination may be better than either treatment alone. The four studies which compared combined cognitive and exposure therapy packages to waiting-list or attention control groups will be examined next.

Butler *et al.* (1984) combined *in vivo* exposure with an anxiety management program consisting of relaxation, distraction, and rational self-talk. Although the anxiety management training was not a purely cognitive intervention, an analysis of which aspect subjects used most revealed that rational self-talk may have been the most important element. Subjects who received the exposure plus anxiety management training were more improved than waiting-list subjects at the end of treatment and continued to improve during the 6-month follow-up period. Mattick and colleagues (1989) reported similar results at posttreatment comparing exposure plus cognitive restructuring to a waiting-list control, with gains maintained through a 3-month follow-up. In one of the few studies to include an attention control condition, Heimberg *et al.* (1990) compared a treatment package called Cognitive-Behavioral Group Therapy (CBGT)—consisting of role-played exposure in group therapy sessions, cognitive restructuring, and homework for *in vivo* exposure—to a credible education–supportive therapy. Subjects in both treatments improved significantly on most measures. However, CBGT subjects were more improved at posttest and 6-month follow-up. Despite significant attrition at a 5-year follow-up, CBGT subjects were more likely to maintain their gains and continued to be more improved than attention control subjects (Heimberg, Salzman, Holt, & Blendell, in press). Hope, Heimberg, and Bruch (1990) reported that the Heimberg *et al.* treatment was also superior to a waiting-list control group.

Nonbehavioral Treatment. Only one study evaluated a nonbehavioral psychotherapy relative to a nonactive treatment control group. The study by Alstrom and colleagues (1984) described above, which included relaxation and prolonged exposure treatment groups, also included a treatment described as "dynamically oriented supportive psychotherapy" (p. 97). As with the behavioral treatments, the supportive psychotherapy was combined with a minimal treatment ("basal therapy") and compared to the minimal treatment alone. Supportive psychotherapy was more effective than basal therapy alone at posttest and 9-month follow-up.

Comments and Discussion. After reviewing these studies, it is time to summarize what we can conclude about which treatments are more effective than no treatment and which may provide more than nonspecific therapy factors such as providing a rationale for the problem.

At this point there is no direct evidence that social skills training is more effective than no treatment for social phobia. Unfortunately, only one study (Marzillier *et al.*, 1976) evaluated the efficacy of social skills training relative to a waiting-list control. Despite lack of differences between the waiting-list and social skills conditions, subjects receiving social skills training did demonstrate significant improvement pre- to posttreatment. As will be discussed in the next section, there is evidence that social skills training is more effective than some other active treatments for at least a subgroup of social phobics. Therefore, one could hypothesize that further research would be supportive of the efficacy of skills training relative to no treatment at all.

The findings are somewhat more promising for the efficacy of systematic desensitization, with one of two studies finding more improvement than a waiting-list control (Kanter & Goldfried, 1979). The failure to find significant differences in the second study may be attributable to excessive attrition and procedural difficulties (Marzillier *et al.*, 1976). On the other hand, the modifications Kanter and Goldfried made in the traditional systematic desensitization protocol may have increased the efficacy of the intervention relative to the procedures used by Marzillier *et al.*.

As with social skills training and desensitization, there is a paucity of studies which evaluated relaxation training. There are no published studies comparing standard progressive relaxation training to a no-treatment control condition with social phobics. However, when compared to a minimal treatment, there was little evidence the relaxation added to the efficacy of the minimal treatment (Alstrom *et al.*, 1984). A modified version of relaxation training, which included practice relaxing in feared situations, does appear to be more beneficial than no treatment (Jerremalm *et al.*, 1986).

Cognitive and exposure interventions have been the most completely evaluated, and all published studies found exposure (four studies) or cognitive therapy (three studies) alone or in combination (four studies) to be more effective than no treatment or attention control interventions. The evidence is strongest for a combined treatment approach because subjects receiving exposure alone showed signs of relapsing during the follow-up period in one study (Mattick *et al.*, 1989), and two of the three "cognitive-alone" treatments included an exposure component (Kanter & Goldfried, 1979; Jerremalm *et al.*, 1986).

In the single study investigating a nonbehavioral treatment, dynamically oriented supportive psychotherapy plus a minimal treatment which included education, self-exposure advice, and anxiolytic medication was more effective than the minimal treatment alone (Alstrom *et al.*, 1984). These findings will be further discussed below because this is also the only study to compare psychological treatments from different theoretical orientations.

Comparison between Behavioral and Cognitive-Behavioral Treatments

Numerous studies have compared the various cognitive-behavioral and behavioral treatments to each other. These treatments have included applied relaxation; social skills training; systematic desensitization; imaginal, role-played and *in vivo* exposure; and variations on cognitive therapy. First, comparisons involving social skills training will be reviewed. Then comparisons including relaxation will be examined, followed by studies which utilized exposure and cognitive interventions.

Seven studies have compared social skills training to another intervention. Two early studies (Marzillier *et al.*, 1976; Shaw, 1979) compared social skills training to systematic desensitization and found the two treatments to be equally effective. However, as noted above, neither active treatment differed substantially from the waiting-list control in one of these studies. In the other study, Shaw reported significant pre- to posttreatment change but did not include a control condition. Shaw also included an imaginal flooding condition which was as effective as social skills training and desensitization. Stravynski *et al.* (1982) found no advantage to adding a cognitive intervention to social skills training.

Several investigators have classified subjects as having primary deficits in performance or social skill versus primary excesses in physiological arousal or subjective anxiety. These studies test the hypothesis that socially inadequate individuals will respond best to social skills training and individuals with excessive anxiety symptoms will respond best to exposure or relaxation. Öst, Jerremalm, and Johansson (1981) found support for this hypothesis. Although both social skills training and applied relaxation (relaxation practiced in phobic situations) were effective, "behavioral reactors," who demonstrated behavioral disruption but little heart rate acceleration in a pretreatment role play, received the most benefit from social skills training. Applied relaxation was somewhat more effective for "physiological reactors" (heart rate acceleration without behavioral disruption at pretest) relative to social skills training. Trower, Yardley, Bryant, and Shaw (1978) also reported that socially inadequate (skills deficit) subjects improved more with social skills training than an anxiety reduction treatment, in this case, systematic desensitization. Trower *et al.*'s socially inadequate subjects were contrasted with the sample of social phobics utilized by Shaw (1979). As noted above, these social phobic (highly anxious but not deficient social skills) subjects responded equally well to social skills training and systematic desensitization. In the final study, which matched treatment strategies to subject characteristics, Wlazlo, Schroeder-Hartwig, Hand, Kaiser, and Munchau (1990) found that social phobic subjects responded equally well to social skills training and *in vivo* exposure but, surprisingly, socially inadequate subjects were somewhat more improved with exposure than social skills training.

Rather than subdividing samples on the basis of social skill, Jerremalm *et al.* (1986) attempted to categorize social phobics as cognitive (excessive irrational thoughts) or physiological reactors and compared applied relaxation to self-instructional training, a cognitive intervention. Unfortunately, the measures used to identify the cognitive reactors proved unreliable, making comparisons between cognitive and physiological reactors difficult to interpret. Their overall findings, however, indicated somewhat more improvement for self-instructional training than applied relaxation. Mersch, Emmelkamp, Bogels, and van der Sleen (1989) partially replicated this study and the one by Öst and colleagues (1981), remedying the difficulty in identifying cognitive reactors. They compared social skills training to rational emotive therapy for subjects identified as cognitive or behavioral reactors. Subjects improved in both conditions with no overall difference between them. There were some trends supporting the hypothesis that behavioral reactors would do better in social skills training. Surprisingly, cognitive reactors also tended to benefit more from skills training than the cognitive intervention. In neither case was the treatment-matching hypothesis strongly supported at posttest. Follow-up data from 14 months posttreatment revealed subjects in both treatments were doing equally well (Mersch, Emmelkamp, & Lips, 1991).

Seven studies have evaluated an exposure and/or cognitive therapy condition, including the one described above under social skills training (Wlazlo *et al.*, 1990). Alstrom *et al.* (1984) found that *in vivo* exposure (combined with imaginal exposure for some subjects) was more effective than traditional relaxation training. In one of the earliest treatment outcome studies for social phobia, Kanter and Goldfried (1979) contrasted a modified version of rational emotive therapy (systematic rational restructuring) to self-control desensitization and the two treatments combined. Much to their surprise, the cognitive intervention alone was the most effective treatment and yielded the greatest generalization to nonsocial situations. The relative efficacy of primarily cognitive interventions was also demonstrated by a study which compared self-instructional training, rational emotive therapy, and *in vivo* and role-played exposure within therapy groups (Emmelkamp, Mersch, Vissia, & van der Helm, 1985). All three treatments were equally effective. Of particular note in this study is the match between treatment modality and response system, with the two cognitive treatments yielding greater reductions in irrational beliefs, and exposure resulting in a greater reduction in pulse rate during a behavioral test.

Finally, several investigators have explored whether there is any advantage to combining exposure and cognitive therapy. Mattick *et al.* (1989) and Mattick and Peters (1988) reported that a combined package was more effective than exposure alone. In Mattick *et al.*, the combined treatment was also compared to cognitive restructuring alone and found to be more effective at posttest and 3-month follow-up. However, subjects who received the cognitive intervention alone appeared to make some additional progress during the follow-up period. Butler and colleagues (1984) also reported an advantage in combining exposure with an anxiety management package (of which the cognitive intervention may have been the most important part). However, Butler *et al.*'s results are somewhat difficult to interpret given that the exposure-alone intervention consisted of exposure and a less credible "filler" to control for the time devoted to the anxiety management package. In contrast, Hope, Heimberg, and Bruch (1990) reported that exposure alone was somewhat more effective than exposure and cognitive restructuring together. Although the combined package was more effective than the waiting-list control, Hope and colleagues noted that subjects receiving this treatment improved substantially less than had been previously demonstrated for the combined package (e.g., Heimberg *et al.*, 1990).

Comments and Discussion. The majority of the comparisons between cognitive-behavioral treatments found both treatments to be equally effective. In the minority of cases in which there was a difference, the following treatments were the most effective: social skills training (two comparisons), applied relaxation (one comparison), cognitive therapy (two comparisons), exposure alone (three comparisons), and exposure plus cognitive therapy (three comparisons). Although at first it may appear that no treatment is consistently the most beneficial, a closer examination helps clarify the picture.

Of particular interest are the data which indicate that treatment efficacy depends in part on the nature of the deficits experienced by the subjects. Subjects with demonstrated behavioral or social skills deficits appear to benefit most from social skills training. Heimberg (1989) questioned whether subjects described as having social skills deficits should be described as social phobics, particularly in research completed prior to the publication of DSM-III. If they were socially inadequate but lacked the cognitive and physiological aspects of fear which make social phobia an anxiety disorder, then treatments such as exposure which focus on fear reduction are less likely to be successful.

Later studies which utilized more clearly defined social phobic samples have tended to examine exposure and cognitive treatments. Cognitive therapy and exposure seem to be effective treatments by themselves. The research by Mattick and colleagues (Mattick and Peters, 1988; Mattick *et al.*, 1989) supports the efficacy of a combined cognitive and exposure package over either treatment alone. However, subjects in these studies were treated for specific fears such as eating, writing, or drinking in public rather than more general interaction fears. It appears that many subjects had more generalized fears but these fears were not targeted in treatment. The superiority of the combined treatment for more generalized fears has not been satisfactorily demonstrated. The two studies which addressed this question (Butler *et al.*, 1984; Hope, Heimberg, and Bruch, 1990) yielded contradictory findings, and the authors of the studies noted some difficulties which may limit the generalizability of their findings.

Pharmacotherapy for Social Phobia

Pharmacotherapy for social phobia has received considerable recent attention. Three main classes of drugs are frequently prescribed: benzodiazepines, beta-adrenergic blockers, and monoamine oxidase inhibitors (MAOIs). Studies in analog populations with more circumscribed phobic reactions suggested that beta-adrenergic blockers might be effective, and clinical trials with mixed phobics indicate that MAOIs might be effective for social phobia. In practice, benzodiazepines have been the most frequently prescribed medication for anxiety disorders, and this may be true for social phobia as well.

Benzodiazepines. The mechanism of action in benzodiazepines is poorly understood, but recent evidence suggests that there is a benzodiazepine receptor system with cortical and limbic system projections. Benzodiazepines vary in the time to maximum dosage response and length of effects. In general, slow response and long-acting benzodiazepines on a set schedule of administration are recommended for phobic disorders (Noyes, 1985). Although this class of medications presents fewer risks than barbiturates, benzodiazepines are known to produce dependence problems and offer the potential for significant abuse. In a study by Fyer *et al.* (1987), over half the patients were unable to discontinue alprazolam (Xanax) when requested to do so, and nearly all patients experienced paniclike attacks after drug discontinuation. In another study (Lydiard, Laraia, Howell, & Ballenger, 1988), one-third of patients became depressed after taking alprazolam. Given the lack of research and the dependence problems associated with long-term use, a trial of benzodiazepines should be carefully considered (or should be carefully integrated into a treatment plan that considers conservative dosage and a timetable for drug discontinuation).

Case studies and open trials suggest that alprazolam, a slower-acting benzodiazepine, might be useful, particularly in the reduction of the arousal and subjective distress associated with phobic responding and anticipatory anxiety. Performance in target situations, however, may be impaired by sedation or motor-coordination side effects. One study using volunteers with musical performance anxiety found diazepam (Valium) to be less effective than the beta-adrenergic blocker Nadolol and to slightly degrade performance (James & Savage, 1984).

In an open trial of alprazolam with 14 social phobics with avoidant personality disorder (APD), Reich, Noyes, and Yates (1989) reported significant improvement in some features of APD (most notably avoidance of interpersonal or everyday activities, fear of embarrassment, and fear of losing control) across 8 weeks of treatment. Seven days after medication was withdrawn, however, all APD features except avoidance of interpersonal activities returned to baseline levels. In a double-blind study described in more detail below (Gelernter *et al.*, 1991), social phobics who received alprazolam improved significantly but not more than subjects who took pill placebo. Alprazolam subjects also tended to relapse when medication was withdrawn.

Beta-Adrenergic Blockers. Beta-adrenergic blocking agents may be effective in the treatment of social phobia when somatic manifestations of anxiety (e.g., sweating, palpitations, trembling, and blushing) are prominent. Beta-blockers interfere with one or two classes of neuroreceptors found in the sympathetic nervous system and in the central nervous system that are associated with somatic symptoms of anxiety (Greenblatt & Shader, 1972; Noyes, 1988).

The beta-adrenergic blocking drugs appear to have certain advantages over the benzodiazepines. These include the lack of addictive potential, nonsedation, and lack of cognitive impairment at doses appropriate for anxiety management (Turner, 1988). The effectiveness of beta-blocking drugs for most anxiety disorders, relative to benzodiazepines, is still questionable (Noyes, 1988), but the specific application of this class of drugs to social phobia does appear to have some merit (Liebowitz *et al.*, 1985). Numerous beta-blockers are available, but atenolol, one of the more cardioselective beta-blockers, is often the preferred medication in this class of drugs (Schneier, Levin, & Liebowitz, 1990). Other advantages of atenolol relative to other beta-blockers include fewer central nervous system side effects and a relatively long half-life that permits less frequent dosing.

The evidence for the effectiveness of beta-blockade treatment of social phobia consists mostly of acute (rather than maintenance) dosage studies in populations such as undergraduate students, musicians, or athletes with stage fright, or performance anxiety (see reviews by Noyes, 1988; Schneier *et al.*, 1990). In general, most studies report a superior subjective response to beta-blockers compared to placebo, but equivocal effect for objective ratings of performance (i.e., quality of recital or speech, or of test or sports score). In the treatment of social phobia, beta-blockers appear promising but may be somewhat less effective than MAOIs. Liebowitz *et al.* (1987) report 9 of 10 patients with at least moderate improvement following an 8-week open trial of atenolol. However, in a controlled, double-blind study of 74 social phobic patients (Liebowitz *et al.*, 1992), the response rate for phenelzine, an MAO inhibitor (64%), was found to be superior to atenolol (30%), which was not significantly different from placebo (23%), over an 8-week trial. Analyses conducted after 16 weeks of treatment showed some increase in effectiveness for atenolol (43% response rate) and some decrease in effectiveness for phenelzine (52%). Phenelzine remained statistically superior to placebo (19%), but atenolol was not different from either phenelzine or placebo. When beta-blockers are compared to benzodiazepines, differing designs, medications, and dosage schedules yield conflicting results across studies.

MAO Inhibitors. The rationale for the use of MAOIs with social phobia stems from successful trials with heterogeneous samples of patients with phobic neuroses and from trials with atypical depression which is characterized by rejection sensitivity. MAOIs inhibit monoamine oxidase, an enzyme that inhibits the production of substances important to the central nervous system, such as dopamine, norepinephrine, serotonin, and tyramine. However, the mechanism of action of MAOIs is still in question (Sheehan & Raj, 1988). The potentially serious side effects (most importantly a hypertensive crisis) associated with this class of drug when mixed with foods containing high concentrations of amines necessitate a tyramine-restricted diet (see Sheehan & Raj, 1988). The resulting precautions and attendant side effects have been thoroughly outlined (e.g., Rabkin, Quitkin, McGrath, Harrison, & Tricamo, 1985) such that patient compliance to the regimen substantially reduces side-effect risk. Other possible side effects—such as orthostatic hypertension, insomnia, weight gain, edema, parathesias, and anorgasmia—sometimes limit the use of MAOIs, but more often these side effects can be controlled by counteractive measures to a degree that is acceptable for the patient. Discontinuation of medication in the heterogeneous phobic samples tended to result in relapse (Solyom *et al.*, 1973; Tyrer, Candy, & Kelly, 1973).

In the United States only three MAOIs are available by prescription: phenelzine sulfate, isocarboxazid, and tranylcypromine sulfate. A number of recent studies have investigated the utility of phenelzine as a treatment for social phobia. Liebowitz and colleagues have conducted several studies showing the benefit of phenelzine (Liebowitz, Fyer, Gorman, Campeas, & Levin, 1986; Liebowitz *et al.*, 1988; Liebowitz *et al.*, 1992) and tranylcypromine (Versiani, Mundim, Nardi, & Liebowitz, 1988). In the previously mentioned study comparing phenelzine and atenolol, Liebowitz *et al.* (1992) reported preliminary results in favor of the MAOI treatment. Schneier *et al.* (1990) suggest that phenelzine may be particularly useful for patients with generalized social phobia compared to patients with a more circumscribed social phobia who may experience more intermittent episodes of anxiety, and the data of Liebowitz *et al.* (1992) provided some support for this contention.

There is very little research on the combination of medication and a psychological treatment compared to either treatment alone. In the only known study, Falloon and colleagues (Falloon, Lloyd, & Harpin, 1981) compared social skills training plus the beta-blocker propranolol (Inderol) to social skills training plus pill placebo. Subjects generally improved with no difference between groups.

Interorientation Comparisons

Perhaps the most interesting treatment outcome research design is one which compares treatments from different theoretical orientations. These studies pose questions such as the relative efficacy of behavior therapy versus psychodynamic psychotherapy or of psychotherapy versus medication. Unfortunately, such studies are relatively rare in the literature and social phobia is no exception. Only three such studies exist, and two of these involve comparisons between medication and cognitive-behavior therapy.

In the study mentioned several times above, Alstrom and colleagues (1984) compared basal therapy (a minimal treatment of education, support, instruction for self-exposure, and unspecified medication) to basal therapy plus dynamically oriented supportive psychotherapy, prolonged *in vivo* exposure, or standard relaxation training. The authors conclude that exposure was the most effective treatment; supportive psychotherapy was somewhat less effective, and relaxation and basal therapy alone were the least effective. Two issues merit consideration when interpreting these results. First, subjects were selected who were deemed "unsuitable for insight-oriented therapy." Although it is unclear exactly what this distinction means, it does seem likely that this sample was less amenable to the supportive psychotherapy than an unselected sample would be. On the other hand, all subjects received instruction for self-exposure, although the extent to which they actually practiced entering feared situations was not reported. It seems unlikely that all of the change seen in the supportive psychotherapy condition was attributable to self-exposure, because these subjects improved more than subjects who received relaxation or basal therapy alone and similar self-exposure instructions. This study, however, tells us little about the efficacy of dynamically oriented supportive psychotherapy "uncontaminated" by behavior therapy.

The two studies to make pharmacotherapy–behavior therapy comparisons both utilized Heimberg's (Heimberg *et al.*, 1990) group therapy package (CBGT) consisting of role-played exposure within therapy groups, cognitive restructuring, and homework for *in vivo* exposure. As noted above, CBGT was more effective than a waiting-list and a credible attention control group in previous studies, although not necessarily more effective than exposure alone (Heimberg *et al.*, 1990; Hope, Heimberg, and Bruch, 1990).

Gelernter and colleagues (1991) compared Heimberg's treatment to phenelzine, alprazolam, and pill placebo. All subjects also received encouragement for self-exposure. Following 12 weeks of active treatment, all treatments, including medications, were withdrawn for the 2-month follow-up period. In general, all subjects improved with very few differences among the groups. There was some evidence that alprazolam subjects were more likely to relapse when medication was withdrawn. Phenelzine subjects evidenced the highest rate of response and tended to maintain their gains without medication; while cognitive-behavioral subjects showed less initial improvement, there were some signs of continuing improvement over the follow-up period. The poorer than expected showing for the cognitive-behavioral intervention may be attributable to the fact that subjects were treated in larger groups for shorter sessions (10 per group, 90-min sessions) than typically used for this treatment package (6–7 per group, 2-hour sessions). The authors attributed the improvement in the placebo group to subjects' self-paced exposure efforts.

Finally, preliminary data are available from a multicenter study conducted by Liebowitz and Heimberg comparing phenelzine, Heimberg's cognitive-behavioral treatment (CBGT), pill placebo, and attention control psychotherapy. Treatment response was determined on the basis of independent assessor ratings. Of 81 subjects who began treatment at either site, 70 completed the 12-week active treatment phase. Among completers, 80% of subjects receiving CBGT and 71% of those receiving phenelzine were classified as positive responders. These rates are significantly higher than those achieved by patients receiving pill placebo (37%) or the attention control treatment (27%), but not significantly different from each other. Data from other measures or from follow-up assessments have not yet been analyzed (Heimberg & Liebowitz, 1992).

Clinically Significant Change

The distinction between statistically significant and clinically significant change is frequently raised in the psychotherapy outcome literature. A few of the studies described above attempted to identify the percentages of subjects who had made clinically significant change. Mattick and colleagues (1989) derived a composite measure of improvement based on clinically significant changes on two self-report measures and a behavioral measure. Using this index, the following percentage of subjects received high or very high improvement ratings at 3-month follow-up: 27% for cognitive therapy alone, 45% for exposure alone, and 72% for the combined cognitive and exposure treatment. Despite large numerical differences, these percentages are not statistically different among the treatment groups. In their earlier study, which included only the combined treatment and exposure conditions, improvement rates were 95% and 56%, respectively. This difference was statistically significant.

In their comparison of CBGT and education plus support (the attention control treatment), Heimberg and colleagues defined clinically significant improvers as subjects who achieved a change of 2 or more points on the 9-point global Clinician's Severity Rating scale and who moved to the nonclinical range of the scale (less than 4) after treatment. By this standard, 81% of subjects in the active treatment were classified as improvers, compared to 47% in the attention control condition at the 6-month follow-up. This difference was statistically significant. Using the same criteria, Hope, Heimberg, and Bruch (1990) reported 36%, 70%, and 0% of combined treatment, exposure alone, and waiting-list subjects, respectively, made clinically significant improvement. The difference between waiting-list and active treatments was statistically significant, but the two active treatments did not differ significantly from each other. Using a similar global rating scale (with 7 rather than 9 points). Alstrom *et al.* (1984) reported the following percentages of subjects that were classified as not at all or only slightly disturbed at 9-month follow-up: prolonged exposure (71%), supportive therapy (15%), relaxation (17%), and basal therapy (13%). These percentages were derived from a table for comparison among studies so statistical analyses are unavailable.

Gelernter *et al.* (1991) used a different strategy for determining clinically significant change. They compared subjects' scores on a self-report measure of avoidance of social phobic situations to normative data. Although the means for all four groups (alprazolam, phenelzine, CBGT, and pill placebo) were two standard deviations above the mean before treatment, all four fell within one standard deviation at posttest and follow-up. Examination of individual subjects' data reveals much greater variability for placebo and alprazolam subjects than for phenelzine and CBGT subjects, suggesting smaller percentages may have made clinically significant change on this measure in the first two groups.

Combining these data with those reported above for medication trials and medication–psychotherapy comparisons, it appears that approximately three-fourths of social phobics make important clinical changes in the best treatments. The next section will focus on prediction of who will make these changes and the nature of their improvement.

Prediction of Treatment Success

Foa and Emmelkamp (1983) noted that one of the most interesting questions in the psychotherapy research is the identification of individuals who fail to make progress in treatment. Unfortunately, this is also one of the least investigated areas. What little is known will be reviewed briefly.

Three separate studies have concluded that the single measure associated with improvement is a reduction in fear of negative evaluation (Hope, Heimberg, and Bruch, 1990; Mattick & Peters, 1988; Mattick *et al.*, (1989). This variable alone accounts for nearly 25% of the variance in end-state functioning, more than change in anxiety ratings or avoidance behavior. This finding provides a nice shorthand for clinicians who can use the Fear of Negative Evaluation Scale (Watson & Friend, 1969) as one index of treatment gains and for prediction of maintenance of those gains following treatment.

Two variables evident prior to treatment may predict treatment outcome. The first, social skills deficits, has already been discussed indirectly above. Although social phobics without social skills deficits may improve in either social skills training or exposure-based interventions (e.g., Trower *et al.*, 1978; Wlazlo *et al.*, 1990), those with skills deficits may do best in a treatment which directly addresses their deficits. Thus social skills deficits may be seen as a predictor of poor treatment success in exposure and cognitive treatments. The second poor prognostic sign is severe depression. Holt, Heimberg, and Hope (1990) reported that depressed subjects made less improvement than nondepressed subjects, regardless of type of treatment. Mild depression, a common sequelae of social phobia, likely will not interfere with treatment and may improve as the social phobia improves.

Conclusions

Research Limitations

In an attempt to make this chapter more practitioner oriented, critical methodological evaluations of the treatment outcome research were limited. Readers who wish to consider a more traditional critical evaluation are referred to Heimberg (1989) and Levin, Schneier and Liebowitz (1989). However, before final recommendations about treatment, some limitations in the studies reviewed above require consideration. First, many of the studies lack adequate control groups. Even some well-established treatments such as social skills training have few comparisons to waiting-list controls and even fewer to attention control groups. Studies which simply compare two or more active treatments can conclude little about the extent to which change can be attributed to the specific techniques, particularly when all treatments appear to be equally effective, as is most often the case. Second, inclusion of some type of exposure, often encouragement for self-paced exposure, appears to be ubiquitous in this literature. Although many authors note it is common sense or standard clinical practice to encourage clients to face their fears, the addition of exposure to medication trials, control conditions, or nonbehavioral treatments obscures interpretation of the results. At the very least, an attempt should be made to assess the extent to which clients engage in exposure.

Several issues are particularly in need of further research. Attempts to match treatments to subject characteristics (e.g., behavioral versus physiological reactors, circumscribed versus generalized fears) have met with some success. Given the heterogeneity of social phobia, more research of this type is needed. Research which does not include some type of subtyping of social phobics as an independent variable should carefully define the sample to help facilitate identification of the group to which the results can be generalized. Another question that remains unresolved is whether combined cognitive and exposure treatments are more effective than either treatment alone. Although Mattick and colleagues (Mattick & Peters, 1988; Mattick *et al.*, 1989) provide consistent evidence for the superiority of combined treatments for more circumscribed social phobias such as eating/drinking/writing in public, more research is needed with generalized fears. Further research is also needed on combining psychological treatments with medication.

Finally, when discussing the research literature, little attention was paid to the format of the treatment—group versus individual. A quick count indicates that social skills training studies tend to use individual treatment and exposure and cognitive studies tend to use group therapy. This is by no means universal. Outside of research settings, it is likely that most social phobics receive individual treatment. However, no study has systematically compared individual versus group formats.

Treatment Recommendations

Given the pervasiveness of exposure instructions across theoretical orientations and treatment modalities, it is somewhat surprising that there is not overwhelming evidence that exposure is the treatment of choice for social phobia. Social phobia, however, is essentially a cognitive disorder. Social phobics' core fear is of negative evaluation, a cognitive construct embedded in the complexities of social relationships. This has lead some leading researchers in the area such as Butler (1989) to propose that cognitive interventions may be particularly useful. However, the research evidence is not overwhelming in this direction either. (Note that purely cognitive interventions are probably more effective for social phobia than for some other anxiety disorders, including panic disorder with agoraphobia.) What then is the treatment of choice for social phobia? It depends on the specific nature of the client's concerns. The following decision tree is recommended.[1]

Once the clinician has arrived at a diagnosis of social phobia for a particular client, the next question is whether a social skills deficit can be identified. This can be a difficult determination because *performance* deficits can occur due to lack of skill or due to the disruptive influence of severe anxiety. There are three ways to help a clinician make this decision. Working on the assumption that if a client can demonstrate the skills under any circumstances, then most likely he or she has most of the requisite skills, the clinician should look for evidence the skills exist. First, can the client demonstrate the skills in very nonthreatening role plays which minimize anxiety? Second, how skilled is the client in interactions with the therapist, particularly after the first few sessions have passed and some habituation has occurred? Third, can the client describe how a third person should behave in a given situation? If this assessment reveals the client does have a social skills deficit, then social skills training is recommended. The advantage of skills training for these types of clients is one of the best documented points in this literature. There are numerous excellent texts on this approach (e.g., Kelly, 1982) for the unfamiliar clinician.

If it appears the client has adequate skills and excessive anxiety is the primary problem, then a treatment plan built around exposure to feared situations is recommended. The research indicates both role-played and *in vivo* exposure should be effective. There is little evidence for the efficacy of purely imaginal exposure, although the findings for obsessive–compulsive disorder suggest that imaginal exposure may be a useful adjunct for situations unavailable through role plays or *in vivo* exposure (Foa, Steketee, & Ozarow, 1985). Research protocols typically use graduated exposure rather than flooding and include homework for *in vivo* exposure, regardless of what type of exposure is conducted in the therapy session. Most good behavioral texts discuss how to conduct exposure. Hope (1993) addresses specific applications to social phobia.

The research findings are unclear about whether adding a cognitive intervention would increase the efficacy of exposure treatment. As noted above, the evidence for a combined approach is most compelling for individuals with discrete fears such as eating/drinking/writing in public. However, there are several reasons why a clinician may want to consider a combined treatment for all social phobics. First, the cognitive intervention may help increase generalizability to other situations (Kanter & Goldfried, 1979). Second, it is unlikely that the addition of cognitive techniques to exposure will reduce the effectiveness of exposure as long as adequate time and attention are devoted to the behavioral intervention, and the combination may improve outcome. Finally, the combined approach has been the most rigorously investigated and fared well in comparison to a credible attention control group and medication.

The research protocols typically consist of 10 to 12 sessions with total clinical

[1]Although all authors (DAH, CSH, and RGH) generally agreed on the recommendations for treatment for social phobia included in this chapter, they disagreed on some points. This disagreement highlights the difficulty in making such recommendations and the need for more research on the efficacy of various therapies for social phobia. In cases of disagreement among the authors, the views presented reflect those primarily of the first author (DAH).

contact ranging from 7.5 to 24 hours (Heimberg, 1989). Thus, clinically significant change for exposure or social skills training should be evident by 17 to 18 hours of treatment, with measurable improvement evident well before that. If improvement is not apparent by this time, consider renegotiating the treatment contract. This could mean a change to another psychological treatment or consideration of pharmacotherapy.

Although there is increasing evidence that pharmacotherapy is beneficial for social phobics, it may not be the first treatment of choice for several reasons. First, studies so far indicate that cognitive-behavioral interventions are likely to be just as effective as medication for many clients. Second, several studies reveal that subjects tend to relapse when removed from medication. This is most likely true for the benzodiazepines and beta-blockers and less true of MAOIs. In contrast, clients receiving most of the psychological treatments maintain gains throughout untreated follow-up, with occasional evidence that additional gains were achieved (presumably because clients continue to use the skills they gained in treatment). Third, the class of medication which may be the most beneficial for individuals with generalized fears, MAOIs, requires a restricted diet to avoid potentially life-threatening side effects. Though these side effects can readily be managed for many people, the risk appears unwarranted if a client is willing to pursue an equally effective psychological treatment. Future research on the new reversible MAOIs which require fewer dietary restrictions and pose less threat for severe side effects may make MAOI treatment more attractive in the near future.

Medication treatment should be considered if a client has made little progress with psychological interventions, is unable to tolerate the anxiety evoked by the treatment, or is unable to assimilate the anxiety reduction skills essential to the treatment. Also, clients may sometimes present with severe but extremely circumscribed fears. The most common of these cases is the public-speaking phobic who handles day-to-day speaking situations adequately but has a particularly difficult event once or twice a year. If the fear is truly limited to those infrequently occurring circumstances, then psychological treatments are likely to be difficult to conduct. Exposure depends on repeated encounters with the feared event. In such cases, a medication such as a beta-blocker may be the most appropriate treatment. It can reduce the excessive arousal without impairing performance, and the client need not devote the time, energy, or money to a more extensive course of therapy.

In summary, social skills training and exposure (probably with cognitive therapy) appear to be the best first choices for the treatment of social phobia. Given the risks associated with pharmacotherapy and lack of evidence that it is more effective than psychological treatments, medication may best be viewed as a back-up plan under most circumstances.

Ethical Issues in Treatment Selection

One of the issues addressed by this volume is whether it is ethical to utilize treatments which are not the ones demonstrated to be the most efficacious for a given disorder. As is true of many disorders, most treatment studies have evaluated cognitive-behavioral therapies or medication. A variety of other interventions from different theoretical orientations may be effective; however, studies supporting their efficacy have not yet been conducted. Therefore, it would seem most ethical to give clients the benefit of what is supported by the research evidence. Or, at the very least, to inform clients of the available treatments and relative success rates in order to assist them in making an informed choice.

At the same time, research is often conducted by narrowing the focus to specific problem areas. Clients, however, often present with a myriad of problems which do not fit neatly into the packages outlined by researchers. An overall treatment plan needs to be determined based on the conceptualization of the case, but the research literature can still guide treatment selection as each individual problem area is addressed. After all, research subjects often have secondary diagnoses which are not the focus of the primary intervention. The research simply evaluates how effective a given treatment is for a particular problem area, often forcing the clinician to draw from several literatures for a comprehensive treatment plan.

References

Alstrom, J. E., Nordlund, C. L., Persson, G., Harding, M., & Ljungqvist, C. (1984). Effects of four treatment methods on social phobic patients not suitable for insight-oriented psychotherapy. *Acta Psychiatrica Scandinavica, 70*, 97–110.

American Psychiatric Association. (1980). *Diagnostic and statistical manual of mental disorders* (3rd ed.). Washington DC: Author.

American Psychiatric Association. (1987). *Diagnostic and statistical manual of mental disorders* (3rd ed.-revised). Washington DC: Author.

Bandura, A. (1977). Self-efficacy: Toward a unifying theory of behavioral change. *Psychological Review, 84*, 191–215.

Barlow, D. H., & Beck, J. G. (1984). The psychosocial treatment of anxiety disorders: Current status, future directions. In J. B. W. Williams & R. L. Spitzer (Eds.), *Psychotherapy research: Where are we and where should we go?*. New York: Guilford.

Beck, A. T., & Emery, G. (1985). *Anxiety disorders and phobias: A cognitive perspective*. New York: Basic Books.

Biran, M., Augusto, F., & Wilson, G. T. (1981). *In vivo* exposure versus cognitive restructuring in the treatment of scriptophobia. *Behaviour Research and Therapy, 19*, 525–532.

Bourdon, K. H., Boyd, J. H., Rae, D. S., Burns, B. J., Thompson, J. W., & Locke, B. Z. (1988). Gender differences in phobias: Results of the ECA Community Survey. *Journal of Anxiety Disorders, 2*, 227–241.

Butler, G. (1989). Issues in the application of cognitive and behavioral strategies to the treatment of social phobia. *Clinical Psychology Review, 9*, 91–106.

Butler, G., Cullington, A., Munby, M., Amies, P., & Gelder, M. (1984). Exposure and anxiety management in the treatment of social phobia. *Journal of Consulting and Clinical Psychology, 52*, 642–650.

Chambless, D. L., Cherney, J., Caputo, G. C., & Rheinstein, B. J. G. (1987). Anxiety disorders and alcoholism: A study with inpatient alcoholics. *Journal of Anxiety Disorders, 1*, 29–40.

Emmelkamp, P. M. G., Mersch, P-P., Vissia, E., & van der Helm, M. (1985). Social phobia: A comparative evaluation of cognitive and behavioral interventions. *Behaviour Research and Therapy, 23*, 365–369.

Falloon, I. R. H., Lloyd, C. G., & Harpin, R. E. (1981). The treatment of social phobia: Real-life rehearsal with non-professional therapists. *Journal of Nervous and Mental Disease, 169*, 180–184.

Foa, E. B., & Emmelkamp, P. M. G. (1983). *Failure in behavior therapy*. New York: Wiley.

Foa, E. B., Steketee, G. S., & Ozarow, B. J. (1985). Behavior therapy with obsessive–compulsives: From theory to treatment. In M. Mavissakalian (Ed.), *Obsessive–compulsive disorders: Psychological and pharmacological treatments*. New York: Plenum.

Frank, J. D. (1982). Therapeutic components shared by all psychotherapies. In J. H. Harvey & M. M. Parks (Eds.), *The Master Lecture Series: Vol. 1. Psychotherapy research and behavior change* (pp. 9–37). Washington, DC: American Psychological Association.

Fyer, A. F., Liebowitz, M. R., Gorman, J., Campeas, R., Levin, A., Davies, S., Goetz, D., & Klein, D. (1987). Discontinuation of alprazolam treatment in panic patients. *American Journal of Psychiatry, 144*, 303–308.

Gelernter, C. S., Uhde, T. W., Cimbolic, P., Arnkoff, D. B., Vittone, B. J., Tancer, M. E., & Bartko, J. J. (1991). Cognitive-behavioral and pharmacological treatment of social phobia. *Archives of General Psychiatry, 48*, 938–945.

Greenblatt, D. J., & Shader, R. I. (1972). On the psychopharmacology of beta-adrenergic blockade. *Current Therapy Research, 14*, 615–625.

Heimberg, R. G. (1989). Cognitive and behavioral treatments for social phobia: A critical analysis. *Clinical Psychology Review, 9*, 107–128.

Heimberg, R. G., Becker, R. E., Goldfinger, K., & Vermilyea, J. A. (1985). Treatment of social phobia by exposure, cognitive restructuring, and homework assignments. *Journal of Nervous and Mental Disease, 173*, 236–245.

Heimberg, R. G., Dodge, C. S., Hope, D. A., Kennedy, C. R., Zollo, L., & Becker, R. E. (1990). Cognitive behavioral group treatment for social phobia: Comparison with a credible placebo control. *Cognitive Therapy and Research, 14*, 1–23.

Heimberg, R. G., & Liebowitz, M. R. (1992, April). *A multi-center comparison of the efficacy of phenelzine and cognitive-behavioral group treatment for social phobia*. Paper presented at the 12th National Conference on Anxiety Disorders, Houston.

Heimberg, R. G., Salzman, D., Holt, C. S., & Blendell, K. (in press). Cognitive behavioral group treatment for social phobia: Effectiveness at five-year follow-up. *Cognitive Therapy and Research.*

Herbert, J. D., Hope, D. A., & Bellack, A. S. (1992). Validity of the distinction between generalized social phobia and avoidant personality disorder. *Journal of Abnormal Psychology, 101*, 332–339.

Holt, C. S., Heimberg, R. G., & Hope, D. A. (1990, November). *Success from the outset: predictors of cognitive-behavioral therapy outcome among social phobics*. Paper presented at the annual meeting of the Association for the Advancement of Behavior Therapy, San Francisco.

Holt, C. S., Heimberg, R. G., & Hope, D. A. (1992). Avoidant personality disorder and the generalized subtype of social phobia. *Journal of Abnormal Psychology, 101*, 318–325.

Holt, C. S., Heimberg, R. G., Hope, D. A., & Liebowitz, M. L. (1992). Situational domains of social phobia. *Journal of Anxiety Disorders, 6*, 63–77.

Hope, D. A. (1993). Conducting exposure-based treatments with social phobics. *The Behavior Therapist, 16*, 7–12.

Hope, D. A., Heimberg, R. G., & Bruch, M. A. (1990, March). *The importance of cognitive interventions in the treatment of social phobia*. Paper presented at the annual meeting of the Phobia Society of America, Washington, DC.

Hope, D. A., Rapee, R. M., Heimberg, R. G., & Dombeck, M. S. (1990). Representations of the self in social phobia: Vulnerability in social interaction. *Cognitive Therapy and Research, 14*, 177–189.

Ishiyama, F. I. (1986). Brief Morita therapy for social anxiety: A single-case study of therapeutic changes. *Canadian Journal of Counseling, 20*, 57–65.

James, I., & Savage, I. (1984). Beneficial effect of nadolol on anxiety induced disturbances of performance in musicians: A comparison with diazepam and placebo. *American Heart Journal, 108*, 1150.

Jerremalm, A., Jansson, L., & Öst, L-G. (1986). Cognitive and physiological reactivity and the effects of different behavioral methods in the treatment of social phobia. *Behaviour Research and Therapy, 24*, 171–180.

Kanter, N. J., & Goldfried, M. R. (1979). Relative effectiveness of rational restructuring and self-control desensitization in the reduction of interpersonal anxiety. *Behavior Therapy, 10*, 472–490.

Kelly, J. A. (1982). *Social skills training: A practical guide for interventions*. New York: Springer-Verlag.

Leary, M. R. (1988). A comprehensive approach to the treatment of social anxieties: The self-presentational model. *Phobia Practice and Research Journal, 1*, 48–57.

Leary, M. R., Kowalski, R. M., & Campbell, C. D. (1988). Self-presentational concerns and social anxiety: The role of generalized impression expectancies. *Journal of Research in Personality, 22*, 308–321.

Levin, A. P., Schneier, F. R., & Liebowitz, M. R. (1989). Social phobia: Biology and pharmacology. *Clinical Psychology Review, 9*, 129–140.

Liebowitz, M. R., Campeas, R., Levin, A. P., Sandberg, D., Hollander, E., & Papp, L. (1987). Pharmacotherapy of social phobia: A condition distinct from panic attacks. *Psychosomatics, 28*, 305–308.

Liebowitz, M. R., Fyer, M. J., Gorman, J. M., Campeas, R., & Levin, A. (1986). Phenelzine in social phobia. *Journal of Clinical Psychopharmacology, 6*, 93–98.

Liebowitz, M. R., Gorman, J. M., Fyer, M. J., Campeas, R. Levin, A., Sandberg, D., Hollander, E., Papp, L., & Goetz, D. (1988). Pharmacotherapy of social phobia: A placebo controlled comparison of phenelzine and atenolol. *Journal of Clinical Psychiatry, 49*, 252–257.

Liebowitz, M. R., Gorman, J. M., Fyer, M. J., & Klein, D. F. (1985). Social phobia: Review of a neglected anxiety disorder. *Archives of General Psychiatry, 42*, 729–736.

Liebowitz, M. R., Schneier, F., Campeas, R., Hollander, E., Hatterer, J., Fyer, A., Gorman, J., Papp, L., Davies, S., Gully, R., & Klein, D. (1992). Phenelzine vs. atenolol in social phobia: A placebo controlled comparison. *Archives of General Psychiatry, 49*, 290–300.

Lydiard, R. B., Laria, M. T., Howell, E. F., & Ballenger, J. C. (1988). Alprazolam in the treatment of social phobia. *Journal of Clinical Psychiatry, 49*, 17–19.

Marzillier, J. S., Lambert, C., & Kellett, J. (1976). A controlled evaluation of systematic desensitization and social skills training for socially inadequate psychiatric patients. *Behaviour Research and Therapy, 14*, 225–238.

Mattia, J. I., Heimberg, R. G., & Hope, D. A. (1991, November). *The revised Stroop color naming task as an indicator of treatment outcome for social phobia.* Paper presented at the annual meeting of the Association for the Advancement of Behavior Therapy, New York.

Mattick, R. P., & Peters, L. (1988). Treatment of severe social phobia: Effects of guided exposure with and without cognitive restructuring. *Journal of Consulting and Clinical Psychology, 56*, 251–260.

Mattick, R. P., Peters, L., & Clarke, J. C. (1989). Exposure and cognitive restructuring for severe social phobia: A controlled study. *Behavior Therapy, 20*, 3–23.

Mersch, P. P. A., Emmelkamp, P. M. G., Bogels, S. M., & van der Sleen, J. (1989). Social phobia: Individual response patterns and the effects of behavioral and cognitive interventions. *Behaviour Research and Therapy, 27*, 421–434.

Mersch, P. P. A., Emmelkamp, P. M. G., & Lips, C. (1991). Social phobia: Individual response patterns and the long-term effects of behavioral and cognitive interventions. A follow-up study. *Behaviour Research and Therapy, 29*, 357–362.

Mullaney, J. A., & Trippett, C. J. (1979). Alcohol dependence and phobias: Clinical description and relevance. *British Journal of Psychiatry, 135*, 563–573.

Myers, J. K., Weissman, M. M., Tischler, G. L., Holzer, C. E., III, Leaf, P. J., Orvaschel, H., Anthony, J. D., Boyd, J. H., Burke, J. D., Jr., Kramer, M., & Stolzman, R. (1984). Six-month prevalence of psychiatric disorders in three communities. *Archives of General Psychiatry, 41*, 959–967.

Noyes, R. M., Jr., (1985). Beta-adrenergic blocking drugs in anxiety and stress. *Psychiatric Clinics of North America, 8*, 119–132.

Noyes, R. J., Jr., (1988). Beta-adrenergic blockers. In C. Last & M. Hersen (Eds.), *Handbook of anxiety disorders* (pp. 445–459). New York: Pergamon Press.

Öst, L-G., Jerremalm, A., & Johansson, J. (1981). Individual response patterns and the effects of different behavioral methods in the treatment of social phobia. *Behavior Research and Therapy, 19*, 1–16.

Rabkin, J. G., Quitkin, F. M., McGrath, P., Harrison, W., & Tricamo, E. (1985). Adverse reactions to monoamine oxidase inhibitors: II. Treatment correlates and clinical management. *Journal of Clinical Psychopharmacology, 5*, 2–9.

Reich, J., Noyes, R. M., Jr., & Yates, W. (1989). Alprazolam treatment of avoidant personality traits in social phobic patients. *Journal of Clinical Psychiatry, 50*, 91–95.

Sanderson, W. C., DiNardo, P. A., Rapee, R. M., & Barlow, D. H. (1990). Syndrome comorbidity in patients diagnosed with a DSM-III-R anxiety disorder. *Journal of Abnormal Psychology, 99*, 308–312.

Schlenker, B. R., & Leary, M. R. (1982). Social anxiety and self-presentation: A conceptualization and model. *Psychological Bulletin, 92*, 641–669.

Schneier, F. R., Levin, A. P., & Liebowitz, M. R. (1990). Pharmacotherapy. In A. S. Bellack & M. Hersen (Eds.), *Handbook of comparative treatments of adult disorders* (pp. 219–239). New York: Wiley.

Schneier, F. R., Spitzer, R. Gibbon, D., Fyer, A., & Liebowitz, M. L. (1991). The relationship of social phobia subtypes and avoidant personality disorder. *Comprehensive Psychiatry, 32*, 1–5.

Shaw, P. (1979). A comparison of three behaviour therapies in the treatment of social phobia. *British Journal of Psychiatry, 134*, 620–623.

Sheehan, D. V., & Raj, A. B. (1988). Monoamine oxidase inhibitors. In C. Last & M. Hersen (Eds.), *Handbook of anxiety disorders* (pp. 478–506). New York: Pergamon Press.

Smail, P., Stockwell, T., Canter, S., & Hodgson, R. (1984). Alcohol dependence and phobic anxiety states: I. A prevalence study. *British Journal of Psychiatry, 144*, 53–57.

Solyom, L., Heseltine, G. F. D., McClure, D. J., Solyom, C., Ledwedge, B., & Steinberg, G. (1973). Behaviour therapy versus drug therapy in the treatment of phobic neurosis. *Canadian Journal of Psychiatry, 18*, 25–31.

Stravynski, A. (1983). Behavioral treatment of psychogenic vomiting in the context of social phobia. *Journal of Nervous and Mental Disease, 171*, 448–451.

Stravynski, A., Marks, I., & Yule, W. (1982). Social skills problems in neurotic outpatients: Social skills training with and without cognitive modification. *Archives of General Psychiatry, 39*, 1378–1385.

Trower, P., & Gilbert, P. (1989). New theoretical conceptions of social anxiety and social phobia. *Clinical Psychology Review, 9*, 19–35.

Trower, P., & Turland, D. (1984). Social phobia. In S. M. Turner (Ed.), *Behavioral theories and treatment of anxiety* (pp. 321–365). New York: Plenum.

Trower, P., Yardley, K., Bryant, B. M., & Shaw, P. (1978). The treatment of social failure. *Behavior Modification, 2*, 41–60.

Turner, P. (1988). *Drug treatment in psychiatry*. London: Routland & Kegan, Inc.

Turner, S. M., Beidel, D. C., Borden, J. W., Stanley, M. A., & Jacob, R. G. (1991). Social phobia: Axis I and II Correlates. *Journal of Abnormal Psychology*, 102–106.

Turner, S. M., Beidel, D. C., Dancu, C. V., & Keys, D. J. (1986). Psychopathology of social phobia and comparison to avoidant personality disorder. *Journal of Abnormal Psychology, 95*, 389–394.

Turner, S. M., Beidel, D. C., & Townsley, R. M. (1992). Social phobia: A comparison of specific and generalized subtypes and avoidant personality disorder. *Journal of Abnormal Psychology, 101*, 326–331.

Tyrer, P., Candy, J., & Kelly, D. (1973). A study of the clinical effects of phenelzine and placebo in the treatment of phobic anxiety. *Psychopharmacology, 32*, 237–254.

Vermilyea, B. B., Barlow, D. H., & O'Brien, G. T. (1984). The importance of assessing treatment integrity: An example in the anxiety disorders. *Journal of Behavioral Assessment, 6*, 1–11.

Versiani, M., Mundim, F. D., Nardi, A. E., & Liebowitz, M. R. (1988). Tranylcypromine in social phobia. *Journal of Clinical Psychopharmacology, 8*, 279–283.

Watson, D., & Friend, R. (1969). Measurement of social-evaluative anxiety. *Journal of Consulting and Clinical Psychology, 33*, 448–457.

Wlazlo, Z., Schroeder-Hartwig, K., Hand, I., Kaiser, G., & Munchau, N. (1990). Exposure *in vivo* vs. social skills training for social phobia: Long-term outcome and differential effects. *Behaviour Research and Therapy, 28*, 181–193.

11

Obsessive–Compulsive Disorder

Gail Steketee and Judy Lam

Described in the psychiatric literature since the nineteenth century, obsessive–compulsive disorder (OCD) could be clearly identified by written accounts centuries earlier. According to present-day psychiatric classification schemes, obsessions are recurrent ideas, thoughts, images or impulses which provoke intense subjective discomfort. Afflicted individuals resist them at first, usually by engaging in some repetitive thoughts or actions designed to reduce the level of discomfort provoked by the obsessions. Rituals take the form of washing or cleaning to remove contamination, checking to verify that no damage has occurred, putting things in precise order, repeating actions to prevent some disaster from occurring, hoarding or saving things to retain important information, as well as various types of mental rituals such as praying, repeating thoughts, and counting. Both obsessions and compulsions are usually recognized by the individual as excessive or unreasonable.

OCD should be distinguished from obsession–compulsive personality disorder (OCPD), which is characterized by orderliness, indecisiveness, perfectionism, and rigidity. Such traits do occur in those with OCD but rarely as a complete syndrome (Joffee, Swinson, & Regan, 1988; Steketee, 1990). OCD does appear to bear a close relationship to hypochondriasis and to bulimia in that these disorders share the symptoms of obsessive concerns about health or weight, followed by ritualized efforts to reduce anxious thoughts through checking, purging, and medical consultations.

Initially considered a rare disorder, current estimates indicate that diagnosable OCD appears in up to 2.5% of the general population (Regier *et al.*, 1988), making it one of the most common psychiatric disorders. It afflicts males nearly as often as females (Rasmussen & Tsuang, 1984), and a considerable range of severity is evident, from minimal interference with daily functioning to extreme disability. Little is known about the course of OCD in the general population, although findings from clinic samples indicate that chronic courses are most typical, occa-

Gail Steketee and **Judy Lam** • School of Social Work, Boston University, Boston, Massachusetts 02215.
This chapter was supported in part by NIMH grant #RO1 MH44190 awarded to the first author.

Handbook of Effective Psychotherapy, edited by Thomas R. Giles. Plenum Press, New York, 1993.

sionally punctuated by periods of remission (Rasmussen & Tsuang, 1984). Patients in most treatment studies report an average duration of symptoms of 10 to 12 years, indicating that many suffered for long periods before obtaining relief.

Psychotherapy strategies for this disorder have included in- and outpatient psychodynamic therapy, supportive or "milieu" therapy, behavioral therapy, and cognitive therapy. Pharmacotherapy approaches have included treatment with tricyclic and especially serotonergic antidepressant drugs. These approaches are derived from psychodynamic, behavioral, cognitive, and biological theories. This chapter will focus on the psychotherapy interventions for adult patients, and will include information about pharmacological treatments only when compared with or added to psychological methods.

Theoretical Models for Therapy

Psychodynamic treatments for OCD are based on the assumption that obsessions and rituals are defensive strategies developed to ward off disturbing impulses, especially phallic tendencies associated with Oedipal wishes which are later replaced by anal sadism. Ego defenses in such individuals most commonly include regression to the anal sadistic level of personality organization, which may produce a severe superego (Fenichel, 1945; Sifneos, 1985), displacement, reaction formation, denial, isolation, undoing, rationalization, and intellectualization (Cawley, 1974; Fenichel, 1945). Treatments based on this theory presume that appropriate interpretative comments by the therapist about early experiences will foster the patient's emotional understanding of the development of the defenses, thereby leading to increased self-esteem, more adaptive interpersonal relationships, and less dependence on the maladaptive obsessional and compulsive symptoms. Though the category of general psychotherapy methods can be broadly defined to include psychoanalysis and its less intensive and usually briefer counterpart, psychodynamic psychotherapy, as well as client-centered, nondirective, counseling and in-patient milieu therapy, there is a notable absence of studies which investigate the effectiveness of these methods.

Behavioral interventions for OCD are based on learning theories explicated by Mowrer (1960) and Dollard and Miller (1950) and refined more recently by others (e.g., Foa & Kozak, 1986; Rachman, 1971). According to this theory, obsessions, like phobias, may be learned from having or observing specific aversive experiences or possibly from acquiring negative information about a situation. Harmless objects (toilets, appliances), as well as thoughts or images (knife, devil), acquire the ability to arouse discomfort (anxiety, guilt) through this association. Any avoidance or escape behaviors which reduce the discomfort are likely to be repeated in future situations. Since many concrete and mental triggers for fear in obsessional patients cannot easily be avoided, rituals are developed to reduce discomfort. Research evidence supports the assumption that obsessions provoke anxiety and that rituals (escape behaviors) reduce it (see Rachman & Hodgson, 1980). Some researchers have suggested that OCD sufferers are unusually sensitive or vulnerable to stress due either to biological sources or to upbringing experiences (e.g., Rachman, 1971; Watts, 1971). Effective treatment, according to a behavioral model, requires a reduction in discomfort associated with obsessions, as well as blocking of rituals which negatively reinforce obsessive fears. Strategies have included exposure methods, such as systematic desensitization, paradoxical intention, satiation/habituation training, and imagined or *in vivo* flooding, as well as blocking strategies, including thought stopping, aversion therapy via electrical shock or other methods, and ritual (response) prevention.

Cognitive theories for OCD have gained some credence in recent years, beginning with assertions that individuals with OCD suffer from erroneous thinking patterns, with overestimation of risk, perfectionistic thinking, and need for certainty (for review, see Steketee & Cleere, 1990). Several investigations have partly supported these hypotheses, finding that obsessive compulsives had difficulty integrating some concepts, underinclusion and overspecification of concepts, reported doubt about their conclusions, and required more repetition of information before making decisions (Persons & Foa, 1984; Reed, 1985; Volans, 1976). Foa and Kozak (1986) also suggested that high arousal, faulty premises, and erroneous rules of inference (e.g., "situations are dangerous unless proven safe") hinder the processing of information needed to reduce obsessions and rituals. Surprisingly, no cognitive methods have been designed specifically for cognitive problems associated with OCD. The few studies of the effects of cognitive therapies have applied existing methods not closely related to the above concepts.

Because we were able to locate only two case reports of family therapy using a systems model for OCD (Churchill, 1986; Hafner, Gilchrist, Bowling, & Kalucy, 1981), we will not discuss this theoretical framework here. To our knowledge, no controlled studies on family therapy for OCD have been published, with the exception of investigations of the usefulness of adding spouse or family assistance to behavioral treatments. The one study of marital therapy for OCD does not follow a family therapy model. We are also omitting discussion of the evidence for biological bases for OCD and the many studies of pharmacological treatments for this disorder. Although a discussion of this topic is outside the scope of this chapter, clinicians and researchers must take into account the probable benefits many of their OCD patients will gain from the use of serotonergic drugs such as clomipramine, fluoxetine, and fluvoxamine (for review, see Jenike, Baer, & Minichiello, 1991; Steketee & Shapiro, 1993). Unfortunately, the effects of these drugs do not appear to last beyond the drug trial (e.g., Marks, Stern, Mawson, Cobb, & McDonald, 1980; Pato, Zohar-Kadouch, Zohar, & Murphy, 1988).

Problems in Reviewing Research on Treatments for OCD

In this chapter our task is to determine from the empirical research evidence which specific treatments are most effective for OCD symptoms beyond the elements common to all these therapies (empathic listening, support, discussion of historical information). Before discussing the findings from single-case and group studies of treatments for OCD, we will highlight some of the difficulties in trying to summarize this research. Problematic in categorizing specific treatments is the wide variability in how they are delivered, as well as in the amount of therapy provided. We will note unusual or potentially problematic choices wherever they appear.

Diagnostic acuity is far from optimal in the research literature on OCD, particularly in early studies. In this review we have included only those studies in which patients appeared by formal diagnosis or by description to have what is currently classified as obsessive–compulsive disorder according to the DSM-III-R. Another persistent problem in comparing studies is the lack of agreement among researchers about the choice of measures for assessing OCD symptoms. Available instruments include standardized assessor-rated measures (Leyton Obsessional Inventory, Yale–Brown Obsessive Compulsive Scale) and self-administered measures (e.g., Maudsley Obsessional–Compulsive Inventory, Compulsive Activity Checklist), as well as Likert scales of target obsessions, compulsions, and avoidance rated by therapist, patient, assessor, or relative. Composites across several symptoms and/or raters are sometimes used. Behavioral measures (approach toward feared situations, time spent thinking obsessively or doing rituals) are employed especially in some cases studies of behavioral treatments. A number of researchers also assessed mood state (depression, anxiety) and general functioning using a variety of instruments, making it difficult at times to determine whether the measure of "anxiety" referred to obsessional fear or to general anxious mood state. Because of space limitations we will not comment on measurement differences across studies unless they render the findings misleading.

Comparing studies which differ in diagnostic definitions, assessment methods, and treatment applications can seem like comparing apples and oranges. In the face of such differences, confidence in conclusions depends on the sheer weight of the evidence, rather than on one or two even carefully controlled trials. As will become apparent, some treatment strategies have been inadequately tested, so that "treatments of choice" for OCD have been partly selected in the absence of adequate comparisons with alternatives.

In our review, we begin with single-case studies and progress to group designs. We have omitted discussion of the numerous studies which provide no scaled measurement and thus no empirical test of a treatment strategy. Studies with no comparisons are summarized very briefly, with more attention given to those containing controlled comparisons (wait period, wait-list group, placebo, treatment components, methods of delivery, and types of treatments).

Single-Subject Designs

Pretest–Posttest, Sequential, and Multiple-Baseline Designs

Included in this section are single-case studies which measured change before and after a treatment, as well as studies which provided limited controls via serial ABA designs and variants of multiple-baseline designs. In the only study examining a nonspecific form of psychotherapy, Gullick and Blanchard (1973) alternated it with behavioral and cognitive methods for a patient with religious obsessions. Treatment periods were too short (as few as two sessions) to adequately determine the separate effects of the various interventions. However, symptoms decreased during two of three applications of psychotherapy alone. All behavioral strategies demonstrated beneficial effects.

Intensive self-monitoring alone eliminated obsessions in one patient (Frederiksen, 1975) and substantially reduced them in another (Tanner, 1971). In the context of exposure and response prevention therapy, self-recording by computer of frequency of checking led to positive gains, but, unfortunately, maintenance was dependent upon continued computer use (Baer, Minichiello, Jenike, & Holland, 1988).

Successful outcomes were achieved with operant techniques employing punishment via electrical shock or snapping a rubber band on the wrist (Bass, 1973) or by listening to an audiotape of compulsive verbalizations (O'Brien & Raynes, 1973). Such aversive methods were often combined with other strategies (relaxation, desensitization, ritual prevention). In a well-controlled case study, Le Boeuf (1974) applied punishment to rituals rather than obsessions. He found that merely delaying washing longer than the length of time recorded at baseline was unproductive, but adding electrical shock to washings that occurred too soon produced a lasting reduction (from 32 to less than 5 per day). Applying another type of blocking method, Yamagami (1971) successfully used variants of the following thought-stopping procedure: After exposure to situations that triggered obsessions and rituals, the therapist shouted "Stop!" at the patient's signal of the obsessional impulse, eventually having the patient say and then merely think the word "Stop!" This method appeared mildly helpful in Gullick and Blanchard's (1973) case of religious obsessions.

In systematic desensitization, the patient's feared situations are arranged from least to most disturbing; each item on the list is repeatedly presented for a few seconds (rarely more than a minute), either in imagination or in practice (*in vivo*), to a patient who is in a very relaxed state until it provokes no further subjective discomfort. An apparently positive outcome was achieved for one woman with OCD, though her self-rating improved less than other phobic patients (Agras *et al.*, 1971). Wickramasekera (1970) treated one man using a baseline, imaginal desensitization, resensitization, and desensitization sequence for jealous obsessions. Considerable improvement was evident during both periods of desensitization for excessive sexual behavior and suspicious behaviors (checking on his wife). The value of desensitization is disputed in Tanner's (1971) single-case study of the separate effects of baseline recording, relaxation, and systematic desensitization for 10 checking behaviors. Desensitization seemed to be unnecessary, since 90% of rituals were reduced by the end of the relaxation period.

Pretest–posttest studies involving nine cases support the efficacy of a different method, exposure *in vivo* combined with response prevention (Farkas & Beck, 1981; Meyer & Levy, 1973; Rainey, 1972). In this treatment, patients are exposed to actual feared obsessive situations for prolonged periods (45 min to 2 hours) and instructed to delay, limit, or eliminate rituals, often under supervision. In the largest of these case studies, Meyer and Levy (1973) reported an average of 80% improvement in self- and assessor-rated rituals for six patients, with benefits maintained up to 6 years later; obsessions were somewhat less affected. Better-controlled case studies have also reported very positive outcomes for cases treated in this manner (Pruitt, Miller, & Smith, 1989).

Imaginal exposure to feared obsessive situations added to this combined treatment produced marked improvement for nine outpatients (Beidel & Bulik, 1990; Boulougouris & Bassiakos, 1973; Cobb & Marks, 1979). Cobb and Marks's (1979) treatment of jealous ruminations and rituals also included marital treatment in some cases; of four patients, three improved in rituals but only one in ruminations, again suggesting a greater effect of combined therapy on rituals than obsessions. The addition of modeling of the exposure by the therapist led to improvement in eight patients whose gains tended to generalize to anxiety, depression, and social adjustment (Catts & McConaghy, 1975; Cooper, 1990; Rowan, Holborn, Walker, & Siddiqui, 1984).

Four reports have provided data on the efficacy of a variant of exposure, audiotaped habituation, in which obsessions are tape-recorded in the patient's voice and replayed repeatedly (Headland & MacDonald, 1987; Salkovskis, 1983; Salkovskis & Westbrook, 1989; Thyer, 1985). Longer taped exposure (90 min) produced more reduction in frequency of ruminations compared with briefer exposure (20 min) (Salkovskis, 1983), and audiotaped exposure proved better than verbalized thoughts (Salkovskis & Westbrook, 1989). Exposure to repeated videotaped verbalizations of obsessions was similarly successful, and effects generalized to untreated OCD symptoms (Milby, Meredith, & Rice, 1981). Several variations in the mode of exposure were studied by Junginger and Ditto (1984), who employed a sequential treatment design. Exposure *in vivo* plus 2-hour response delay combined with verbal exposure to feared consequences led to near elimination of checking behavior, which was maintained at 7 months follow-up.

In a study of variants of ritual prevention, Junginger and Turner (1987) investigated response delay in which rituals are postponed for increasingly longer periods. Four weeks of exercise (increased activity) reduced anxiety and depression but not obsessional thinking and checking rituals, which were subsequently eliminated by 23 weeks of self-controlled response delay. However, as obsessions declined, depression and anxiety increased, possibly a consequence of the client's experience of "nothing on my mind." Without follow-up data, the persistence of the positive effects on obsessions in the presence of highly negative mood state remains questionable.

Salkovskis and Warwick (1985) used cognitive therapy to alter unrealistic beliefs when exposure therapy failed to resolve the contamination fears of a patient worried about skin cancer. Though the attribution of the successful outcome to the cognitive therapy has been disputed (e.g., Gurnani & Wang, 1987), its addition appeared to enable the patient to benefit from exposure treatment, and it may have implications for treatment of those with fixed, unreasonable obsessive beliefs (overvalued ideas).

Dismantling Designs and Comparisons between Treatments

Two case studies explored the specific efforts of exposure and of response prevention. Mills, Agras, Barlow, and Mills (1973) conducted carefully controlled studies of five inpatient OCD cases to examine the separate effects of exposure and response prevention. They found that response prevention reduced the frequency of rituals and, to a lesser extent, urges to wash. Supervised response prevention had a greater impact than instructions alone. By contrast, exposure alone led to an *increase* in rituals. Generalization to untreated rituals was demonstrated in one case. In a similar well-controlled series of three inpatient case studies, Turner, Hersen, Bellack, and Wells (1979) demonstrated the beneficial effects of combined exposure and ritual prevention in one study, and of ritual prevention alone in the other two. Though no appreciable effect was evident from adding flooding in cases two and three, exposure was not added in either case until long periods of response prevention had already reduced rituals to very low levels, leaving little room for change. Unfortunately, measures of obsessions were not reported. Beneficial effects appeared to generalize to other symptoms, including weight and anxiety, and to persist at follow-up.

Single-Case Comparisons between Behavioral Treatments

Only a few case studies have compared different treatments. Stern (1978) conducted two pilot studies of 11 "pure obsessionals," comparing thought stopping, relaxation, satiation (prolonged exposure to obsessions), and antidepressant drug treatments. Thought stopping, satiation, and antidepressants were only slightly helpful, and relaxation showed no benefits. For another patient with obsessions and rituals, Meredith and Milby (1978) employed a sequential treatment, multiple-response design to observe the effects of several treatments on various target problems. Desensitization led to only mild improvement in one mother's fears of leaving her child and associated rituals. Greater benefits were achieved by cognitive treatment via rational emotive therapy combined with disputation of erroneous beliefs and self-control of rituals. A 2-year follow-up indicated good maintenance of gains and generalization to mood and marital satisfaction.

Group Studies: Treatment Comparisons with Nonspecific Effects

Our review of the OCD literature indicates that no comparisons of psychodynamic or family systems treatments to wait-list control, to placebo, or to other therapies have been published. Since the only study of marital therapy did not appear to follow a strict family therapy model, it is discussed later in relation to behavioral treatment. Uncontrolled research on psychodynamic methods is summarized below.

Sifneos (1985) has examined the usefulness of short-term anxiety-provoking dynamic psychotherapy, a systematic effort by the therapist to interpret the patient's underlying conflicts and Oedipal wishes to produce insight, anxiety, and symptom resolution. Sifneos reported good outcomes after an unspecified follow-up period for 10 patients, using nonstandardized (8-point) scales to assess symptoms, interpersonal relations, understanding, problem solving, new learning, work performance, self-esteem, new attitudes, and resolution of the specific factors underlying the difficulties. Two independent assessors reported that symptoms were resolved for five patients, much improved for four others, and not changed for the one who withdrew from the study. Based on the two representative case descriptions, however, these patients showed only mild symptoms akin to ruminations or worries that did not appear to meet DSM-III criteria for OCD.

Black (1974) provides a comprehensive review of 16 early studies examining the short- and long-term outcome of patients treated in or out of the hospital with whatever psychotherapeutic methods the clinic or hospital typically employed. These uncontrolled studies suffer from multiple problems, including inconsistent diagnostic procedures, treatments, and measurements and the use of retrospective data and inferences from hospital charts. With respect to symptom change, Black concluded that the average improvement for outpatients or mixed in- and outpatients after 1 to 26 years was approximately 60%, and for inpatients (1 to 35 years) it was 46%. Although the majority of outpatients regained presymptomatic adjustment levels according to one study (Grimshaw, 1965), only 20% of the inpatient group were able to lead a "normal" social life (Kringlen, 1965).

Cawley (1974) also summarized findings from uncontrolled follow-up studies of psychoanalysis and psychotherapy patients, noting the bias in these studies to select patients deemed most likely to benefit. Two studies included data on obsessives or "compulsion neurotics" with uncertain diagnostic criteria. Figures were 59% improved or much improved after psychotherapy, with 52% maintaining gains at follow-up (Luff & Garrod, 1935), and 63% improved after analysis (after a dropout rate of 27%) (Knight, 1941). Despite the somewhat positive figures, Cawley (1974) concluded from these studies and other available evidence that "there is no grounds for feeling optimistic about the place of psychoanalysis or other types of formal psychotherapy in the treatment of obsessional disorders" (pp. 285–286).

Pretest–Posttest Designs and Limited-Control Designs

Like single-subject designs, most uncontrolled group studies using different behavioral strategies demonstrated beneficial effects. Solyom, Garza-Perez, Ledwidge, and Solyom (1972) conducted an early study of paradoxical intention in which eight participants were instructed to dwell on obsessive thoughts and try to convince themselves of the validity of feared consequences. They reported an improvement rate of 50% in the target thoughts, with an estimated specific effect of 40%. Solyom, Zamanzadeh, Ledwidge, and Kenny (1971) examined aversion relief in which an audiotape of silence was followed by shock; pressing a button ended the shock and began a tape of self-narrated obsessions. Of 15 patients, 47% were much improved, and 27% improved on obsessions, with some improvement in general functioning.

As in single-case studies, therapist-directed exposure and supervised response prevention was found to be a highly effective treatment combination in several uncontrolled group studies. Treating 15 inpatients, Meyer, Levy, and Schnurer (1974) found 67% very much improved on target symptoms and 33% improved after treatment. At follow-up of 6 months to 6 years, figures were nearly identical, but half of the improved group (17%) had relapsed. This tendency of partially improved patients to relapse has also been reported by others (e.g., Foa *et al.*, 1983). A much less strict self-imposed, unsupervised exposure and response prevention method led to very good results in two studies (Hoogduin & Duivenvoorden, 1988; Hoogduin & Hoogduin, 1984). About 80% of patients were much or very much improved.

Several other studies involving over 100 patients have included exposure and ritual prevention among a variety of treatments applied on a case-by-case basis (Kirk, 1983; Marks, Bird, & Lindley, 1978; Marks, Hallam, Connolly, & Philpott, 1977; Pradhan *et al.*, 1984). All of these studies reported symptom improvements comparable to those given above, with 75% maintaining gains. Generalization to work adjustment was also evident in the Marks *et al.* studies. Hand and Tichatzki (1978) are the only researchers who investigated the effectiveness of behavioral group treatment. Their outpatient model involved three phases. Phase 1 required 12 weeks of 2- to 3-hour group meetings twice weekly and five *in vivo* practice home visits by the therapist in the presence of a family member and a peer. Phase 2 consisted of 6 weekly sessions in which patients were trained to conduct group sessions. Phase 3, a structured follow-up, included 12 weekly meetings to establish self-help skills. Fourteen patients in three successive groups showed good results with this method. In Group 1, five of six patients improved. For Groups 2 and 3, all eight patients reported symptom reductions ranging from 50% to 90%. Overall, significant improvements were evident on two of the Maudsley–Oxford scales, suggesting that group therapy helped to manage anxiety and to reduce daily life restrictions (but not leisure activities or unspecific complaints), though most patients still had some OCD symptoms.

Limited controlled comparisons are available for thought stopping, aversion, and exposure and ritual prevention. Nammalvar and Venkoba Rao (1983) compared progressive muscular relaxation (control treatment) with thought stopping (TS) for 17 patients with obsessional thoughts in a sequential treatment design. Direct treatment for compulsions was not provided. Frequency of obsessions and subjective distress was significantly reduced only after the second TS phase (65% improved markedly, 17.5% minimally, and 17.5% not at all) and was essentially maintained at a 1- to 4-year follow-up. Manifest anxiety and depression scores also showed improvement, but measures of rituals were not taken. Unfortunately, due to the sequential nature of the design, the only conclusion that can be drawn is that TS is effective for controlling obsessive thoughts when preceded by relaxation. A better-controlled within-subjects test was conducted by Stern, Lipsedge, and Marks (1973), who randomly alternated TS for taped obsessional thoughts with TS for neutral thoughts, which served as a control treatment. The value of TS was not supported since there were no differences between treatments on OCD measures and psychophysiology, and only four of eleven subjects (36%) were much improved, three (27%) slightly, and three (27%) not at all. The authors suggested that therapist-administered TS might have been more powerful.

Kenny, Mowbray, and Lalani (1978) applied electrical aversion ("faradic disruption") to obsessive thoughts, comparing six treated patients with four wait-list controls. Aversion led to more improvement in target symptoms (four much improved and one improved) compared to no changes for wait-list subjects. After 1 year, three of the four patients had maintained their gains. Aversion treatment effects generalized somewhat to untreated OCD symptoms and to overall adjustment.

Foa and Goldstein (1978) tested the effects of 2 weeks of information gathering compared to 2 weeks of *in vivo* and imaginal exposure with supervised response prevention for 21 OCD patients. No changes in symptoms were evident during the first 2 weeks, whereas significant improvements on most OCD symptoms were evident after 10 daily 2-hour sessions of exposure and response prevention. On nonstandardized measures of target symptoms, an impressive 81% were much or very much improved and 14% were improved. Data reported at follow-up 3 months to 3 years later indicated that only 8% relapsed. Effects generalized somewhat to mood state and social adjustment. As noted in some studies above, compulsions responded more than obsessions. This study's intensive treatment trial had the highest success rate of all but Meyer *et al.*'s 1974 report. Studies of exposure and ritual prevention by other researchers indicated that 65% to 80% were improved or much improved (e.g., Emmelkamp, Hoekstra, & Visser, 1985; Marks, Hodgson, & Rachman, 1975).

Placebo Comparisons

Of all the treatments for OCD, only exposure and response prevention has been compared with a placebo treatment, relaxation. Unfortunately, since researchers did not include any assessment of the credibility of treatment procedures in these early studies, the possibility that the superior performance of exposure therapy could be due to this factor cannot be ruled out. In the first of a series of studies, Rachman, Hodgson, and Marks (1971) compared the effectiveness of modeling and of exposure *in vivo* (both with response prevention) to relaxation (control condition). Ten inpatients received 15 sessions of relaxation before being randomly assigned to 15 sessions of either participant modeling (observing a therapist engage in feared activities and following suit) or flooding alone. Both behavioral treatments produced significantly more improvement in OCD symptoms than relaxation. In a second study, with five additional patients, modeling plus flooding was again found superior to the relaxation control (Hodgson, Rachman, & Marks, 1972). A third study compared passive and participant modeling to relaxation control in a similarly designed study of 10 patients (Roper, Rachman, & Marks, 1975). As in the first study, both exposure treatment conditions were better than the relaxation control.

Comparisons between Behavioral Treatments

So far, comparisons between different types of behavioral treatments have all involved thought stopping and some form of prolonged exposure. In a crossover design, Hackmann and McLean (1975) compared four twice-weekly sessions of flooding plus modeling, presumably without response prevention, with the same number of thought-stopping sessions for 10 outpatients. Both treatments proved equally effective, but as predicted, flooding led to more overall improvement than thought stopping and specifically reduced avoidance behavior. Flooding was more effective than thought stopping in five cases, equivalent in two, and less effective in three. However, there was also a tendency for the first treatment to be more successful, regardless of type. The degree of improvement achieved in so few sessions is noteworthy: 80% experienced improvement, 10% minimal improvement, and 10% no change. However, gains did not generalize to non-OCD symptoms or overall functioning. In a very similar comparison, Likierman and Rachman (1982) also contrasted four sessions of "habituation training" (relaxation and flooding/satiation) with thought stopping in 12 patients. In this study, however, there were no significant differences between groups, nor did either treatment significantly reduce obsessional symptoms, suggesting that this brief treatment was not sufficient to produce substantial relief of OCD symptoms.

Sookman and Solyom (1977) also studied the effects of thought stopping, comparing it with a variant—desensitization plus thought stopping—and with two other behavioral treatments: (1) aversion relief and (2) combined flooding in imagery and *in vivo* with response prevention instructions. In this study, thought stopping was also applied not only to obsessions but also to rituals when appropriate. All treatments were administered for 50 one-hour sessions twice weekly to 33 subjects matched prior to assignment to treatments. Interestingly, thought stopping alone and flooding were most effective, each leading to 50% reduction in OCD symptoms, whereas aversion relief and desensitization plus thought stopping led to reductions of only 5% and 22%, respectively. Some differential effects on symptoms were apparent: Rituals responded best to thought stopping, and obsessive ruminations and impulses improved more with flooding treatment. This finding is somewhat comparable to later researchers' reports that blocking strategies such as response prevention have a greater impact on rituals, whereas exposure methods have more of an effect on the obsessions (e.g., Foa, Steketee, Grayson, Turner, & Latimer, 1984; Foa, Steketee, & Milby, 1980; Turner *et al.*, 1979).

Comparisons between Components and Variants of Exposure and Response Prevention

Other studies which have compared treatments have tended to be efforts to identify the most effective manner for delivery of combined exposure and response prevention for OCD. The studies discussed below examined the form of exposure (imaginal, *in vivo*, modeling) and rate of exposure (gradual, flooding) and, to a very limited extent, the strictness of response prevention, though this was confounded with other design variations.

Dismantling Designs. In the first of a series of related studies using dismantling designs, Foa, Steketee, and Milby (1980) studied 16 patients with washing rituals. Subjects were randomly assigned to 10 daily 2-hour sessions of either exposure alone or response prevention alone, both followed by combined treatment. Significant improvement was apparent in all conditions on target symptoms, but exposure improved subjective anxiety more, whereas response prevention reduced ritualized behavior more. Because of its crossover design, this study did not allow inferences about the long-term effects of components or of combined treatment.

To address this problem, a second study serially assigned 32 subjects to exposure only, response prevention only, or the two combined (Foa *et al.*, 1984). All received 15 sessions over a 3-week period followed by two lengthy home visits during the fourth week. The results of this study were consistent with those reported in the earlier one: Prolonged exposure affected primarily obsessive anxiety, response prevention reduced rituals, and both were necessary for maximum reduction of symptoms. The authors also reported a need for maintenance programs since partial relapse was evident for several patients, especially those in the single-component treatments, and particularly on obsessions.

A third study collected 72 patients from earlier studies to investigate the overall effectiveness of particular treatment components (imaginal exposure, *in vivo* exposure, response prevention) compared with combined methods (Foa, Grayson, Steketee, Doppelt, Turner, & Latimer, 1982). Combined exposure and ritual prevention treatments effected significantly more benefits both at posttreatment and at follow-up; single-component treatments resulted in partial treatment gains that proved unstable over time.

Modalities of Exposure. Two studies contrasted imaginal and practice exposure without including ritual prevention. In an early controlled comparison of the effect of long versus short, imagined versus *in vivo* flooding, 12 OCD patients were serially assigned to four sequential experimental conditions of a balanced Latin-square design (Rabavilas, Boulougouris, & Stefanis, 1976); that is, every patient received every treatment, and the order of treatments was varied across patients. In general, exposure was effective in relieving OCD symptoms, with no differences between actual and fantasied exposure. Longer exposures were superior to shorter ones, especially for real-life confrontation.

Results consistent with those reported in the study above come from research on 19 checkers which compared 15 sessions of imaginal flooding to *in vivo* exposure, both without ritual prevention (Foa, Steketee, & Grayson, 1985). There were no differences between groups; both showed significant improvements on 11 of the 12 standardized OCD scales, though gains were less impressive than those achieved for subjects receiving exposure with prevention of rituals.

To examine the effect of adding imaginal exposure to combined response prevention and *in vivo* treatment, Foa and her colleagues compared seven checkers who received all three methods with eight who did not have imaginal exposure (Foa, Steketee, Turner, & Fisher, 1980). The authors speculated that checkers, with their persistent fears of the catastrophic consequences of failing to check properly, might respond better to imaginal treatment in which such fears could be more readily incorporated. Both groups improved but did not differ significantly from each other at posttreatment. However, at follow-up, the subjects in the group that received both types of exposure were better able to maintain their gains on obsessions, compulsions, urges to ritualize, and overall OCD symptoms.

To further investigate the specific contribution of adding imaginal exposure, Steketee, Foa, and Grayson (1982) studied 49 OCD inpatients and outpatients. Adding imaginal treatment led to slightly better short- and long-term outcomes. In a larger sample of 72 patients mentioned earlier, Foa *et al.* (1983) noted that treatment that included imaginal exposure resulted in a higher proportion of "much improved" patients (71% versus 48%), indicating that for some patients imaginal exposure may be an important addition.

Variants of Exposure. Several researchers sought to identify variations in delivery of exposure and response prevention which might improve outcome. In particular, the rate of exposure, presence of a model, degree of therapist control, and partner or familial assistance were examined.

Earlier in the placebo comparisons section, we reported findings by Rachman and his colleagues regarding comparisons of exposure treatment to a control condition of relaxation (Hodgson *et al.*, 1972; Rachman *et al.*, 1971; Rachman *et al.*, 1973). In examining the effect of modeling, these researchers also found that modeling and flooding did not differ significantly from each other. Combining the two methods was somewhat more beneficial than applying either alone. Participant modeling (observation plus direct exposure) was more effective than passively observing a model doing exposure (Roper *et al.*, 1975). The apparent clinical importance of home treatment (also used by Foa and colleagues) was noted and incorporated as part of therapy in several of these studies.

Boersma, Den Hengst, Dekker, and Emmelkamp (1976) randomly assigned 13 OCD patients to gradual versus rapid exposure (flooding) and modeling versus no modeling. No significant differences were found between any of these variants. Significant clinical improvements appeared to result from mechanisms common to all four experimental conditions, that is, exposure and blocking of rituals.

Heyse (1975) varied both the modeling and the strictness of response prevention. Twenty-four inpatients received 4 weeks of either exposure and strictly supervised response prevention or therapist-modeled exposure and less strict response prevention. Again, no significant differences were found between conditions; about two-thirds of patients improved. However, patients who received modeling demonstrated some superiority in social adjustment. According to the above research, then, therapist modeling of exposures does not add significantly to exposure without modeling, though it may be quite helpful clinically for individual patients.

The contribution of therapist presence was studied by Emmelkamp and Kraanen (1977). Exposure *in vivo* administered by the therapist was compared to patient-controlled exposure, both with ritual prevention. Both conditions had significant and equivalent positive effects on patients' posttreatment and follow-up (1 to 3.5 months), ratings of OCD symptoms, depression, and anxious mood. However, the self-controlled treatment required only half the therapy time (10 hours versus 20 hours over 5 weeks) and was therefore more cost effective.

Family-Assisted Exposure. Three studies have examined the effects of including a family member in the therapy as an "adjunct therapist." Emmelkamp and De Lange (1983) randomly assigned 12 married OCD patients to self-controlled exposure or partner-assisted exposure. As with other variations discussed above, both conditions resulted in significant improvements in OCD symptoms which further generalized to anxious mood and depression. The partner-assisted group showed greater improvement than the self-controlled group at posttest, but the difference in effectiveness was not sustained at the 1-month and 6-month follow-ups due to continued improvement in the latter group.

A larger investigation of the above variants was completed by Emmelkamp, de Haan, and Hoogduin (1990) 7 years later. In this study, 50 DSM-III-diagnosed OCD outpatients were randomly assigned to either self-controlled or partner-assisted treatment for eight sessions over 5 weeks. Again, both treatments were equally effective, this time at posttest as well as follow-up. Furthermore, marital distress was found unrelated to treatment outcome on standardized OCD and mood inventories. Interestingly, the marital partners also showed improvements on most of the measures (Symptom Checklist-90, anxiety, anger, and marital satisfaction).

Along similar lines, Mehta (1990) randomly assigned 30 DSM-III OCD outpatients to either treatment with a family member as "cotherapist" or treatment alone. The basic treatment included 24 sessions of self-monitoring, relaxation, systematic desensitization, exposure, and response prevention over a 12-week period, more than double the amount of therapy applied by Emmelkamp and colleagues. Contrary to findings in the above studies, significantly greater improvement was found at posttreatment and follow-up for the family-assisted treatment on standardized measures of OCD symptoms, as well as anxiety, depression, and social adjustment. Clinical observations indicated that firm and nonanxious family members were more successful than ones who were inconsistent and tense.

Interorientation Comparisons

Few comparisons have been made between treatment methods for OCD representing different theoretical models. To our knowledge, no comparisons of behavioral methods with psychodynamic treatments or with strict family systems interventions have been conducted. So far, most of the contrasts have been between the behavioral exposure and response prevention method, cognitive treatment, marital therapy (not a systemic model), and pharmacotherapy.

Exposure versus Cognitive Therapies

In an early attempt to test the efficacy of one form of cognitive therapy, Emmelkamp, van der Helm, van Zanten, and Plochg (1980) studied the contribution of self-instructional training to exposure and response prevention by randomly assigning 15 OCD patients either to exposure alone or to exposure preceded by self-instructional training. Subjects from both groups benefited equally, showing clinically significant improvements on OCD measures (average ranged from 41% to 78%). Thus this cognitive procedure did not add to the efficacy of gradual exposure and response prevention. The effects of treatment generalized to ratings of anxious mood and depression with most gains maintained at the 6-month follow-up.

In a second study of cognitive therapy, Emmelkamp, Visser, and Hoekstra (1988) randomly assigned 18 OCD patients either to self-controlled exposure and response prevention or to rational emotive therapy (RET). Both treatments produced significant changes in most measures of OCD symptoms, with improvements largely maintained 6 months later. Rates of improvement were 78% at posttest; continued gains by patients led to 94% improvement at follow-up. However, as in several earlier studies, follow-up data should be interpreted conservatively since several patients received additional treatment as needed. Subjective ratings of anxiety and depression also improved with both methods, though RET demonstrated some superiority over exposure for the latter. It is noteworthy that for this study, the investigators developed treatment manuals, monitored treatment integrity and compliance, and used standardized measures.

Exposure versus Marital Therapy

In a crossover design, Cobb, McDonald, Marks, and Stern (1980) compared the differential effects of exposure and marital therapy on marital problems as well as OCD symptoms. Twelve couples with severe marital problems and one partner with OCD symptoms were randomly assigned to 10 weekly 1-hour sessions of either marital or OCD treatment during phase 1, followed by 3 months of no treatment, and then by 10 sessions of the alternative treatment during phase 2. The authors reported that exposure treatment using the nonsymptomatic partner as a cotherapist produced significant improvement in both the OCD and the marital targets, whereas marital therapy alone effected changes only in the marital targets. Improvements were maintained at 13-month follow-up. Though exposure is recommended over marital therapy, the possible advantages of combining the two types of treatment merits further investigation (cf. Cobb & Marks, 1979).

Exposure versus Pharmacological Treatment

At the present time, three drugs, all serotonergic in their action, have proven effective in relieving OCD symptoms: clomipramine, fluoxetine, and fluvoxamine.

Several studies have compared these medications to variants of the exposure and response prevention method. We will omit studies of drugs which have no demonstrated efficacy for OCD (e.g., imipramine).

Investigators in England have studied the separate and combined effects of clomipramine (CMI) and exposure and response prevention in two controlled trials using double-blind assessments. In the first study (Marks *et al.*, 1980), 40 inpatient OCD subjects (excluding those with primary depression) were randomly assigned to placebo or CMI (weeks 1 to 4) and then to relaxation or exposure and ritual prevention (weeks 4 to 7). All patients received exposure therapy from weeks 7 to 10. CMI produced significant improvement in rituals, mood and social adjustment, but only in those who were initially depressed. Maximum benefit from the drug was not achieved until week 10, indicating that a trial of only 4 weeks was insufficient to determine the full effect of CMI. Relapse tended to follow drug withdrawal. As observed in earlier studies, relaxation was ineffective, whereas exposure led to substantial improvement, again, more in rituals than in mood state. Gains were maintained 1 year later. The combination of CMI and exposure had a slight additive effect and appeared to improve compliance with behavioral treatment. Follow-up findings 6 years later indicated that results were essentially maintained, except for general anxiety, which returned to mild to moderate pretreatment levels (O'Sullivan, Noshirvani, Marks, Monteiro, & Lelliott, 1991).

A second study used a complex randomized design for 49 OCD inpatients to compare CMI with placebo under self-controlled exposure (and ritual prevention) or "antiexposure" instructions (Marks *et al.*, 1988). After 8 weeks, therapist-assisted exposure and response prevention was then added for half the subjects to test its effects relative to self-exposure. CMI and self-exposure led to more improvement after 7 weeks than placebo and self-exposure for rituals and depression (but not for obsessions, anxiety, or general adjustment), but this advantage disappeared after 15 more weeks of therapy. CMI without exposure was generally equivalent to exposure-only treatment. Not surprisingly, self-exposure was much more effective for OCD symptoms than antiexposure instructions, and this benefit generalized to some extent to social adjustment, but not to mood state. Therapist-assisted exposure added marginal benefit. The earlier finding that only depressed OCD patients responded to CMI was not replicated here.

In a study of fluoxetine (FXT), Turner, Beidel, Stanley, and Jacob (1988) compared 14 weeks of FXT to 10 weeks of exposure and response prevention, which always followed drug therapy. Treatments were applied sequentially in a small sample of five DSM-III-diagnosed outpatient OCD ritualizers. FXT improved depression and anxiety, but not OCD symptoms, whereas behavioral treatment led to substantial clinical improvement in OCD symptoms and to some extent in depression. As in the first Marks *et al.* (1980) study, medication had an effect primarily for patients with greater initial depression and anxiety. By contrast, the effect of behavior therapy was independent of mood state.

A controlled study of fluvoxamine (FVM) and exposure with response prevention treatment was conducted in France with DSM-III-diagnosed OCD outpatients (Cottraux *et al.*, 1989). Subjects were randomly assigned to FVM with relaxation and no exposure, FVM plus imaginal and *in vivo* exposure with ritual prevention, and placebo plus the same behavioral treatment. Subjects in all three groups improved significantly, with a slight advantage for drug plus exposure at week 24, which largely disappeared by week 48. Gains were maintained at week 48. FVM led to more improvement in depression than either placebo or exposure, and, again, initial depression was associated with somewhat better outcome for the drug-treated patients only.

Further studying the relative efficacy of behavioral intervention and drug treatment for OCD, Christensen and colleagues conducted a meta-analysis of effect sizes for tricyclic antidepressant drugs and behavioral treatments with OCD (Christensen, Dadzi-Pavlovic, Andrews, & Mattick, 1987). They concluded from their analyses that patients with obsessions only responded less well to treatment than those with rituals. Behavioral treatment effects appeared stable at follow-up; such data were not available for drug treatments. According to their findings, drug and exposure therapies did not differ significantly, and both were superior to nonspecific treatments. Unfortunately, the criteria for the selection of studies for their comparison were quite broad, resulting in inclusion of treatment methods which were not adequately representative of either the pharmacological or the behavioral treatments of choice for OCD. A more appropriate meta-analysis would require a comparison of serotonergic antidepressants with demonstrated efficacy for OCD (clomipramine, fluvoxamine, fluoxetine) and behavioral treatments combining exposure and ritual prevention.

Outcome Parameters

Apart from the specific effects of a treatment method on target OCD symptoms, additional measures of the efficacy of an intervention can be derived from examining its impact on other problems (mood, functioning, etc.), its efficiency in producing change, and the probability that patients will elect or remain in the therapy for an adequate trial.

Generalization of Gains

Findings regarding the generalization of treatment effects to other areas of functioning are summarized in Table 11.1. Only seven studies reported on the impact of treatments to untreated OCD symptoms. As evident from the table, the minimal evidence available does not support generalization to similar but untreated symptoms for thought stopping and aversion methods, and is somewhat equivocal for exposure and response prevention. However, two single-case studies have demonstrated that exposure and prevention reduced treated symptoms, with clear generalization of effects to untreated symptoms (Hayashida, 1982; Moergen, Maier, Brown, & Pollard, 1987).

Many more studies examined generalization to mood and functioning, but nearly all pertain to variants of exposure treatments. No conclusions can be drawn from research on other behavioral methods, since only three studies reported on depression and only two on anxiety, with no evidence of any consistent pattern. Findings on measures of mood state following exposure and response prevention treatment in numerous studies, typically support a generalization of the beneficial effect to depression and especially to general anxiety. However, in studies which compared exposure therapy to drugs, only the medicated patients experienced significant or substantial relief from depressed mood. Further confusing the issue is Emmelkamp *et al.*'s (1988) study indicating that cognitive therapy (RET) produced improvement in depression, whereas exposure did not. Still, the weight of the evidence supports the benefits of exposure treatment for mood state.

The beneficial effects of exposure on general functioning are also strongly supported (see Table 11.1). Findings are somewhat inconsistent, however, since some investigators measured only one or two aspects of functioning (e.g., work or relationships) and others assessed several. General functioning of OCD patients improved more when exposure was combined with modeling (Heyse, 1975), with family assistance (Mehta, 1990), and with medication (Marks *et al.*, 1980). With respect to other behavioral treatments, thought stopping produced no obvious benefits, whereas both desensitization and aversion therapy generated improvement in general functioning. Aversion *relief*, however, did not improve functioning (Sookman & Solyom, 1977).

Efficiency of Treatments

Group studies provide little useful information about the optimal number of therapy sessions or weeks of treatment required, since the number is usually arbitrarily selected by the investigator and rarely adjusted to the needs of individual patients. In some ways, single-case studies may provide a better estimate, since intensity and duration of treatments are usually matched to patients' needs. Further, the efficiency of a treatment may not be closely associated with its effectiveness. In reviewing the duration of treatment across the different behavioral treatment methods, it is apparent that thought stopping was quite efficient, though ineffective, often requiring only 4 sessions over 2 to 4 weeks, though one case study used 17 sessions and another group trial applied 50 sessions. The most time-consuming treatment was aversion therapy, with a range of 18 to 47 sessions

Table 11.1. Number of Studies Showing Generalization of Therapy Effects to Other Problems

Treatment	OCD symptoms	Depression	Anxiety	Functioning
Thought stopping				
Yes	1 (1)	1 (11)	—	—
No	1 (10)	—	1 (10)	2 (18)
Aversion therapy				
Yes	1 (1)	—	—	2 (8)
No	1 (6)	—	1 (6)	1 (8) relief
Covert modeling				
Yes	1 (1)	—	—	—
No	—	1 (1)	—	—
Desensitization				
Yes	—	1 (17)	1 (17)	3 (10)
No	—	—	—	—
Exposure/prevention				
Yes	4 (15)	18 (170)	18 (254)	17 (297)
No	1 (10)	7 (99)	4 (61)	3 (63)
Cognitive therapy +/− exposure				
Yes	—	3 (25)	3 (25)	1 (1)
No	—	—	—	—

Note. Numbers in parentheses are numbers of patients in the studies.

over 13 to 60 weeks. Desensitization typically required an average of 25 sessions in as many weeks. By contrast, exposure and response prevention has been administered in 10 to 20 sessions applied over 4 to 12 weeks (though 5 of 12 case studies required more time); thus, a greater frequency of sessions (2 to 5 times per week) is typical of this therapy. As O'Sullivan *et al.* (1991) observed, better long-term gains were associated with longer trials of exposure therapy. This method so far best combines efficiency and effectiveness.

Refusal and Dropout Rates

No studies of behavioral treatments other than exposure and ritual prevention or cognitive therapy reported on refusal and dropout rates. Thus, we can only comment on the question of the acceptability of these two methods. According to 17 studies, of 297 participants in treatments containing exposure and response prevention, only 6.3% refused such therapy and only 8.6% dropped out. The low dropout rate is consistent with the clinical impression of several researchers. However, the much higher rejection rates of 20% to 30% for studies of rigorous and anxiety-provoking exposure and response prevention (e.g., Foa *et al.*, 1984, 1985; Marks *et al.*, 1975) suggest that refusal rates for this intensive therapy may be considerably higher. With regard to cognitive treatments, Emmelkamp *et al.*'s two studies involving 33 patients showed a very low refusal rate (2.6%) but a slightly higher dropout rate (10.5%). The additional cooperation required for exposure therapy with partner assistance (62 subjects in two studies) produced more refusals (10.5%) but about the same number of dropouts (7.9%). Adding drugs to the behavioral regimen appears to lead to much more rejection; in the Marks *et al.* (1988) study of 49 completers, 22 patients had refused drugs, whereas only 8 had declined behavioral treatment.

Prognostic Factors

It is not surprising that with the majority of research on treatment of OCD devoted to studying exposure and ritual prevention, efforts to identify prognostic factors have focused nearly exclusively on this therapeutic method. Below we present findings from studies using statistical methods to identify predictors of outcome for exposure and ritual prevention, as well as those using prospective designs to compare patients on variables of interest (e.g., high versus low depression, adolescents versus adults).

Demographic Variables. Although nearly all studies have observed that age at time of treatment did not predict outcome (e.g., Boulougouris, 1977; Hoogduin & Duivenvoorden, 1988; Rachman *et al.*, 1973), Foa *et al.* (1983) did find that younger adult patients fared better. Adolescents, however, appear to have more difficulty. In a prospective study, Cox, Merkel, and Pollard (1987) reported that inpatient exposure and response prevention administered to 13 adults and 13 matched adolescents led to improvement in both groups, but adults improved significantly more than adolescents, who tended to withdraw prematurely from treatment. In several studies examining other biographical factors, gender, marital status, intelligence, and education level were not predictive of gains.

Aspects of OCD. Predictive studies were nearly unanimous in finding that neither duration of illness nor severity predicted outcome. Some studies suggested that patients with contamination fears and washing rituals had a better prognosis than those with checking rituals (Boulougouris, 1977; Rachman *et al.*, 1973), though Foa and her colleagues failed to find such a relationship (Foa & Goldstein, 1978; Foa *et al.*, 1983). Patients with pure obsessions (or perhaps cognitive rituals) do appear to fare more poorly than those with overt rituals (Steketee & Cleere, 1990; see Salkovskis and Westbrook, 1989, for treatment strategies to address obsessives with mental rituals).

Cognitive Factors. Low motivation and failure to comply with instructions has led to poor outcome according to several studies (e.g., Cobb & Marks, 1979; Hoogduin & Duivenvoorden, 1988; O'Sullivan *et al.*, 1991; Rachman & Hodgson, 1980). Although Foa (1979) has suggested that fixed beliefs ("overvalued ideation") predicted poor outcome, subsequent studies have failed to find a significant association (e.g., Foa *et al.*, 1983; Hoogduin & Duivenvoorden, 1988). The effect of behavioral treatment on the fixity of overvalued beliefs has not been adequately studied.

Mood State. Early studies suggested that high initial depression was predictive of treatment failure (e.g., Foa *et al.*, 1983; Marks *et al.*, 1980), but more recent evidence consistently contradicts this finding (e.g., Emmelkamp *et al.*, 1985; Hoogduin & Duivenvoorden, 1988; O'Sullivan *et al.*, 1991). Indeed, findings from a prospective comparison by Foa, Kozak, Steketee, and McCarthy (1992) of depressed and nondepressed OCD patients who received either antidepressant medication or placebo prior to behavior therapy indicated that depressed patients did not fare better than nondepressed ones and that amelioration of depression via drugs had no impact on treatment outcome. With regard to general anxiety prior to therapy, the weight of the evidence indicates no association with outcome (e.g., Boulougouris, 1977; Emmelkamp *et al.*, 1985; O'Sullivan *et al.*, 1991). Interestingly, Steketee (1993) observed that high levels of anxiety and depression *after* therapy were the strongest predictors of poor outcome.

Interpersonal Factors. Among social variables, OCD patients with more satisfactory marriages improved more than patients with less satisfactory marriages (Hafner, 1982), but as noted above, spouse-assisted exposure therapy did not lead to better outcome than unassisted treatment, though family treatment did. General social support was not predictive. However, patients fared worse at follow-up if they came from families with critical or angry loved ones who believed that patients could control their symptoms if they chose to (Steketee, 1993). It seems clear that support from immediate family members is likely to be helpful in ensuring continued treatment benefit.

Personality Variables. Diagnosis of unspecified personality disorder or of obsessive–compulsive personality disorder does not appear to predict outcome (Baer & Jenike, 1990; Steketee, 1990). Likewise, in a prospective study, Rabavilas, Boulougouris, Perissaki, and Stefanis (1979) did not find significant differences in outcome between patients who had or did not have premorbid obsessional personality traits, although, surprisingly, on some measures the obsessional group improved more. Certain personality disorders and traits, however, do appear to bode ill for behavioral treatment outcome; these include schizotypal personality disorder (Minichiello, Baer, & Jenike, 1987) and passive–aggressive traits (Steketee, 1990).

Other Variables. In a path analysis of several variables, Foa *et al.* (1983) noted that more reactive patients tended to habituate less during, as well as between, exposure sessions. All three factors were associated with poorer outcome. Both Foa *et al.* (1983) and O'Sullivan *et al.* (1991) have observed that greater posttest gains on OCD measures (i.e., at least 67% improvement) reduced the risk of relapse at follow-up. However, data by Emmelkamp *et al.* (1985) did not support these findings: Of 18 patients rated only improved (31% to 69%) at posttest, 13 continued to improve further at follow-up.

Conclusions

Our review of the empirical literature on OCD revealed that treatments based strictly on psychodynamic or family systems theories have not been tested in controlled trials and that comparisons between these therapy methods and behavioral interventions have been inadequately researched. Of all the behavioral strategies, variants of exposure and response prevention were most studied, generating more than 20 case studies and 30 group investigations in the past 20 years. At least half of the group studies contained methodologically rigorous designs, including random, matched, or serial assignment to control or other treatment comparisons and multiple measures of outcome.

Most researchers were probably motivated to study this method by the consistently positive results from case studies and group comparisons showing that 65% to 85% of patients improved in OCD symptoms, as well as in mood and general functioning. It seems abundantly clear from the findings reported here that the combined use of exposure to feared situations and blocking of rituals is the current treatment of choice for OCD. Although there is clearly room for more research on other methods, it seems unlikely that other treatments, such as family therapy, psychodynamic therapy, or other behavioral methods, are likely to match the magnitude of the benefits derived from exposure and response prevention.

Studies which examined variations in the delivery of therapy and prognostic factors have some specific implications for how to administer behavioral treatment for OCD. Exposure and response prevention appears to be appropriate for both adolescents and adults, though treatment for the former is liable to require special consideration of developmental issues (e.g., struggle for independence) in this age group. No special attention appears needed for males versus females, married versus unmarried patients, or for differences in intellectual or educational level. Similarly, specialized treatment for depressed or anxious patients seems unnecessary, with the possible exception of the very seriously depressed who are either unresponsive or overly reactive to exposure; for this group, beginning with antidepressant medications may be helpful. It seems clear that certain personality characteristics, especially schizotypal and possibly passive–aggressive ones, portend less benefit from therapy. How to address such problems is unknown at this time and difficult to foresee, particularly since beginning the therapy for OCD symptoms with efforts to alter personality disorders is likely to be extremely time-consuming and have an uncertain outcome.

Findings regarding fixed irrational obsessional beliefs are conflicting and unsatisfying. Many investigators of drug or behavioral treatment remain convinced by clinical experience that overvalued obsessions interfere with patients' progress. Better agreement regarding the nature and especially the measurement of this phenomenon are essential for clarity regarding its predictive ability and response to drugs, exposure treatment, or other strategies such as cognitive therapy. Similarly, the value of cognitive treatments for OCD, alone or added to exposure and ritual prevention, remains unclear. Only three investigations have been conducted, all by Emmelkamp and colleagues, with only one showing benefits from RET. Since efforts to measure beliefs and attitudes typical of OCD patients and possible problematic for outcome are lacking, attempts to treat presumed cognitive problems in these patients puts the cart before the horse (cf. Gurnani & Wang, 1987). First we must measure and identify problematic cognitions, and only then strategize about how to change them.

Although there is limited information, as yet, regarding familial support, the above findings suggest that treatment progresses more satisfactorily when loved ones are reasonably tolerant and supportive of their afflicted family members. Similarly, although spouse assistance in therapy did not affect treatment outcome, it may prove helpful in extending the therapist's ability to apply exposure and ritual prevention, but very likely, only for those with supportive partners. Further investigation of such familial issues is ongoing at our clinic at present and should provide some indicators regarding whether particular familial interaction patterns are prognostic.

Clearly, future research in this area will benefit from the use of the DSM-III-R diagnostic criteria, standardized measures of OCD symptoms (especially the Yale–Brown Obsessive Compulsive Checklist and scales), of depressed mood unconfounded with anxious mood (e.g., Beck Depression Inventory), of general anxious mood (e.g., Beck Anxiety Inventory), and of general functioning (e.g., Social Adjustment Scales—Self-Report). Assessment of the comparability of interventions vis-à-vis patients' confidence in their efficacy has been lacking in research to date. Well-designed and controlled studies with the elements mentioned above will facilitate comparison across investigations.

Guides to aid the clinician in treating OCD are available in Steketee and Foa (1985) and in Steketee and White (1990). The latter book was designed as a psychoeducational and self-help guide for patients and family members, as well as a basic clinical text. A more complete guide for mental health practitioners is in progress (Steketee, in press). These books provide detailed information about planning and carrying out exposure in practice for individuals who have a variety of obsessive fears. Instructions and examples of imagined exposure are detailed, and guidelines are provided for deciding when to employ this method. Strategies for preventing compulsions are presented, along with specific suggestions for blocking different types of behavioral rituals (e.g., washing, checking, repeating) and covert ones (mental compulsions). In addition to these writings, workshops for clinicians in behavioral treatment of OCD are available at the annual meetings of the Association for the Advancement of Behavior Therapy (AABT), 18 W. 36th St., New York, NY 10018. Information and referral services for prospective patients can may be obtained from AABT and from the OC Foundation, 9 Depot Street, Milford, CT 06460. The latter organization also publishes an informative newsletter on a variety of issues related to obsessive–compulsive disorder.

References

Agras, W. S., Leitenberg, H., Barlow, D. H., Curtis, N-A., Edwards, J., & Wright, D. (1971). Relaxation in systematic desensitization. *Archives of General Psychiatry, 25*, 511–513.

Baer, L., & Jenike, M. A. (1990). Personality disorders in obsessive compulsive disorder. In M. A. Jenike, L. Baer, & W. E. Minichiello (Eds.), *Obsessive compulsive disorder: Theory and management* (pp. 76–88). Chicago: Year Book Medical Publishers.

Baer, L., Minichiello, W. E., Jenike, M. A., & Holland, A. (1988). Use of a portable computer program to assist behavioral treatment in a case of obsessive compulsive disorder. *Journal of Behavior Therapy and Psychiatry, 19*, 237–240.

Bass, B. A. (1973). An unusual behavioral technique for treating obsessive ruminations. *Psychotherapy: Theory, Research and Practice, 10*, 191–192.

Beidel, D. C., & Bulik, C. M. (1990). Flooding and response prevention as a treatment for bowel obsessions. *Journal of Anxiety Disorders, 4*, 247–256.

Black, A. (1974). The natural history of obsessional neurosis. In H. R. Beech (Ed.), *Obsessional states* (pp. 19–54). London: Methuen.

Boersma, K., Den Hengst, S., Dekker, J., & Emmelkamp, P. M. G. (1976).Exposure and response prevention: A comparison with obsessive compulsive patients. *Behaviour Research and Therapy, 14*, 19–24.

Boulougouris, J. C. (1977). Variables affecting the behaviour modification of obsessive-compulsive patients treated by flooding. In J. C. Boulougouris & A. D. Rabavilas (Eds.), *The treatment of phobic and obsessive-compulsive disorder* (pp. 73–84). Oxford: Pergamon Press.

Boulougouris, J. C., & Bassiakos, L. (1973). Prolonged flooding in cases with obsessive compulsive neurosis. *Behaviour Research and Therapy, 11*, 227–231.

Catts, S., & McConaghy, N. (1975). Ritual prevention in the treatment of obsessive-compulsive neurosis. *Australian and New Zealand Journal of Psychiatry, 9*, 37–41.

Cawley, R. (1974). Psychotherapy and obsessional disorders. In H. R. Beech (Ed.), *Obsessional states* (pp. 259–290). London: Methuen.

Christensen, H., Dadzi-Pavlovic, D., Andrews, G., & Mattick, R. (1987). Behavior therapy and tricyclic medication in the treatment of obsessive-compulsive disorder: A quantitative review. *Journal of Consulting and Clinical Psychology, 55*, 701–711.

Churchill, J. E. (1986). Hypnotherapy and conjoint family therapy: A viable treatment combination. *American Journal of Clinical Hypnosis, 28*, 170–176.

Cobb, J., McDonald, R., Marks, I. M., & Stern, R. (1980). Marital versus exposure therapy: Psychological treatments of co-existing marital and phobic obsessive problems. *Behavioural Analysis and Modification, 4*, 3–16.

Cobb, J. P., & Marks, I. M. (1979). Morbid jealousy featuring as obsessive-compulsive neurosis: Treatment by behavioural psychotherapy. *British Journal of Psychiatry, 134*, 301–305.

Cooper, M. (1990). Treatment of a client with obsessive-compulsive disorder. *Social Work Research and Abstracts, 26*, 32.

Cottraux, J., Mollard, E., Bouvard, M., Marks, I., Sluys, M., Nury, A. M., Douge, R., & Cialdella, P. (1989). A controlled study of fluvoxamine and exposure in obsessive compulsive disorder. *International Clinical Psychopharmacology, 5*, 1–14.

Cox, G.L., Merkel, W. T., & Pollard, C. A. (1987, November). *Age-related differences in response to exposure and response prevention: A comparison of adolescents and adults with OCD*. Paper presented at the annual meeting of the Association for the Advancement of Behavior Therapy, Boston, MA.

Dollard, J., & Miller, N. E. (1950). *Personality and psychotherapy: An analysis in terms of learning, thinking and culture*. New York: McGraw-Hill.

Emmelkamp, P. M. G., de Haan, E., & Hoogduin, C. A. L. (1990). Marital adjustment and obsessive-compulsive disorder. *British Journal of Psychiatry, 156*, 55–60.

Emmelkamp, P. M. G., & De Lange, I. (1983). Spouse involvement in the treatment of obsessive-compulsive patients. *Behaviour Research and Therapy, 21*, 341–346.

Emmelkamp, P. M. G., Hoekstra, R. J., & Visser, S. (1985). The behavioral treatment of OCD: Prediction of outcome at 3.5 years follow-up. In P. Pichot, P. Berner, R. Wolf, & K. Thau (Eds.), *Psychiatry: The state of the art* (pp. 265–270). New York: Plenum.

Emmelkamp, P. M. G., & Kraanen, J. (1977). Therapist-controlled exposure *in vivo* versus self-controlled exposure *in vivo*: A comparison with obsessive-compulsive patients. *Behaviour Research and Therapy, 15*, 491–495.

Emmelkamp, P. M. G., van der Helm, M., van Zanten, B. L., & Plochg, I. (1980). Contributions of self-instructional training to the effectiveness of exposure *in vivo*: A comparison with obsessive compulsive patients. *Behaviour Research and Therapy, 18*, 61–66.

Emmelkamp, P. M. G., Visser, S., & Hoekstra, R. J. (1988). Cognitive therapy vs. exposure *in vivo* in the treatment of obsessive-compulsives. *Cognitive Therapy and Research, 12*, 103–114.

Farkas, G. M., & Beck, S. (1981). Exposure and response prevention of morbid ruminations and compulsive avoidance. *Behaviour Research and Therapy, 19*, 257–261.

Fenichel, O. (1945). *The psychoanalytic theory of neurosis*. New York: Norton.

Foa, E. B. (1979). Failure in treating obsessive-compulsives. *Behaviour Research and Therapy, 17*, 169–179.

Foa, E. B., & Goldstein, A. (1978). Continuous exposure and complete response prevention of obsessive-compulsive disorder. *Behavior Therapy, 9*, 821–829.

Foa, E. B., Grayson, J. B., Steketee, G., Doppelt, H. G., Turner, R. M., & Latimer, P. R. (1983). Success and failure in the behavioral treatment of obsessive-compulsives. *Journal of Consulting and Clinical Psychology, 51*, 287–297.

Foa, E. B., & Kozak, M. J. (1986). Emotional processing of fear: exposure to corrective information. *Psychological Bulletin, 99*, 20–35.

Foa, E. B., Steketee, G., & Grayson, J. B. (1985). Imaginal and *in vivo* exposure: A comparison with obsessive-compulsive checkers. *Behavior Therapy, 16*, 292–302.

Foa, E. B., Steketee, G., Grayson, J. B., Turner, R. M., & Latimer, P. R. (1984). Deliberate exposure and blocking of obsessive-compulsive rituals: Immediate and long term effects. *Behavior Therapy, 15*, 450–472.

Foa, E. B., Steketee, G., & Milby, J. B. (1980). Differential effects of exposure and response prevention in obsessive compulsive washers. *Journal of Consulting and Clinical Psychology, 48*, 71–79.

Foa, E. B., Steketee, G., Turner, R. M., & Fischer, S. C. (1980). Effects of imaginal exposure to feared disasters in obsessive compulsive checkers. *Behaviour Research and Therapy, 18*, 449–455.

Frederiksen, L. W. (1975). Treatment of ruminative thinking by self-monitoring. *Journal of Behavior Therapy and Experimental Psychiatry, 6*, 258–259.

Grimshaw, L. (1965). The outcome of obsessional disorder: A follow-up study of 100 cases. *British Journal of Psychiatry, 111*, 1051–1056.

Gullick, E. L., & Blanchard, E. B. (1973). The use of psychotherapy and behavior therapy in the treatment of an obsessional disorder: An experimental case study. *The Journal of Nervous and Mental Disease, 156*, 427–431.

Gurnani, P. O., & Wang, M. (1987). [Letter to the Editor]. *Behaviour Psychotherapy, 15*, 101–103.

Hackmann, A., & McLean, C. (1975). A comparison of flooding and thought stopping in the treatment of obsessional neurosis. *Behaviour Research and Therapy, 13*, 263–269.

Hafner, R. J. (1982). Marital interaction in persisting obsessive-compulsive disorders. *Australian and New Zealand Journal of Psychiatry, 16*, 171–178.

Hafner, R. J., Gilchrist, P., Bowling, J., & Kalucy, R. (1981). The treatment of obsessional neurosis in a family setting. *Australian and New Zealand Journal of Psychiatry, 15*, 145–151.

Hand, I., & Tichatzki, M. (1978). Behavioral group therapy for obsessions and compulsions: First results of a pilot study. In S. Bates, W. S. Dockens, K. G. Gotestam, L. Melin, & P. O. Sjoden (Eds.), *Trends in behavior therapy* (pp. 269–297). New York: Academic Press.

Hayashida, M. (1982). Successful response prevention of ritual producing increase then decrease of untreated rituals. *Journal of Behavior Therapy and Experimental Psychiatry, 13*, 225–228.

Headland, K., & MacDonald, B. (1987). Rapid audio-tape treatment of obsessional ruminations: A case report. *Behavioural Psychotherapy, 15*, 188–192.

Heyse, H. (1975). Response prevention and modeling in the treatment of obsessive-compulsive neurosis: A study of 24 patients. In J. C. Brengelmann, J. T. Quinn, P. I. J. Graham, J. J. M. Harbison, & H. McAllister (Eds.), *Progress in behavior therapy* (pp. 53–58). New York: Springer-Verlag.

Hodgson, R. J., Rachman, S., & Marks, I. M. (1972). The treatment of chronic obsessive-compulsive neurosis: Follow-up and further findings. *Behaviour Research and Therapy, 10,* 181–189.

Hoogduin, C. A. L., & Duivenvoorden, H. J. (1988). A decision model in the treatment of obsessive-compulsive neuroses. *British Journal of Psychiatry, 152,* 516–521.

Hoogduin, C. A. L., & Hoogduin, W. A. (1984). The outpatient treatment of patients with an obsessional-compulsive disorder. *Behaviour Research and Therapy, 22,* 455–459.

Jenike, M. A., Baer, L., & Minichiello, W. E. (Eds.). (1991). *Obsessive compulsive disorder: Theory and management.* Chicago: Year Book Medical Publishers.

Joffee, R. T., Swinson, R. P., & Regan, J. J. (1988). Personality features of obsessive-compulsive disorder. *American Journal of Psychiatry, 145,* 1127–1129.

Junginger, J., & Ditto, B. (1984). Multitreatment of obsessive-compulsive checking in a geriatric patient. *Behavior Modification, 8,* 379–390.

Junginger, J., & Turner, S. M. (1987). Spontaneous exposure and "self-control" in the treatment of compulsive checking. *Journal of Behavior Therapy and Experimental Psychiatry, 18,* 115–119.

Kenny, F. T., Mowbray, R. M., & Lalani, S. (1978). Faradic disruption of obsessive ideation in the treatment of obsessive neurosis: A controlled study. *Behavior Therapy, 9,* 209–221.

Kirk, J. W. (1983). Behavioural treatment of obsessional-compulsive patients in routine clinical practice. *Behaviour Research and Therapy, 21,* 57–62.

Knight, R. P. (1941). Evaluation of results of psychoanalytic therapy. *American Journal of Psychiatry, 98,* 434–446.

Kringlen, E. (1965). Obsessional neurotics: A long-term follow-up. *British Journal of Psychiatry, 111,* 709–722.

Le Boeuf, A. (1974). An automated aversion device in the treatment of a compulsive handwashing ritual. *Journal of Behavior Therapy and Experimental Psychiatry, 5,* 267–270.

Likierman, H., & Rachman, S. (1982). Obsessions: An experimental investigation of thought-stopping and habituation training. *Behavioural Psychotherapy, 10,* 324–338.

Luff, M. C., & Garrod, M. (1935). After-results of psychotherapy in 500 cases. *British Medical Journal, 2,* 54–59.

Marks, I. M., Bird, J., & Lindley, P. (1978). Behavioral nurse therapists. *Behavioural Psychotherapy, 6,* 25–35.

Marks, I. M., Hallam, R. S., Connolly, J., & Philpott, R. (1977). *Nursing in behavioral psychotherapy.* London: Royal College of Nursing of the United Kingdom.

Marks, I. M., Hodgson, R., & Rachman, S. (1975). Treatment of chronic obsessive-compulsive neurosis by *in vivo* exposure, a two-year follow-up and issues in treatment. *British Journal of Psychiatry, 127,* 349–364.

Marks, I. M., Lelliott, P., Basoglu, M., Noshirvani, H., Monteiro, W., Cohen, D., & Kasvikis, Y. (1988). Clomipramine, self-exposure and therapist-aided exposure for obsessive compulsive rituals. *British Journal of Psychiatry, 152,* 522–534.

Marks, I. M., Stern, R. S., Mawson, D., Cobb, J., & McDonald, R. (1980). Clomipramine and exposure for obsessive-compulsive rituals. *British Journal of Psychiatry, 136,* 1–25.

Mehta, M. (1990). A comparative study of family-based and patient-based behavioral management in obsessive-compulsive disorder. *British Journal of Psychiatry, 157,* 133–135.

Meredith, R. L., & Milby, J. B. (1978). *Multi-modal conceptualization of obsessive-compulsive neurosis: Theoretical perspective and case presentation.* Paper presented at the Southeastern Psychological Association meeting, Hollywood, FL.

Meyer, V., & Levy, R. (1973). Modification of behavior in obsessive-compulsive disorders. In H. E. Adams & P. Unikel (Eds.), *Issues and trends in behavior therapy* (pp. 77–137). Springfield, IL: Thomas.

Meyer, V., Levy, R., & Schnurer, A. (1974). A behavioral treatment of obsessive-compulsive disorders. In H. R. Beech (Ed.), *Obsessional states* (pp. 233–258). London: Methuen.

Milby, J. B., Meredith, R. L., & Rice, J. (1981). Videotaped exposure: A new treatment for obsessive-compulsive disorders. *Journal of Behavior Therapy and Experimental Psychiatry, 12,* 249–255.

Mills, H. L., Agras, W. S., Barlow, D. H., & Mills, J. R. (1973). Compulsive rituals treated by response prevention. *Archives of General Psychiatry, 28,* 524–529.

Minichiello, W., Baer, L., & Jenike, M. A. (1987). Schizotypal personality disorder: A poor prognostic indicator for behavior therapy in the treatment of obsessive-compulsive disorder. *Journal of Anxiety Disorders, 1,* 273–276.

Moergen, S., Maier, M., Brown, S., & Pollard, C. A. (1987). Habituation to fear stimuli in a case of obsessive-compulsive disorder: Examining the generalization process. *Journal of Behavior Therapy and Experimental Psychiatry, 18,* 65–70.

Mowrer, O. H. (1960). *Learning theory and behavior.* New York: Wiley.

Nammalvar, N., & Venkoba Rao, A. (1983). Obsessive compulsive behaviours—A therapeutic study with thought stopping procedure. *Indian Journal of Psychiatry, 25*, 52–56.

O'Brien, J. S., & Raynes, A. E. (1973). Treatment of compulsive verbal behavior with response contingent punishment and relaxation. *Journal of Behavior Therapy and Experimental Psychiatry, 4*, 347–352.

O'Sullivan, G., Noshirvani, H., Marks, I., Monteiro, W., & Lelliott, P. (1991). Six-year follow-up after exposure and clomipramine therapy for obsessive compulsive disorder. *Journal of Clinical Psychiatry, 52*, 150–155.

Pato, M. T., Zohar-Kadouch, R., Zohar, J., & Murphy, D. (1988). Return of symptoms after discontinuation of clomipramine in patients with obsessive-compulsive disorder. *American Journal of Psychiatry, 145*, 1521–1527.

Persons, J. B., & Foa, E. B. (1984). Processing of fearful and neutral information by obsessive-compulsives. *Behaviour Research and Therapy, 22*, 259–265.

Pradhan, P. V., Ayyar, K. S., Munjal, P. L. D., Gopalani, J. H., Mundra, A. V., Doshi, J., & Bagadia, V. N. (1984). Obsessive compulsive neurosis: Treatment of 28 cases by behaviour therapy. *Indian Journal of Psychiatry, 26*, 71–75.

Pruitt, S. D., Miller, W. R., & Smith, J. E. (1989). Outpatient behavioral treatment of severe obsessive-compulsive disorder: Using paraprofessional resources. *Journal of Anxiety Disorders, 3*, 179–186.

Rabavilas, A. D., Boulougouris, J. C., Perissaki, C., & Stefanis, C. (1979). Pre-morbid personality traits and responsiveness to flooding in obsessive-compulsive patients. *Behaviour Research and Therapy, 17*, 575–580.

Rabavilas, A. D., Boulougouris, J. C., & Stefanis, C. (1976). Duration of flooding sessions in the treatment of obsessive-compulsive patients. *Behaviour Research and Therapy, 14*, 349–355.

Rachman, S. (1971). Obsessional ruminations. *Behaviour Research and Therapy, 9*, 229–235.

Rachman, S., & Hodgson, R. (1980). *Obsessions and compulsions*. New York: Prentice-Hall.

Rachman, S., Hodgson, R., & Marks, I. M. (1971). The treatment of chronic obsessive-compulsive neurosis. *Behaviour Research and Therapy, 9*, 237–247.

Rachman, S., Marks, I. M., & Hodgson, R. (1973). The treatment of obsessive-compulsive neurotics by modeling and flooding *in vivo*. *Behaviour Research and Therapy, 11*, 463–471.

Rainey, C. A. (1972). An obsessive-compulsive neurosis treated by flooding *in vivo*. *Journal of Behavior Therapy and Experimental Psychiatry, 3*, 117–121.

Rasmussen, S. A., & Tsuang, M. T. (1984). Epidemiology of obsessive compulsive disorder: A review. *Journal of Clinical Psychiatry, 45*, 450–457.

Reed, G. F. (1985). *Obsessional experience and compulsive behavior*. Orlando, FL: Academic Press.

Regier, D. A., Boyd, J. H., Burke, J. D., Rae, D. S., Myers, J. K., Kramer, M., Robins, L. N., George, L. K., Karno, M., & Locke, B. Z. (1988). One-month prevalence of mental disorders in the United States. *Archives of General Psychiatry, 45*, 977–986.

Roper, G., Rachman, S., & Marks, I. M. (1975). Passive and participant modeling in exposure treatment of obsessive-compulsive neurotics. *Behaviour Research and Therapy, 13*, 271–279.

Rowan, V. C., Holborn, S. W., Walker, J. R., & Siddiqui, A-R. (1984). A rapid multi-component treatment for an obsessive- compulsive disorder. *Journal of Behavior Therapy and Experimental Psychiatry, 15*, 347–352.

Salkovskis, P. M. (1983). Treatment of an obsessional patient using habituation to audiotaped ruminations. *British Journal of Clinical Psychology, 22*, 311–313.

Salkovskis, P. M., & Warwick, H. M. C. (1985). Cognitive therapy of obsessive-compulsive disorder: Treating treatment failures. *Behavioral Psychotherapy, 13*, 243–255.

Salkovskis, P. M., & Westbrook, D. (1989). Behavior therapy and obsessional ruminations: Can failure be turned into success? *Behavior Research and Therapy, 27*, 149–160.

Sifneos, P. E. (1985). Short-term dynamic psychotherapy for patients suffering from an obsessive-compulsive disorder. In M. Mavissakalian, S. M. Turner, & L. Michelson (Eds.), *Obsessive-compulsive disorder* (pp. 131–154). New York: Plenum.

Solyom, L., Garza-Perez, J., Ledwidge, & Solyom, C. (1972). Paradoxical intention in the treatment of obsessive thoughts: A pilot study. *Comprehensive Psychiatry, 13*, 291–297.

Solyom, L., Zamanzadeh, D., Ledwidge, B., & Kenny, F. (1971). Aversion relief treatment of obsessive neurosis. In R. D. Rubin (Ed.), *Advances in behaviour therapy* (pp. 93–109). London: Academic Press.

Sookman, D., & Solyom, L. (1977). The effectiveness of four behaviour therapies in the treatment of obsessive neurosis. In J. C. Boulougouris, & A. D. Rabavilas (Eds.), *The treatment of phobic and obsessive-compulsive disorders* (pp. 85–100). Oxford: Pergamon Press.

Steketee, G. (1993). Social support and treatment outcome of obsessive-compulsive disorder at 9-month follow-up. *Behavioural Psychotherapy, 21*, 81–95.

Steketee, G. (1990). Personality traits and disorders in obsessive compulsive patients. *Journal of Anxiety Disorders, 4*, 351–364.

Steketee, G. (in press). *Treatment of obsessive-compulsive disorder.* New York: Guilford.

Steketee, G., & Cleere, L. (1990). Obsessive-compulsive disorders. In A. S. Bellack, M. Hersen, & A. E. Kazdin (Eds.), *International handbook of behavior modification and therapy* (pp. 307–332). New York: Plenum.

Steketee, G., & Foa, E. B. (1985). Obsessive-compulsive disorder. In D. H. Barlow (Ed.), *Clinical handbook of psychological disorders* (pp. 69–144). New York: Guilford.

Steketee, G. S., Foa, E. B., & Grayson, J. B. (1982). Recent advances in the behavioral treatment of obsessive-compulsives. *Archives of General Psychiatry, 39*, 1365–1371.

Steketee, G., & Shapiro, L. (1993). Obsessive-compulsive disorder. In A. S. Bellack & M. Hersen (Eds.), *Handbook of behavior therapy in the psychiatric setting* (pp. 199–227). New York: Plenum.

Steketee, G., & White, K. (1990). *When once is not enough.* Oakland, CA: New Harbinger Press.

Stern, R. S. (1978). Obsessive thoughts: The problem of therapy. *British Journal of Psychiatry, 132*, 200–205.

Stern, R. S., Lipsedge, M. S., & Marks, I. M. (1973). Electro-aversion therapy of chronic alcoholism. *Behaviour Research and Therapy, 2*, 663–665.

Tanner, B. A. (1971). A case report on the use of relaxation and systematic desensitization to control multiple compulsive behaviors. *Journal of Behavior Therapy and Experimental Psychiatry, 2*, 267–272.

Thyer, B. A. (1985). Audiotaped exposure therapy in a case of obsessional neurosis. *Journal of Behavior Therapy and Experimental Psychiatry, 16*, 271–274.

Turner, S. M., Beidel, D. C., Stanley, M. A., & Jacob, R. G. (1988). A comparison of fluoxetine, flooding, and response prevention in the treatment of obsessive compulsive disorder. *Journal of Anxiety Disorders, 2*, 219–225.

Turner, S. M., Hersen, M., Bellack, A. S., & Wells, K. C. (1979). Behavioral treatment of obsessive-compulsive neurosis. *Behaviour Research and Therapy, 17*, 95–106.

Volans, P. J. (1976). Styles of decision-making and probability appraisal in selected obsessional and phobic patients. *British Journal of Social and Clinical Psychology, 15*, 305–317.

Watts, F. N. (1971). Habituation model of systematic desensitization. *Psychological Bulletin, 86*, 627–637.

Wickramasekera, I. (1970). Desensitization, re-sensitization and desensitization again: A preliminary study. *Journal of Behavior Therapy and Experimental Psychiatry, 1*, 257–262.

Yamagami, T. (1971). The treatment of an obsession by thought-stopping. *Journal of Behavior Therapy and Experimental Psychiatry, 2*, 133–135.

12

Treatment of Bulimia Nervosa

Harold Leitenberg

Introduction

Although symptoms of bulimia have been described for centuries (Parry-Jones & Parry-Jones, 1991), in modern times bulimia nervosa was first defined as a syndrome distinct from anorexia nervosa in the late 1970s (Boskind-Lodahl & White, 1978; Russell, 1979). Bulimia nervosa refers to a severe eating disorder in which normal-weight individuals, the vast majority women, habitually vomit or abuse laxatives after binge eating or after eating even minimal amounts of "forbidden" foods. Vomiting is self-induced, and the mean purging frequency per week reported in the treatment literature is usually between 10 and 15 times. The major complaint of patients with bulimia nervosa is that they cannot control their eating, that they binge eat and therefore "have to" vomit or otherwise purge to prevent themselves from becoming fat. People with this disorder typically have a negative body image and feel that various parts of their body are too fat even if they are in the lower end of the normal weight range. Most importantly they are terrified of gaining any weight and believe they cannot eat normally without purging or they will inexorably and very rapidly become obese.

The diagnostic criteria for bulimia nervosa according to DSM-III-R (American Psychiatric Association, 1987) are

1. Recurrent episodes of binge eating (rapid consumption of a large amount of food in a discrete period of time)
2. A feeling of lack of control over eating behavior during the eating binges
3. Regular practice of at least one of the following:
   (a) self-induced vomiting,
   (b) use of laxatives or diuretics,
   (c) strict dieting or fasting,
   (d) vigorous exercise in order to prevent weight gain

Harold Leitenberg • Department of Psychology, University of Vermont, Burlington, Vermont 05405.

Handbook of Effective Psychotherapy, edited by Thomas R. Giles. Plenum Press, New York, 1993.

4. A minimum average of two binge-eating episodes a week for at least 3 months
5. Persistent overconcern with body shape and weight

A major problem with these criteria is that they fail to distinguish between those individuals who purge after binge eating and those who do not purge. These groups are very different from each other. For example, in a recent study we found that normal-weight purging bulimics were much more disturbed than were nonpurging bulimics on measures of eating behavior, psychological adjustment, body image, depression, and eating attitudes (Willmuth, Leitenberg, Rosen, & Cado, 1988). Purging and nonpurging bulimics may also differ in the etiology and course of their disorder, and the most effective type of treatment may turn out to be different. In any case, the treatment studies of bulimia nervosa almost exclusively involve patients who self-induce vomiting after eating. In point of fact, there are probably very few normal-weight women who meet the other criteria for bulimia nervosa but who do not vomit. Or if they do exist, they seldom seek treatment (Willmuth *et al.*, 1988). Bulimia without purging, on the other hand, is more common in obese individuals.

Recent surveys conducted in the United States and in England suggest that the prevalence rate for bulimia nervosa involving purging behavior is around 1% to 4% in adult women (Clement & Hawkins, 1980; Cooper & Fairburn, 1983; Cooper, Charnock, & Taylor, 1987; Crowther, Chernyk, Hahn, Hedeen, & Zaynor, 1983; Drewnowski, Hopkins, & Kessler, 1988; Fairburn & Beglin, 1990; Halmi, Falk, & Schwartz, 1981; Hart & Ollendick, 1985; Pope, Hudson, & Yurgelun-Todd, 1984; Pyle, Neuman, Halvorson, & Mitchell, 1991; Rand & Kuldan, 1992; Schotte & Stunkard, 1987). The prevalence in high school samples in the United States also appears to be around 3% of the female sample (Johnson, Tobin, & Lipkin, 1989). Approximately 95% to 97% of all patients diagnosed with bulimia nervosa are women, and 3% to 5% are men. There is also some evidence that the prevalence may be higher in white women than in black women in the United States and in Great Britain (Dolan, 1991; Rosen & Gross, 1987).

Bulimia nervosa appears to be a chronic disorder. For example, a number of recent treatment studies report that a mean of 5 or more years elapsed between onset and the time therapy was sought (e.g., Conners, Johnson, & Stuckey, 1984; Giles, Young, & Young, 1981; Johnson, Schlundt, & Jarrell, 1986; Kirkley, Schneider, Agras, & Bachman, 1985; Leitenberg, Rosen, Gross, Nudelman, & Vara, 1988; Yates & Sambrailo, 1984).

In addition to the specific symptoms associated with their eating disorder, bulimia nervosa patients have often been noted to have a large number of other associated psychological and social problems, including low self-esteem, depression, guilt, obsessive ruminations and anxiety, difficulty concentrating, alcohol and drug abuse, theft, and family conflict (Mitchell & Pyle, 1982). Physical problems, particularly bloating, constipation, other gastrointestinal complications, dental enamel erosion, and parotid gland enlargement, are also often a consequence of this disorder, but serious life-threatening concerns, such as electrolyte imbalance, appear to occur in less than 5% of the cases as long as normal weight is maintained (Jacobs & Schneider, 1985).

Because occasional episodes of binge eating and vomiting are also observed in approximately 30% of anorexia nervosa patients (Gandour, 1984) and because fear of weight gain is evident in both disorders, some important distinctions between bulimia nervosa and anorexia are sometimes overlooked. For example:

1. Bulimia nervosa refers to normal-weight individuals who generally do eat, however chaotically, whereas anorexia nervosa refers to emaciated individuals who are engaged almost exclusively in self-starvation.
2. Bulimia nervosa patients are usually trying to achieve some stereotyped and idealized conception of a perfect feminine and sexually attractive appearance. In fact, they have an exaggerated need to please and obtain approval from others in these areas. In contrast, anorexic patients seem to be trying to prevent themselves from looking sexually attractive. They are supposedly trying to reject or deny their adult sexuality.
3. Bulimia nervosa patients tend to be older than anorexia nervosa patients (low twenties versus low teens).
4. Bulimia nervosa is a secretive disorder, whereas the signs of self-starvation in the anorexic are quite obvious and the center of attention by others.
5. Bulimia nervosa patients are less likely than anorexia nervosa patients to minimize or deny their problem.
6. Finally, bulimia nervosa patients feel their eating is out of control, whereas anorexic patients feel in perfect control.

As with most complex behavior disorders, there is probably no single cause of bulimia nervosa. Instead, there are many interacting risk factors. Most often cited in the literature are cultural pressures on women to be slim (e.g., Orbach, 1978); the desire to achieve some idealized image of the perfect body in order to compensate for low self-esteem and fears of rejection (e.g., Boskind-Lodahl & White, 1978); negative mood states including depression (e.g., Hudson, Pope, & Jonas, 1983); interpersonal stress with poorly developed problem-solving and assertion skills (e.g., Wolchik, Weiss, & Katzman, 1986); poor eating and weight control habits including, especially, the attempt to adhere to an unrealistically rigid and drastically restrained diet (e.g., Johnson *et al.*, 1986); and a host of distorted cognitions about nutrition, weight, and appearance (Fairburn, 1981, 1985; Fairburn, Kirk, O'Connor, & Cooper, 1986; Garner, 1986). It should be noted that anecdotal reports of a history of sexual abuse in this population are not uncommon. However, controlled research suggests that the frequency of such abuse is not greater in bulimia nervosa subjects than in other clinical samples (Coovert, Kinder, & Thompson, 1989).

Figure 12.1 provides a framework for explaining the complexity of these interacting influences and pathways. At the broadest level of analysis (see the lower right-hand corner), societal values are clearly implicated. In our current youth-fixated and relatively affluent times, there is tremendous pressure on women to be slim. Obviously this alone cannot account for bulimia nervosa, otherwise all women, not just 1–3% would be afflicted. However, if a woman, for whatever reason (see lower-left corner of Figure 12.1), also has extremely low self-esteem and strong fears of rejection, and has a negative body image and body dissatisfaction, it is not difficult to see how she would develop the view that only a perfectly slim body will ensure acceptance. She can easily believe that if her appearance is just right, no one will know how bad a person she really is. Hence, self-worth becomes dependent on achieving a "perfect" body, with a resulting morbid fear of weight gain.

Binge eating is usually accounted for in two different ways. These are both indicated in the left side of Figure 12.1. The first factor pertains to the chain of low self-esteem, life stressors, poor coping skills, and the resulting host of dysphoric feelings that are evoked. One hypothesis is that many women who binge eat do so in order to escape, to "space out," anesthetize, or self-nurture themselves against these negative feeling states. The second hypothesis that is often considered has to do with the unrealistically rigid and drastic diets these women attempt to adhere to in order to regulate their weight and compensate for their negative body image. When this fails, the patient gives up and binge eats (Wardle & Ileinhart, 1981). Such a pattern of binge eating after dieting is analogous to the counterregulatory eating of chronic dieters who are temporarily forced to break their restraint in the laboratory (Herman & Polivy, 1980). According to both of these conceptions binge eating is triggered by either antecedent event: dysphoric feelings or lapses from a rigid diet.

Without in any way discounting the importance of all of these factors, we have noted in previous articles (Leitenberg, Gross, Peterson, & Rosen, 1984; Leitenberg & Rosen, 1986; Rosen & Leitenberg, 1982, 1985) that these explanations neglect the special and central role that self-induced vomiting plays in this disorder as distinguished from other eating disorders. One of the defining characteristics of bulimia nervosa, according to Russell (1979), is a morbid fear of weight gain. By itself, however, dread of weight gain cannot fully account for the vicious cycle of repetitive binge eating and vomiting. In fact, one of the most obvious questions is: If bulimia nervosa patients are so terrified about weight gain, why do they binge eat? Why are they not anorexic instead? The answer for most is that they would seldom binge eat if they did not plan in advance to vomit afterwards. The self-nurturing, anesthetizing effects of binge eating is usually realized in bulimia nervosa patients only because of the freedom from anxiety about weight gain

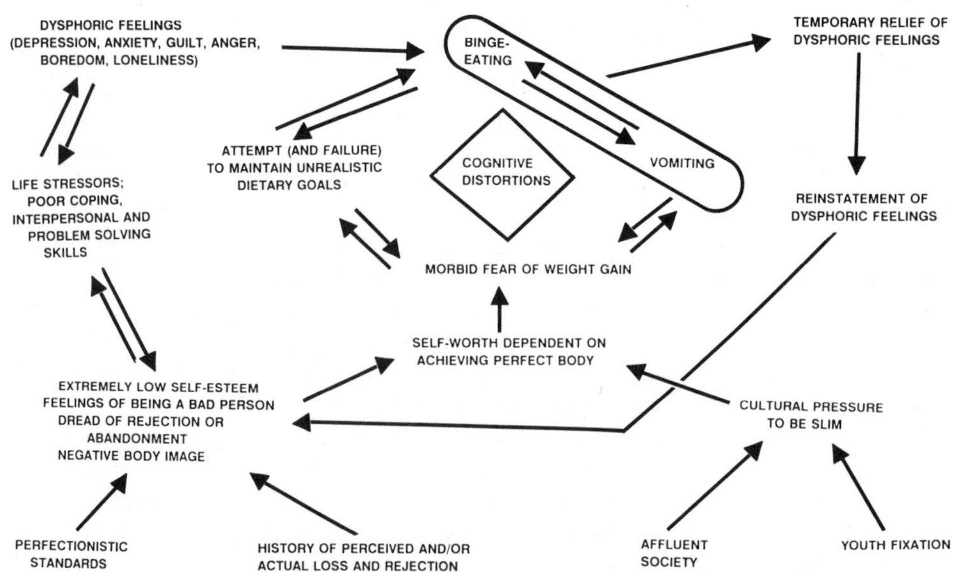

Figure 12.1. Interacting risk factors for bulimia nervosa.

provided by the anticipation of vomiting. In fact, if circumstances are such that they cannot vomit immediately afterwards, women suffering from bulimia nervosa usually eat very little and much less than do control subjects (Rosen, Leitenberg, Fondacaro, Gross, & Willmuth, 1985).

We tested how much food 20 bulimia nervosa subjects would be willing to eat if they knew they could not vomit afterwards and compared this amount to what 20 normal controls were willing to eat. The first test situation was a standard multi-course dinner of about 700 to 800 calories, the second was a pasta dish of about 600 calories, and the third involved three 1-ounce candy bars. Subjects were instructed "to eat as much of the test meal as you comfortably can, not to push yourself to eat more than is comfortable." The bulimia nervosa subjects had also been told that they should not vomit within 1 hour before eating and within 2 hours after eating. The results showed that women with bulimia nervosa will not eat normal amounts of food if they are unable to vomit afterwards. The normal controls ate about 70%of each of the three test meal situations. In contrast, for the large dinner, the bulimia nervosa subjects ate 27% of the total calories available; for the pasta meal they ate only 15% (a few forkfuls); and as for the candy, they ate only 2% (about one bite of one candy bar).

Normally, however, the freedom to vomit is usually present and the decision to do so usually precedes the decision to binge eat. Even small amounts of food are perceived as "bad" or "too much" and trigger self-reported feelings of anxiety (albeit not necessarily any physiological arousal; see Leitenberg *et al.*, 1984; Williamson, Kelley, Davis, Ruggiero, & Veitia, 1985; Wilson, Rossiter, Kleinfield, & Lindholm, 1986) and thoughts of massive weight gain. The feelings of anxiety can be controlled by deciding to vomit, thus removing further inhibitions against a binge. We have suggested that vomiting serves an anxiety-reducing function in bulimia nervosa akin to compulsive hand washing and checking rituals in obsessive–compulsive neuroses (Leitenberg *et al.*, 1984; Rosen & Leitenberg, 1982). For bulimia nervosa patients, eating most foods is in some ways parallel to bringing obsessive–compulsive patients into contact with substances they believe to be contaminating. A wide variety of foods of normal quantity are considered unsafe, repulsive, and fattening. Bulimia nervosa patients believe that if they eat normal amounts of food without vomiting they will become obese and as a result will be rejected and never achieve love, success, and happiness. Vomiting is the ritual that they believe protects them from these terrifying consequences. Vomiting has also been shown to relieve negative feelings of anger, inadequacy, and lack of control (Johnson & Larson, 1982), and in the usual progression of this disorder, once self-induced vomiting is learned, binge eating typically becomes more severe and frequent (Abraham & Beaumont, 1982). In short, this analysis suggests that once the bulimia nervosa syndrome is fully established, binge eating may be more a consequence of vomiting than vomiting is a consequence of binge eating. To reiterate, however, this is not to deny that the motivation to binge for other reasons—prior restrained eating, spacing out, coping with stress, and so forth—is not present with a vengeance in bulimia nervosa patients. In fact, it is. We are simply arguing that if they did not plan to vomit, most women with bulimia nervosa would be too afraid to binge eat. There are, of course, some exceptions (Steere & Cooper, 1988).

Considering that bulimia nervosa in normal-weight women was first defined in the research literature only a little over 10 years ago, a large number of studies on descriptive psychopathology, etiology, assessment, and treatment of this disorder has accumulated. The focus of the remainder of this chapter, however, is solely on a review of the empirical literature on treatment outcome. There are many forms of treatment provided to bulimia nervosa patients. The list seems endless. Whatever therapy one can think of is probably available in the community for patients with this disorder. Some of the more common treatment modalities are Overeaters Anonymous, nutritional counseling, dance therapy, group therapy, feminist therapy, psychoanalytic therapy, family therapy, cognitive-behavior therapy, and pharmacotherapy. Virtually all of the controlled research, however, has been with cognitive-behavior therapy and pharmacotherapy. Hence this chapter will focus primarily on an evaluation of the effectiveness of these two treatment modalities and especially on cognitive-behavior therapy.

The first section of this review describes what cognitive-behavior therapy for bulimia nervosa entails and summarizes initial findings from single-case experimental studies and uncontrolled clinical trials. The second section reviews studies that compared cognitive-behavior therapy to waiting-list controls. Third, studies comparing cognitive-behavior therapy to other psychological treatments will be described. Fourth, studies that examined different variations of cognitive-behavior therapy will be considered. Fifth, studies comparing cognitive-behavior therapy to pharmacotherapy will be evaluated. A sixth section will review the few evaluations I was able to locate of other psychological treatments for bulimia nervosa. Finally, a brief conclusions section will be provided.

Description of Cognitive-Behavior Therapy for Bulimia Nervosa and Initial Findings from Uncontrolled and Within-Subjects Experimental Designs

Fairburn (1981) in Oxford, England, developed a systematic cognitive-behavioral treatment package for bulimia nervosa. His program consists of a number of different cognitive therapy and behavior therapy components. Fairburn (1985) describes the therapy as taking place in three stages. The first stage is designed to modify bulimic eating behavior with strategies commonly used in the behavioral treatment of obesity. Included in this stage are instructions to keep a daily detailed self-monitoring record of eating and vomiting behavior, provision of information about the mechanisms of weight regulation and about the negative consequences of attempting to maintain a strict diet and of binge eating followed by self-induced vomiting. Patients are encouraged to establish a pattern of regular eating of three or four meals each day, plus one or two planned snacks, regardless of the amount eaten. Stimulus control procedures are instituted, as is a weekly schedule of taking one's weight. Patients are asked to construct a list of pleasurable activities that they can engage in between meals to reduce the likelihood of binge eating. Fairburn says that vomiting *per se* does not have to be tackled directly, but patients are instructed to eat only those foods that they are prepared not to vomit and to engage in distracting activities for about an hour if they have an urge to vomit. During this first stage, an attempt is also made to interview friends and relatives with the aim of bringing the problem out into the open and enlisting their cooperation with the patient's treatment.

In the second stage, after there is some improvement in binge eating and vomiting, the major focus of therapy is placed on helping the patient deal with situations that trigger binge eating. There is a heavy emphasis on cognitive therapy to modify dysfunctional and irrational beliefs pertaining to weight, eating, and body image. In addition, patients are taught problem-solving techniques in order to improve the way they cope with stressful events that have been associated with binge eating. The idea is to provide some effective substitute to binge eating and vomiting. In the third stage, which is shorter than the others, treatment focuses on cognitive factors that might lead to relapse with plans for dealing with a relapse should one occur. This treatment package was delivered over 18 weeks with twice-weekly sessions in the first month, weekly sessions in the next 2 months, and biweekly sessions in the last 6 weeks.

Based on research first conducted at the University of Vermont (Leitenberg *et al.*, 1984; Rosen & Leitenberg, 1982, 1985), an exposure plus response prevention format for the treatment of bulimia nervosa is also sometimes used. We thought that if patients were exposed to eating normal foods while vomiting was blocked, they would discover that their anxiety could be reduced without recourse to vomiting. We also thought that this technique would provide them with the opportunity to learn that eating normal foods without vomiting would not lead to the extreme weight gains that they predicted. Moreover, many of the other distorted cognitions associated with this disorder (Fairburn, 1985; Garner, 1986) might be more amenable to change if they could be elicited and challenged while bulimia nervosa patients were actually experiencing anxiety: that is, while eating frightening foods (exposure) in the presence of a therapist with vomiting prevented (response prevention). As the literature on the cognitive-behavioral treatment of anxiety disorders suggests, whether or not distorted cognitions are an important characteristic of the disorder or whether or not cognitive processes are important mediators of behavioral change, the most effective method of achieving both cognitive and behavioral change is via a performance-based therapy protocol that involves active and repeated practice in approaching feared situations (Bandura, 1982; Biran & Wilson, 1981; Ellis, 1979; Emmelkamp, Kuipers, & Eggeraat, 1978; Williams & Rappaport, 1983).

During each exposure plus response prevention treatment session, the patient is encouraged to eat an amount of food that causes a strong urge to vomit, beyond the point at which vomiting would ordinarily occur. The patient knows in advance that she will not be allowed to vomit and that the therapist will stay with her until the urge to vomit is under control. The patient is told that treatment would be most beneficial if vomiting did not occur within 2 hours after the end of any treatment session—so as to allow enough time for the anxiety to be reduced without recourse to vomiting—and that it is best to stay with the therapist until she feels she can safely leave without vomiting afterwards. At the beginning of therapy, 1½- to 2-hour sessions are usually needed for the patient to eat and gain control over the anxiety and to allow time to process not only her feelings about what she has eaten in the session but also time to review the at-home eating records. Subsequently, sessions can be reduced to 1 to 1½ hours. The types of foods used in therapy sessions are those that are found to be the most anxiety provoking during pretreatment evaluation. It is probably best to use a variety of frightening foods. For example, under the category of snack food, a patient might need to alternately practice with ice cream, cake, candy, and a variety of chips, if she usually vomits after eating each one.

The amount of food presented to the patient in the therapy session should typically be a "normal" amount or only slightly above the range most people could eat comfortably. It is not necessary for the patient to binge eat in the session in order to become anxious. In the absence of vomiting, even small quantities of food that are typically defined by patients as "too much" provoke intense anxiety. Initially, the patient needs to eat only very slight amounts to feel extreme anxiety (e.g., five french fries or two forkfuls of pie). As therapy progresses, the patient should be encouraged to eat even more, although still for the most part within normal limits. For example, two to three slices of pizza, a submarine sandwich, or three cups of macaroni and cheese will provide the patient with more than enough frightening food with which to practice without being excessive. An occasional session of binge eating might eventually also be introduced. The order in which different foods are used depends on how much anxiety they provoke. The more frightening eating situations should be introduced after the patient has adapted to less frightening ones.

While the patient is eating and after she has finished, the therapist directs the patient's attention to the thoughts and sensations underlying the anxiety that is provoked by the exposure plus response prevention procedure. Sometimes the patient will voluntarily verbalize various distorted and anxiety-provoking cognitions about food, eating, vomiting, weight, body image, and interpersonal relationships that are tied to the urge to vomit. At other times, the therapist has to probe to elicit these thoughts. It is important that maladaptive cognitions be brought to the surface so that they may be challenged during the therapy session.

These cognitions are not different from those described by Fairburn (1985) and Garner (1986). They simply may be easier to elicit and modify, however, under the anxiety-provoking conditions of eating without vomiting. The exposure session is more affectively charged and is firsthand compared to recounts of eating episodes that occur outside of therapy sessions. This increases the likelihood of accurately identifying those beliefs that underlie a particular patient's anxiety and desire to vomit. In fact, these irrational cognitions are sometimes stimulated only by the anxiety associated with eating frightening foods. Patients can be perfectly rational about food and body shape when they are not eating, but this does not easily transfer to the emotional state evoked by eating. Another potential advantage of the exposure plus response prevention format is that it enables the therapist to immediately rather than retroactively challenge distorted cognitions.

Otherwise, exposure plus response prevention therapy of bulimia nervosa is very similar to the cognitive-behavior therapy procedures described by Fairburn (1981, 1985). Self-monitoring is used, regular meals are scheduled, antecedent events that trigger binge eating and vomiting episodes are identified, and suggestions for stimulus control and alternative means of coping with these stressors are explored.

The initial findings of uncontrolled clinical trials and some single-case experimental analyses of cognitive-behavioral treatment of bulimia nervosa were encouraging. Fairburn (1981) first reported on the results for a consecutive series of 11 patients. Of the 11 patients, 9 reduced binge-eating and purging episodes to less than once a month at the end of treatment. Fairburn also mentioned that there was a reduction in abnormal attitudes toward food, eating, weight, and body shape. A

1-year follow-up was available for six patients. One had relapsed, one had completely stopped all binge eating and vomiting, and the other four reported only an occasional lapse every 2 or 3 months at times of severe stress.

Conners *et al.* (1984) described a 10-week "psychoeducational" group treatment of 20 bulimia nervosa patients. There were twelve 2-hour treatment sessions. Information on the set-point theory of weight regulation and the sociocultural and emotional causes of bulimia were provided. Self-monitoring was instituted and the antecedents of particular binge–purge episodes were explored. Techniques that group members had found useful for avoiding binges were discussed. Short-term contracts were arranged for eating regular meals, engaging in exercise, and for other goals that directly focused on eating behavior. Assertion training, relaxation, and cognitive-restructuring techniques were also employed. At 10-week follow-up, there was a 70% mean reduction in binge–purge episodes, and 17 out of the 20 subjects had improved on this measure. Improvement was also noted on measures of assertion and self-concept. However, only 3 subjects had stopped vomiting. Also, body image had not improved.

Schneider and Agras (1985) used a cognitive-behavioral group treatment program with 13 bulimia nervosa subjects (only 11, however, were engaged in vomiting behavior) delivered over 16 weeks. In the first stage, methods used to control binge eating included prescription of regular balanced meals, progressive increments in delaying binge eating, arranging alternative activities incompatible with binge eating, stimulus control, and self-monitoring. In the second stage, irrational beliefs related to binge eating and vomiting were challenged and "forbidden foods" were introduced to the diet at home. Interpersonal problem solving, assertiveness training, and relaxation were added to promote better alternatives for handling events surrounding binge-eating episodes. At posttreatment there was a 90% reduction in vomiting, and 54% of the subjects were not vomiting at all. At 6-month follow-up, vomiting frequency was reduced by 84%, relative to pretreatment levels, but only 38% of the subjects were not vomiting at all. Improvements were also noted on measures of depression, eating attitudes, and assertiveness.

The early results of adding an exposure plus response prevention format in the treatment of bulimia nervosa were also encouraging (Leitenberg *et al.*, 1984; Rosen & Leitenberg, 1982). Using single-case experimental analyses, we were able to show that the ability to eat anxiety-provoking foods without vomiting increased as each type of food was treated in sequence (Rosen & Leitenberg, 1982). We also found that, within sessions, self-reported anxiety and the urge to vomit increased while subjects were eating, but then subsequently declined even though subjects were not able to vomit. Across treatment sessions the mean amount of calories consumed increased, anxiety and the urge to vomit decreased, and negative self-statements about eating problems, appearance, and weight decreased (Leitenberg *et al.*, 1984). Out of the six patients in this initial series, vomiting decreased 89% and was eliminated entirely for three subjects (another subject vomited only 1 day in the 3-week follow-up assessment period). There were also improvements in eating attitudes, body image, self-esteem, and depression.

Subsequently, Giles *et al.* (1985) reported promising findings in an open clinical trial with 34 bulimia nervosa patients. Of these, 41% had been anorexic when they were in their teens, and 68% had undergone prior unsuccessful treatment for bulimia nervosa. After a mean of only 11 treatment sessions, 20 of these patients had at least an 80% reduction in binge–purge episodes per week, and another 2 showed a reduction of between 50% and 79%. At follow-up, 14 of these 22 patients (41% of the total sample of 34) had completely stopped vomiting after eating and were otherwise eating normally. In addition, depression scores and dysfunctional attitudes about eating declined to a normal range.

Another uncontrolled clinical trial of cognitive-behavioral therapy with exposure plus response was reported by Wilson, Rossiter, Lindholm, and Tebbutt (1986). Their sample consisted of 40 consecutive subjects who were provided with cognitive restructuring first, then exposure plus response prevention and dietary management for a total of 16 sessions. At posttreatment, 65% showed considerable improvement, defined by at least a 75% reduction in binge eating and vomiting, and 50% had completely stopped binge eating and vomiting. These results included 14 treatment dropouts who were assumed to be treatment failures. The mean reduction in vomiting was actually 93% in just those who completed treatment. An unusually systematic effort was made to help the clients maintain treatment gains. Relapse prevention strategies for coping with high-risk situations were rehearsed. Clients were contacted by phone each month for the first year of follow-up and given support and encouragement and additional therapy sessions if necessary. At 1-year follow-up, 53% of these 40 subjects were eating normally without any vomiting episodes. They had also improved on measures of depression, psychopathology, assertiveness, self-efficacy, body image, concern with thinness, and personality characteristics associated with eating disorders.

Comparison to Waiting-List Controls

A number of studies have compared a cognitive-behavior therapy condition to a waiting-list control condition. In a study reported by Lacey (1983), 15 subjects were assigned to a behaviorally oriented group treatment program and 15 were assigned to a waiting-list control. Patients in the treatment condition were seen in groups of five. They signed a contract stating that they would follow a structured diet of limited carbohydrate intake and three meals per day. (After learning of this contract, 19% of the initial volunteers refused to participate in treatment.) At the outset of treatment, patients also contracted to stop binge eating and vomiting eventually. The author says that treatment sessions focused on identifying alternative methods of handling interpersonal stressors that triggered binge eating, and that "insight-oriented" therapy was provided for issues pertaining to family conflict. The waiting-list controls showed no improvement. For treated subjects, however, there was a 96% reduction in vomiting at posttreatment, and 83% had stopped vomiting completely. In the year after treatment (waiting-list subjects had been treated in the interim), 8 patients out of 30 were reported to have had a few bulimic episodes, whereas the others did not vomit at all.

In another study comparing cognitive-behavior therapy to a waiting-list control, Lee and Rush (1986) employed a sample of 30 patients who met DSM-III criteria for bulimia. However, 5 were not involved in any purging behavior (no vomiting or laxative abuse). Treatment was provided twice weekly in groups of 7 or 8 subjects for only 6 weeks. Treatment included education about weight regulation, scheduling of regular meals, cognitive restructuring of irrational beliefs about weight and eating, and prescription of various behavioral self-control strategies to modify binge-eating behavior at home. Only 8 subjects completed treatment (at least 11 of 12 sessions); 3 discontinued after 8 or 9 sessions, and 4 subjects discontinued after 4, 5, or 7 sessions. The results, however, are reported for 14 out of the 15 treatment subjects. The waiting-list controls showed little improvement, and the treated subjects had significantly better outcomes. Nevertheless, the amount of improvement was still not very great. Only 2 out of 14 treated subjects had completely stopped vomiting, and only 7 out of 14 had decreased their vomiting frequency by more than 50%.

Wolchik *et al.* (1986) provided treatment to 11 bulimic subjects over a 7-week period and compared outcomes to a waiting-list control group of 7 subjects. It is not clear how many subjects were vomiting, but in a table summarizing the number of purges per month for each subject (which could be laxatives or vomiting or both), 2 of the 11 subjects were not purging at all, and another 2 were not purging more than once a week at most. there were two individual treatment sessions and seven group treatment sessions. Treatment focused primarily on decreasing depression, enhancing self-esteem, increasing assertiveness, and improving body image. Although therapy included information regarding weight regulation, use of self-monitoring, prescription of three meals a day, cognitive restructuring of irrational beliefs about weight, and an attempt to teach alternative methods of dealing with stressors associated with binge eating, the authors stressed that behavioral techniques to control eating and vomiting were downplayed relative to the effort to increase personal competence.

The overall effects for treated subjects were not substantial. Purging decreased only 60% in the treatment subjects and one of the eight who were regular purgers at pretreatment had stopped this behavior at posttreatment. In fact, the decrease in purging for the treatment group was not statistically significant. At follow-up, only two of the eight treated subjects abstained from vomiting. Body image was improved equally in both the treatment and the waiting-list control condition. On self-esteem and depression measures, however, the treatment group improved significantly more than the waiting-list control group.

The first between-group controlled evaluation of cognitive-behavioral treatment with exposure plus response prevention was reported by Ordman and Kirschenbaum (1985). They compared treatment to a waiting-list control condition in 20 bulimia nervosa subjects. A total of 10 subjects were put on a waiting list after receiving a minimal intervention of three sessions for collecting baseline measures and encouraging them to practice eating at home without vomiting. The other 10 subjects received a mean of 15 treatment sessions involving cognitive-behavior therapy and exposure plus response prevention. On average, however, the subjects had only two sessions of supervised exposure plus response prevention, although they were also asked to conduct exposure plus response prevention practice exercises on their own at home. The waiting-list group showed a 29% reduction in vomiting, whereas there was a 75% decrease in the treatment condition. Treated subjects also showed significantly greater improvement in the amount of food they could eat in test meals without vomiting, and on measures of eating attitudes, body image, and depression. On the more negative side, only two of the treated subjects (20%) had stopped vomiting completely, and there was no long-term follow-up.

In a more recent study, two cognitive-behavior therapy conditions with exposure and response prevention and one without were compared to a waiting-list control group (Leitenberg *et al.*, 1988). The subcomparisons between the different cognitive-behavior therapy groups will be described in a later section, but for now the comparison of interest is between each of the cognitive-behavior therapy groups and the waiting-list control. There were a total of 47 subjects, 11 in one group and 12 in the other three. The mean age of the sample was 26, and 53% had been in treatment before. The mean duration of the disorder was 6.94 years, and the pretreatment mean vomiting frequency was 12.13 per week. Subjects were seen in groups of three for a total of 24 sessions scheduled over 14 weeks. All three treatment groups improved significantly more than did the waiting-list control on measures of eating behavior, vomiting, eating attitudes, body image, self-esteem, and depression.

In another recent study, several different cognitive-behavior therapy groups were compared to a waiting-list control group (Freeman, Barry, Dunkeld-Turnbull, & Henderson, 1988). There were a total of 92 bulimia nervosa subjects distributed across three different cognitive-behavior therapy conditions and the waiting-list control group. Therapy was provided in 15 weekly 1-hour sessions, and at the end of therapy each treatment group had significantly improved relative to the waiting-list controls. Of treated subjects, 77% were reported to have ceased binge eating. Scores on questionnaires of eating attitudes and self-esteem and depression also showed significant improvement relative to the waiting-list controls.

Agras, Schneider, Arnow, Raeburn, and Telch (1989) also recently compared several different cognitive-behavior therapy conditions with a waiting-list control group. Patients received 14 individual treatment sessions over a 4-month period. The full package cognitive-behavior therapy group improved significantly more than the waiting-list control group on eating and purging behavior and depression. These investigators have also shown that cognitive-behavioral treatment for non-purging bulimics is more effective than a waiting-list control (Telch, Agras, Rossiter, Wilfley, & Kenardy, 1990).

Two recent controlled studies with relatively large samples have shown that behavior therapy for bulimia nervosa, with or without a cognitive restructuring component, is more effective than a waiting-list control (Freeman, Barry, Dunkeld-Turnbull, & Henderson, 1988; Wolf & Crowther, 1992).

In summary, nine studies have compared cognitive-behavioral treatment of bulimia nervosa to a waiting-list control, and in each case subjects in the cognitive-behavior therapy condition improved significantly more than subjects in the waiting-list condition. This was generally not only true for primary measures of eating and purging behavior but for measures of eating attitudes, body image, and more global measures of psychological and social adjustment including, with one exception, depression. Interestingly, the authors of the one study which showed the least difference in purging behavior of treated subjects relative to the waiting-list control stated that they downplayed the behavioral techniques to control eating and vomiting.

Comparison to Other Psychotherapy Conditions

In the first controlled study to compare cognitive-behavior therapy to another form of psychotherapy, Kirkley *et al.* (1985) compared cognitive-behavioral group therapy to nondirective group therapy with 28 bulimia nervosa patients. The cognitive-behavioral condition was modeled after Fairburn (1985) and nearly identical to the treatment program described in the Schneider and Agras (1985) article. Subjects in the nondirective group discussed food choices, eating and vomiting behavior, role of stress in their disorder, and beliefs about forbidden food, but they were not instructed on how to alter any behavior or beliefs. Emphasis was placed instead on self-discovery, self-disclosure, and understanding one's bulimia. Multiple outcome measures were employed. There were 5 dropouts in the nondirective condition compared to 1 in the cognitive-behavior therapy condition, and the results were presented for the 13 subjects in the cognitive-behavioral condition and the 9 subjects in the nondirective condition who completed treatment. It should be noted that these were subjects who had been suffering with bulimia nervosa for a long time—the means were 9 and 10 years, respectively. At posttreatment the cognitive-behavioral group's vomiting frequency had declined from a mean of 13.62 incidents per week to less than once a week (95% reduction). The nondirective group had declined from 13 to 4 incidents (69% reduction). This difference was statistically significant. In addition, at a 3-month follow-up, 38% of the subjects in the cognitive therapy condition had completely stopped vomiting compared to 11% of the subjects in the nondirective condition. This difference was not statistically significant, however. Both groups also improved equally on measures of depression, anxiety, and attitudes about eating.

In a later study, Fairburn, Kirk, O'Connor, and Cooper (1986) assigned 24 subjects to either cognitive-behavior therapy or short-term structured psychotherapy. The cognitive-behavioral treatment was as described earlier (Fairburn, 1981, 1985). The structured psychotherapy was based on Bruch's writings about psychotherapy for anorexia nervosa. It focused on identifying the underlying feelings and problems that triggered bulimia symptoms, and an effort was made to show how binge eating fails to solve these problems. Patients were encouraged to develop their own new solutions. The distinction between treatment conditions may have been somewhat blurred, however, because education regarding weight regulation and the effects of dieting and purging was also provided and some self-monitoring took place. No other specific behavioral or cognitive modification techniques were used. Both treatments lasted 18 weeks; two subjects from each condition failed to complete treatment and were dropped from the study.

Outcome was assessed using multiple measures at posttreatment and at 4-, 8-, and 12-month follow-ups. There were large and similar reductions in vomiting in both groups; 93% and 100% for cognitive-behavior therapy at posttreatment and at 1-year follow-up, respectively, and 88% and 92% for structured psychotherapy. Equivalent improvements in eating attitudes and psychopathology were also achieved in both conditions. At 1-year follow-up, however, 55% of the cognitive-behavioral therapy subjects, compared to only 27% of the short-term psychotherapy subjects, had completely stopped vomiting. Moreover, when the outcome measures were combined to yield a global rating of improvement, the cognitive-behavioral condition proved superior at posttreatment and throughout the follow-up.

In a recent study, Fairburn *et al.* (1991) compared cognitive-behavioral therapy to interpersonal therapy (Klerman, Weissman, Rounsaville, & Chevron, 1984). A total of 75 bulimia nervosa patients participated in this study. Although there was a simplified behavior therapy condition as well as the standard cognitive-behavioral therapy package, only the comparison of the latter with interpersonal therapy will be considered in this section. Therapy was provided on an individual basis for 19 sessions over 18 weeks, twice a week in the first month, weekly for the next two months, and every other week during the final 6 weeks. The cognitive-behavior therapy condition was as described earlier by Fairburn (1981, 1985). In the interpersonal psychotherapy condition, therapy focused on the interpersonal problems involved in the development and maintenance of the disorder. No attention was paid to the patients' eating behavior or attitudes to shape and weight, and there was no self-monitoring of eating and purging behavior. At the end of treatment the cognitive-behavior therapy condition was more effective in reducing purging, increasing nonpurged food intake, and improving attitudes toward body shape and weight. At a 12-month follow-up, however, these differences were no longer evident (Fairburn, Jones, Peveler, Hope, & O'Connor, in press). There was also no difference between the groups on the amount of improvement in general psychopathology and depression at the end of treatment or at follow-up.

In summary, these studies suggest that cognitive-behavior therapy is somewhat more effective than nondirective therapy and short-term psychodynamic therapy in changing the core symptoms of bulimia nervosa and is at least equally effective in facilitating improvement in depression and other more global outcome measures. The comparison to interpersonal psychotherapy is less clear. Cognitive-behavior therapy was more effective than interpersonal psychotherapy at the end of treatment but at follow-up the two groups no longer significantly differed.

Component Analyses of Cognitive-Behavior Therapy

Studies have begun to investigate the contribution of different components of cognitive-behavior therapy for bulimia nervosa. One series of investigations compared cognitive-behavior therapy with and without exposure plus response prevention. Rossiter and Wilson (1985) first made this comparison using a within-subjects reversal or crossover design in four bulimia nervosa patients. Although not all of the experimental phases could be completed in each subject, there was a trend favoring the package of cognitive-behavior therapy with exposure plus response prevention.

In a later study, nine subjects were assigned to a cognitive-behavior therapy condition without exposure plus response prevention, and eight subjects were assigned to cognitive-behavior therapy with exposure plus response prevention (Wilson, Rossiter, Kleinfield, & Lindholm, 1986). In the latter condition, the exposure plus response prevention procedure was introduced only in the fifth session (in all there were 16 treatment sessions). Two subjects dropped out of each condition before the two treatments diverged. At posttreatment, 71% of the subjects who received exposure plus response prevention sessions had completely ceased binge eating and vomiting compared to only 33% of the cognitive-behavior therapy group without exposure plus response prevention. At 1-year follow-up six of the seven patients who had originally received exposure plus response prevention sessions were still abstaining from binge eating and vomiting, whereas only one of the two subjects who had responded positively to cognitive-behavior therapy alone was able to maintain her improvement.

Another controlled evaluation of the exposure plus response prevention approach to treatment of bulimia nervosa involved a comparison of three treatment conditions and a waiting-list control group (Leitenberg *et al.*, 1988). The three treatment conditions were (1) exposure plus response prevention conducted in a single setting (clinic), (2) exposure plus response prevention conducted in multiple settings (clinic, patients' homes, and restaurants), and (3) cognitive-behavior therapy without exposure plus response prevention.

Outcome was evaluated at posttreatment for all four conditions, including the waiting-list control group, and at 6-month follow-up for just the three treatment conditions. The three treatment groups improved significantly on almost all of the outcome measures, whereas the waiting-list control group showed little change. All three treatment groups improved significantly more than did the waiting-list control on measures of eating behavior, vomiting, eating attitudes, body image, self-esteem, and depression. At follow-up there was a statistically significant greater reduction in vomiting behavior for the two exposure plus response prevention groups relative to the no-exposure condition. However, on most other measures, the degree of improvement from pretreatment to follow-up was the same for all three treatment groups, and the two exposure groups did not show a significant difference.

Agras *et al.* (1989) made a similar comparison between cognitive-behavior therapy with and without exposure plus response prevention. In contrast to the findings of Wilson *et al.* (1986) and Leitenberg *et al.* (1988), however, the addition of therapist-assisted exposure plus response prevention led to poorer results both at outcome and at follow-up. There were a number of procedural differences between the Agras *et al.*, Leitenberg *et al.*, and Wilson *et al.* studies which probably account for the different findings.

Perhaps the most significant difference is that in the Leitenberg *et al.* (1988) study, therapy sessions were usually 2 hours in length; in the Wilson *et al.* (1986) study, therapy sessions were 90 min in length. By contrast, in the Agras *et al.* (1989) study, therapy sessions were only 1 hour. As Agras *et al.* indicate, "the response-prevention procedure, because it was time-consuming, shortened the participants' exposure to some of the basic procedures involved in cognitive-behavioral treatment, thus reducing treatment efficacy" (p. 220). However, the exposure plus response prevention procedure was designed to supplement, not replace, the standard cognitive-behavioral treatment paradigm (Leitenberg & Rosen, 1989). It is unlikely the two procedures could be effectively combined in 50 to 60 min, especially in the first 2 months after the exposure plus response prevention procedure is introduced. Just as therapist-assisted exposure in the treatment of agoraphobia should not be limited in duration to the routine of the 50-min hour, the addition of therapist-assisted exposure plus response prevention to the treatment of bulimia nervosa should not be limited in this manner. Adequate time must be allowed for discussion of the pattern of eating exhibited between treatment sessions, including distorted cognitions and antecedent events associated with skipped meals and binge–purge episodes. It would indeed be a mistake if treatment sessions dealt exclusively with feelings and thoughts evoked by eating feared foods in the sessions. This would mean that essential material associated with pathological eating behavior during the week could not be covered. We have found that as treatment progresses, less anxiety is induced by eating feared foods in therapy sessions (Leitenberg, Gross, Peterson, & Rosen, 1984). As a result, the length of each therapy session can gradually be reduced.

Another important methodological difference between these studies is that in the Agras *et al.* (1989) study, the exposure plus response prevention procedure was not introduced until the seventh session (halfway through the scheduled 15 sessions of treatment). By contrast, it was introduced in the second session in the Leitenberg *et al.* (1988) study and in the fifth session in the Wilson *et al.* (1986) study. Aside from the issue of whether or not a long-delayed introduction leads to too few exposure plus response prevention sessions (23 in the Leitenberg *et al.* study vs. only 7 in the Agras *et al.* study), a question can be raised about what impact such a delayed introduction has to the credibility of the technique. No credibility ratings were reported in the Agras *et al.* study, whereas in both the Leitenberg *et al.* and Wilson *et al.* studies, patients' credibility ratings of the treatments being compared were the same.

Still more recently, Wilson, Eldredge, Smith, and Niles (1991) compared cognitive-behavior therapy with and without an in-session exposure and response prevention component. They found both treatments to be equally effective. Unfortunately exposure and response prevention was not introduced until sometime between the 10th and 13th treatment session. As a result the two groups received unequal lengths of the two treatments, making the comparison suspect. Moreover, if one wanted to test the benefits of adding only a few in-treatment sessions of exposure plus response prevention, the best time would presumably be early in treatment when the fear of eating without purging is greatest.

In short, it is still uncertain whether or not exposure plus response prevention provides a sufficiently more positive outcome to the cognitive-behavior therapy package to warrant the extra effort involved. At the least, however, in those subjects who are not able to resume eating much food at home without vomiting, exposure plus response prevention in therapy sessions is a technique which appears worth trying.

The Agras *et al.* (1989) study also examined whether or not an abbreviated behavioral condition did as well as the standard cognitive-behavior therapy package. In this condition self-monitoring records were reviewed to discover antecedents to binge–purge episodes. However, no specific behavior-change procedures were taught to patients, and as a result it was not as effective as the full treatment in reducing purging behavior or depression.

There are mixed results in regard to the need to explicitly engage in cognitive restructuring. Freeman *et al.* (1988) found that eliminating this focus did not change outcomes. Fairburn *et al.* (1991) also found that solely emphasizing regaining control over eating and purging produced just as much change as the full cognitive-behavior therapy protocol on measures of binge eating, purging, and social and psychological adjustment. However, distorted attitudes toward shape, weight, and dieting were more effectively changed by including the cognitive focus. Wolf and Crowther (1992) found that a behavioral condition without cognitive restructuring produced a greater reduction in binge eating at follow-up, whereas the combined condition produced greater reductions in general psychological symptoms of distress and in preoccupation with dieting.

Yates and Sambrailo (1984) compared what might be considered two different portions of the typical cognitive-behavioral package for treatment of bulimia nervosa. In one condition, 12 subjects were trained in assertiveness, relaxation, and modification of self-defeating thoughts regarding weight and self-worth. In the other condition, which also contained 12 subjects, the focus was on self-control techniques, including stimulus control, instructions to delay eating following the urge to binge, and instructions to schedule alternative activities at normal binge-eating times. Treatment lasted for only 6 weeks for both conditions, however, and although there was significant improvement on various measures for both groups, the gains were not that substantial and there was no significant difference between the two treatment groups. Only 16 subjects completed treatment, and only 7 subjects appeared to show any improvement. Overall, there was only a 31% decrease in vomiting at posttreatment. Only one subject stopped vomiting completely at posttreatment, and that person relapsed at a 6-week follow-up.

Olmsted *et al.* (1991) examined the effectiveness of a brief psychoeducational group intervention relative to standard individual cognitive-behavior therapy. The full treatment did better in reducing both binge and purge frequency, especially for those patients who exhibited the greatest disturbance at pretreatment.

In summary, it so far appears as if the full cognitive-behavioral treatment is slightly more effective than any one of its individual components that have been experimentally analyzed. And as for exposure plus response prevention, the results are mixed; as a result there is a question as to whether the potential gain is worth the added cost in session duration. The answer to this question may depend on the degree of anxiety a patient exhibits about resuming eating feared foods at home. If it is extreme, which has been our experience, then adding exposure plus response prevention to the therapy session may be indicated.

Empirical Evaluations of Other Psychological Treatments of Bulimia Nervosa

As mentioned in the introduction, although there are numerous psychological treatments provided in the community for bulimia nervosa, only cognitive-behavior therapy has been systematically evaluated in controlled research. There were only two outcome studies of other therapies that I found. One was uncontrolled and one controlled.

One study involved 92 bulimia nervosa subjects who received time-limited "psychodynamic" group treatment with some cognitive-behavioral components (Frommer, Ames, Gibson, & Davis, 1987). Treatment is described as primarily psychodynamically oriented using a

> supportive-interactional model in which the content of the group process shifts among individual dynamic issues, group dynamics, and specific cognitive-behavioral interventions in response to the needs of the individual group and its members. Although the groups are neither prescriptive in approach nor prestructured in format, didactic material is offered and strategies for behavior change are discussed. (Frommer *et al.*, 1987, p. 471)

Therapists had advanced training in family, group, and psychoanalytic treatment, but apparently little training in cognitive-behavioral treatment. Treatment was provided to groups of 5 subjects at a time for 12 weekly 1-hour sessions. For the 71 subjects who were vomiting at pretreatment (21 of the 92 original subjects purged in some other unspecified manner), the mean vomiting frequency per week declined from a pretreatment level of 10.35 to 8.85. This is only about a 10% reduction. Moreover, when subjects were categorized into mild, moderate, and severe groups, based on pretreatment levels of 1 to 3, 4 to 7, and 8 or more weekly vomiting frequencies, only the severe group showed any significant improvement, from a pretreatment mean of 16.87 to a posttreatment mean of 12.10 vomiting episodes. The mild group, however, showed a significant increase in vomiting episodes after treatment, from a pretreatment mean of 2.13 to a posttreatment mean of 4.33. The moderate group remained essentially unchanged: The pretreatment mean was 5.50 and the posttreatment mean was 6.13.

Equally negative findings were reported by Russell, Szmuckler, Zare, and Eisler (1987) in a comparison of family therapy and individual psychotherapy for 23 bulimia nervosa patients. Prior to discharge from hospital these patients were randomly assigned to receive either individual psychotherapy or family therapy for the next year as outpatients. Individual psychotherapy was described as a control therapy, which was not designed to follow a strict psychoanalytic format but instead was "supportive, educational, and problem-centered with elements of cognitive, interpretive, and strategic therapies" (Russell *et al.*, 1987, p. 1049). The family therapy involved the entire family and assessed family structure and alliances.

> The most common interventions involved the parents' management of the patients' symptoms and other aspects of her life, emphasizing the need for parental cooperation, mutual support, consistency, and resoluteness. The therapist used a variety of techniques of persuasion and suggestion, including rationalizations, parables, paradoxes, personal authority, psychodynamic interpretations, behavioral strategies, manipulations, and homework. (p. 1049)

The results were not good for either treatment. Seventy-eight percent of the bulimia nervosa subjects were considered to have a poor outcome, and there was no difference in outcome between treatment conditions.

Pharmacotherapy versus Cognitive-Behavioral Treatment of Bulimia Nervosa

The only alternative form of treatment of bulimia nervosa which has received relatively extensive controlled evaluation is pharmacotherapy. Ten controlled drug studies have been conducted to evaluate the effectiveness of antidepressant medications relative to placebo in the treatment of bulimia nervosa (Agras, Dorian, Kirkely, Arnow, & Bachman, 1987; Barlow, Blouin, Blouin, Perez, 1988; Fluoxetine Bulimia Nervosa Collaborative Study Group, 1992; Horne *et al.*, 1988; Hughes, Wells, Cunningham, & Ilstrup, 1986; Mitchell & Groat, 1984; Mitchell *et al.*, 1990; Pope, Hudson, Jonas, & Yurgelun-Todd, 1983; Pope, Keck, McElroy, & Hudson, 1989; Sabine, Yonace, Farrington, Barratt, & Wakeling, 1983; Walsh, Stewart, Roose, Gladis, & Glassman, 1984; Walsh, Hadison, Devlin, Gladis, & Roose, 1991). Seven out of these ten studies found that bulimia nervosa patients were significantly more improved with the active drug than with the placebo (Barlow *et al.*, 1988; Fluoxetine Study, 1992; Hughes *et al.*, 1986; Mitchell *et al.*, 1990; Pope *et al.*, 1983; Pope *et al.*, 1989; Walsh *et al.*, 1984; Walsh *et al.*, 1991), and another reported a significant difference 6 weeks into treatment but not at 16 weeks (Agras *et al.*, 1987). For the studies that report these data, the average reduction in bulimic episodes for subjects receiving antidepressant medication was about 64%, and 31% completely stopped purging and vomiting—outcomes that are slightly poorer than those obtained with cognitive-behavior therapy. One important difference, however, is that the drug studies typically measured short-term outcomes while patients were still receiving medication, whereas most of the cognitive-behavior therapy studies evaluated outcomes at follow-up after treatment was discontinued. Clinical reports suggest that a substantial relapse will occur when medication is discontinued (Pope, Hudson, Jonas, & Yurgelun-Todd, 1985), and more recent research has confirmed this (Pyle *et al.*, 1990; Walsh *et al.*, 1991).

A comparison of the effectiveness of one of the major antidepressants, imipramine, with cognitive-behavior therapy has recently been published (Mitchell *et al.*, 1990). There were 171 bulimia nervosa subjects randomly assigned to four treatment conditions: imipramine alone, imipramine combined with cognitive-behavior therapy, placebo, and cognitive-behavior therapy combined with placebo. Cognitive-behavior therapy was delivered in a group format. In the first 2 weeks (preparatory phase), subjects were seen for two 2-hour sessions per week. During weeks 3 to 7 (interruption phase), subjects were initially seen five nights a week for 3 hours each night. The frequency of sessions was reduced during the next 3 weeks from four to two sessions each week. Exposure plus response prevention was included throughout this phase. During the last month (stabilization phase), there was a single 1½-hour session each week. On measures of eating behavior (binge-eating and vomiting episodes per week), cognitive-behavior therapy was more effective than imipramine, even though imipramine was more effective than placebo. Moreover, imipramine combined with cognitive-behavior therapy was not more effective in changing binge-eating and purging behavior than cognitive-behavior therapy alone. Both the cognitive-behavior therapy group and the imipramine group improved on measures of depression and anxiety with no significant difference between them. Accordingly these authors concluded that cognitive-behavior therapy was more effective than antidepressant medication in the treatment of bulimia nervosa and there was no benefit to combining the two forms of treatment.

A second study examined the relative effectiveness of another antidepressant medication, desipramine, compared to cognitive-behavior therapy (Agras *et al.*, 1992). There were five groups: Desipramine alone (for either 16 or 24 weeks); desipramine combined with cognitive-behavior therapy (for either 16 or 24 weeks); and cognitive-behavior therapy alone (for 16 weeks, plus three additional sessions at weeks 20, 24, and 28). There was no placebo group. Two assessments were conducted, one at 16 weeks and one at 32 weeks after all treatments had been discontinued. At 16 weeks, both the cognitive-behavior therapy alone and combined treatment conditions showed significantly greater reductions in binge eating and purging than the desipramine alone condition; there was no significant difference between the cognitive-behavior therapy alone condition and the combined conditions. These results are thus very similar to those of Mitchell *et al.* (1990). At 32 weeks, the 24-week combined condition showed significantly greater reductions in binge eating and purging than the 16-week medication alone condition. The cognitive-behavior therapy alone condition, however, was no longer significantly different from the 16-week medication alone condition. The authors therefore concluded that a combination of medication and cognitive-behavior therapy may be the preferred treatment for bulimia nervosa. However, although their results support the conclusion that the combined condition is superior to medication alone, they do not support the conclusion that the combined condition is superior to cognitive-behavior therapy alone. The combined condition did not significantly differ from the cognitive-behavior therapy alone group at any time on binge eating or purging behavior.

We also recently conducted a study comparing desipramine with cognitive-behavior therapy (Leitenberg *et al.*, in press). There were three conditions: cognitive-behavior therapy alone, desipramine alone, and cognitive-behavior therapy combined with desipramine. The cognitive-behavior therapy condition was provided on an individual basis for 20 weeks and included exposure plus response prevention beginning with week 2. We originally planned to assign 12 bulimia nervosa subjects to each condition, but the results were so consistently poor for the desipramine-alone condition that we felt ethically obligated to stop the study after only seven subjects had been assigned to each treatment condition. Four subjects in the desipramine condition dropped out in the first month, and the three who completed treatment showed little benefit. In contrast, there was only one dropout from the cognitive-behavior therapy alone condition. Five out of the six subjects who completed this treatment had completely stopped vomiting at the end of treatment, and the remaining subject vomited only once during the 2-week end-of-treatment assessment phase. There was also no indication on any of the outcome measures—binge–purge episodes, attitudes toward eating, weight, and body shape, depression, psychological distress as measured by the Brief Symptom Inventory, or self-esteem—of any benefit from combining desipramine with cognitive-behavior therapy. If anything the trend was in the reverse direction on measures of binge eating and purging, with subjects in the combined drug and cognitive-behavior therapy condition doing somewhat worse than those who received just cognitive-behavior therapy.

Rossiter, Agras, Losch, & Telch (1988) reported that patients with bulimia nervosa who decrease their purging behavior in response to antidepressant medication nevertheless continue to eat in a restricted fashion. By contrast, patients who received cognitive-behavior therapy increased their nonpurged energy intake. Based on this finding, Craighead and Agras (1991) have recently suggested that these two treatments may not be compatible for bulimia nervosa. Certainly Mitchell *et al.*'s (1990) results with imipramine and our results with desipramine lend no support to combining these two treatments as a matter of routine. Based on the results of these studies it would seem that cognitive-behavior therapy alone should be the treatment of first choice for bulimia nervosa. If a subject fails to respond, then one of the antidepressants might be considered since they have been shown to be more effective than placebo.

Conclusions

Bulimia nervosa was first identified as a distinct eating disorder in normal-weight women only a little over a decade ago. It is remarkable how much research has already been conducted on cognitive-behavioral treatment of this disorder. Equally remarkable is the sparsity of controlled research on other psychotherapeutic approaches to this disorder. The results so far are encouraging, albeit far from optimal. Cognitive-behavioral therapy has been shown to be more effective than no treatment in a series of studies. A positive impact was observed not only on binge-eating and purging behavior but also on attitudes toward food, weight, body shape, and appearance and on broad-based measures of social and psychological adjustment including depression. Cognitive-behavior therapy was also shown to be somewhat more effective than either nondirective therapy, interpersonal therapy, or short-term psychodynamically oriented individual psychotherapy. Finally, in the few comparison studies that have been conducted, cognitive-behavior therapy has been shown to be more effective than pharmacotherapy, which in turn is more effective than placebo.

There is not much information about which patient variables might predict outcome. Because of the small sample sizes in most of the treatment studies this question has seldom been examined adequately. Some of the more obvious possible prognostic indicators, such as frequency of purging, do not appear to reliably predict response to treatment. What have so far appeared in the literature as predictors of poorer outcome are low self-esteem (Fairburn, Kirk, O'Connor, Anastasiades, & Cooper, 1987), dissatisfaction with body image (Freeman, Beach, Davis, & Solyom, 1985), concurrent diagnosis of borderline personality disorder (Johnson, Tobin, & Dennis, 1990), and a family history of anorexia nervosa (Lacey, 1983).

Despite the overall positive findings of the relative effectiveness of cognitive-behavior therapy in the treatment of bulimia nervosa, it should be observed that only approximately 30–60% of patients receiving this treatment completely cease vomiting after treatment is terminated and at follow-up. Thus there is still room for considerable improvement.

References

Abraham, S. F., & Beaumont, P. J. V. (1982). How patients describe bulimia or binge-eating. *Psychological Medicine, 12*, 625–635.

Agras, W. S., Dorian, B., Kirkley, B. G., Arnow, B., & Bachman, J. (1987). Imipramine in the treatment of bulimia: A double-blind controlled study. *International Journal of Eating Disorders, 6*, 29–38.

Agras, W. S., Schneider, J. A., Arnow, B., Raeburn, S. D., & Telch, C. F. (1989). Cognitive-behavioral and response prevention treatments for bulimia nervosa. *Journal of Consulting and Clinical Psychology, 57*, 215–221.

Agras, W. S., Rossiter, E. M., Arnow, B., Schneider, J. A., Telch, C. F., Raeburn, S. D., Bruce, B., Perl, M., & Koran, L. M. (1992). Pharmacologic and cognitive-behavioral treatment for bulimia nervosa: A controlled comparison. *American Journal of Psychiatry, 149*, 82–87.

American Psychiatric Association. (1987). *Diagnostic and statistical manual of mental disorders* (3rd ed.-revised). Washington, DC: Author.

Bandura, A. (1982). Self-efficacy mechanisms in human agency. *American Psychologist, 37*, 122–147.

Barlow, J., Blouin, J., Blouin, A., & Perez, E. (1988). Treatment of bulimia with desipramine: A double-blind crossover study. *Canadian Journal of Psychiatry, 33*, 129–133.

Biran, M., & Wilson, T. (1981). Treatment of phobic disorders using cognitive and exposure methods: A self-efficacy analysis. *Journal of Consulting and Clinical Psychology, 19*, 886–899.

Boskind-Lodahl, M., & White, W. C. (1978). The definition and treatment of bulimiarexia in college women—A pilot study. *Journal of American College Health Association, 27*, 84–86.

Clement, P. F., & Hawkins, R. C. (1980). *Pathways to bulimia: Personality correlates, prevalence and a conceptual model.* Paper presented at the annual meeting of the Association for the Advancement of Behavior Therapy, New York.

Conners, M. E., Johnson, C. L., & Stuckey, M. K. (1984). Treatment of bulimia with brief psychoeducational group therapy. *American Journal of Psychiatry, 141*, 1512–1516.

Cooper, P. J., Charnock, D. J., & Taylor, M. J. (1987). The prevalence of bulimia nervosa: A replication study. *British Journal of Psychiatry, 151*, 684–686.

Cooper, P. J., & Fairburn, C. G. (1983). Binge-eating and self-induced vomiting in the community: A preliminary study. *British Journal of Psychiatry, 142*, 139–144.

Coovert, D. L., Kinder, B. N., & Thompson, J. K. (1989). The psychosexual aspects of anorexia nervosa and bulimia nervosa: A review of the literature. *Clinical Psychology Review, 9*, 169–180.

Craighead, L. W., & Agras, W. S. (1991). Mechanisms of action in cognitive-behavioral and pharmacological interventions for obesity and bulimia nervosa. *Journal of Consulting and Clinical Psychology, 59*, 115–125.

Crowther, J. H., Chernyk, B., Hahn, M., Hedeen, C., & Zaynor, L. (1983). *The prevalence of binge-eating and bulimia in a normal college population.* Paper presented at the annual meeting of the Midwestern Psychological Association, Chicago.

Dolan, B. (1991). Cross-cultural aspects of anorexia nervosa and bulimia: A review. *International Journal of Eating Disorders, 10*, 67–78.

Drewnowski, A., Hopkins, S. A., & Kessler, R. L., (1988). The prevalence of bulimia nervosa in the U.S. college student population. *American Journal of Public Health, 78*(10), 1322–1325.

Ellis, A. (1979). A note on the treatment of agoraphobics with cognitive modification versus prolonged exposure in vivo. *Behaviour Research and Therapy, 17*, 162–164.

Emmelkamp, P. M. G., Kuipers, A., & Eggeraat, J. (1978). Cognitive modification versus prolonged exposure in vivo; A comparison with agoraphobics. *Behaviour Research and Therapy, 16*, 33–41.

Fairburn, C. G. (1981). A cognitive behavioural approach to the treatment of bulimia. *Psychological Medicine, 11*, 707–711.

Fairburn, C. G. (1985). Cognitive-behavioral treatment for bulimia. In D. M. Garner & P. E. Garfinkel (Eds.), *Handbook of psychotherapy for anorexia nervosa and bulimia* (pp. 160–192). New York: Guilford.

Fairburn, C. G., & Beglin, S. J. (1990). Studies of the epidemiology of bulimia nervosa. *American Journal of Psychiatry, 127*, 401–408.

Fairburn, C. G., Jones, R., Peveler, R. C., Carr, S. J., Solomon, R. A., O'Connor, M., Burton, J., & Hope, R. A. (1991). Three psychological treatments for bulimia nervosa: A comparative trial. *Archives of General Psychiatry, 48*, 463–469.

Fairburn, C. G., Jones, R., Peveler, R. C., Hope, R. A., & O'Connor, M. (in press). Psychotherapy and bulimia nervosa: The longer-term effects of interpersonal psychotherapy, behavior therapy and cognitive behavior therapy. *Archives of General Psychiatry.*

Fairburn, C. G., Kirk, J., O'Connor, M., Anastasiades, P., & Cooper, P. J. (1987). Prognostic factors in bulimia nervosa. *British Journal of Clinical Psychology, 26*, 223–224.

Fairburn, C. G., Kirk, J., O'Connor, M., & Cooper, P. J. (1986). A comparison of two psychological treatments for bulimia nervosa. *Behaviour Research and Therapy, 24*, 629–643.

Fairburn, C. G., Peveler, R. C., Jones, R., Hope, R. A., & Doll, H. A. (in press). Predictors of twelve-month outcome in bulimia nervosa and the influence of attitudes to shape and weight. *Journal of Consulting and Clinical Psychology.*

Fluoxetine Bulimia Nervosa Collaborative Study Group (1992). Fluoxetine in the treatment of bulimia nervosa. *Archives of General Psychiatry, 49*, 139–147.

Freeman, C. P. L., Barry, F., Dunkeld-Turnbull, J., & Henderson, A. (1988). Controlled trial of psychotherapy for bulimia nervosa. *British Medical Journal, 296*, 521–526.

Freeman, R. J., Beach, B., Davis, R., & Solyom, L. (1985). The prediction of relapse in bulimia nervosa. *Journal of Psychiatric Research, 19*, 349–353.

Frommer, M. S., Ames, J. R., Gibson, J. W., & Davis, W. N. (1987). Patterns of symptom change in the short-term group treatment of bulimia. *International Journal of Eating Disorders, 6*, 469–476.

Gandour, M. J. (1984). Bulimia: Clinical description, assessment, etiology, and treatment. *International Journal of Eating Disorders, 3*, 3–38.

Garner, D. M. (1986). Cognitive therapy for bulimia nervosa. In S. C. Feinstein, A. H. Estman, J. G. Looney, A. Z. Schwartzberg, & M. Sugar (Eds.), *Adolescent psychiatry: Developmental and clinical studies* (Vol. 13, pp. 358–390). Chicago: University of Chicago Press.

Giles, T. R., Young, R. R., & Young, D. E. (1985). Behavioral treatment of severe bulimia. *Behavior Therapy, 16*, 393–405.

Halmi, K. A., Falk, J. R., & Schwartz, E. (1981). Binge eating and vomiting: A survey of a college population. *Psychological Medicine, 11*, 697–706.

Hart, K. J., & Ollendick, T. H. (1985). Prevalence of bulimia in working and university women. *American Journal of Psychiatry, 142*, 851–854.

Herman, C. P., & Polivy, J. (1980). Restrained eating. In A. J. Stunkard (Ed.), *Obesity* (pp. 208–225). Philadelphia: Saunders.

Hudson, J. I., Pope, H. G., & Jonas, J. M. (1983). Treatment of bulimia with antidepressants: Theoretical considerations and clinical findings. In A. J. Stunkard, & E. Stellar (Eds.), *Eating and its disorders* (pp. 259–273). New York: Raven.

Hughes, P. L., Wells, L. A., Cunningham, C. J., & Ilstrup, D. M. (1986). Treating bulimia with desipramine. *Archives of General Psychiatry, 43*, 182–186.

Jacobs, M. B., & Schneider, J. A. (1985). Medical complications of bulimia: A prospective evaluation. *Quarterly Journal of Medicine, 54*, 177–186.

Johnson, C., Tobin, D. L., & Dennis, A. (1990). Differences in treatment outcome between borderline and nonborderline bulimics at one-year follow-up. *International Journal of Eating Disorders, 9*, 617–627.

Johnson, C., Tobin, D. L., & Lipkin, J. (1989). Epidemiologic changes in bulimic behavior among female adolescents over a 5-year period. *International Journal of Eating Disorders, 8*, 647–655.

Johnson, D., & Larson, R. (1982). Bulimia: an analysis of moods and behavior. *Psychosomatic Medicine, 44*, 341–351.

Johnson, W. G., Schlundt, D. G., & Jarrell, M. P. (1986). Exposure with response prevention, training in energy balance, and problem solving therapy for bulimia nervosa. *International Journal of Eating Disorders, 5*, 35–45.

Kirkley, B. G., Schneider, J. A., Agras, W. S., & Bachman, J. A. (1985). Comparison of two group treatments for bulimia. *Journal of Consulting and Clinical Psychology, 53*, 43–48.

Klerman, G. L., Weissman, M. M., Rounsaville, B. J., & Chevron, E. S. (1984). *Interpersonal psychotherapy of depression*. New York: Basic Books.

Lacey, J. H. (1983). Bulimia nervosa, binge eating, and psychogenic vomiting: A controlled treatment study and long term outcome. *British Medical Journal, 286*, 1609–1613.

Lee, N. F., & Rush, A. J. (1986). Cognitive-behavioral group therapy for bulimia. *International Journal of Eating Disorders, 5*, 599–615.

Leitenberg, H., Gross, J., Peterson, J., & Rosen, J. C. (1984). Analysis of an anxiety model and the process of change during exposure plus response prevention treatment of bulimia nervosa. *Behavior Therapy, 15*, 3–20.

Leitenberg, H., & Rosen, J. C. (1986). A behavioral approach to treatment of bulimia nervosa. In S. C. Feinstein, A. H. Esman, J. G. Looney, A. Z. Schwartzberg, & M. Sugar (Eds.), *Adolescent psychiatry: Developmental and clinical studies* (Vol. 13, pp. 333–357). Chicago: University of Chicago Press.

Leitenberg, H., & Rosen, J. (1989). Cognitive-behavioral therapy with and without exposure plus response prevention in the treatment of bulimia nervosa: Comment on Agras, Schneider, Arnow, Raeburn, and Telch. *Journal of Consulting and Clinical Psychology, 57*, 776–777.

Leitenberg, H., Rosen, M. C., Gross, J., Nudelman, S., & Vara, L. S. (1988). Exposure plus response prevention treatment of bulimia nervosa: A controlled evaluation. *Journal of Consulting and Clinical Psychology, 56*, 535–541.

Leitenberg, H., Rosen, J. C., Wolf, J., Vara, L. S., Detzer, M., & Srebnik, D. (in press). Comparison of cognitive behavior therapy and desipramine in the treatment of bulimia nervosa. *Behaviour Research and Therapy.*

Mitchell, J. E., & Groat, R. (1984). A placebo-controlled, double-blind trial of amitriptyline in bulimia. *Journal of Clinical Psychopharmacology, 4*, 186–193.

Mitchell, J. E., & Pyle, R. L. (1982). The bulimia syndrome in normal weight individuals: A review. *International Journal of Eating Disorders, 2*, 60–73.

Mitchell, J. E., Pyle, R. L., Eckert, E. D., Hatsukami, D., Pomeroy, C., & Zimmerman, R. (1990). A comparison study of antidepressants and structured group therapy in the treatment of bulimia nervosa. *Archives of General Psychiatry, 47*, 149–157.

Olmsted, M. P., Davis, R., Rochert, W., Irvine, M. J., Eagle, M., & Garner, D. M. (1991). Efficacy of a brief group psychoeducational intervention for bulimia nervosa. *Behaviour Research and Therapy, 29*, 71–83.

Orbach, S. (1978). *Fat is a feminist issue*. New York: Paddington Press.

Ordman, A. M., & Kirschenbaum, D. S. (1985). Cognitive-behavioral therapy for bulimia: An initial outcome study. *Journal of Consulting and Clinical Psychology, 53*, 305–313.

Parry-Jones, B., & Parry-Jones, W. L. I. (1991). Bulimia: An archival review of its history in psychosomatic medicine. *International Journal of Eating Disorders, 10*, 129–143.

Pope, H. G., Hudson, J. I., Jonas, J. M., & Yurgelun-Todd, D. (1983). Bulimia treated with imipramine: A placebo-controlled, double-blind study. *American Journal of Psychiatry, 140*, 554–558.

Pope, H. G., Hudson, J. I., Jonas, J. M., & Yurgelun-Todd, D. (1985). Antidepressant treatment of bulimia: A two-year follow-up study. *Journal of Clinical Psychopharmacology, 5*, 320–327.

Pope, H. G., Hudson, J. I., & Yurgelun-Todd, D. (1984). Anorexia nervosa and bulimia among 300 suburban women shoppers. *American Journal of Psychiatry, 141*, 292–294.

Pope, H. G., Keck, P. E., McElroy, S. L., & Hudson, J. I. (1989). A placebo-controlled study of trazodone in bulimia nervosa. *Journal of Clinical Psychopharmacology, 9*, 254–259.

Pyle, R. L., Mitchell, J. E., Eckert, E. D., Hatsukami, D., Pomeroy, C., & Zimmerman, R. (1990). Maintenance treatment and 6-month outcome for bulimia patients who respond to initial treatment. *American Journal of Psychiatry, 147*, 871–875.

Pyle, R. L., Neuman, P. A., Halvorson, P. A., & Mitchell, J. E. (1991). An ongoing cross-sectional study of the prevalence of eating disorders in freshman college students. *International Journal of Eating Disorders, 10*, 667–677.

Rand, C. S. W., & Kuldan, J. M. (1992). Epidemiology of bulimia and symptoms in a general population: Sex, age, race, and socioeconomic status. *International Journal of Eating Disorders, 11*, 37–44.

Rosen, J. C., Gross, J. (1987). Prevalence of weight reducing and weight gaining in adolescent girls and boys. *Health Psychology, 6*, 131–147.

Rosen, J. C., & Leitenberg, H. (1982). Bulimia nervosa: Treatment with exposure and response prevention. *Behavior Therapy, 13*, 117–124.

Rosen, J. C., & Leitenberg, H. (1985). Exposure plus response prevention treatment of bulimia. In D. M. Garner & P. E. Garfinkel (Eds.), *A handbook of psychotherapy for anorexia nervosa and bulimia* (pp. 193–209). New York: Guilford Press.

Rosen, J. C., Leitenberg, H., Fondacaro, K. M., Gross, J., & Willmuth, M. E. (1985). Standardized test meals in assessment of eating behavior in bulimia nervosa: Consumption of feared foods when vomiting is prevented. *International Journal of Eating Disorders, 4*, 59–70.

Rossiter, E. M., Agras, W. S., Losch, M., & Telch, C. F. (1988). Changes in self-reported food intake in bulimics as a consequence of antidepressant treatment. *International Journal of Eating Disorders, 7*, 779–789.

Rossiter, E., & Wilson, G. T. (1985). Cognitive restructuring and response prevention in the treatment of bulimia nervosa. *Behaviour Research and Therapy, 23*, 349–360.

Russell, G. F. M. (1979). Bulimia nervosa: An ominous variant of anorexia nervosa. *Psychological Medicine, 9*, 429–448.

Russell, G. F. M., Szmuckler, G. I., Zare, C., & Eisler, I. (1987). An evaluation of family therapy in anorexia nervosa and bulimia nervosa. *Archives of General Psychiatry, 44*, 1047–1056.

Sabine, E. J., Yonace, A., Farrington, A. J., Barratt, K. H., & Wakeling, A. (1983). Bulimia nervosa: A placebo controlled double-blind therapeutic trial of Mianserin. *British Journal of Clinical Pharmacology, 15*, 195–202.

Schneider, J. A., & Agras, W. S. (1985). A cognitive behavioural group treatment of bulimia. *British Journal of Psychiatry, 146*, 66–69.

Schotte, D. E., & Stunkard, A. J. (1987). Bulimia versus bulimic behaviors on a college campus. *The Journal of the American Medical Association, 258*, 1213–1215.

Steere, J., & Cooper, P. J. (1988). The anxiety reduction model of bulimia nervosa: Contrary case reports. *International Journal of Eating Disorders, 7*, 385–391.

Telch, C. F., Agras, W. S., Rossiter, E. M., Wilfley, D., & Kenardy, J. (1990). Group cognitive-behavioral treatment for the nonpurging bulimic: An initial evaluation. *Journal of Consulting and Clinical Psychology, 58*, 629–635.

Walsh, B. T., Hadigan, C. M., Devlin, M. J., Gladis, M., & Roose, S. P. (1991). Long-term outcome of antidepressant treatment for bulimia nervosa. *American Journal of Psychiatry, 148*, 1206–1212.

Walsh, B. T., Stewart, J. W., Roose, S. P., Gladis, M., & Glassman, A. H. (1984). Treatment of bulimia with phenelzine: A double-blind, placebo controlled study. *Archives of General Psychiatry, 41*, 1105–1109.

Wardle, J., & Ileinhart, J. (1981). Binge eating: A theoretical review. *British Journal of Clinical Psychology, 20*, 97–109.

Williams, S. L., & Rappaport, A. (1983). Cognitive treatment in the natural environment for agoraphobia. *Behavior Therapy, 14*, 299–313.

Williamson, D. A., Kelley, M. L., Davis, C. J., Ruggiero, L., & Veitia, M. C. (1985). The psychophysiology of bulimia. *Advances in Behaviour Research and Therapy, 7*, 163–172.

Willmuth, M. E., Leitenberg, H., Rosen, J. C., & Cado, S. (1988). A comparison of purging and nonpurging normal weight bulimics. *International Journal of Eating Disorders, 7*, 825–835.

Wilson, G. T., Eldredge, K. L., Smith, D., & Niles, B. (1991). Cognitive-behavioral treatment with and without response prevention for bulimia. *Behaviour Research and Therapy, 29*, 575–583.

Wilson, G. T., Rossiter, E., Kleinfield, E. I., & Lindholm, L. (1986). Cognitive-behavioral treatment of bulimia nervosa: A controlled evaluation. *Behaviour Research and Therapy, 24*, 277–288.

Wilson, G. T., Rossiter, E., Lindholm, L., & Tebbutt, J. (1986). *Cognitive behavioral treatment of bulimia nervosa: Clinical issues and findings*. Unpublished manuscript, Rutgers University.

Wolchik, S. A., Weiss, L., & Katzman, M. K. (1986). An empirically validated, short-term psychoeducational group treatment program for bulimia. *International Journal of Eating Disorders, 5*, 21–34.

Wolf, E. M., & Crowther, J. H. (1992). An evaluation of behavioral and cognitive-behavioral group interventions for the treatment of bulimia nervosa in women. *International Journal of Eating Disorders, 11*, 3–15.

Yates, A. J., & Sambrailo, F. (1984). Bulimia nervosa: A descriptive and therapeutic study. *Behaviour Research and Therapy, 22*, 503–517.

13

Outcome of Psychotherapy for Unipolar Depression

Jacqueline B. Persons

Introduction

Clinical depression is a significant mental health and social problem. One in eight individuals is expected to require treatment for depression during his or her lifetime (Secunda, Katz, Friedman, & Schuyler, 1973). Seventy-five percent of psychiatric hospitalizations are due to depression (Secunda *et al.*, 1973). Depressed individuals have poorer health, poorer social functioning (Wells *et al.*, 1989), and higher mortality (Murphy, Monson, Olivier, Sobol, & Leighton, 1987) than non-depressed individuals. Increased mortality is apparently due to higher rates of suicide and accidents for young people and higher rates of chronic medical illness for older ones (Murphy *et al.*, 1987). Depression is a recurrent disorder; participants in a National Institute of Mental Health/National Institutes of Health (NIMH/NIH) conference estimated that 50% of depressed patients relapse within 2 years of recovery from their initial episode (NIMH/NIH, 1985).

Many psychotherapies have been used to treat depression, some developed specifically for depression and others adapted for it. The oldest, and probably the most frequently used clinically, is the psychodynamic approach, developed for treatment of nearly any neurotic difficulty. Psychodynamic therapies are typically long-term therapies in which the therapist plays a relatively passive role, encouraging the patient's free association and obtaining of insight about unconscious conflicts. Recently, a psychodynamic approach developed specifically for the treatment of depression—interpersonal therapy—was described by Klerman, Weissman, Rounsaville, and Chevron (1984). Interpersonal therapy, which draws on the ideas of Adolph Meyer, John Bowlby, and Harry Stack Sullivan, emphasizes the importance of the depressed person's interpersonal environment. The goal of treatment is to alleviate symptoms by helping the patient become more effective in dealing with interpersonal losses and stresses. In contrast with more traditional

Jacqueline B. Persons • Department of Psychiatry, University of California, San Francisco, San Francisco, California 94143.

Handbook of Effective Psychotherapy, edited by Thomas R. Giles. Plenum Press, New York, 1993.

psychodynamic therapies, it is time limited, deals with current—not past—relationships, and is concerned with interpersonal—not intrapsychic—phenomena.

Many cognitive, behavioral, and cognitive-behavioral approaches to depression have been developed. Perhaps the most prominent of these is the cognitive therapy developed by Aaron T. Beck and his colleagues (Beck, Rush, Shaw, & Emery, 1979), which proposes that depression is due to irrational, maladaptive thinking and can be treated by teaching patients to think in more adaptive, rational ways. Behavioral theories of depression propose that depression stems from a dearth of positive reinforcers and from poor interpersonal skills (Lewinsohn, Hoberman, & Hautzinger, 1985), from deficits in problem-solving skills (D'Zurilla, 1986), or from deficits in self-control skills (Rehm, 1977). These models have led to interventions designed to address the proposed deficiencies. Other therapeutic modalities, including the humanistic/Rogerian and existential models, are used by clinicians to treat depression although they were not developed specifically for that problem.

This review examines the efficacy of psychodynamic approaches of various sorts, cognitive and behavioral therapies, and pharmacotherapy in the treatment of depression. Although other psychotherapeutic models, including the humanistic/Rogerian and existential approaches are undoubtedly used to treat depression, almost no empirical evidence examines their efficacy. Although cognitive-behavioral approaches are probably not the most common ones used by clinicians, these therapies dominate the empirical outcome literature; as a result, they dominate this review as well.

This is not an exhaustive review. I focus on large and/or conceptually important studies. Other reviews are provided by Dobson (1989), Hollon, Shelton, and Loosen (1991), and Miller and Berman (1983), among others.

This review examines single-case studies, comparisons of psychotherapy with placebo, dismantling studies, between-orientation comparisons, and comparisons with pharmacotherapy. It does not compare active treatments with no treatment control conditions for two reasons. First, it has been repeatedly demonstrated and is generally accepted that psychotherapies for depression are superior to no treatment (cf. de Jong, Treiber, & Henrich, 1986; Reynolds & Coats, 1986; Rude, 1986; Shaw, 1977; Taylor & Marshall, 1977; Thompson, Gallagher, & Breckenridge, 1987). Second, the option of "no treatment" is not an ethical alternative for providers or an acceptable one for consumers.

Single Subject Designs

Because there are so many large, controlled outcome studies that deserve attention, only one single-case study of particular theoretical interest is examined here. McKnight, Nelson, Hayes, and Jarrett (1984) tested the hypothesis that treatment interventions that focus on an individual's area of deficit are more effective than interventions that do not. Nine depressed women were treated: three who had social skills deficits, three who had cognitive distortions, and three who had both. Subjects received alternating sessions of social skills training (SST) and cognitive restructuring (CT) (four sessions of each treatment); responses to each type of intervention were measured at the beginning of the following sessions. McKnight *et al.* (1984) reported that subjects with social skills deficits benefited more from SST than from CT, and subjects with cognitive deficits benefited more from CT than from SST. Subjects with both deficits benefited from both treatments, but SST produced more improvement in social skills than did CT, and CT produced more cognitive change than did SST. Thus, overall results indicate no clear superiority for either treatment but suggest that one treatment can be superior to another for a particular patient, depending on the nature of the patient's difficulties. I will return to this idea.

Despite the interest of the findings, several weaknesses of this study must be acknowledged. As the authors acknowledge, it is impossible to measure effects of one treatment uncontaminated by the other; sessions have effects that extend over time and are not simply localized to the beginning of the next session. Second, although the authors show that subjects receiving SST in the previous session do show lower depression scores than when they received CT in the previous session, no statistical tests were carried out; the investigators simply examined whether or not the depression score following the SST session was lower than the depression score following the CT session. Although this frequently happened, it is not clear that the magnitude of these effects was either statistically or clinically significant. Demand characteristics may also have been a problem. Subjects may have felt a demand to report improvement on social skills following SST sessions and improvement on cognitions following CT sessions.

In a larger-scale test of the same hypothesis examined by McKnight *et al.*, Rude (1986) failed to show, in a crossover design, that individuals low on assertion benefited more from assertiveness training than from a cognitive self-control treatment, or that individuals low on cognitive self-control benefited more from cognitive self-control treatment than from assertiveness training. Perhaps Rude's failure to replicate McKnight *et al.* (1984) is due to the fact that she used median splits on cognitive and assertiveness measures to define high and low cognitive and assertiveness functioning; means of the high and low groups were not very different—the groups overlapped quite a lot. In contrast, McKnight *et al.* (1984) screened 45 depressed subjects to select 3 who had social skills but not cognitive deficits, 3 who had cognitive but not social skills deficits, and 3 who had both. The interest of the McKnight *et al.* study is the finding that individualized matching of intervention to problem seemed to produce superior results.

Treatment Comparisons Demonstrating Nonspecific Effects

This section examines comparisons of active treatments with credible placebos, and comparisons of treatments that are equal except for the presence of a particular treatment component in one condition but not the other (dismantling studies). These two types of studies address both the issue of efficacy and the issue of mechanisms of action. If treatment *X* is superior to a placebo or to another treatment that is the same except for one missing component (dismantling studies), then the argument can be made that the superiority of treatment *X* is not due to nonspecific effects like the therapeutic relationship or expectations of change, but to the unique treatment or treatment component that is specific to treatment *X*.

The most important study in this group, because it is the largest and one of the most recent, is the National Institute of Mental Health Treatment of Depression Collaborative Research Program (Elkin *et al.*, 1989), or, as it is called here, the

Collaborative Study. In addition to the Collaborative Study, I focus on studies that provide the strongest evidence I found for nonspecific factors.

Studies Comparing Psychotherapy and Placebo

The Collaborative Study (Elkin *et al.*, 1989) provides data relevant to three comparisons this chapter addresses: comparison of psychotherapies with placebo, comparisons between psychotherapies, and comparisons between psychotherapies and medication. This section describes the study and the results of the psychotherapy versus placebo comparisons. Results relevant to the other comparisons will be described later.

The Collaborative Study randomly assigned 250 depressed patients to one of four treatments: interpersonal therapy (IPT), cognitive-behavior therapy (CBT), imipramine plus clinical management, and medication placebo plus clinical management. IPT was conducted as described by Klerman *et al.* (1984) and CBT was conducted as described by Beck *et al.* (1979). The medication and pill placebo treatments consisted of imipramine or pill placebo and brief weekly clinical management visits with a psychiatrist who provided support and encouragement; the clinical management component "approximated a 'minimal supportive therapy' condition" (p. 973). All treatments were 16 to 20 sessions in length. Psychotherapy sessions were 50 min long, and the initial clinical management session was 45 to 60 min long; subsequent sessions were 20 to 30 min long.

Four outcome variables were collected. Two were patient-rated measures (Beck Depression Inventory [BDI] and Hopkins Symptom Checklist-90 Total Score [HSCL-90] and two were clinician-rated measures (Hamilton Rating Scale for Depression [HRS-D] and Global Assessment Scale [GAS]). Three samples were studied: all patients entering treatment, patients receiving at least 3.5 weeks of treatment, and completers. Paired *t* tests showed significant improvement for all groups, including placebo, for all four outcome measures in all three samples.

Outcome was studied using analysis of covariance (ANCOVA), with treatment site (treatment occurred at one of three sites), pretreatment score on the outcome variable, and marital status generally serving as covariates. Twelve ANCOVAs (four dependent measures, three samples) were conducted, followed by paired comparisons. None of these analyses showed statistically significant differences between either of the psychotherapies and the placebo condition.

Separate analyses compared the proportion of patients in each group reaching a specified recovery criterion on the HRSD (score of 6 or less) or the BDI (score of 9 or less). There were no statistically significant differences between psychotherapy and placebo when the BDI criterion was used, and only one statistically significant difference between psychotherapy and placebo when the HRS-D criterion was used: IPT was superior to placebo for HRS-D in the 239 sample of patients entering treatment; CBT fell in between and was not statistically different from either imipramine or placebo.

Secondary analyses examined outcome as a function of initial severity of depression. Patients were viewed as severely depressed if they scored 20 or greater on their rescreening HRSD or 50 or less on the GAS. ANCOVAs, with severity as a covariate, were carried out for all outcome measures for all samples, using both severity cutting scores. Treatments rarely differed for less severely depressed patients, but they did differ for more severely depressed patients. Pairwise comparisons showed that IPT was significantly more effective than placebo in several analyses, using both HRS-D and GAS scores to index severity. CBT was not superior to placebo in any analyses.

Attrition rates for the four treatments were: IPT, 23%; CBT, 32%; imipramine, 33%; placebo, 40%. These differences were not statistically significant. In a preliminary report of follow-up findings, Shea (1990) reported that relapse (defined as receiving 3 weeks or more of treatment) was lower for CBT patients than for patients in any other group during the 18-month follow-up period.

Overall, with regard to the comparison of psychotherapy versus placebo, IPT was superior to placebo in a few analyses of outcome, particularly when severity was used as a covariate. CBT was superior to placebo only in a preliminary report of relapse. Results of this important study are discouraging for the psychotherapies. Perhaps the placebo condition was a powerful one. However, psychotherapists would like to think that their active treatments, based on specific mechanisms, are more effective than nonspecific placebos.

Nezu (1986) compared problem-solving therapy (PST) with a placebo "problem-focused" therapy (PFT). In the PFT placebo, participants discussed problems but were not taught problem-solving strategies as in the active treatment. Both treatments were conducted in groups. The PST group did significantly better than the PFT group at posttreatment and 6-month follow-up on the BDI, the Depression scale of the MMPI (MMPI-D), and a problem-solving measure, but not on a measure of locus of control. The treatments did not differ in attrition.

This is an interesting demonstration of a specific effect of a treatment as compared to a powerful placebo. Results are enhanced by the finding that problem solving improved in the PST but not the placebo group, supporting the proposed mechanism of the treatment. Weaknesses include the small size of the study (20 subjects) and the fact that it was conducted by adherents of the treatment demonstrated to be superior.

McLean and Hakstian (1979) randomly assigned 196 depressed patients to 10 weeks of behavior therapy, nondirective psychotherapy, amitriptyline, or relaxation therapy. The relaxation treatment was intended to serve as a placebo control. The current discussion focuses on the comparison of the two active treatments (behavior therapy and nondirective psychotherapy) to relaxation. The other comparisons will be discussed later.

Nondirective psychotherapy was a psychodynamic treatment modeled on the work of Marmor and Wolberg; behavior therapy focused on coping techniques, with particular emphasis on development of prosocial behavior; relaxation included deep muscle relaxation training and an explanation of depressive symptoms as due to muscle tension. In all conditions, patients were encouraged to bring their spouse or partner to sessions.

Posttreatment assessment was done by mail. The investigators focused on results for 10 outcome measures, including the BDI and several components obtained from a factor analysis of items from a depression scale constructed by the authors. Behavior therapy was superior to placebo on 9 of 10 measures at posttreatment, on 1 measure (social functioning) at 3-month follow-up, and on 3 measures (social functioning, personal activity, and mood), at 2.25-year follow-up (McLean & Hakstian, 1990). Nondirective psychotherapy did not differ from relaxation on any outcome measure at any assessment point. Behavior therapy was superior to placebo in dropout frequency (5% for behavior therapy and 26% for relaxation) but nondirective psychotherapy was not (30%). Groups did not differ in the proportion of patients seeking further treatment during the 2.25-year follow-up period.

Overall, this study shows a slight superiority for one of the two therapeutic modalities studied (behavior therapy but not nondirective psychotherapy). Interpretation of this finding is complicated by the fact that the study was carried out by adherents of behavior therapy and by the fact that relaxation might arguably be viewed as an active treatment rather than a placebo (cf. Reynolds & Coats, 1986; Wilson, 1982).

Although I have presented only three studies, these are the strongest ones I could find. Overall, results of psychotherapy versus placebo comparisons are disappointing. It is difficult to find a study showing strong superiority of any psychotherapy over a credible placebo. There are hints that differences are more likely to appear during the follow-up period (cf. Shea, 1990; Wilson, 1982) or in attrition (McLean & Hakstian, 1979) than in measures of posttreatment outcome.

Dismantling Studies

If treatment *A* differs from treatment *B* only in having component *Z*, and treatment *A* is more effective than treatment *B*, we infer that component *Z*, is an active treatment mechanism that produced the incremental benefit of treatment *A*. Thus, dismantling studies examine effects of treatment due to specific mechanisms.

Nezu and Perri (1989) compared problem-solving therapy (PST) with a version of the therapy that omitted training in the problem-orientation component of the treatment. Although subjects in the abbreviated problem-solving therapy (APST) received training in problem-solving skills, they did not receive training in the first component of the problem-solving process, problem-orientation, designed "to facilitate an individual's motivation both to actually apply the four problem-solving skills and to feel self-efficacious in doing so" (p. 408).

PST and APST treatments were conducted in 10 weekly group sessions. PST was superior to APST on the BDI, HRS-D, the Problem Check List, and two scales of the Problem-Solving Inventory (PSI), but not in the approach–avoidance style scale of the PSI. There was no differential attrition. Results were stable at 6-month follow-up assessment.

This is a theoretically very interesting result. Weaknesses of the study include its small size, the fact that the study was conducted by the developers of the therapy, and—as the authors point out—the fact that problem-solving skills were measured only by self-report.

De Jong, Treiber, and Henrich (1986) compared cognitive restructuring (CR) and cognitive restructuring plus behavioral treatment (Comb). A specific active effect of the behavioral component would be demonstrated in the finding that Comb is superior to CR.

Subjects were severely and chronically depressed inpatients; treatment lasted approximately 2 to 3 months. An attempt was made to equalize the treatment time in the CR and Comb conditions. CR involved 45 to 50 fifty-minute individual sessions. Comb involved 20 to 25 individual sessions focusing on activity scheduling and cognitive restructuring and 10 to 12 ninety-minute group sessions focusing on social competence training. In addition, Comb patients were encouraged to participate in the activities on the inpatient unit.

Results differed depending on the outcome measures. A small superiority for the Comb treatment appeared when self-report outcome measures were examined. Comb was superior to CR on the BDI, the Reinforcement Survey Schedule, and the Dysfunctional Attitude Scale (DAS), but not on the HRS-D, the Inpatient Multidimensional Psychiatric Scale, or the U-questionnaire measuring social competence and social anxiety. Of the 33 patients, 25 completed the treatment; the groups did not differ in attrition. Follow-up data on the BDI and HRS-D collected 6 to 12 months later for 70% of subjects indicated that gains were relatively stable.

Taylor and Marshall (1977) also examined the effects of a combined cognitive plus behavioral treatment. They compared cognitive therapy (CT), behavior therapy (BT), and CT plus BT with a waiting-list control for the treatment of mild to moderate depression. Again, the specific-effects hypothesis predicts superior results for the combined treatment.

Twenty-eight women were recruited for the study; all received six 40-min sessions conducted by the same therapist. At the end of treatment, patients in the three active treatments were significantly more improved than waiting-list controls. Patients in the CT and BT conditions did not differ from each other; patients in the combined treatment were significantly more improved than either CT or BT patients on one of the three outcome measures (BDI) at posttreatment and on two of three outcome measures (BDI and Visual Analogue Scale but not Dempsey's D-30 of the MMPI) at 5-week follow-up. The generalizability of this study is limited by the fact that only women were treated and treatment and follow-up periods were brief.

Both de Jong *et al.* (1986) and Taylor and Marshall (1977) show a slight benefit for combined cognitive and behavioral treatment. However, other studies, including the large, carefully done study by Rehm *et al.* (1987), show no benefit to combining cognitive and behavioral treatments. In their review, Miller and Berman (1983) concluded there was no enhanced effect for combined cognitive-behavioral treatments. Thus, evidence supporting the benefits of combined cognitive and behavioral treatments is small.

Miller, Norman, Keitner, Bishop, and Dow (1989), in the treatment of 47 depressed inpatients, tested the hypothesis that the addition of cognitive therapy (CT) or social skills training (SST) to standard hospital treatment (milieu, medication, and medication management) will produce a superior result.

All patients received just over 3 weeks of inpatient treatment, followed by 20 weeks of outpatient treatment. Patients receiving standard treatment met with their psychiatrist for medication management sessions daily during the inpatient phase and approximately six to eight times during the 20-week outpatient phase of treatment. Patients receiving CT or SST met for 50-min therapy sessions daily with their psychiatrist starting in the second week of their hospital stay and weekly during the 20-week outpatient phase.

The medication treatment was conducted in an unusual way that approximates the way medications are prescribed in the "real world." Physicians chose between amitriptyline and desipramine and could use other medications (neuroleptics, antianxiety medications) as they wished. If the patient did not respond to a dose of 250 mg or greater for 3 weeks or could not tolerate this dose, then another antidepressant of the treating psychiatrist's choice could be tried or a suboptimal dose could be used. If a patient did not respond to adequate trials of three antidepressants or was unable to tolerate them, the psychiatrist had the option to discontinue medications.

There were four outcome measures: BDI, Modified HRS-D, Modified Scale for Suicidal Ideation (SSI), and SCL-90. There were no differences between groups on any of the measures during the hospital phase of treatment, but differences between groups did appear during outpatient treatment. SST patients showed significantly lower scores than standard treatment patients on the BDI and the SCL-90 (treatment completers). CT patients fell in between; their scores did not differ significantly from SST or from standard treatment. A higher proportion of CT patients were classified as "responders" on the SCL-90 (50% or more improvement) than patients in the standard treatment; SST fell between CT and standard treatment and did not differ from either.

Of the 46 patients beginning treatment, 14 did not complete it. Dropout rates were 41% for the standard treatment, 33% for CT, and 14% for SST. When the CT and SST groups are combined, there is a statistically significant difference between standard treatment and combined treatment.

A 1-year follow-up report (Miller, Norman, & Keitner, 1989) compares the CT and SST groups (combined into one group) with the standard treatment group. Although groups did not differ in proportion seeking additional treatment, proportion rehospitalized, or depression level at follow-up, there was a statistically significantly greater proportion of combined treatment patients (versus standard treatment) who were classified as having achieved remission. Remission was defined as meeting criteria for recovery during the active treatment phase (Modified HRSD < 7, BDI < 9, and SSI score < 7) and failure to meet criteria for relapse (Modified HRS-D > 17, BDI > 16, SSI > 7, or rehospitalization) during the follow-up phase.

This study shows some benefits of adding cognitive or behavioral treatment to standard hospital treatment. Strengths of this study are its inclusion of severely depressed and suicidal patients that are excluded from most outpatient outcome studies and the high level of experience of the therapists. Weaknesses include the fact that research assistants were not blind to treatment condition and the fact that the medication protocol, although appealing from the point of view of ecological validity, resulted in 18% of patients having dosages below 150 mg and 16% having no medications at all at the end of treatment. (Although the low medication dosages may be viewed as a weakness, it is not clear what the alternative to this strategy is; it is not appealing to exclude these patients from the protocol.)

Many other studies have examined the benefits of adding psychotherapy to medication treatment. Results have been mixed. Several studies found no benefit to combining psychotherapy and pharmacotherapy (Beck, Hollon, Young, Bedrosian, and Budenz, 1985, and Murphy, Simons, Wetzel, and Lustman, 1984, in studies of cognitive therapy; Hersen, Bellack, Himmelhoch, and Thase, 1984, in a study of social skills training; Covi and Lipman, 1987, in a comparison of CBT plus imipramine with CBT alone; Roth, Bielski, Jones, Parker, and Osborn, 1982, in a comparison of self-control therapy and self-control therapy plus desipramine). Wilson (1982) found no benefit of combining amitriptyline with pleasant events therapy or relaxation therapy versus doing these therapies with placebo.

Some studies show a small benefit of adding psychotherapy to antidepressant medication. Blackburn, Bishop, Glen, Whalley, and Christie (1981) found that CT plus antidepressant medication was superior to antidepressant medication alone (but not to CT alone) on one (anxiety) of seven outcome measures in the hospital sample and one (HRS-D) of seven measures in the general practice sample. Hollon *et al.* (1992) found that CT plus imipramine was superior to imipramine (but not to CT) on the MMPI-D and the Raskin Three-Area Depression Scale but not on the HRSD or BDI. Weissman, Klerman, Prusoff, Sholomskas, and Padian (1981) found combined treatment to be superior to interpersonal therapy or amitriptyline alone at posttreatment but not at 1-year follow-up. In a meta-analysis, Conte, Plutchik, Wild, and Karasu (1986) reported that combined psychotherapy–pharmacotherapy treatments appeared only slightly superior to psychotherapy alone or pharmacotherapy alone, although they were significantly superior to placebo alone. Hollon *et al.* (1991) drew a similar conclusion in a recent review.

Several elegant dismantling studies have been conducted by Rehm and his colleagues to determine the active components of his self-control therapy for depression. Disappointingly, these studies show that single components are as effective as multiple components (Kornblith, Rehm, O'Hara, Lamparski, 1983; Rehm & Kornblith, 1979; Rehm *et al.*, 1981).

Conclusions

Overall, results of both placebo and dismantling studies indicate that although it is sometimes possible to demonstrate specific effects of treatments or treatment components, these effects are not large or easy to obtain. These findings are disappointing. What do they mean?

The conclusion I draw is that psychotherapies for depression need strengthening. If therapies were more powerful, it would be easier to demonstrate their efficacy in placebo and dismantling studies. Current treatments have (at least) three types of weaknesses: (1) many patients drop out prematurely, (2) many fail to respond, and (3) many relapse. In a review of controlled outcome studies of depression, Simons, Levine, Lustman, and Murphy (1984) reported attrition rates ranging from 20% to 47%. Simons, Murphy, Levine, and Wetzel (1986), in their outcome study of cognitive therapy and pharmacotherapy for depression, classified 26, or 41%, of the 70 patients completing treatment as nonresponders. Of the treatment responders in that study, 36% relapsed during a 1-year follow-up interval. These rates for attrition, failure to respond, and relapse appear to be typical.

I suggest two strategies for strengthening treatments. One is the idea illustrated by the McKnight *et al.* (1984) study described above; that is, individualize treatment for each case. Instead, controlled outcome studies utilize standardized treatment protocols. Although individualization of the protocol undoubtedly occurs, this individualization is done on an ad hoc basis, rather than systematically, on the basis of results of an individualized assessment procedure. The individualized, or idiographic strategy, which I call the case formulation approach, is not an original idea; the concept of carrying out an individualized treatment based on the results of an individualized assessment is at the heart of all approaches to psychotherapy, ranging from behavior therapy to modern psychoanalytic approaches (Persons, 1991). If controlled outcome studies utilized this strategy, it might be possible to reduce dropout, improve the response rate, and prevent relapse.

Another strategy for strengthening treatments was proposed by Miranda

(1992). She is studying the effects of adding a "case management" component to cognitive-behavior therapy for depression. Patients receiving the case management component meet with a social worker to alleviate the environmental and external stresses in the patient's life circumstances that may contribute to depression and make it difficult for the patient to benefit from treatment. This type of intervention may be particularly important for disadvantaged populations, who do not respond as well as other populations to the usual cognitive-behavioral treatment (Organista, Munoz, & Gonzalez, in press).

Interorientation Comparisons

This section addresses the question: Is one treatment more effective than another? I focus on psychoanalytic and traditional insight-oriented therapies because they are the oldest and continue to be the most widely used treatments. I present comparisons of these treatments with cognitive and behavioral therapies. Although the comparison of psychoanalytic and insight-oriented therapies with cognitive or behavioral treatments is not the only comparison of interest (I would like to see comparisons between psychodynamic and humanistic therapies, for example), these are the only comparisons that have been studied empirically.

Outcome Studies

This discussion of the NIMH Collaborative Study focuses on the comparison of the cognitive-behavioral (CBT) and interpersonal (IPT) conditions. When the therapies were compared, there were no statistically significant differences between them on any of the outcome measures in any of the samples, including the criterion recovery measures and the analyses which classified patients as less or more severely depressed. The only difference between the therapies appeared in a preliminary report of the follow-up period: Fewer CBT patients than IPT patients sought additional treatment (Shea, 1990).

Covi and Lipman (1987) provided a preliminary report of results of an outcome study comparing group CBT, group CBT plus imipramine, and "the traditional interpersonal type of group psychotherapy" (p. 173) in the treatment of depressed outpatients. Treatment lasted 15 weeks. Six outcome measures were collected—three physician-rated measures (HRS-D, SCL-90, Global Improvement Scale [GIS]) and three patient-rated measures (BDI, SCL-90, GIS). Seventy subjects began treatment and 53 completed it; the treatment groups did not differ in attrition rate. Results presented in Covi and Lipman (1987) appear to be end-point analyses for a sample of 70 patients (presumably the same 70 who began the study, though this is not stated) who completed at least a minimal amount of therapy; "most of these . . . patients completed at least 1 month of group therapy (five sessions)" (p. 175).

The present discussion focuses on the comparison of CBT and psychodynamic therapy. A dramatic difference between these two groups is seen on the BDI; only 5% of psychodynamic patients (1 of 20) were nondepressed (BDI < 10) at the end of treatment, whereas 52% (14 of 27) of CBT patients met this criterion. Results for other measures, however, are less dramatic (or unavailable). The groups did not differ on the HRSD. CBT was superior to the psychodynamic treatment on one of four subscales of the physician-rated SCL-90; results for the patient-rated SCL-90 were not presented but were described as similar. No results for the physician-rated or patient-rated GIS were presented. Follow-up data were not fully presented, but there was some evidence of superiority of CBT to the psychodynamic treatment on the HRS-D and the BDI 9 months after treatment ended. This study does appear to show a superiority of CBT over psychodynamic psychotherapy; however, the preliminary nature of the report of the results tempers this conclusion.

Graff, Whitehead, and LeCompte (1986) compared CBT and "supportive insight" treatments to two control conditions (waiting-list, minimal contact) in the treatment of divorced women. Although subjects were not selected on the basis of clinical depression, mean pretreatment BDI scores were high (30.1 and 27.0 for the CBT and insight-support groups, respectively). Patients received approximately 12 hours of CBT or approximately 20 hours of insight-supportive therapy. There were four outcome measures: Eysenck neuroticism scale, BDI, Lubin Depression Checklist, and Rosenberg Self-Esteem Inventory. At posttreatment, the CBT group was superior to the insight-support group on the neuroticism scale; at 4-month follow-up, the CBT group was superior to the insight-support group on neuroticism, self-esteem, and state depression.

Gallagher and Thompson (1982) randomly assigned 30 elderly depressed patients to cognitive, behavioral, or short-term insight therapy, the cognitive treatment based on Beck, the behavioral treatment based on Lewinsohn, and the insight therapy based on Bellak and Small (1965). Patients were treated for 16 sessions over a 12-week period. Patients in all groups showed substantial benefits, and there were no differences between treatments as assessed with the HRSD, BDI, or Zung Self-Rating Depression Scale at posttreatment. However, at 1-year follow-up, both cognitive and behaviorally treated patients were superior to the insight-treated patients (on the BDI, the HRSD, and RDC criteria for major depressive disorder, but not the Zung), but not different from each other. Attrition data were not presented.

Two studies of suicidal behavior compared psychodynamic and nondirective/supportive approaches with behavioral ones. Liberman and Eckman (1981) compared behavior therapy and insight-oriented therapy in the treatment of individuals who had received medical treatment for a suicide attempt. All patients began treatment with a 10-day inpatient hospitalization. During that time, behavior therapy patients received 17 hours of social skills training, 10 hours of anxiety management training, and 5 hours of family negotiation and contingency contracting (32 hours total). Insight-oriented psychotherapy patients received 17 hours of individual psychotherapy, 10 hours of psychodrama and group therapy, and 5 hours of family therapy (32 hours total). In addition, all patients participated in the milieu treatment on the inpatient unit, which included a token economy. Upon discharge, patients were treated in a local community mental health clinic or by a private therapist of the patient's choice; this was treatment-as-usual in the community.

Outcome measures were the Zung Self-Rating Depression Scale, BDI, Fear Survey Schedule (FSS), Reinforcement Survey Schedule, an assertiveness questionnaire, and the Depression scale of the MMPI; these measures were obtained at pretreatment, posttreatment, and at 2, 6, 12, 24, and 36 weeks following discharge.

At posttreatment, behavior therapy patients were superior to insight-oriented therapy patients on all six outcome measures. The superiority of the behavior therapy treatment was largely maintained over the 9-month follow-up period. There were six outcome measures collected at each of five follow-up assessment times; the behavior therapy group showed greater improvement on 22 of the 30 assessments. Behavior therapy patients also were superior to insight-oriented patients on several follow-up measures of suicidal ideation and behavior. This study provides one of the strongest demonstrations available in the literature of the superiority of one treatment over another—in this case, the superiority of behavior therapy to insight-oriented therapy in the treatment of suicidal behavior. An important limitation of the study, as the authors acknowledge, is its small number of subjects (24 patients, 12 in each condition).

Lerner and Clum (1990) compared problem-solving therapy (based on D'Zurilla's model) and supportive therapy, which "consisted of empathic listening on the part of the therapist and the facilitation of sharing of experiences within the group" (pp. 406–407) in the treatment of suicidal adolescents. Treatments were conducted in groups which met for 10 sessions over a 5- to 7-week period. There were six outcome measures (Modified Scale for Suicidal Ideations [MSSI], Modified Means–Ends Problem-Solving Procedure [Modified MEPS], Problem-Solving Inventory [PSI], BDI, Hopelessness Scale [HS], and UCLA Loneliness Scale). The problem-solving treatment was superior to the supportive treatment on two measures (BDI, PSI) at posttreatment and on three measures (BDI, HS, UCLA Loneliness Scale) at 3-month follow-up. As the authors note, the small sample size (18 subjects completed the study) and brief follow-up period are limitations of this study.

In addition to the studies reviewed here, most of which show differences between psychodynamic/nondirective and cognitive/behavioral treatments, several other studies fail to find such differences. Hersen *et al.* (1984) found no difference between social skills training and time-limited dynamic therapy; interpretation of results from this study are complicated by the fact that all psychotherapy patients also received amitriptyline or placebo. Kornblith *et al.* (1983) found several variants of self-control therapy equal in efficacy to psychodynamic therapy. Fleming and Thornton (1980) found cognitive and behavioral group workshops to be equal to nondirective group therapy. Thompson *et al.* (1987; 2-year follow-up results reported by Gallagher-Thompson, Hanley-Peterson, and Thompson, 1990) found no differences between cognitive, behavioral, and short-term psychodynamic therapies for depressed elders. Steuer *et al.* (1984) found that cognitive-behavioral group treatment was superior to psychodynamic group treatment of depression in elderly patients. However, the effect appeared on only one of four outcome measures (BDI but not HRS-D, HRS-Anxiety, or Zung Self-Rating Depression Scale), and Steuer *et al.* argued that the superiority of the cognitive-behavioral treatment on the BDI (8.70 vs. 11.60) was statistically but not clinically significant).

Conclusions

My reading of the literature comparing cognitive-behavioral and psychodynamic/insight treatments leads me to two conclusions. First, there is some, but certainly not overwhelming, evidence of the superiority of cognitive and behavioral treatments (considered a generic class) to the traditional psychodynamic, insight-oriented treatments (also considered a generic class) (see also Dobson, 1989, who drew a similar conclusion).

Of course, considering all of the traditional psychodynamic, nondirective, insight-oriented therapies as a generic class is unsatisfying and not very informative. However, with the exception of the recently developed interpersonal therapy (IPT), there is almost no evidence of the efficacy of *any particular* psychodynamic/insight/supportive treatment. With the exception of IPT, it does not appear to be possible to locate more than one study of any particular variety of psychodynamic or insight-oriented therapy. This leads me to my second conclusion: We need more empirical work examining the efficacy of psychodynamic approaches to the treatment of depression. We need evidence about the efficacy of the traditional approaches, as well as evidence about some of the newer approaches, including those developed by Horowitz *et al.* (1984), Luborsky (1984), Strupp and Binder (1984), Weiss, Sampson, and the Mount Zion Psychotherapy Research Group (1986), and others.

Pharmacotherapy

Before psychotherapies for depression were developed (at least, before cognitive and behavioral therapies were developed and before other psychotherapies began to be empirically evaluated), a large literature had shown antidepressant medications to be more effective than no treatment (Klein & Davis, 1969; Morris & Beck, 1974). These medications were, and continue to be, widely used in the treatment of unipolar depression. For this reason, comparisons of psychotherapies with medication treatment are particularly important. If any psychotherapies can be shown to be equal to or superior to antidepressant medication—a known effective treatment—then their efficacy will be firmly established (Basham, 1986).

The only studies of this question examine interpersonal therapy or some variety of a cognitive-behavioral treatment. Of the large number of recent studies, two stand out in importance. The study comparing cognitive therapy and imipramine conducted by Rush, Beck, Kovacs and Hollon (1977) and published in the first issue of *Cognitive Therapy and Research* is historically important because it is the first to show that a psychotherapeutic approach was superior to medications. The Collaborative Study is important for its size, comprehensiveness, and recency. Following a detailed description of these two studies, some of the other studies of this question will be reviewed very briefly. A recent thoughtful review of the studies comparing cognitive therapy and pharmacotherapy was provided by Hollon *et al.* (1991).

Rush, Beck, Kovacs, and Hollon (1977)

Forty-one patients with unipolar depression were randomly assigned to 12 weeks of treatment with cognitive therapy (CT) or imipramine. CT patients received a maximum of 20 sessions. Pharmacotherapy consisted of weekly 20-min sessions for a maximum of 12 sessions; the last 2 weeks of treatment were used to taper and discontinue the medication.

Although both treatments produced significant declines in depression, patients treated with CT improved more than those treated with imipramine, as measured both by self-report (BDI) and clinician ratings (HRS-D). Fewer patients dropped out of CT (one) than pharmacotherapy (eight). Naturalistic follow-up data collected 1 year later (Kovacs, Rush, Beck, & Hollon, 1981) showed that the CT group still scored significantly lower statistically than the drug group on the BDI and the Hopelessness Scale; however, the groups did not differ on three clinician-rated scales (Hamilton Psychiatric Rating Scales for Depression and Anxiety and the Raskin Three-Area Depression Scale). Five patients in each condition sought treatment during the follow-up period, apparently not a statistically significant difference.

This study, particularly the drug treatment, has been criticized for several reasons. Dosages were low (maximum dosage was 200 mg daily); tapering the medication treatment at week 10 may have tilted results against the effectiveness of the drug treatment; and the drug patients had less therapist contact than CT patients; however, this last difference could be viewed as inherent to the treatment rather than a design flaw. Also, the study was conducted at a center for cognitive therapy, and assessors were not blind to treatment (Hollon *et al.*, 1991). Another aspect of the protocol may have had the effect of *favoring* the drug treatment. Patients were excluded from participation in the study if they reported a prior poor response to antidepressant medication—but not if they reported a prior poor response to psychotherapy. Hollon, an author of the Rush *et al.* (1977) study, recently stated, ". . . although this study is typically interpreted as suggesting an advantage for cognitive therapy over pharmacotherapy, we consider the execution of that latter modality to have been sufficiently flawed to negate this finding" (Hollon *et al.*, 1991, p. 91).

The Collaborative Study

Although the Collaborative Study showed several statistically significant differences between imipramine and placebo, it showed few differences between imipramine and either of the two psychotherapies studied (CBT and IPT). (Imipramine dose was 150–300 mg per day, and serum levels were monitored.) There were no statistically significant differences between the drug treatment and either psychotherapy treatment when outcome was examined using the four outcome measures and the criterion for recovery scores. One difference between imipramine and psychotherapy did emerge when more severely depressed patients were examined separated: Imipramine was superior to CBT in the sample of patients completing 3.5 sessions using the criterion of proportion of patients reaching a score of 6 or less on the HRSD. There were no differences between groups in attrition, but there was a difference in relapse, with CBT patients less likely to seek treatment during the follow-up period (Shea, 1990).

Other Studies

My reading of the remainder of the literature comparing psychotherapy and medication indicates that most studies show equal posttreatment outcomes when cognitive-behavioral treatments and medications are compared (Blackburn *et al.*, 1981 [in the outpatient sample]; Hersen *et al.*, 1984; Hollon *et al.*, 1992; Murphy *et al.*, 1984) and when IPT and medications are compared (DiMascio *et al.*, 1979, with 1-year follow-up data reported by Weissman *et al.*, 1981). Only two studies other than Rush *et al.* (1977) have reported that psychotherapy is superior to pharmacotherapy. Blackburn *et al.* (1981) reported that cognitive therapy was superior to pharmacotherapy in the general practice sample. However, Hollon *et al.* (1991) argue, quite convincingly, that the pharmacotherapy treatment was inadequate in this study (the response rate among general practice patients was very low [14% to 16%] compared to rates reported in most other studies [60% to 75%]). Weissman *et al.* (1981) found interpersonal therapy equal to amitriptyline at the end of 16 weeks of treatment but superior to amitriptyline on several measures of social functioning (but not on the Raskin, HRSD, GAS, or SCL-90) 1 year later.

Several studies show that cognitive therapy is more effective than pharmacotherapy at preventing relapse (Blackburn *et al.*, 1986; Evans *et al.*, 1992; Shea, 1990; Simons *et al.*, 1986). Similarly, the 1-year follow-up report of the Rush *et al.* (1977) study showed that patients treated with cognitive therapy were less depressed than patients treated with medication (Kovacs *et al.*, 1981). Recent studies suggest that the relapse-prevention effect of cognitive therapy can be achieved via prolonged medication treatment at the same dose used to treat the acute episode (Evans *et al.*, 1992; Frank *et al.*, 1990). Frank *et al.* (1990) also showed that monthly interpersonal therapy sessions following acute treatment with antidepressant medication had a relapse-prevention effect.

Outcome Parameters

For studies reviewed here, three outcome parameters are reported: posttreatment outcome, attrition, and follow-up. Although posttreatment outcome is obviously important, the other measures are important as well. If patients drop out of treatment, they are unlikely to benefit from it. If they relapse within 1 or 2 years of completing treatment, the treatment must be viewed as less effective than otherwise.

On more than one occasion, differences between treatments that were not apparent at posttreatment outcome appeared at follow-up. The most important example of this occurred in the comparison of psychotherapy and antidepressant medication. Although cognitive therapy and medication rarely differ at posttreatment, clear differences (in favor of cognitive therapy) emerge when relapse is examined.

Conclusions

This review of the outcome of psychotherapy for depression reports several major findings. First, psychotherapies were occasionally but not frequently superior to placebo, and it was disappointingly difficult to demonstrate effects of dismantling studies. My conclusion is that psychotherapies for depression need strengthening. This is particularly true for more severely depressed and chronic patients (Elkin *et al.*, 1989; Fennell & Teasdale, 1982) and for disadvantaged medical patients (Organista *et al.*, in press). I propose strengthening treatment by individualizing treatment based on a case formulation. To test the hypothesis that the case formulation approach produces a stronger treatment, the case formulation treatment could be directly compared to the standardized protocol approach currently used in outcome research (Persons, 1991).

Second, interorientation comparisons show some, but not overwhelming, evidence of superiority of cognitive-behavioral to nondirective, insight-oriented psychodynamic therapies considered as a generic class. There is a dearth of evidence examining the efficacy of the widely used insight-oriented, psychodynamic therapies in the treatment of depression.

Third, comparisons of psychotherapy and pharmacotherapy indicate that cognitive therapy and interpersonal therapy are generally equal to pharmacotherapy at posttreatment outcome; however, several studies indicate that cognitive therapy is superior in preventing relapse. There is some evidence of a small benefit to combined pharmacotherapy and psychotherapy treatment.

A final note: The studies reviewed here are controlled outcome studies conducted in research settings. The patients participating in these studies and the treatment methods used to treat them differ considerably from the patients seen by practicing clinicians and the treatment procedures utilized by these clinicians. A handful of empirical studies of the efficacy of psychotherapies as used in clinical practice have been conducted (McLean, Ogston, & Grauer, 1973; Persons, Burns, & Perloff, 1988; Teasdale, Fennell, Hibbert, & Amies, 1984), but many more are needed.

References

Basham, R. B. (1986). Scientific and practical advantages of comparative design in psychotherapy outcome research. *Journal of Consulting and Clinical Psychology, 54*, 88–94.

Beck, A. T., Hollon, S. D., Young, J. E., Bedrosian, R. C., & Budenz, D. (1985). Treatment of depression with cognitive therapy and amitriptyline. *Archives of General Psychiatry, 42*, 142–148.

Beck, A. T., Rush, A. J., Shaw, B. F., & Emery, G. (1979). *Cognitive therapy of depression.* New York: Guilford.

Bellack, L., & Small, L. (1965). *Emergency psychotherapy and brief psychotherapy.* New York: Grune & Stratton.

Blackburn, I. M., Bishop, S., Glen, A. I. M., Whalley, L. J., & Christie, J. E. (1981). The efficacy of cognitive therapy in depression: A treatment trial using cognitive therapy and pharmacotherapy, each alone and in combination. *British Journal of Psychiatry, 139*, 181–189.

Blackburn, I. M., Eunson, K. M., & Bishop, S. (1986). A two-year naturalistic follow-up of depressed patients treated with cognitive therapy, pharmacotherapy and a combination of both. *Journal of Affective Disorders, 10*, 67–75.

Conte, H. R., Plutchik, R., Wild, K. V., & Karasu, T. B. (1986). Combined psychotherapy and pharmacotherapy for depression. *Archives of General Psychiatry, 43*, 471–479.

Covi, L., & Lipman, R. S. (1987). Cognitive-behavioral group psychotherapy combined with imipramine in major depression. *Psychopharmacological Bulletin, 23*, 173–176.

de Jong, R., Treiber, R., & Henrich, G. (1986). Effectiveness of two psychological treatments for inpatients with severe and chronic depression. *Cognitive Therapy and Research, 10*, 645–663.

DiMascio, A., Weissman, M. M., Prusoff, B. A., Neu, C., Zwilling, M., & Klerman, G. L. (1979). Differential symptom reduction by drugs and psychotherapy in acute depression. *Archives of General Psychiatry, 36*, 1450–1456.

Dobson, K. S. (1989). A meta-analysis of the efficacy of cognitive therapy for depression. *Journal of Consulting and Clinical Psychology, 57*, 414–419.

D'Zurilla, T. J. (1986). *Problem-solving therapy: A social competence approach to clinical intervention.* New York: Springer.

Elkin, I., Shea, M. T., Watkins, J. T., Imber, S. D., Sotsky, S. M., Collins, J. F., Glass, D. R., Pilkonis, P. A., Leber, W. R., Docherty, J. P., Fiester, S. J., & Parloff, M. B. (1989). National Institute of Mental Health Treatment of Depression Collaborative Research Program: General effectiveness of treatments. *Archives of General Psychiatry, 46*, 971–982.

Evans, M. D., Hollon, S. D., DeRubeis, R. J., Piasecki, J. M., Grove, W. M., Garvey, M. J., & Tuason, M. D. (1992). Differential relapse following cognitive therapy and pharmacotherapy for depression. *Archives of General Psychiatry, 49*, 802–808.

Fennell, M. J. V., & Teasdale, J. D. (1982). Cognitive therapy with chronic, drug-refractory depressed outpatients: A note of caution. *Cognitive Therapy and Research, 6*, 455–460.

Fleming, B. M., & Thornton, D. W. (1980). Coping skills training as a component in the short-term treatment of depression. *Journal of Consulting and Clinical Psychology, 48*, 652–654.

Frank, E., Kupfer, D. J., Perel, J. M., Cornes, C., Jarrett, D. B., Mallinger, A. G., Thase, M. E., McEachran, A. B., Grochocinski, V. J. (1990). Three-year outcomes for maintenance therapies in recurrent depression. *Archives of General Psychiatry, 47*, 1093–1099.

Gallagher, D. E., & Thompson, L. W. (1982). Treatment of major depressive disorder in older adult outpatients with brief psychotherapies. *Psychotherapy, 19*, 482–490.

Gallagher-Thompson, D., Hanley-Peterson, P., & Thompson, L. W. (1990). Maintenance of gains versus relapse following brief psychotherapy for depression. *Journal of Consulting and Clinical Psychology, 58*, 371–374.

Graff, R. W., Whitehead, G. I., III, & LeCompte, M. (1986). Group treatment with divorced women using cognitive-behavioral and supportive-insight methods. *Journal of Counseling Psychology, 33*, 276–281.

Hersen, M., Bellack, A. S., Himmelhoch, J. M., & Thase, M. E. (1984). Effects of social skill training, amitriptyline, and psychotherapy in unipolar depressed women. *Behavior Therapy, 15*, 21–40.

Hollon, S. D., DeRubeis, R. J., Evans, M. D., Wiemer, M. J., Garvey, M. J., Grove, W. M., & Tuason, V. B. (1992). Cognitive-therapy and pharmacotherapy for depression: Singly and in combination. *Archives of General Psychiatry, 46*, 774–781.

Hollon, S. D., Shelton, R. C., & Loosen, P. T. (1991). Cognitive therapy and pharmacotherapy for depression. *Journal of Consulting and Clinical Psychology, 59*, 88–99.

Horowitz, M., Marmar, C., Krupnick, J., Wilner, N., Kaltreider, N., & Wallerstein, R. (1984). *Personality styles and brief psychotherapy*. New York: Basic Books.

Klein, D. F., & Davis, J. M. (1969). *Diagnosis and drug treatment of psychiatric disorders*. Baltimore: Williams & Wilkins.

Klerman, G. L., Weissman, M. M., Rounsaville, B. J., & Chevron, E. S. (1984). *Interpersonal psychotherapy for depression*. New York: Basic Books.

Kornblith, S. J., Rehm, L. P., O'Hara, M. W., & Lamparski, D. M. (1983). The contribution of self-reinforcement training and behavioral assignments to the efficacy of self-control therapy for depression. *Cognitive Therapy and Research, 7*, 499–528.

Kovacs, M., Rush, A. J., Beck, A. T., & Hollon, S. D. (1981). Depressed outpatients treated with cognitive therapy or pharmacotherapy. *Archives of General Psychiatry, 38*, 33–41.

Lerner, M. S., & Clum, G. A. (1990). Treatment of suicide ideators: A problem-solving approach. *Behavior Therapy, 21*, 403–411.

Lewinsohn, P. M., Hoberman, T., & Hautzinger, M. (1985). An integrative theory of depression. In S. Reiss & R. Bootzin (Eds.), *Theoretical issues in behavior therapy*. New York: Academic Press.

Liberman, R. P., & Eckman, T. (1981). Behavior therapy vs. insight-oriented therapy for repeated suicide attempters. *Archives of General Psychiatry, 38*, 1126–1130.

Luborsky, L. (1984). *Principles of psychoanalytic psychotherapy: A manual for supportive-expressive treatment*. New York: Basic Books.

McLean, P. D., & Hakstian, A. R. (1979). Clinical depression: Comparative efficacy of outpatient treatments. *Journal of Consulting and Clinical Psychology, 47*, 818–836.

McLean, P. D., & Hakstian, A. R. (1990). Relative endurance of unipolar depression treatment effects: Longitudinal follow-up. *Journal of Consulting and Clinical Psychology, 58*, 482–488.

McLean, P. D., Ogston, K., & Grauer, L. (1973). A behavioral approach to the treatment of depression. *Journal of Behavior Therapy and Experimental Psychiatry, 4*, 323–330.

McKnight, D. L., Nelson, R. O., Hayes, S. C., & Jarrett, R. B. (1984). Importance of treating individually assessed response classes in the amelioration of depression. *Behavior Therapy, 15*, 315–335.

Miller, I. W., Norman, W. H., & Keitner, G. I. (1989). Cognitive-behavioral treatment of depressed inpatients: Six- and twelve-month followup. *American Journal of Psychiatry, 146*, 1274–1279.

Miller, I. W., Norman, W. H., Keitner, G. I., Bishop, S. B., & Dow, M. G. (1989). Cognitive-behavioral treatment of depressed inpatients. *Behavior Therapy, 20*, 25–47.

Miller, R. C., & Berman, J. S. (1983). The efficacy of cognitive behavior therapies: A quantitative review of the research evidence. *Psychological Bulletin, 94*, 39–53.

Miranda, J. (1992, June). *Treatment of depression in disadvantaged medical patients.* Paper presented at meetings of Society for Psychotherapy Research, Berkeley, CA.

Morris, J. B., & Beck, A. T. (1974). The efficacy of antidepressant drugs: A review of research (1958–1972). *Archives of General Psychiatry, 30,* 667–674.

Murphy, G. E., Simons, A. D., Wetzel, R. D., & Lustman, P. J. (1984). Cognitive therapy and pharmacotherapy. *Archives of General Psychiatry, 41,* 33–41.

Murphy, J. M., Monson, R. R. Olivier, D. C., Sobol, A. M., & Leighton, A. H. (1987). Affective disorders and mortality. *Archives of General Psychiatry, 44,* 473–480.

National Institute of Mental Health/National Institutes of Health (NIMH/NIH). (1985). Mood disorders: Pharmacological prevention of recurrences. *American Journal of Psychiatry, 142,* 469–476.

Nezu, A. M. (1986). Efficacy of a social problem-solving therapy approach for unipolar depression. *Journal of Consulting and Clinical Psychology, 54,* 196–202.

Nezu, A. M., & Perri, M. G. (1989). Social problem-solving therapy for unipolar depression: An initial dismantling investigation. *Journal of Consulting and Clinical Psychology, 57,* 408–413.

Organista, K. C., Munoz, R., & Gonzalez, G. (in press). Cognitive-behavioral therapy for depression in low-income and minority medical patients: Description of a program and exploratory analysis. *Cognitive Therapy and Research.*

Persons, J. B. (1991). Psychotherapy outcome studies do not accurately represent current models of psychotherapy: A proposed remedy. *American Psychologist, 46,* 99–106.

Persons, J. B., Burns, D. D., & Perloff, J. M. (1988). Predictors of dropout and outcome in cognitive therapy for depression in a private practice setting. *Cognitive Therapy and Research, 12,* 557–575.

Rehm, L. P. (1977). A self-control model of depression. *Behavior Therapy, 8,* 787–804.

Rehm, L. P., Kaslow, N. J., & Rabin, A. S. (1987). Cognitive and behavioral targets in a self-control therapy program for depression. *Journal of Consulting and Clinical Psychology, 55,* 60–67.

Rehm, L. P., & Kornblith, S. J. (1979). Behavior therapy for depression: A review of recent developments. In M. Hersen, R. M. Eisler, & P. M. Miller (Eds.), *Progress in behavior modification* (Vol. 7). New York: Academic Press.

Rehm, L. P., Kornblith, S. J., O'Hara, M. W., Lamparski, D. M., Romano, J. M., & Volkin, J. (1981). An evaluation of major components in a self-control behavior therapy program for depression. *Behavior Modification, 5,* 459–489.

Reynolds, W. M., & Coats, K. I. (1986). A comparison of cognitive-behavioral therapy and relaxation training for the treatment of depression in adolescents. *Journal of Consulting and Clinical Psychology, 54,* 653–660.

Roth, D., Bielski, R., Jones, M., Parker, W., & Osborn, G. (1982). A comparison of self-control therapy and combined self-control therapy and antidepressant medication in the treatment of depression. *Behavior Therapy, 13,* 133–144.

Rude, S. S. (1986). Relative benefits of assertion or cognitive self-control treatment for depression as a function of proficiency in each domain. *Journal of Consulting and Clinical Psychology, 54,* 390–394.

Rush, A. J., Beck, A. T., Kovacs, M., & Hollon, S. (1977). Comparative efficacy of cognitive therapy and pharmacotherapy in the treatment of depressed outpatients. *Cognitive Therapy and Research, 1,* 17–38.

Secunda, S. K., Katz, M., Friedman, R., & Schuler, D. (1973). *Special report: The depressive disorders* (National Institute of Mental Health). Washington, DC: U.S. Government Printing Office.

Shaw, B. F. (1977). Comparison of cognitive therapy and behavior therapy in the treatment of depression. *Journal of Consulting and Clinical Psychology, 45,* 543–551.

Shea, M. T. (1990, June). *NIMH Treatment of Depression Collaborative Research Program: Followup findings.* Paper presented at the meeting of the Society for Psychotherapy Research, Wintergreen, VA.

Simons, A. D., Levine, J. L., Lustman, P. J., & Murphy, G. E. (1984). Patient attrition in a comparative outcome study of depression. *Journal of Affective Disorders, 6,* 163–173.

Simons, A. D., Murphy, G. E., Levine, J. L., & Wetzel, R. D. (1986). Cognitive therapy and pharmacotherapy for depression. *Archives of General Psychiatry, 43,* 43–48.

Steuer, J. L., Mintz, J., Hammen, C. L., Hill, M. A., Jarvik, L. F., McCarley, T., Motoike, P., & Rosen, R. (1984). Cognitive-behavioral and psychodynamic group psychotherapy in treatment of geriatric depression. *Journal of Consulting and Clinical Psychology, 52,* 180–189.

Strupp, H. H., & Binder, J. L. (1984). *Psychotherapy in a new key: A guide to time-limited dynamic psychotherapy.* New York: Basic Books.

Taylor, F. G., & Marshall, W. L. (1977). Experimental analysis of a cognitive-behavioral therapy for depression. *Cognitive Therapy and Research, 1,* 59–72.

Teasdale, J. D., Fennell, M. J. V., Hibbert, G. A., & Amies, P. L. (1984). Cognitive therapy for major depressive disorder in primary care. *British Journal of Psychiatry, 144*, 400–406.

Thompson, L. W., Gallagher, D., & Breckenridge, J. S. (1987). Comparative effectiveness of psychotherapies for depressed elders. *Journal of Consulting and Clinical Psychology, 55*, 385–390.

Weiss, J., Sampson, H., & the Mount Zion Psychotherapy Research Group. (1986). *The psychoanalytic process: Theory, clinical observation and empirical research.* New York: Guilford.

Weissman, M. M., Klerman, G. L., Prusoff, B. A., Sholomskas, D., & Padian, N. (1981). Depressed outpatients: Results one year after treatment with drugs and/or interpersonal psychotherapy. *Archives of General Psychiatry, 38*, 51–55.

Wells, K. B., Stewart, A., Hays, R. D., Burnam, M. A., Rogers, W., Daniels, M., Berry, S., Greenfield, S., & Ware, J. (1989). The functioning and well-being of depressed patients: Results from the Medical Outcomes Study. *Journal of the American Medical Association, 262*, 914–919.

Wilson, P. H. (1982). Combined pharmacological and behavioural treatment of depression. *Behaviour Research and Therapy, 20*, 173–184.

14

Efficacy of Psychotherapy for Schizophrenia

Kim T. Mueser and Shirley M. Glynn

Introduction

Schizophrenia is one of the most debilitating adult mental illnesses. More psychiatric hospital beds are occupied by persons with schizophrenia than any other psychiatric disorder, and the illness accounts for the majority of admissions to psychiatric hospitals. Over the past 35 years, significant gains have been made in both the pharmacological and psychosocial treatment of schizophrenia. Despite these gains, the effects of the illness continue to be pervasive and chronic. The limited efficacy of currently available treatments for schizophrenia is illustrated by the high rate of relapse for outpatients living in the community and the poor social functioning of most patients. Because schizophrenia tends to be a socially impairing and chronic illness, even in patients who receive optimal treatment, distinguishing effective from ineffective treatments can be difficult in clinical practice. For this reason, it is vital for clinical decision making to be guided by the results of appropriately controlled and executed outcome studies that examine the efficacy of various treatment approaches. The present chapter evaluates the evidence supporting the effectiveness of different types of psychotherapeutic treatment for schizophrenia in order to aid clinicians in selecting interventions with the most promise. Prior to reviewing the treatment outcome research on schizophrenia, an overview of the illness is provided and a conceptual model for guiding treatment is described.

Kim T. Mueser • Department of Psychiatry, Medical College of Pennsylvania at Eastern Pennsylvania Psychiatric Institute, Philadelphia, Pennsylvania 19129. **Shirley M. Glynn** • West Los Angeles VA Medical Center (Brentwood Division) and University of California, Los Angeles, Los Angeles, California 90073.

Handbook of Effective Psychotherapy, edited by Thomas R. Giles. Plenum Press, New York, 1993.

Overview of Schizophrenia

Prevalence, Onset, and Course of Illness

The lifetime prevalence of schizophrenia in the general population is approximately 1%. The illness usually develops in late adolescence or early adulthood, between the ages of 16 and 30 years old. Childhood onset of schizophrenia before the age of 10 is rare, as is its emergence after age 35. Once a person has developed schizophrenia, the course of the illness is usually chronic across the adult life span, with gradual improvements, and in some cases total remissions, later in life (Ciompi, 1980; Harding, Brooks, Ashikaga, Strauss, & Breier, 1987). Females tend to have a later onset and a more benign course of schizophrenia than males (Angermeyer & Kuhn, 1988).

The causes of schizophrenia are unknown, but current theories suggest the illness is biological in nature and that environmental stress contributes to the onset of symptoms and symptom relapses (Liberman & Mueser, 1989). There is evidence that the vulnerability to schizophrenia is influenced by genetic factors (Holzman & Matthysse, 1990), but most individuals who develop the illness have no afflicted family members.

Symptomatology

Schizophrenia usually develops over a period of several months to a few years, during which time *prodromal symptoms* appear, such as social withdrawal, decreased spontaneity and interests, and perceptual and cognitive aberrations. Frequently, even before the onset of prodromal symptoms, the preschizophrenic person has poorer premorbid social and sexual adjustment than others (Zigler & Glick, 1986). Once the illness has fully developed there is a wide range of symptoms that may be present at varying levels of severity, including negative, positive, and affective symptoms.

Negative symptoms are defined by the absence or paucity of behaviors, mood states, or cognitions ordinarily present in healthy individuals. Common negative symptoms include blunted (or flattened) affect, alogia (reduced amount of speech or poverty of content), emotional withdrawal, apathy, social withdrawal, attention impairment, and motor and psychomotor retardation. Severe negative symptoms are strongly associated with poor social functioning and are weakly related to social skill deficits (Bellack, Morrison, Wixted, & Mueser, 1990). These symptoms are relatively stable over time (Lewine, 1990; Mueser, Douglas, Bellack, & Morrison, 1991). Despite overlap between some negative symptoms and depression (e.g., decreased interests), prominent negative symptoms occur in schizophrenia independent of depression. While each of the negative symptoms can have a particularly pernicious effect on outcome, attentional impairments are especially insidious and may require systematic modifications of psychotherapeutic techniques. Patients who evidence severe deficits in attention and concentration often have difficulty with more abstract reasoning, and thus may be especially poor candidates for cognitive or psychodynamic therapies, which rely more heavily on conceptualization and/or interpretation.

Positive symptoms, in contrast to negative symptoms, are defined as the presence of thoughts or behaviors that are ordinarily absent in healthy persons.

The most common positive symptoms include hallucinations and delusions. Examples of other positive symptoms are loose associations, word salad, stereotypical behaviors, mannerisms, and posturing. Positive symptoms are less stable than negative symptoms over time, and exacerbations of positive symptoms frequently require rehospitalizations for acute treatment. Because relapses of positive symptoms are associated with a marked worsening in social functioning and negative symptoms, lowering patients' vulnerability to relapses of positive symptoms is an important goal of pharmacological and psychotherapeutic interventions for schizophrenia.

In addition to negative and positive symptoms, affective symptoms such as depression, anxiety, and anger are common in schizophrenia. Most patients experience bouts of severe depression, which often presage relapses (Ventura, Nuechterlein, Lukoff, & Hardesty, 1989). Approximately 50% of schizophrenics attempt suicide at some time during their lives, with a 10% rate or mortality (Roy, 1986). Affective symptoms in schizophrenia tend to be related to high levels of unremitting positive symptoms (Mueser, Douglas *et al.*, 1991) and lead patients to develop personal coping strategies to manage these distressful experiences (Falloon & Talbot, 1981).

Stress–Vulnerability–Coping Skills Model of Schizophrenia

A variety of different stress–vulnerability models have been proposed to account for the episodic course of schizophrenia (Ciompi, 1987). These models share the basic assumptions that the presence and severity of schizophrenic symptoms are the result of the combined influences of *psychobiological vulnerability* and *environmental stress*. Biological vulnerability is believed to be determined early in life by genetic and other biological factors, although substance abuse may increase vulnerability to psychosis. Environmental stressors, such as life events (e.g., the death of a significant other), exposure to high levels of negative ambient emotion (i.e., "expressed emotion"; Parker & Hadzi-Pavlovic, 1990), and lack of meaningful structure impinge on vulnerability to increase risk of relapse and rehospitalization. *Coping skills* (e.g., social skills) serve to reduce the noxiousness of stressors on the individual, thereby lowering vulnerability to stress-induced relapses (Liberman & Mueser, 1989).

There are several implications of the stress–vulnerability model for the treatment of schizophrenia. Generally, the model suggests that the outcome of the illness can be improved by either reducing vulnerability, reducing environmental stress, or enhancing coping skills. Most currently available treatments for schizophrenia share one or more of these goals. Thus, biological vulnerability can be lessened by providing antipsychotic medications and decreasing substance abuse. Family interventions have been developed with the primary aim of reducing environmental stress. Individual treatment approaches, such as social skills training, tend to focus mainly on improving patients' coping skills.

The Assessment of Outcome

The symptoms of schizophrenia vary widely across different individuals, but all patients experience problems initiating and maintaining meaningful interpersonal relationships, meeting socially defined roles (e.g., student, homemaker, wage earner), and maintaining self-care skills (e.g., grooming and hygiene). In order to evaluate the efficacy of treatments for schizophrenia, assessments need to be conducted across the different domains of functioning typically impaired by the illness (Avison & Speechley, 1987; Strauss & Carpenter, 1972). These domains, and representative instruments used to measure them, are briefly reviewed below.

Symptomatology and Relapses

Symptomatology is most commonly assessed using semistructured interviews such as the Brief Psychiatric Rating Scale (Overall & Gorham, 1962), the Scale for the Assessment of Negative Symptoms (Andreasen & Olsen, 1982), and the Positive and Negative Syndrome Scale (Kay, Fiszbein, & Opler, 1987). While affective symptoms can be assessed via interviews with the patient, self-report scales (e.g., Symptom Checklist-90; Derogatis, 1977) are also useful, and they have the advantage of avoiding possible rating confounds due to blunted affect or discrepancies between patient verbal report and behavioral presentation.

Many treatment studies of schizophrenia have focused solely on comparing the cumulative relapse rates of psychotic symptoms across different interventions. Relapse is usually defined as either the reemergence of psychotic symptoms in a person who was previously free of those symptoms, or a significant worsening of symptoms in a continuously symptomatic person. While reliance on relapse rates alone as a measure of the outcome of schizophrenia has been criticized as too narrow (Falloon, 1984), it does provide a useful index of the course of psychotic symptoms. Relapses of psychotic symptoms frequently require rehospitalizations, but there is an imperfect relationship between relapse and rehospitalization. Some relapses can be treated effectively on an outpatient basis, especially when they are detected rapidly. Rehospitalizations can occur in response to situational crises, such as housing instability, even when there has not been a symptom relapse. Thus, the amount of time spent in the hospital is an important outcome measure related to relapse rate.

Social Adjustment and Quality of Life

Social adjustment refers to the patient's ability to meet role expectations, whereas quality of life is the subjective enjoyment of different aspects of living (e.g., leisure activities, living situation). Social adjustment can be most reliably measured with a structured interview with the patient and/or significant other (e.g., the Social Adjustment Scale-II; Schooler, Hogarty, & Weissman, 1979) or, when the patient is in the hospital or a supervised living arrangement, with behavioral observations (e.g., Social Performance Schedule; Wykes & Sturt, 1986). Vocational functioning is an important consideration for those patients who are able to sustain sheltered, part-time, or full-time employment. Both the ability of patients to perform a job, including volunteer work, and the number of days worked are relevant measures of vocational functioning.

Many schizophrenic persons' quality of life is particularly poor. Substandard or no housing, limited access to medical care, poor nutrition, few friendships, and limited finances would be expected to take a heavy toll on any person; concurrent psychiatric difficulties only compound the situation. Quality of life, which might best be conceptualized as the individual's satisfaction with the life he or she is living, is an important, but too often neglected, outcome measure in intervention research with the seriously psychiatrically ill. Few treatment studies to date have reported data on subjective assessments of quality of life, although the recent publication of a scale (Lehman, 1988) to assess this construct may help remedy this situation.

Treatment of Schizophrenia

Pharmacological Treatment

The discovery of antipsychotic medications almost 40 years ago revolutionized the treatment of schizophrenia, enabling the majority of patients to be treated as outpatients in the community. Numerous double-blind controlled studies have been conducted that attest to the efficacy of antipsychotic medications for schizophrenic patients. Antipsychotics serve two primary purposes in the treatment of schizophrenia. First, they reduce acute symptoms that appear during an exacerbation, including both positive and negative symptoms (Meltzer, 1985). Second, the prophylactic administration of antipsychotics after a relapse lowers the probability of subsequent relapses by 30–60% (Davis, 1975; Kane, 1989). Recent research indicates that very low dosages of antipsychotic medication are effective at lowering risk of relapse (Van Putten & Marder, 1986), suggesting that patients' vulnerability to long-term side effects of these medications (e.g., tardive dyskinesia) can be reduced. Furthermore, recent advances in the development of atypical antipsychotic medications (e.g., clozapine) hold promise for improving the functioning of patients who are treatment refractory to the standard antipsychotics (Meltzer, 1990). Nevertheless, the antipsychotics are not a cure for schizophrenia, and significant residual symptoms usually persist between episodes, resulting in severe impairments in social functioning. For these reasons, antipsychotic medications are a mainstay in all treatment programs for schizophrenia, but there is still a great need for effective psychotherapeutic interventions that impact on the pervasive deficits of schizophrenia.

Comprehensive Treatment

The multiple impairments of schizophrenia necessitate a range of different services. In the absence of other interventions, psychotherapy cannot have a lasting impact on the course of the illness. Therefore, research on the efficacy of psychotherapy needs to be conducted in the context of a comprehensive treatment program for schizophrenia. Bellack and Mueser (1986) have proposed that the comprehensive intervention in schizophrenia requires the provision of three types of integrated services: treatment (e.g., medication, psychotherapy), rehabilitation (e.g., job skills training), and social services (e.g., income, housing).

Methodological Requirements for Psychotherapy Research

Many studies have been conducted on the effects of psychotherapy for schizophrenia. However, relatively little research has met the methodological requirements for psychotherapy outcome research in schizophrenia, including diagnostic assessment, assignment of patients to treatment groups, and assessment of domains of functioning.

Diagnostic Assessment

In order to demonstrate the effects of a particular form of psychotherapy for schizophrenia, a standardized assessment instrument must be used to verify that the patients have the illness. Prior to DSM-III, diagnostic criteria for schizophrenia were highly subjective and lacked clear behavioral definitions of symptoms, resulting in poor reliability between different diagnosticians. As more objective diagnostic systems have emerged, standardized structured interviews have been validated to assure high reliability in diagnosis (Matarazzo, 1983). The most widely used instruments are the Structured Clinical Interview for DSM-III-R (Spitzer & Williams, 1985), the Schedule for Affective Disorders and Schizophrenia (Endicott & Spitzer, 1978), and the Present State Examination (Wing, Cooper, & Sartorius, 1974). Use of a standardized instrument to establish a diagnosis of schizophrenia is an important consideration when evaluating outcome research on the treatment of schizophrenia.

Assignment to Treatment Groups

Many different psychotherapeutic techniques for schizophrenia have been developed and refined using single-case study designs, including both behavioral and psychodynamic approaches. The close scrutiny of individual cases permits a more detailed analysis of changes in constructs which are hypothesized to underlie improvements in functioning (e.g., increases in deficient social skills are postulated to result from social skills training). However, single-case reports are less useful for demonstrating the effects of treatment on other aspects of functioning in schizophrenia, such as social adjustment, which has a highly variable course in untreated patients. Group design studies that randomly assign patients to treatment groups provide the most valuable information on the efficacy of psychotherapy for schizophrenia. Nonrandom assignment of patients to treatments is problematic because patient selection factors can bias the results in favor of or against the intervention.

Assessment of Domains of Functioning

In order to evaluate different psychotherapy approaches for schizophrenia, relevant domains of functioning need to be assessed, including social and vocational adjustment, symptomatology, subjective quality of life, and time spent in the hospital. To demonstrate the efficacy of an intervention, it is not sufficient to show that patients improve in theoretical constructs related to the treatment technique (e.g., social skill, ego strength). Rather, it must be shown that the treatment results in better functioning in commonly accepted outcome measures (e.g., symptoms, social adjustment, etc.).

Individual and Group Psychotherapy Approaches

The effectiveness of a variety of different individual and group psychotherapies for schizophrenia has been studied, with the majority of research devoted to psychodynamic or behavioral methods. We review here data supporting the efficacy of these interventions, with a primary emphasis on the controlled studies.

Psychodynamic Treatments

The psychodynamic treatment of schizophrenia has had a long and controversial history. While Freud and his more orthodox followers believed that schizophrenics were not suitable for psychoanalysis, there are many others who have strongly advocated for psychodynamic treatment (e.g., Fromm-Reichmann, 1950; Pao, 1979; Rosen, 1947; Searles, 1965). Psychodynamic theories have played an important role in the clinical conceptualization of schizophrenia throughout the twentieth century and continue to serve as an impetus to research in this area (e.g., Silverman & Lachmann, 1985). For decades psychodynamic psychotherapy was the dominant treatment approach, but recent evidence has questioned the efficacy of this intervention for schizophrenia (May, 1968, 1984). Psychodynamic treatment continues to be a common, but not dominant, intervention for schizophrenia, even in the absence of data supporting its efficacy (Mueser & Berenbaum, 1990).

Controlled Studies. Four controlled studies have examined the efficacy of psychodynamic therapy for schizophrenia (Grinspoon, Ewalt, & Shader, 1972; Gunderson *et al.*, 1984; Karon & VandenBos, 1972, 1975; May, 1968; Stanton *et al.*, 1984). The methodological characteristics of these studies and their results are summarized in Table 14.1.

Three of the four studies found no benefits of psychodynamic therapy, when given either alone or in combination with antipsychotic medication (Grinspoon *et al.*, 1972; Gunderson *et al.*, 1984; May, 1968). Grinspoon's study was unique in that the study population consisted of chronic inpatient schizophrenics. While no positive effects of psychodynamic treatment were found by Grinspoon, problems with the nonrandom assignment of patients to treatment groups limit the conclusions that can be reached about this study. In contrast to Grinspoon *et al.* (1972), May's study was conducted on first-admission schizophrenics, although the results also failed to support the efficacy of psychodynamic treatment. May's (1968) study was methodologically sound, although the inexperience of the psychotherapists has been criticized by Karon and VandenBos (1970; but cf. Tuma & May, 1974).

The Gunderson and Stanton collaborative study (Gunderson *et al.*, 1984; Stanton *et al.*, 1984) was unique in that it used only experienced therapists to provide the psychodynamic treatment, and it compared that treatment with an alternative treatment: "reality-adaptive supportive therapy." There was a consistent pattern of results favoring the reality-adaptive therapy over psychodynamic treatment. Patients who received the former treatment had lower rates of rehospitalization, as well as superior vocational adjustment, and, to a lesser extent, better social functioning than psychodynamically treated patients. There were no differences between the groups in symptomatology over the 2-year treatment period. The only methodological limitation of this study was the absence of a standard treatment, medication-only control group. Since the effectiveness of neither psychodynamic nor reality-adaptive therapy is known, the lack of a control group leaves open the question as to the effectiveness of either treatment compared to no psychosocial treatment.

Table 14.1. Characteristics and Results of Controlled Psychodynamic Treatment Studies[a]

	May (1968)	Karon & VandenBos (1972, 1975)	Grinspoon *et al.* (1972)	Gunderson *et al.* (1984)
Random assignment	Yes[b]	Yes	No[c]	Yes
Number of prior hospitalizations	0	0.3	27	0.9
Treatment groups (*N*)	PD (46) PD-D (44) D (48) M (43) ECT (47)	PD (12)[d] PD-D (12) D (12)	PD (10) PD-D (10) D (21)	PD-D (43) RAS-D (52)
Frequency and duration of treatment	2 hrs/wk for 1 yr	PD: 5 hrs/wk then 1 hr/wk for 20 months PD-D: 3 hrs/wk then 1 hr/wk for 20 months	2 hrs/wk for 2 yrs	PD-D 2 hrs/wk for 2 yrs RAS-D 0.6 hrs/wk for 2 yrs
Symptomatology	D = PD-D > ECT > PD = M	PD ≥ PD-D > D	D = PD-D > PD	RAS-D = PD-D
Relapse or rehospitalization	D = PD-D = ECT > PD = M	For experienced therapists: PD = PD-D > D For inexperienced therapists: PD > PD-D = D		RAS-D > PD-D
Social adjustment			D = PD-D > PD	RAS-D ≥ PD-D
Vocational adjustment				RAS-D > PD-D
Methodological weaknesses	Inexperienced therapists	Only 2 experienced therapists Nonrandom assignment to experienced or inexperienced therpists Drug-only group transferred to different hospital	Nonrandom assignment to treatment groups Drug-only treatment given in different environment Patients very chronic	High dropout rate (42%) Absence of drug-only control group

Note. PD = psychodynamic; D = drugs; PD-D = psychodynamic plus drugs; RAS = reality-adaptive, supportive psychotherapy. ECT = Electroconvulsive Therapy; M = Milieu Therapy.

[a]For further methodological details on these studies, see Mueser and Berenbaum (1990).

[b]Patients were randomly assigned to PD, PD-D, and D groups, but were not randomly assigned to experienced or inexperienced therapists.

[c]Patients in the D group were those who elected to remain at the state hospital and were compared with the PD and PD-D groups, which were composed of those patients who consented to be transferred to a clinical research center for treatment.

[d]The PD group was treated with active psychoanalytic psychotherapy, whereas PD-D was treated with ego-analytic psychoanalytic psychotherapy.

The study by Karon and VandenBos (1972, 1975) reported the astounding result that psychodynamic treatment, both with and without drugs, was superior to treatment with antipsychotic medications alone. A complex interaction was also found between therapist experience and outcome, with concomitant medication interfering with the effects of psychodynamic therapy for inexperienced, but not experienced, therapists. However, several methodological flaws limit the generalizability of these results. First, patients receiving the drug-only treatment were transferred to another hospital, which could have resulted in less effective pharmacological or case management than patients who received therapy. Second, there was a confound between therapist experience and treatment modality. Half of the patients who received only psychodynamic treatment were treated by one experienced therapist, and half of the patients who received psychodynamic treatment with drugs were treated by a different experienced therapist, with the remaining patients receiving treatment from inexperienced therapists. Thus, the interaction between therapist experience and concomitant pharmacological treatment may simply reflect differences between these therapists, rather than the therapist experience. Furthermore, the type of psychodynamic treatment differed between the no-drug group ("active psychoanalytic psychotherapy") and the drug group ("ego-analytic psychoanalytic psychotherapy"). Overall, it is impossible to determine whether the positive results of this study resulted from differences in treatment facilities, therapists, or psychodynamic treatment approaches.

Naturalistic Studies. Two naturalistic reports have described the results of long-term psychodynamic treatment for large samples of schizophrenic patients. Stone (1986) followed up 72 schizophrenics who had received an average of 12.3 months of intensive psychodynamic therapy at the New York State Psychiatric Institute. Ten to twenty years later, more than half of these patients were substantially dysfunctional, and 20% had committed suicide, approximately twice the rate of suicide in the population of schizophrenics (Drake & Cotton, 1986).

McGlashan (1984a, 1984b) reported on the outcomes of schizophrenic patients treated at Chestnut Lodge, a long-term private residential facility that specializes in psychoanalytic treatment. Of 163 patients treated at the Lodge over an average of 3 years, two-thirds were functioning marginally or worse 15 years later. The apparent failure of this group of patients to benefit from intensive psychoanalytic treatment led McGlashan to conclude that with respect to psychotherapy for schizophrenia, "Unfortunately, we still have not improved much on Kraepelin's work" (McGlashan, 1984b, p. 600).

Evaluation of Psychodynamic Treatments. In summary, neither the controlled outcome studies of psychodynamic psychotherapy nor naturalistic research on its long-term effects provide much support for its efficacy in schizophrenia. The only study that found positive effects for psychodynamic treatment was that of Karon and VandenBos (1972, 1975), whose sample size was relatively small (12 patients per group), and whose study design contained significant methodological flaws. The replicability of the results obtained by Karon and VandenBos are also dubious considering the failure of any additional supportive data from controlled studies to be published in the 20 years since this study was conducted.

The negative results of most studies of psychodynamic treatment for schizophrenia raise the intriguing question of whether this approach can have deleterious effects on this population. Strupp, Hadley, and Gomes-Schwartz (1977) have pointed out that psychotherapy can have negative, rather than positive, effects. Drake and Sedere (1986) have reviewed research indicating that intensive treatments can have a harmful impact on the course of schizophrenia. Stone (1986) has suggested that psychodynamic psychotherapy can harm schizophrenics by exposing them to memories and insights that they are unable to handle emotionally. The high suicide rate in the naturalistic study conducted by Stone (1986) is in line with this hypothesis, although the lack of a control group limits the conclusions that can be drawn about the study. In Gunderson *et al.*'s (1984) collaborative study, the amount of time that patients remained in psychodynamic treatment tended to be *negatively* correlated with outcome (i.e., patients who received *more* treatment did poorly), in contrast to time spent in reality-adaptive, supportive therapy, which was positively correlated with outcome. While these data only raise the possibility that psychodynamic psychotherapy can have a negative impact on schizophrenia, they are generally supportive of other research that indicates that this approach has not been demonstrated to be efficacious.

Social Learning Theory Interventions

Since the publication of Ayllon and Azrin's (1968) seminal book on the token economy for chronic psychiatric patients, there has been a proliferation of social learning-based treatments for schizophrenia. Most early social learning interventions for schizophrenia were based on the token economy (for a review, see Glynn, 1990), but by the 1970s social skills training had become the focus of extensive research. The token economy appears to be the treatment of choice for chronic, treatment-refractory inpatients (Paul & Lentz, 1977). However, most schizophrenics require outpatient interventions that can be provided on a group or individual basis, such as social skills training.

Social Skills Training. The fundamental premise of social skills training is that the social impairments of schizophrenia can be rectified through systematically teaching the behavioral components of social skill (e.g., appropriate voice tone and loudness, gaze, verbal content). Teaching is conducted through a combination of therapist modeling (i.e., demonstration of the skill), patient behavioral rehearsal (i.e., role playing), positive and corrective feedback, and homework assignments to program generalization of the skill to the natural environment. Targeted social skills span a wide range of adaptive interpersonal and self-care behaviors, including the expression of feelings, conflict resolution skills, and medication management. While social skills training has been applied extensively to schizophrenics, the social skills model makes no specific assumptions about the origins of skill deficits, and the approach has been used with a variety of clinical populations (Liberman, DeRisi, & Mueser, 1989).

As the lack of efficacy of psychodynamic treatments for schizophrenia has become recognized, the role of social skills training as a viable alternative has grown. A survey conducted by Taylor and Dowell (1986) indicated that over 50% of board-and-care homes for chronic mental patients provide social skills training to their clients. Unfortunately, this same survey also found that most board-and-care operators had a poor understanding of the principles of social skills training. It is likely that many treatment settings claiming to conduct social skills training fail to adhere to the core ingredients of treatment, including demonstration, behavioral rehearsal, feedback, and homework. Nevertheless, the body of research on social skills training has grown in recent years, and evidence suggests that this approach may be beneficial for schizophrenia.

Research on Social Skills Training. Many studies have been published on social skills training with schizophrenics and other patients with chronic psychiatric disorders. Methodological limitations, such as lack of random assignment of patients to treatment groups, inadequate diagnostic information on patients, and failure to attend to concomitant medications, plagued much of the early research on social skills training. Some studies have aimed primarily at determining whether patients with schizophrenia are capable of acquiring and maintaining new social skills, but have not examined the effects of skills training on other domains of functioning in schizophrenia. Despite these limitations, extensive research on social skills training has converged on several results regarding the feasibility and effects of training with schizophrenics (Benton & Schroeder, 1990; Donahoe & Driesenga, 1988; Halford & Hays, 1991):

1. Schizophrenics can be taught a wide range of social skills, including skills for initiating and maintaining conversations, making friends, expressing feelings, assertiveness, conflict resolution, and medication management.
2. There is limited evidence suggesting that patients can transfer social skills taught in the training setting to the natural environment. However, the amount of skill generalization is limited by the complexity of the targeted skill and the degree of cognitive impairment present in the patient.
3. Patients who receive social skills training usually experience reductions in anxiety in social situations.
4. Social skills training can be successfully conducted in a variety of settings (e.g., inpatient, day treatment programs, community rehabilitation residences), either individually or in groups, for brief or long periods of time (i.e., durations ranging from 2 weeks to 2 years), by a number of different professionals and paraprofessionals (e.g., psychologists, nurses, psychiatric aids, activities therapists).

In short, extensive experience with social skills training indicates that it can readily be delivered to schizophrenic patients.

Despite the positive results of studies that demonstrate learning effects from social skills training and the feasibility of the treatment, less controlled research has been conducted on the effects of skills training on social adjustment and symptomatology in schizophrenia (e.g., social functioning, symptoms). Ultimately, the efficacy of an psychotherapeutic intervention must be determined by its ability to improve those impairments most characteristic of schizophrenia. The studies most relevant to the clinical efficacy of social skills training are reviewed below.

Controlled Outcome Research on Social Skills Training. Three controlled studies have been conducted on social skills training for schizophrenic patients that have assessed the impact of treatment on social adjustment, symptomatology, and/or relapse. Each study employed careful diagnostic assessments using semistructured interviews, an improvement over most previous studies on social skills training. The methodological characteristics of these studies and their results are summarized in Table 14.2.

Bellack, Turner, Hersen, and Luber (1984) examined the efficacy of skills training in a group of schizophrenic patients who had recently received inpatient treatment for an acute symptom exacerbation. All patients participated in a day treatment program, with a subsample of patients randomly assigned to additional social skills training conducted three times per week for 3 months. The results of the study indicated that 6 months after the initiation of treatment, patients who received skills training had maintained their improvements in symptomatology

Table 14.2. Characteristics and Results of Controlled Social Skills Training Studies

	Bellack *et al.* (1984)	Liberman *et al.* (1986)	Hogarty *et al.* (1986, 1987, 1991)
Random assignment	Yes	Yes	Yes
Number of prior hospitalizations	4.9	?	2.7
Treatment groups (*N*)	SST (29)[a] C (14)	SST (14)[b] HHT (14)	SST (23)[c] FP (22) SST & FP (23) C (35)
Frequency and duration of treatment	3 hrs/wk for 3 months	Group: 10 hrs/wk for 9 weeks Multiple Family[d]: 1 hr/wk for 9 weeks	SST: weekly for 1 yr then biweekly for 1 yr FP: weekly, monthly for 2 yrs
Symptomatology	At 6 months[e]: SST > C	SST > HHT	SST = SST & FP = FP = C[f,g]
Relapse or rehospitalization	At 12 months: SST = C	2 yr relapse rate: SST: 42% SST: 50% HHT: 79%	2 yr relapse rate: FP: 32% SST & FP: 25% C: 66%
Social adjustment		ST > HHT	SST & FP ⩾ FP ⩾ SST ⩾ C[f]
Vocational adjustment		SST = HHT	FP = FP & SST > SST = C[f]
Methodological weaknesses	Brief treatment, lack of long-term follow-up data	Absence of drug-only control group Individual and family treatment methods confounded. Males only included	All patients in high expressed emotion households Follow-up assessments on nonrelapsed patients only

Note. SST = social skills training; C = control treatment (e.g., case management); HHT = holistic health treatment; FP = family psychoeducation. Patients in all studies were maintained on antipsychotic medications.

[a]All patients participated in a day hospital program.

[b]Treatment was provided on an inpatient basis, after which patients were discharged into the community.

[c]All patients were living with high expressed emotion (EE) relatives.

[d]Families of patients who received SST were treated with behavioral family therapy (Falloon, Boyd, & McGill, 1984), whereas families of patients who received HHT were treated with dynamic family therapy that included mental health education and supportive interventions for coping with mental illness (Wallace & Liberman, 1985).

[e]Six-month follow-up data available on only 27/43 (63%) patients.

[f]Follow-up data on symptoms, social adjustment, and vocational adjustment available only on nonrelapsed patients.

[g]There was a trend for patients in the FP and SST & FP groups to have less social withdrawal at 2 years, but there were no other symptom differences.

that had occurred over the first 3 months of treatment, whereas the symptoms of patients who had not received skills training deteriorated from 3 to 6 months post-hospital discharge. Information on social functioning was not obtained, and too few patients were available for the 1-year assessment. However, 1-year hospitalization rates did not differ between the two groups. This study provides some support for the effectiveness of social skills training, but it is limited by the narrow range of assessment, brief treatment duration, and lack of long-term follow-up data.

Liberman, Mueser, and Wallace (1986; Wallace & Liberman, 1985) examined the effects of an intensive social skills training program compared to an equally intensive "holistic health treatment" program (e.g., exercise, yoga) for inpatient schizophrenics awaiting discharge into the community. The treatments were provided 2 hours per day, 5 days per week for 9 weeks, and patients were followed up periodically over a 2-year period. In addition to daily training sessions, both groups of patients also participated in regular trips into the community to prepare them for community life after discharge. Families of patients who received social skills training also received 9 weekly sessions of behavioral family therapy, whereas families of patients in the holistic health treatment received an educational-dynamic form of therapy. As evident from Table 14.2, the social skills training patients were more adjusted and less symptomatic at the 2-year follow-up. However, the experimental design employed limits the conclusions that can be drawn from this study. The absence of a standard psychosocial treatment group (e.g., inpatient treatment with only medication and activities) makes it impossible to determine whether both treatments were effective or ineffective relative to ordinary approaches to treatment. Further, the provision of different forms of family intervention to patients receiving different group interventions confounds family treatment with group treatment. Thus, the superior outcome of patients who received social skills training could have been due to the effects of behavioral family therapy rather than skills training. Despite these limitations, this study supports the hypothesis that social skills training may improve the outcome of schizophrenia.

Hogarty and his colleagues have conducted the largest study of social skills training for schizophrenia, which compared skills training with family psychoeducation over 2 years (Hogarty, Anderson, & Reiss, 1987; Hogarty *et al.*, 1986; Hogarty *et al.*, 1991). Outpatients who had recently been treated for an acute symptom exacerbation were assigned to 2 years of social skills training, family psychoeducation, skills training and family psychoeducation, or standard treatment (medication, case management, day treatment). All patients were living with high expressed emotion (EE) family members or in regular contact with high-EE relatives, and they were therefore at increased risk for a symptom relapse. In contrast to the Bellack *et al.* (1984) and Liberman *et al.* (1986) studies, patients were treated individually with social skills training, rather than in groups. Overall, the pattern of results supported the efficacy of the family treatment over social skills training, which was better than the control treatment. As with the previous studies reviewed, the experimental design constrained the generalizability of the results, particularly for the social skills intervention. First, follow-up assessments at 1 and 2 years after treatment initiation were conducted only on nonrelapsed patients. This resulted in small sample sizes for the follow-up assessments and precludes a test of whether skills training improved social functioning independent of relapse. Second, all patients were living with high-EE relatives, and the ambient tension to which patients were exposed may have limited the ability of patients who received only social skills training to benefit from this treatment. This study leaves open the question of whether skills training would be more effective if it were provided to patients living in less stressful environments.

Future Directions for Social Learning Interventions. The controlled studies on social skills training for schizophrenia provide some support for its efficacy. However, the methodological limitations of each study render it difficult to determine the impact of skills training on social adjustment and quality of life, the areas that this intervention is believed to influence most directly. Two of the three controlled studies examined relatively brief social skills training treatments provided in a group format (i.e., 3 months or less; Bellack *et al.*, 1984; Liberman *et al.*, 1986). Given the chronic nature of schizophrenia, it is unlikely that social skills training will have a lasting effect unless the treatment is provided for longer periods of time. Additionally, there may be some patients who benefit from social skills training given on a long-term, rather than time-limited, basis. In research conducted in our clinic, we have found that patients with memory impairments acquire social skills at a slower rate but are able to maintain these skills at follow-up (Mueser, Bellack, Douglas, & Wade, 1991). Patients with chronic psychotic symptoms, by contrast, acquired skills at the same rate as nonpsychotic patients but were unable to retain their skills at follow-up (Mueser, Kosmidis, & Sayers, 1992). These results are in line with the hypothesis that many schizophrenic patients require lengthy social learning interventions, and that maintenance of targeted skills may be a problem in some cases.

Future research on the efficacy of social skills training needs to examine treatment provided over a longer period of time to patients not living in high-EE family households. The question of whether skills training should be provided individually (Hogarty *et al.*, 1986) or on a group basis (Bellack *et al.*, 1984; Liberman *et al.*, 1986) has also not been addressed, raising the question of whether treatment format needs to be matched with individual patient characteristics. Another unresolved issue about social skills training concerns the relationship between gains in social skills, environmental variables known to impact on the course of schizophrenia (e.g., stress, substance abuse), and outcome of the illness. According to the stress–vulnerability model, improvements in social skill mediate the noxious effects of stressors, yet previous social skills research has not examined whether skills training confers protection against such stressors. Last, more attention should be given to the identification of patient variables that are predictive of response to social skills training. Such information will enable clinicians to make differential treatment recommendations and will provide valuable information regarding the mechanisms underlying social skills training. While a definitive answer regarding the efficacy of social skills training for schizophrenia is not presently available, research conducted thus far has been encouraging.

Other Psychotherapy Approaches

In addition to social learning and psychodynamic interventions, the efficacy of a variety of other psychotherapy approaches for schizophrenia has been explored in a limited number of studies. Most of these studies have lacked the diagnostic and methodological rigor necessary for outcome research. However, several well-controlled studies of other psychotherapy methods have been conducted, which we briefly review here.

Fairweather, Simon, Gebhard, Weingarten, and Reahl (1960) are credited with conducting the first controlled study of psychotherapy for schizophrenia. These investigators examined the effects of individual and group psychotherapy provided for an average of 4 to 5 months to patients with short- or long-term psychoses. Few differences were found between the treatment groups at posttreatment and 6-month follow-up, and patients with long-term psychoses benefited the least from psychotherapy. Diagnostic uncertainty, the unspecified nature of the psychotherapy method, and the failure to control for pharmacological treatment across treatment groups limit the conclusions that can be drawn from this study (Stanton *et al.*, 1984).

Rogers, Gendlin, Kiesler, and Traux (1967) examined the effects of client-centered therapy provided by chronic schizophrenic inpatients over long periods of time—up to 2 years. At the follow-up assessment, the patients who had received therapy showed only minimal improvements compared to patients who received standard treatment. However, the experience of the therapists varied widely, and pharmacological treatment was not standardized across treatment groups.

Two studies conducted by Hogarty and his colleagues have examined the effects of major role therapy, an approach to therapy involving individual casework and vocational counseling, in combination with different pharmacological treatments for stabilized schizophrenic outpatients. In the first study, patients were randomly assigned to receive antipsychotic medication alone, therapy alone, both treatments, or neither treatment over a 2-year study period (Hogarty & Goldberg, 1973; Hogarty, Goldberg, Schooler, & Ulrich, 1974; Hogarty, Goldberg, & Schooler, 1974). Antipsychotic drug therapy protected patients from relapses over the 2-year period, but major role therapy did not. Among nonrelapsed patients there was an intriguing interaction between therapy and medication. Nonrelapsed patients who received both therapy and medication or patients who received *neither* medication nor therapy had better social functioning than patients who received either therapy or medication alone. This interaction is difficult to interpret since data on nonrelapsed patients were not available.

In a subsequent study, Hogarty and colleagues (1979) compared the effects of major role therapy on patients receiving either oral antipsychotic medication (fluphenazine hydrochloride) or injectable depot antipsychotics (fluphenazine decanoate) over a 2-year period. There were no main effects for either therapy or drug type. However, there was a trend for patients who received therapy and depot medication to relapse the most, with the relapse rate of patients who received no therapy falling in between the two groups. This peculiar result is difficult to account for considering the absence of differences in relapse rates between the two medication groups.

In summary, controlled studies of other individual therapy approaches for schizophrenia have not yielded consistent results supporting the efficacy of these interventions. The lack of significant effects for these therapies on the course and outcome of schizophrenia suggests that the illness is unlikely to improve from nonspecific factors inherent to therapy such as the provision of warmth, empathy, and the like. This conclusion obviates the need for "placebo"-controlled psychotherapy outcome studies in schizophrenia (i.e., studies that control for the amount of therapist contact with the patient) and indicates that "standard" treatment (e.g., medication and case management) is the most relevant control group for this population.

Family Therapy

In view of the limited data available substantiating the efficacy of individual psychotherapy, the preponderance of rigorously conducted studies demonstrating the benefits of family therapy for persons with schizophrenia is especially welcome. A confluence of critical historical and scientific factors no doubt contribute to the growing interest in this area. The prominence of the deinstitutionalization movement and the commitment to community care included the expectation that family members would now shoulder more of the burden for caring for their mentally ill relatives. Caring for the mentally ill can be a challenging, onerous, and demanding task, however, and family members became quite vocal in their need for support and aid. In addition, the past 25 years have witnessed a revolution in the conceptualization of psychological interventions. While dynamically based treatments tend to be long term, intensive, less structured, and focused on the inner workings of the individual, more recently developed interventions are frequently shorter, more structured, and problem focused, and thus lend themselves easily to use in a family format.

Perhaps most importantly, a series of studies in the 1970s and 1980s demonstrated that family attitudes assessed at the time of a symptom exacerbation of a schizophrenic person predicted his or her relapse during the subsequent 9 months (Brown, Birley & Wing, 1972; Vaughn & Leff, 1976a; Vaughn, Snyder, Jones, Freeman, & Falloon, 1984; see Parker & Hadzi-Pavlovic, 1990, for a recent review). These family attitudes are assessed using the Camberwell Family Interview (CFI; Vaughn & Leff, 1976b), a 90-min assessment conducted with the relative while the patient is absent. The CFI is a semistructured interview focused on obtaining a brief chronology of the patient's illness in addition to the specifics of his or her behavior, and the relative's response to it, in the 3 months prior to the index hospitalization. Interviews are scored for (1) number of critical comments, (2) number of positive comments, (3) hostile attitudes, (4) warmth, and (5) overinvolvement. Higher levels of critical comments, hostility, and overinvolvement (high "expressed emotion," or EE), which is likely normative among Anglos in the United States (Vaughn *et al.*, 1984), appear to reflect the extraordinary toll that caring for a mentally ill relative exacts. High EE is associated with increased rates of relapse, although the directionality of this relation is controversial (Glynn *et al.*, 1990). Nevertheless, studies demonstrating the importance of ambient stress—as indicated by EE—on prognosis in schizophrenia quickly evolved into investigations of whether the more facilitative low-EE family attitudes and behaviors could be taught.

Although the emphasis here is on highlighting empirically tested psychotherapeutic family interventions in schizophrenia, it is important to recognize that some authors have reported successful treatment of limited numbers of cases using techniques and approaches which have not been submitted to rigorous evaluation. For example, benefits of structural family therapy and strategic family therapy have been reported in single-case descriptions (Madanes, 1983). However, the difficulty of interpreting these types of findings, given possible confounds resulting from subject selection factors, therapeutic expectancy (the Hawthorne effect), and natural recovery processes, precludes discussion of them here.

In all, eight family studies meet at least minimum experimental design standards, including random assignment of rigorously diagnosed recently exacerbated schizophrenic subjects to carefully developed and reliably conducted treatment interventions (Falloon *et al.*, 1982; Glick *et al.*, 1985; Goldstein, Rodnick, Evans, May, & Steinberg, 1978; Hogarty *et al.*, 1986; Kottgen, Sonnichsen, Mollenhauer, Jurth, 1984; Leff, Kuipers, Berkowitz, Eberlein-Vries, & Sturgeon, 1982; Randolph *et al.*, 1991; Tarrier *et al.*, 1988). All study designs involved embedding the family intervention in a comprehensive treatment program including psychiatric medication administration. Most, but not all, also utilized outcome assessors blind to treatment group assignment. Importantly, these studies differed on a variety of dimensions, including location of intervention (home, inpatient, or outpatient clinic), modality (single family treatment vs. multiple family groups), intervention duration (6 weeks to 2 years), the inclusion of the ill relative in sessions, and the degree of formal structure in the intervention. With the exception of the psychodynamically oriented treatment conducted by Kottgen *et al.*, these studies have established that family-based interventions can have a significant, positive impact on many patients with schizophrenia and, frequently, on their relatives as well. The consistency of these positive findings is particularly striking in light of the variations in the treatments provided and the methodological difficulties in the investigations. An overview and critique of each of these studies will be presented below (see also Tables 14.3–14.5), followed by a brief discussion of the research issues still to be addressed in this important area of treatment innovation.

Psychoanalytic Approaches

Kottgen *et al.* (1984) tested the efficacy of psychodynamically oriented group therapy with schizophrenic patients and their relatives. High-EE families were randomly assigned to either group therapy or a customary care condition; low-EE families were eligible to receive only customary care. In the relative treatment condition, patients and their families met in separate small groups. To investigate optimal group scheduling, some sessions were scheduled weekly and some were scheduled monthly. The treatment objectives included (1) "working through" recent hurtful situations, (2) reducing mutual prejudices and negative expectations, (3) delving into the origins of the patient's and relative's critical and hostile overinvolvement, (4) alleviating family isolation, (5) relieving feelings of guilt, shame, and inadequacy, (6) encouraging autonomy, and (7) reducing chronic stress situations. A critical treatment objective was to help relatives understand the mechanisms underlying their own behavior, with the assumption that making these intelligible would lead to positive change.

In view of the previously discussed negative findings regarding psychodynamic psychotherapy for persons with schizophrenia, it is perhaps not surprising that this approach offered little as a family intervention. Less than half of the relatives and patients attended at least 75% of the scheduled sessions. Approximately half of the relatives in both the control and therapy groups who were initially high EE changed to low EE at 18-month follow-up; psychodynamic group treatment was not differentially effective at reducing EE. Finally, there were no statistically significant differences in relapse rates in the three groups. Since therapy groups were poorly attended, it is difficult to determine whether the null effect resulted from an ineffective treatment or too limited exposure to a potentially effective treatment. Small sample size may have also presented a problem, especially because the random assignment was violated in an unreported number of cases where transportation posed difficulties. In summary, the results of this investigation on family-based psychodynamic treatment are disappointing.

Table 14.3. Characteristics and Results of Controlled Family Studies[a,b]

	Kottgen *et al.* (1984)	Goldstein *et al.* (1978)	Glick *et al.* (1985)
Number of prior hospitalizations	69% first admission	69% first admission	$\bar{x}$ = 2.0
Treatment groups (*N*)	FT (high EE-15) CC (high EE-14) CC (low EE-20)	Mod dose/FT (25) Mod dose/no FT (28) Low dose/FT (27) Low dose/no FT (24)	FT (37) CC (55)
Type of family treatment	Separate psychodynamic patient and relative groups	Crisis-oriented; identify and plan for stressors	Crisis-oriented; identify and plan for stressors
Session frequency and duration[c]	Weekly or monthly up to 2 years	6 weekly sessions	$\bar{x}$ = 8.6 sessions over 5 week inpatient stay
Early outcome Psychotic relapse/ exacerbation	FT = CC (high EE) FT = CC (low EE)	Mod dose/FT > Mod dose/no FT = Low dose/FT > Low dose/no FT	Females: FT/good premorbid > all others Males: FT = CC[d]
Social/vocational functioning			
Follow-up Psychotic relapse/ exacerbation (follow-up duration)	FT = CC (high EE) FT = CC (low EE) (24 months)	Mod dose/FT > Mode dose/no FT > Low dose/FT = Low dose/no FT (6 months)	Females: FT/poor premorbid > all others Males: FT = CC (18 months)
Social/vocational functioning			Females: FT/poor premorbid > all others Males: FT = CC
Methodological weaknesses	Loose operationalization of therapy; poor attendance	Relapse defined as rehospitalization; brief treatment	Brief treatment; FT & medication changes confounded; treatment integrity an issue

Note FT = family therapy; CC = customary care; EE = expressed emotion; Ed only = 2 education sessions only; ICM = individual case management.
[a]The Hogarty *et al.* (1986, 1991) study is presented in Table 14.2.
[b]All studies involve random assignment of subjects to outpatient treatment unless described otherwise.
[c]All family treatments begin with educaiton about illness, which may involve 1–2 additional initial sessions.
[d]Unlike the other studies, Glick *et al.* (1985) present symptom status but do not include data on "relapse" or specifically operationalized exacerbations.

Four sets of investigators have explored the impact of psychoeducational family interventions on outcome in schizophrenia (Glick *et al.*, 1985; Goldstein *et al.*, 1978; Hogarty *et al.*, 1986; Leff *et al.*, 1982). The results have generally been positive, although the brevity of some of these interventions is associated with more modest benefits. These interventions share the "vulnerability–stress–coping" conceptualization of mental illness described above and have the goal of minimizing stress in the family in order to reduce the patients' symptoms and increase their social functioning. These programs begin with one to two educational sessions to provide basic information on the etiology, treatment, phenomenology, and prognosis in schizophrenia; some of these treatments included the patient in these sessions while others did not. Conveying accurate information about schizophrenia is considered to be a necessary treatment component, but it is important to recognize that education alone has not been found to yield significant improvement in schizophrenia (Tarrier *et al.*, 1988), and many authors have been quite elegant in highlighting the limitations of free-standing educational programs for severe psychiatric illness (e.g., Tarrier & Barrowclough, 1986).

Subsequent to the formal educational sessions, these programs differ in the

Table 14.4. Characteristics and Results of Controlled Family Studies[a]

	Leff *et al.* (1982, 1985)	Falloon *et al.* (1982, 1985)
Number of prior hospitalizations	$\bar{x} = 2.3$	$\bar{x} = 3.0$
Treatment groups (*N*)	FT (12) CC (12)	FT (18) ICM (18)
Type of family treatment	Relatives' group to model low-EE coping; pragmatic (dynamic and/or behavioral) individual family work	Home-based communication and problem-solving training
Session frequency and duration[b]	9 months biweekly relative groups and varied number of individual family sessions	3 months biweekly, 6 months biweekly, 15 monthly
Early outcome Psychotic relapse/exacerbation (duration)	FT > CC	FT > ICM
Social/vocational functioning		FT > ICM
Follow-up Psychotic relapse/exacerbation (duration)	FT > CC (24 months)	FT > ICM (24 months)
Social/vocational functioning		FT > ICM (24 months)
Methodological weaknesses[c]	Small sample size; assessors not blind; differential attrition/follow-up	ICM not home-based

Note. See Table 14.3 for explanation of abbreviations.
[a]All studies involve random assignment of subjects to outpatient treatment unless described otherwise.
[b]All family treatments begin with education about illness, which may involve 1–2 additional initial sessions.
[c]Falloon *et al.* (1982, 1985) had clinical management responsibilities permitting close monitoring of patient status during follow-up period.

methods utilized to reduce family stress. The Goldstein *et al.* intervention, which was conducted on an outpatient basis with first- and second-break patients and their families, was brief (6 sessions) and was designed to help the family identify the stressors precipitating the psychotic exacerbation, minimize those stressors, and to plan for anticipated stressors in the near future. In conjunction with assignment to either the family therapy or customary care control group, subjects were also randomly assigned to receive either moderate or small doses of fluphenazine decanoate. At 6 weeks, the results demonstrated that subjects in the moderate-dose/family therapy group had significantly fewer relapses than those in the low-dose/no family therapy group, with the two intermediate groups (low dose/family therapy and moderate dose/no family therapy) not differing statistically from either of the extreme groups. At 6 months, there was a marginal effect of the family therapy across the two dosage levels ($p < .1$), with subsequent analyses indicating a positive effect for family therapy in the moderate-dose condition, but not in the low-dose condition. Thus, these results suggested that family therapy, provided in

Table 14.5. Characteristics and Results of Controlled Family Studies[a]

	Randolph *et al.* (1991)	Tarrier *et al.* (1988, 1989)
Number of prior hospitalizations	$\bar{x} = 4.5$	$\bar{x} = 2.8$
Treatment groups (*N*)	FT (21) CC (20)	FT (high EE-enactive-16; symbolic-16) Ed only (high EE-16; low EE-9); CC (high EE-10; low EE-10)
Type of family treatment	Clinic-based communication and problem-solving training	Stress management and goal-setting training
Session frequency and duration[b]	3 months weekly, 3 months biweekly, 6 monthly	3 stress management and 8 goal-setting sessions over 9 months
Early outcome		
Psychotic relapse/ exacerbation	FT > CC	FT > Ed = CC Low EE > High EE
Social/vocational functioning		
Follow-up		
Psychotic relapse/ exacerbation (duration)		FT > Ed = CC Low EE > High EE (24 months)
Social/vocational functioning		
Methodological weaknesses[c]	Subject selection may limit generalizability	Integrity of two family treatments an issue; floor effects

Note. See Table 14.3 for explanation of abbreviations.
[a]All studies involve random assignment of subjects to outpatient treatment unless described otherwise.
[b]All family treatments begin with education about illness, which may involve 1–2 additional initial sessions.
[c]Randolph *et al.* (1991) had clinical management responsibilities permitting close monitoring of patient status during follow-up period.

the context of adequate antipsychotic medication, maximized the likelihood of positive outcomes. One difficulty in interpreting these findings, however, is that relapse was defined as a major medication adjustment and/or readmission to the hospital. Since a variety of factors independent of symptomatic status, including absence of suitable other housing or a family's need for respite care, can influence admission decisions, relapse results can be more clearly interpreted when they are defined by symptom severity. Other difficulties in understanding the findings result from the failure to present social adjustment outcome and the lack of control on data collection and subject treatment during the follow-up period.

The Glick *et al.* intervention (Glick *et al.*, 1985; Glick *et al.*, 1990; Haas *et al.*, 1988; Spencer *et al.*, 1988) was very similar to the one developed by Goldstein *et al.*. However, the Glick intervention varied on three critical dimensions—it was conducted on an inpatient basis, it was offered to subjects with other psychiatric diagnoses as well as schizophrenia, and the outcome variable of interest was not "relapse" *per se*, but symptom level at specified time points, as assessed on a number of psychiatric measurement scales. Patients were randomly assigned to receive customary care either with or without the addition of the family intervention. Family members attended an average of 8.6 (mode = 6) sessions. Among the schizophrenic sample at discharge, females with a good premorbid adjustment benefited from the therapy, but there were no effects for females with poor premorbid adjustment or the overall male sample. At 18 months, the findings had reversed for females; there was a trend for participation in family therapy to reduce symptomatology and improve family role functioning among women with poor premorbid adjustment. The family therapy had little impact on males or females with good premorbid adjustment, however. Glick and his associates have clearly articulated the limitations of their study, including the small number of sessions, the frequent confounding of medication adjustments and therapy activity inherent in an acute setting, the difficulty of maintaining fidelity to a treatment protocol when it is embedded in a comprehensive inpatient milieu program, and the failure to collect longitudinal data on relapse during the follow-up period (Haas *et al.*, 1988). Given these problems, interpretation of their modest results is difficult.

In contrast to the Goldstein *et al.* (1978) and Glick *et al.* (1985) studies just discussed, the Leff *et al.* (1982, 1985) and Hogarty *et al.* (1986, 1991) interventions had broader treatment goals and were conducted over an extended period of time. Both of these projects included only patients from high-EE families in their samples and specified the reduction of EE as a primary treatment objective. The studies differed, however, in how they sought to achieve this goal. In the Leff *et al.* study, the primary therapeutic agent was at least 9 months' participation in groups composed of high- and low-EE relatives which were intended to help the high-EE relatives model low-EE attitudes and behaviors; participation in these groups was supplemented by a limited number of individual family sessions held with the patient in the home. Patients were randomly assigned to receive customary care either with or without the addition of this multicomponent family treatment. As hypothesized, patients from the family therapy condition demonstrated significantly fewer relapses than those in the customary care only condition, both at 9 months and at 2-year follow-up. Anecdotal evidence also indicated that the patients from the family therapy condition achieved more improved social functioning than those receiving only customary care. Seventy-three percent of the therapy families changed from high to low EE during the study; no patient relapsed in families achieving this change in attitude.

While the findings of the Leff *et al.* (1982) study are impressive, methodological weaknesses make interpretation of some results difficult. Patients' symptom status was evaluated by clinicians who were not blind to treatment condition. In addition, the relatives' group component of the therapy evolved quite differently from what had initially been conceptualized. While the investigators had hoped that contact with low-EE relatives would promote more benign attitudes and behaviors among high-EE relatives, most low-EE relatives dropped out early in treatment, reporting that they did not feel the need for a relatives' group; by default, the intervention evolved into a high-EE relatives' group with much greater need for the facilitator to provide instruction and support for attitude changes. Interpreting the follow-up data is complicated in this study, because a greater proportion of the control relatives refused further assessments, possibly skewing the results. In addition, two suicides in the family treatment condition during follow-up were considered as "nonrelapses" because they did not appear to result from psychosis. If these were reclassified as "relapses" then the trend for fewer relapses in the family condition (40%) compared to the customary care condition (78%) would no longer be statistically significant.

As discussed previously, the efficacy of individual social skills training and family therapy was investigated in the Hogarty *et al.* (1986, 1991) study. Subjects were randomly assigned to received either none, one, or both of the two treatments. The family therapy, which included the patient, was conducted individually over a 2-year period, with sessions planned biweekly over the first year, then monthly thereafter. Primary family therapeutic techniques included advice giving, reframing, helping set realistic expectations, and assigning successive homework activities to help the patient achieve social and vocational independence (Anderson, Reiss, & Hogarty, 1986). Work in the first year was devoted to stress reduction, symptom management, and relapse prevention, while the second year was typically focused on enhancing social functioning and autonomy.

The first-year results indicated that both the individual and family treatment were equally successful at reducing relapse rates and that the combined condition was most efficacious. The second-year results suggested that the benefits of the individual social skills training were attenuated; only the family therapy continued to demonstrate significant differences over customary care. While the results of the Hogarty *et al.* (1986, 1991) investigations are dramatic, they must be interpreted with some caution. As mentioned previously, patients who relapsed during the study were excluded from subsequent data analysis, which unexpectedly led to unbalanced cell sizes. For example, because of differential relapse, there was a substantial disparity in number of survivors available for analyses of social adjustment in year 2 in the combined (n = 12) versus the social skills training (n = 7) versus the family therapy (n = 15) versus the control conditions (n = 6). These group size differences may have obscured any positive results on social adjustment, independent from relapse, accruing from the social skills training condition. Another concern in this study is the nonblind judgment of relapse. Finally, while the protocol called for declining contact and eventual termination in year 2, the needs of the patients were deemed to preclude a systematic reduction in services, which resulted in the continuation of treatment at year-1 levels until month 21.

Similar to the psychoeducational interventions discussed above, the behavioral interventions also subscribe to the vulnerability–stress–coping model outlined above. However, the behavioral approach emphasizes skill acquisition to manage stress and incorporates the use of traditional behavioral techniques, including modeling, coaching, prompting, behavioral rehearsal, and the assignment and review of homework, to achieve this goal. Appropriate pharmacological treatment and successful stress management are considered the cornerstones of rehabilitation in the behavioral approach. To encourage medication compliance and the development of a collaborative relationship with the treating psychiatrist, these interventions also typically begin with two or three educational sessions about schizophrenia and its treatment. Subsequent to this education, a series of sessions including the patient and his or her relatives are conducted. While the basic philosophy and techniques of the Falloon *et al.* (1982) and Tarrier *et al.* (1988) interventions are similar, the content of individual sessions differs. The specific techniques and empirical support for the two interventions are presented below.

The Falloon *et al.* (1982, 1985; Falloon, McGill, Boyd, Pederson, 1987; Falloon & Pederson, 1985) intervention involves home-based training in communication and problem solving preceded by a thorough behavioral assessment. The ultimate objective of the intervention is to help families manage stress successfully through effective problem solving. While arriving at satisfactory solutions to problems during the therapy is desirable, the paramount goal is to teach the family a *method* for solving problems. Typically, four to six sessions are devoted to communication skills training (i.e., active listening, expressing positive feelings, making positive requests, and expressing negative feelings). In-session behavioral rehearsal, facilitated through coaching and prompting, shaping, and positive reinforcement, is supplemented with daily homework assignments to promote generalization.

Special attention is focused on remediating specific deficits which have been identified in the initial behavioral analysis or during ongoing assessment. After families have demonstrated mastery of the communication skills, the therapist transitions to formal problem solving, using the 6-step technique outlined by D'Zurilla & Goldfried (1971). Families are taught to (1) define the problem or goal, (2) generate solutions, (3) evaluate solutions, (4) select the best solution(s), (5) plan for and implement the solution, and (6) review the implemented solution and modify as necessary. To promote generalization, families are instructed to schedule continuing weekly "executive sessions" in which they apply the problem-solving techniques to the real-world difficulties they are facing. The development of problem-solving skills is the primary therapeutic objective for the family work. Nevertheless, the therapist can augment this instruction with the use of other techniques (e.g., relaxation training, the development of a token economy) to intervene on more intractable problems that may not lend themselves as readily to remediation through problem solving.

The efficacy of behavioral family therapy in schizophrenia has been demonstrated in two studies to date. In the initial study, Falloon and colleagues randomly assigned 36 patients and their families to receive either home-based behavioral family therapy or individual therapy on a declining contact basis over a 2-year period. In comparison to the individual treatment, the family therapy resulted in fewer relapses, greater rates of remission, fewer and shorter hospitalizations, improved social functioning, and reduced family burden and distress. In spite of being home based, the family therapy was more cost-efficient that the individual therapy, when the reduced need for hospitalization was taken into account (Liberman, Cardin, McGill, Falloon, & Evans, 1987). While the Falloon *et al.* (1982) study is quite sound methodologically, its strong emphasis on problem-solving training has been critiqued by Bellack, Morrison, and Mueser (1989), who correctly note that not all life challenges lend themselves to solutions utilizing such a technique.

The initial Falloon *et al.* (1982, 1985) results generated a great deal of research enthusiasm, with the National Institute of Mental Health currently completing a five-site collaborative study investigating the utility of behavioral family therapy in conjunction with three different medication strategies (high, low, and targeted dose) (Schooler & Keith, 1985). In a replication and extension of Falloon's work, Randolph *et al.* (1991) recently reported that *clinic-based* behavioral family therapy reduced 1-year relapse rates among veterans with schizophrenia; furthermore, this reduction in relapse was observed in patients from both high- and low-EE families. One complication in interpreting the Randolph *et al.* (1991) findings, however, is the observation that most of the potential candidates for the protocol were excluded because of minimal family contact or compromised diagnoses due to drug use (Eth *et al.*, 1991). The relevance of empirically based interventions to the typical "real-world" clinical population in a public or VA outpatient setting remains to be determined.

One critical research issue involves determining whether formal skills training, including behavioral rehearsal, is required to achieve the benefits of behavioral family therapy. Effective skills training requires a high level of specialized technical expertise, which many clinicians lack. If formal behavioral instruction is not required to accrue benefits from family therapy, than the treatment may gain wider acceptance among "frontline" mental health professionals. Tarrier and his associates (1988, 1989) have begun to explore this issue. These investigators randomly assigned patients from high-EE families to receive either customary care, or family education alone, or family therapy. In addition to education, the family therapy included training in stress management and goal setting and achievement. The researchers systematically varied whether the family therapy included only discussion and didactic training (i.e., "symbolic" work) or also included formal skills training and behavioral rehearsal (i.e., "enactive" work). They found no differences between the relapse rates in the customary care and educational only conditions, and reduced relapse rates in the two family therapy conditions. Interestingly, relapse rates in the two family therapy conditions did not differ, suggesting that formal skills training *per se* may add little to an overall structured approach to working with the families of persons with schizophrenia. However, Tarrier and Barrowclough (1990) have suggested that the failure to find differences in the two treatment groups may be due to floor effects (i.e., very low relapse rates) and unanticipated contamination of the two conditions. Further work on the necessity of skills training for effective behavioral family therapy is still required.

Unanswered Questions

Many important issues still need to be addressed in the area of family treatment for schizophrenia. There are a variety of different family-based therapeutic modalities that have resulted in significant benefits for schizophrenic patients. The time for a comparative study, testing the relative efficacy of these different modalities, is clearly imminent. A second topic of interest involves determining the durability of therapeutic effects. Both Falloon *et al.* (1982) and Hogarty *et al.* (1986) offered treatment throughout their 2-year follow-up period, eliminating the possibility of determining whether effects were sustained once treatment had been completed. Hogarty *et al.* (1991) anecdotally reported that most of their subjects, regardless of their treatment group assignment, had been readmitted in the 7 years after their study had been completed. However, no study to date has carefully monitored patients during follow-up *after* family treatment has been completed. Fortunately, the Randolph *et al.* (1991) VA study and the NIMH studies mentioned previously are designed to permit exploration of this issue. Finally, an equally compelling theoretical concern involves determining whether these interventions achieve their benefits through the mechanisms proposed by the developers. For example, behavioral family therapy is hypothesized to achieve its effects by enhancing effective problem solving, yet no study to date has shown that changes in specific problem-solving skills accrue from participation in the treatment, or that these changes are associated with patient improvement. It may be, however, that the therapy achieves its effects by engendering realistic expectations of the patient on the part of the relatives, which then lowers family EE levels, thus yielding improved prognosis. Further work in this area is needed.

Summary and Conclusions

The past 20 years have witnessed a tremendous growth in research on the efficacy of psychotherapy for schizophrenia, with mounting evidence suggesting that some interventions may improve the outcome of this chronic illness. At present, the evidence from controlled studies supporting the efficacy of psychodynamic or other nonbehavioral individual treatment approaches (e.g., client-centered therapy) is minimal, and sufficient research has been conducted in this area to recommend against these forms of treatment for schizophrenia. More encouraging results have emerged from social learning treatments for schizophrenia. The token economy still appears to be the treatment of choice for chronic schizophrenic inpatients, although only a few rigorous studies have been conducted, and ethical and legal concerns have recently limited the adoption of token economy programs. While some controlled research has examined the effects of social skills training for patients awaiting discharge in the hospital or living in the community, the results have been encouraging and suggest that skills training may be a potentially useful approach. A definitive conclusion regarding the efficacy of social skills training cannot be made at this time because of the methodological limitations of prior research. The strongest support for effective psychotherapeutic treatment for schizophrenia has been for family therapy. Over the past decade several controlled studies have demonstrated the beneficial efforts of both behavioral and educational family therapy models for schizophrenia on long-term (i.e., 2-year) outcome of the illness. While comparative studies of these two models have yet to be conducted and the mechanisms underlying the effects of the treatments remain in question, family intervention designed to inform family members about the nature of the illness and teach strategies to lower ambient levels of stress is the most empirically validated form of psychotherapy for schizophrenia. Research on the psychotherapeutic treatment of schizophrenia has made important gains in recent years. These exciting innovations hold promise for our ability to more effectively treat and improve the quality of lives of persons with this devastating illness.

References

Anderson, C. M., Reiss, D. J., & Hogarty, G. E. (1986). *Schizophrenia and the family*. New York: Guilford Press.

Andreasen, N. C., & Olsen, S. (1982). Negative vs positive schizophrenia: Definition and validation. *Archives of General Psychiatry, 39*, 789–794.

Angermeyer, M. C., & Kuhn, L. (1988). Gender difference in age at onset of schizophrenia: An overview. *European Archives of Psychiatry and Neurological Sciences, 237*, 351–364.

Avison, W. R., & Speechley, K. N. (1987). The discharged psychiatric patient: A review of social, social-psychological, and psychiatric correlates of outcome. *American Journal of Psychiatry, 144*, 10–18.

Ayllon, T., & Azrin, N. (1968). *The token economy: A motivation system for therapy and rehabilitation*. Appleton-Century-Crofts.

Bellack, A. S., Morrison, R. L., & Mueser, K. T. (1989). Social problem solving in schizophrenia. *Schizophrenia Bulletin, 15*, 101–116.

Bellack, A. S., Morrison, R. L., Wixted, J. T., & Mueser, K. T. (1990). An analysis of social competence in schizophrenia. *British Journal of Psychiatry, 156*, 809–818.

Bellack, A. S., & Mueser, K. T. (1986). A comprehensive treatment program for schizophrenia and chronic mental illness. *Community and Mental Health Journal, 22*, 175–189.

Bellack, A. S., Turner, S. M., Hersen, M., & Luber, R. F. (1984). An examination of the efficacy of social skills training for chronic schizophrenic patients. *Hospital and Community Psychiatry, 35*, 1023–1028.

Benton, M. K., & Schroeder, H. E. (1990). Social skills training with schizophrenics: A meta-analytic evaluation. *Journal of Consulting and Clinical Psychology, 58*, 741–747.

Brown, G. W., Birley, J. L. T., & Wing, J. K. (1972). Influence of family life on the course of schizophrenic disorders: A replication. *British Journal of Psychiatry, 121*, 241–258.

Ciompi, L. (1980). The natural history of schizophrenia in the long-term. *British Journal of Psychiatry, 136*, 413–420.

Ciompi, L. (1987). Toward a coherent multidimensional understanding and therapy of schizophrenia: Converging new concepts. In J. S. Strauss, W. Boker, & H. D. Brenner (Eds.), *Psychosocial treatment of schizophrenia* (pp. 48–62). Toronto: Hans Huber Publishers.

Davis, J. M. (1975). Overview: Maintenance therapy in psychiatry: I. Schizophrenia. *American Journal of Psychiatry, 132*, 1237–1245.

Derogatis, L. R. (1977). *SCL-90-R* (revised version). Baltimore: Johns Hopkins University School of Medicine.

Donahoe, C. P., & Driesenga, S. A. (1988). A review of social skills training with chronic mental patients. In M. Hersen, R. M. Eisler, & P. M. Miller (Eds.), *Progress in behavior modification* (pp. 131–164). Newbury Park, CA: Sage.

Drake, R. E., & Cotton, P. G. (1986). Depression, hopelessness and suicide in chronic schizophrenia. *British Journal of Psychiatry, 148*, 554–559.

Drake, R. E., & Sedere, L. I. (1986). The adverse effects of intensive treatment of chronic schizophrenia. *Comprehensive Psychiatry, 27*, 313–326.

D'Zurilla, T., & Goldfried, M. (1971). Problem solving and behavioral modification. *Journal of Abnormal Psychology, 78*, 197–226.

Endicott, J., & Spitzer, R. L. (1978). A diagnostic interview: The schedule for affective disorders and schizophrenia. *Archives of General Psychiatry, 35*, 837–844.

Eth, S., Randolph, E., Glynn, S., Paz, G., Leong, G., & Van Vort, W. (1991, May). *Family therapy for schizophrenia: Who participates?* Paper presented at the meeting of the American Psychiatric Association, New Orleans, LA.

Fairweather, G. W., Simon, R., Gebhard, M. E., Weingarten, E., & Reahl, J. E. (1960). Relative effectiveness of psychotherapeutic programs: A multicriteria comparison of four programs for three different patient groups. *Psychological Monographs, 74*, 1–26.

Falloon, I. R. H. (1984). Relapse: A reappraisal of assessment of outcome in schizophrenia. *Schizophrenia Bulletin, 10*, 293–299.

Falloon, I., Boyd, J., McGill, C., Razani, J., Moss, H., & Gilderman, A. (1982). Family management in the prevention of exacerbations of schizophrenia. *New England Journal of Medicine, 306*, 1437–1440.

Falloon, I., Boyd, J., McGill, C., Williamson, M., Razani, J., Moss, H., & Gilderman, A. (1985). Family management in the prevention of morbidity of schizophrenia: Clinical outcome of a two-year longitudinal study. *Archives of General Psychiatry, 42*, 887–896.

Falloon, I. R. H., Boyd, J. L., & McGill, C. W. (1984). *Family care of schizophrenia.* New York: Guilford.

Falloon, I., McGill, C., Boyd, J., & Pederson, J. (1987). Family management in the prevention of morbidity of schizophrenia: Social outcome of a two-year longitudinal study. *Psychological Medicine, 17*, 59–66.

Falloon, I., & Pederson, J. (1985). Family management in the prevention of morbidity of schizophrenia: The adjustment of the family unit. *British Journal of Psychiatry, 147*, 156–163.

Falloon, I. R. H., & Talbot, R. E. (1981). Persistent auditory hallucinations: Coping mechanisms and implications for management. *Psychological Medicine, 11*, 329–339.

Fromm-Reichmann, F. (1950). *Principles of intensive psychotherapy.* Chicago: University of Chicago Press.

Glick, I., Clarkin, J., Spencer, J., Haas, G., Lewis, A., Peyser, J., DeMane, N., Good-Ellis, M., Harris, E., & Lestelle, V. (1985). A controlled evaluation of inpatient family intervention: I. Preliminary results of a 6-month follow-up. *Archives of General Psychiatry, 42*, 882–886.

Glick, I., Spencer, J., Clarkin, J., Haas, G., Lewis, A., Peyser, J., DeMane, N., Good-Ellis, M., Harris, E., & Lestelle, V. (1990). A randomized clinical trial of inpatient family intervention: IV. Follow-up results for subjects with schizophrenia. *Schizophrenia Research, 3*, 187–200.

Glynn, S. M. (1990). Token economy approaches for psychiatric patients: Progress and pitfalls over 25 years. *Behavior Modification, 14*, 383–407.

Glynn, S., Randolph, E., Eth, S., Paz, G., Leong, G., Shaner, A., & Strachan, A. (1990). Patient psychopathology and expressed emotion in schizophrenia. *British Journal of Psychiatry, 157*, 877–880.

Goldstein, M., Rodnick, E., Evans, J., May, P., & Steinberg, M. (1978). Drug and family therapy in the aftercare of acute schizophrenics. *Archives of General Psychiatry, 35*, 1169–1177.

Grinspoon, L., Ewalt, J. R., & Shader, R. I. (1972). *Schizophrenia: Pharmacotherapy and psychotherapy.* Baltimore: Williams & Wilkins.

Gunderson, J. G., Frank, A., Katz, H. M., Vannicelli, M. L., Frosch, J. P., Knapp, P. H. (1984). Effects of psychotherapy in schizophrenia: II. Comparative outcome of two forms of treatment. *Schizophrenia Bulletin, 10*, 564–598.

Haas, G., Glick, I., Clarkin, J., Spencer, J., Lewis, A., Peyser, J., DeMane, N., Good-Ellis, M., Harris, E., & Lestelle, V. (1988). Inpatient family intervention: A randomized clinical trial: II. Results at hospital discharge. *Archives of General Psychiatry, 48*, 217–224.

Halford, W. K., & Hayes, R. (1991). Psychological rehabilitation of chronic schizophrenic patients: Recent findings on social skills training and family psychoeducation. *Clinical Psychology Review, 11*, 23–44.

Harding, C. M., Brooks, G. W., Ashikaga, T., Strauss, J. S., & Breier, A. (1987). The Vermont longitudinal study of persons with severe mental illness, I: Methodology, study sample, and overall status 32 years later. *American Journal of Psychiatry, 144*, 718–726.

Hogarty, G. E., Anderson, C. M., & Reiss, D. J. (1987). Family psychoeducation, social skills training, and medication in schizophrenia: The long and short of it. *Psychopharmacology Bulletin, 23*, 12–13.

Hogarty, G. E., Anderson, C. M., Reiss, D. J., Kornblith, S. J., Greenwald, D. P., Javna, C. D., & Madonia, M. J. (1986). Family psycho-education, social skills training and maintenance chemotherapy: I. One year effects of a controlled study on relapse and expressed emotion. *Archives of General Psychiatry, 45*, 797–805.

Hogarty, G., Anderson, C., Reiss, D., Kornblith, S., Greenwald, D., Ulrich, R., & Carter, M. (1991). Family psychoeducation, social skills training, and maintenance chemotherapy in the aftercare treatment of schizophrenia: II. Two-year effects of a controlled study on relapse and adjustment. *Archives of General Psychiatry, 48*, 340–347.

Hogarty, G. E., & Goldberg, S. C. (1973). Drug and sociotherapy in the aftercare of schizophrenic patients: III. Adjustment of non relapsed patients. *Archives of General Psychiatry, 28*, 54–63.

Hogarty, G. E., Goldberg, S. C., & Schooler, N. R. (1974). Drug and sociotherapy in the aftercare of schizophrenic patients. *Archives of General Psychiatry, 31*, 609–618.

Hogarty, G. E., Goldberg, S. C., Schooler, N. R., & Ulrich, R. F. (1974). Drug and sociotherapy in the aftercare of schizophrenic patients: II. Two-year relapse rates. *Archives of General Psychiatry, 31*, 603–608.

Hogarty, G. E., Schooler, N. R., Ulrich, R., Mussare, F., Ferro, P., & Herron, E. (1979). Fluphenazine and social therapy in the aftercare of schizophrenic patients. *Archives of General Psychiatry, 36*, 1283–1294.

Holtzman, P. S., & Matthysse, S. (1990). The genetics of schizophrenia: A review. *Psychological Science, 1*, 279–286.

Kane, J. M. (1989). Innovations in the psychopharmacologic treatment of schizophrenia. In A. S. Bellack (Ed.), *A clinical guide for the treatment of schizophrenia* (pp. 43–75). New York: Plenum.

Karon, B. P., & VandenBos, G. R. (1970). Experience, medication and the effectiveness of psychotherapy with schizophrenics: A note on Drs. May and Tuma's conclusions. *British Journal of Psychiatry, 116*, 427–428.

Karon, B. P., & VandenBos, G. R. (1972). The consequences of psychotherapy for schizophrenic patients. *Psychotherapy: Theory, Research and Practice, 9*, 111–119.

Karon, B. P., & VandenBos, G. R. (1975). Issues in current research on psychotherapy vs. medication in treatment of schizophrenics. *Psychotherapy: Theory, Research and Practice, 12*, 143–148.

Kay, S. R., Fiszbein, A., & Opler, L. A. (1987). The positive and negative syndrome scale (PANSS) for schizophrenia. *Schizophrenia Bulletin, 13*, 261–276.

Keith, S. J., Bellack, A., Frances, A., Mance, R., Matthews, S., & the Treatment Strategies in Schizophrenia Study Group. (1989). The influence of diagnosis and family treatment on acute treatment response and short-term outcome in schizophrenia. *Psychopharmacology Bulletin, 25*, 336–339.

Kottgen, C., Sonnichsen, I., Mollenhauer, K., & Jurth, R. (1984). Group therapy with families of schizophrenic patients: Results of the Hamburg Camberwell-Family-Interview Study III. *International Journal of Family Psychiatry, 5*, 83–94.

Leff, J., Kuipers, L., Berkowitz, R., Eberlein-Vries, R., & Sturgeon, D. (1982). A controlled trial of social intervention in the families of schizophrenic patients. *British Journal of Psychiatry, 141*, 121–134.

Leff, J., Kuipers, L., Berkowitz, R., & Sturgeon, D. (1985). A controlled trial of social intervention in the families of schizophrenic patients: Two year follow-up. *British Journal of Psychiatry, 146*, 594–600.

Lehman, A. F. (1988). A quality of life interview for the chronically mentally ill. *Evaluation and Program Planning, 11*, 51–62.

Lewine, R. R. J. (1990). A discriminant validity study of negative symptoms with a special focus on depression and antipsychotic medication. *American Journal of Psychiatry, 147*, 1463–1466.

Liberman, R., Cardin, V., McGill, C., Falloon, I. I., Evans, C. (1987). Behavioral family management of schizophrenia: Clinical outcome and costs. *Psychiatric Annals, 17*, 610–619.

Liberman, R. P., DeRisi, W. J., & Mueser, K. T. (1989). *Social skills training for psychiatric patients*. Boston: Allyn and Bacon.

Liberman, R. P., & Mueser, K. T. (1989). Schizophrenia: Psychosocial treatment. In H. I. Kaplan & B. J. Sadock (Eds.), *Comprehensive textbook of psychiatry/V* (pp. 792–806). Baltimore: Williams & Wilkins.

Liberman, R. P., Mueser, K. T., & Wallace, C. J. (1986). Social skills training for schizophrenic individuals at risk for relapse. *American Journal of Psychiatry, 143*, 523–526.

Madanes, C. (1983). Strategic therapy of schizophrenia. In W. McFarlane (Ed.), *Family therapy in schizophrenia* (pp. 209–225). New York: Guilford Press.

Matarazzo, J. D. (1983). The reliability of psychiatric and psychological diagnosis. *Clinical Psychology Review, 3*, 103–145.

May, P. R. A. (1968). *Treatment of schizophrenia: A comparative study of five treatment methods*. New York: Science House.

May, P. R. A. (1984). A step forward in research on psychotherapy of schizophrenia. *Schizophrenia Bulletin, 10*, 604–607.

McGlashan, T. H. (1984a). The Chestnut Lodge follow-up study I. Follow-up methodology and study sample. *Archives of General Psychiatry, 41*, 475–585.

McGlashan, T. H. (1984b). The Chestnut Lodge follow-up study II. Long-term outcome of schizophrenia and the affective disorders. *Archives of General Psychiatry, 41*, 586–601.

Meltzer, H. Y. (1985). Dopamine and negative symptoms in schizophrenia: Critique of the type I-II hypothesis. In M. Alpert (Ed.), *Controversies in schizophrenia* (pp. 110–136). New York: Guilford Press.

Meltzer, H. Y. (1990). Clozapine: Mechanism of action in relation to its clinical advantages. In A. Kales, C. N. Stefanis, & J. Talbott (Eds.), *Recent advances in schizophrenia* (pp. 237–256). New York: Springer-Verlag.

Mueser, K. T., Bellack, A. S., Douglas, M. S., & Wade, J. H. (1991). Prediction of social skill acquisition in schizophrenic and major affective disorder patients from memory and symptomatology. *Psychiatry Research, 37*, 218–296.

Mueser, K. T., & Berenbaum, H. (1990). Psychodynamic treatment of schizophrenia: Is there a future? *Psychological Medicine, 20*, 253–262.

Mueser, K. T., Douglas, M. S., Bellack, A. S., & Morrison, R. L. (1991). Assessment of enduring deficit and negative symptom subtypes in schizophrenia. *Schizophrenia Bulletin, 17*, 565–582.

Mueser, K. T. Kosmidis, M. H., & Sayers, M. D. (1992). Symptomatology and the prediction of social skills acquisition in schizophrenia. *Schizophrenia Research, 8*, 59–68.

Overall, J. E., & Gorham, D. R. (1962). The Brief Psychiatric Rating Scale. *Psychological Reports, 18*, 799–812.

Pao, P. N. (1979). *Schizophrenic disorders: Theory and treatment from a psychodynamic point of view*. New York: International Universities Press.

Parker, G., & Hadzi-Pavlovic, D. (1990). Expressed emotion as a predictor of schizophrenic relapse: An analysis of aggregated data. *Psychological Medicine, 20*, 961–965.

Paul, G. L., & Lentz, R. J. (1977). *Psychosocial treatment of chronic mental patients: Milieu versus social-learning programs*. Cambridge, MA: Harvard University Press.

Randolph, E., Eth, S., Glynn, S., Leong, G., Paz, G., & Shaner, A. (1991, May). *Behavioral family therapy: One year outcome results*. Paper presented at the meeting of the American Psychiatric Association, New Orleans, LA.

Rogers, C. R., Gendlin, E. G., Kiesler, D. J., & Traux, C. B. (1967). *The therapeutic relationship and its impact: Study of psychotherapy with schizophrenics*. Madison: University of Wisconsin Press.

Rosen, J. (1947). The treatment of schizophrenic psychosis by direct analytic therapy. *Psychiatric Quarterly, 21*, 3–37.

Roy, A. (1986). Suicide in schizophrenia. In A. Roy (Ed.), *Suicide* (pp. 97–112). Baltimore: Williams & Wilkins.

Schooler, N., Hogarty, G., & Weissman, M. (1979). Social Adjustment Scale II (SAS-II). In W. A. Hargreaves, C. C. Atkisson, & J. E. Sorenson (Eds.), *Resource materials for community mental health program evaluations* (pp. 290–303) (DHEW Publication No. ADM 79328. Rockville, MD: Department of Health, Education, and Welfare.

Schooler, N. R., Keith, S. J., Severe, J. B., Matthews, S., & the Treatment Strategies in Schizophrenia Collaborative Study Group. (1989). Acute treatment response and short-term outcome in schizophrenia: First results of the NIMH Treatment Strategies in Schizophrenia study. *Psychopharmacology Bulletin, 25*, 331–335.

Searles, H. F. (1965). *Collected papers on schizophrenia and related subjects*. New York: International Universities Press.

Silverman, L. H., & Lachmann, F. M. (1985). The therapeutic properties of unconscious oneness fantasies: Evidence and treatment implications. *Contemporary Psychoanalysis, 21*, 91–115.

Spencer, J., Glick, I., Haas, G., Clarkin, J., Lewis, A., Peyser, J., DeMane, N., Good-Ellis, M., Harris, E., & Lestelle, V. (1988). A randomized clinical trial of inpatient family intervention: III. Effects at 6-month and 18-month follow-ups. *American Journal of Psychiatry, 145*, 1115–1121.

Spitzer, R. L., & Williams, J. B. W. (1985). *Instruction manual for the structured clinical interview for DSM-III*. New York: New York State Psychiatric Institute, Biometrics Research Department.

Stanton, A. H., Gunderson, J. G., Knapp, P. H., Frank, A. F., Vannicelli, M. L., Schnitzer, R., & Rosenthal, R. (1984). Effects of psychotherapy in schizophrenia: I. Design and implementation of a controlled study. *Schizophrenia Bulletin, 10*, 520–563.

Stone, M. H. (1986). Exploratory psychotherapy in schizophrenia-spectrum patients. *Bulletin of the Menninger Clinic, 50*, 287–306.

Strauss, J. S., & Carpenter, W. T. (1972). The prediction of outcome in schizophrenia: I. Characteristics of outcome. *Archives of General Psychiatry, 27*, 739–746.

Strupp, H. H., Hadley, S. W., & Gomes-Schwartz, B. (1977). *Psychotherapy for better or worse*. New York: Jason Aronson.

Tarrier, N., & Barrowclough, C. (1986). Providing information to relatives about schizophrenia: Some comments. *British Journal of Psychiatry, 149*, 458–463.

Tarrier, N., & Barrowclough, C. (1990). Family interventions for schizophrenia. *Behavior Modification, 14*, 408–440.

Tarrier, N., Barrowclough, C., Vaughn, C. Bamrah, J., Porceddu, K., Watts, S., & Freeman, H. (1988). The community management of schizophrenia: A controlled trial of a behavioral intervention with families to reduce relapse. *British Journal of Psychiatry, 153*, 532–542.

Tarrier, N., Barrowclough, C., Vaughn, C. Bamrah, J., Porceddu, K., Watts, S., & Freeman, H. (1989). Community management of schizophrenia: A two-year follow-up of a behavioral intervention with families. *British Journal of Psychiatry, 154*, 625–628.

Taylor, A., & Dowell, D. A. (1986). Social skills training in board and care homes. *Psychosocial Rehabilitation Bulletin, 10*, 55–69.

Tuma, A. H., & May, P. R. A. (1974). Psychotherapy, drugs and therapist experience in the treatment of schizophrenia: A critique of the Michigan State project. *Psychotherapy: Theory, Research and Practice, 12*, 138–142.

Van Putten, T., & Marder, S. R. (1986). Low-dose treatment strategies. *Journal of Clinical Psychiatry, 47*, 12–16.

Vaughn, C., & Leff, J. (1976a). The influence of family and social factors on the course of psychiatric illness. *American Journal of Psychiatry, 129*, 125–137.

Vaughn, C., & Leff, J. (1976b). The measurement of expressed emotion in the families of psychiatric patients. *British Journal of Psychiatry, 15*, 157–165.

Vaughn, C., Snyder, K., Jones, S., Freeman, W., & Falloon, I. (1984). Family factors in schizophrenia relapse. *Archives of General Psychiatry, 41*, 1169–1177.

Ventura, J., Nuechterlein, K. H., Lukoff, D., & Hardesty, J. P. (1989). A prospective study of stressful life events and schizophrenia relapse. *Journal of Abnormal Psychology, 98*, 407–411.

Wallace, C. J., & Liberman, R. P. (1985). Social skills training for patients with schizophrenia: A controlled clinical trial. *Psychiatry Research, 15*, 239–247.

Wing, J. K., Cooper, J. E., & Sartorius, N. (1974). *The measurement and classification of psychiatric symptoms*. London: Cambridge University Press.

Wykes, T., & Sturt, E. (1986). The measurement of social behaviour in psychiatric patients: An assessment of the reliability and validity of the SBS schedule. *British Journal of Psychiatry, 148*, 1–11.

Zigler, E., & Glick, M. (1986). *A developmental approach to adult psychopathology*. New York: Wiley.

15

Comparative Treatments for Borderline Personality Disorder

Theory and Research

Darren A. Tutek and Marsha M. Linehan

Interest in and concern about borderline personality disorder (BPD) have escalated rapidly since the introduction of the disorder into the *Diagnostic and Statistical Manual of Mental Disorders*, published by the American Psychiatric Association (APA) in 1980. A quick perusal of psychological and psychiatric journals reveals the plethora of articles on this topic. At present, it is the most widely researched personality disorder. A recent literature review of journal articles on personality disorders has shown that over 40% were devoted exclusively to research on BPD (Widiger & Frances, 1989). The popularity of BPD has spurred numerous articles, book chapters, and books on the diagnosis, behavioral patterns, epidemiology, and etiology of this disorder. Unfortunately, research on treatment theory and outcome for BPD has been sparse and generally not subject to stringent empirical examination. The lack of quality treatment research on BPD can be attributed to a myriad of factors, including poorly defined constructs for the etiology and diagnosis of BPD, the difficult nature of treating borderline patients, and the numerous shortcomings that obfuscate clinical research. Consequently, much of what we know today about treatment of borderlines is based on particular theoretical guidelines, unsystematic observation, retrospective studies, and clinical lore. This chapter will attempt to consolidate much of the research literature on treatment theory and outcome for borderline personality disorder.

Darren A. Tutek and **Marsha M. Linehan** • Department of Psychology, University of Washington, Seattle, Washington 98195.

Handbook of Effective Psychotherapy, edited by Thomas R. Giles. Plenum Press, New York, 1993.

Diagnosis and Behavioral Patterns

Although the history of the "borderline" concept has been rife with political, economic, and medical connotations for several decades, the term has traditionally been used to describe patients that were inherently difficult to treat with either psychotherapy or biomedical approaches (Kroll, 1988). The specific criteria for borderline personality disorder have only recently been operationalized (DSM-III and DSM-III-R; APA, 1980, 1987). Although some of these criteria for BPD are expected to be slightly modified for DSM-IV, the basic definition of the diagnosis remains the same. Borderline personality disorder is typically characterized by pervasive patterns of instability in various areas of psychosocial functioning, including difficulties with affect regulation, interpersonal problem solving and relationships, and control of self-destructive and impulsive behavior. A diagnosis of BPD requires that the individual meet at least five of the following DSM-III-R criteria (APA, 1987)

1. A pattern of intense and unstable interpersonal relationships
2. Impulsive and/or reckless behaviors (not including suicidal behaviors) that are potentially self-damaging
3. Marked affective instability characterized by extreme mood shifts in relatively short periods of time
4. Intense, inappropriate and/or uncontrollable anger
5. Recurrent suicidal and/or parasuicidal behaviors
6. Marked and persistent identity disturbances
7. Chronic feelings of boredom and emptiness
8. Frantic efforts to avoid real or imagined abandonment

Numerous empirical studies (e.g., Clarkin *et al.*, 1983; Gardner, Leibenluft, O'Leary, & Cowdry, 1991; Marziali *et al.*, 1984; McGlashan, 1987; Modestin, 1987; Perry & Klerman, 1980; Snyder & Pitts, 1985) have sought to validate these criteria to some degree, although there is still disagreement about the nature of the borderline diagnosis. Two major issues concerning the diagnosis involve the validity and reliability of the diagnosis and the consistent overlap of BPD with a variety of other Axis I and Axis II disorders. By using the DSM-III polythetic system to diagnose BPD, there are 56 different ways an individual may meet criteria for BPD. Consequently, the heterogeneity of the borderline diagnosis creates numerous diagnostic, research, and treatment issues.

Furthermore, the diagnosis of BPD is often complicated by comorbidity with other disorders. A recent study reported that out of 180 patients diagnosed with BPD, 91% had one additional diagnosis and 42% had two or more additional diagnoses (Fyer, Frances, Sullivan, Hurt, & Clarkin, 1988). Among these comorbid diagnoses, affective disorders are most prevalent (Manos, Vasilopoulou, & Sotiriou, 1987; Zimmerman, Pfohl, Coryell, Stangl, & Corenthal, 1988), with 40% to 60% of BPD patients meeting criteria for some form of affective disorder (Gunderson & Elliott, 1985). This high comorbidity rate has led many researchers to postulate that BPD may actually be a variant or consequence of the mood disorders (Gunderson & Elliott, 1985). The "affectophile" (Kroll, 1988) approach to BPD characterizes the disorder as a pervasive personality style that reflects the underlying mood disorder, and since BPD is viewed as primarily an affective disorder, pharmacological treatment is deemed superior to relieving the behavioral patterns of BPD. Other frequent comorbid diagnoses often include anxiety disorders, eating disorders, psychoses, and other personality disorders, particularly narcissistic, antisocial, and schizotypal personality disorders (McGlashan & Heinssen, 1989; Rosenberger & Miller, 1989; Serban, Conte, & Plutchik, 1987). Many of these overlapping disorders reflect the DSM-III criteria for BPD, including affect, impulsivity, self-damaging behaviors, and interpersonal dysfunctions. The high comorbidity rate of BPD with other Axis I and Axis II disorders has both complicated research in terms of design limitations and generalizations of findings, and hindered the development of efficacious treatment approaches to the disorder.

Several other features of BPD have been investigated in the research literature and deserve special attention. Recent research has indicated a high correlation between BPD and childhood sexual and physical abuse. The risk for sexual abuse is approximately two to three times greater for females than males (Finkelhor, 1979). The prevalence of childhood sexual abuse in the histories of women meeting criteria for BPD is such that it simply cannot be ignored as an important, and perhaps crucial, factor in the etiology of the disorder. Of 12 hospitalized borderline patients assessed by Stone (1981), 75% reported a history of incest. In another study (Bryer, Nelson, Miller, & Kroll, 1987), childhood sexual abuse was reported by 86% of borderline inpatients compared to 21% of other psychiatric inpatients. Among borderline outpatients, 67% to 76% report childhood sexual abuse (Herman, 1986; Herman, Perry, & van der Kolk, 1989; Shearer *et al.*, 1990; Wagner & Linehan, in press). This is in contrast to a 26% rate among nonborderline outpatients (Herman *et al.*, 1989). Ogata *et al.* (1989) report that 71% of borderline patients reported a history of sexual abuse compared to 22% of major depressive disorder control patients. Wagner and Linehan (in press) also found that past sexual abuse predicted more medically serious parasuicidal behavior in women diagnosed with BPD.

Although in epidemiological data, girls are at no higher risk for physical abuse than are boys, rates of reported childhood physical abuse are higher among borderline patients (71%) than among nonborderline patients (Herman *et al.*, 1989). In addition, Herman *et al.* reported that 62% of their borderline patients had witnessed domestic violence during childhood compared to 30% of nonborderline outpatients. There is also a positive correlation between physical and sexual abuse (Westen *et al.*, 1990), suggesting that those at risk for sexual abuse are at higher risk for physical abuse also. Bryer *et al.* (1987), however, found that whereas early sexual abuse predicted the borderline diagnosis, the combination of physical and sexual abuse did not. Ogata *et al.* (1989) also report similar rates of physical abuse in borderline and depressed patients. Thus, it may be that sexual abuse, in contrast to other types of abuse, is uniquely associated with BPD. Much more research is needed here to clarify this relationship. Overall, the high frequency of past childhood abuse in borderline patients necessitates that at least part of the treatment of this disorder focus on posttraumatic stress symptoms (Perry, Herman, van der Kolk, & Hoke, 1990; Linehan, 1993a).

Another behavioral pattern of BPD that has received considerable attention in the research literature is suicidal and parasuicidal behavior. Gunderson (1984) has called this the "behavioral specialty" of the disorder. *Parasuicide* refers to any intentional, acute, self-injurious behavior with or without suicidal intent, including both suicide attempts and self-mutilative behaviors. The high prevalence of parasuicidal behavior in borderlines has been noted by many researchers (Clarkin *et al.*, 1983; Gardner & Cowdry, 1985; Liebenluft, Gardner, & Cowdry, 1987; Raczek, True, & Friend, 1989) and is indeed a highly indicative criterion for meeting the DSM-III borderline diagnosis. Suicidal behavior is the one criterion that differentiates BPD from other personality disorders (Morey, 1988). The role and function of parasuicidal behavior in borderline individuals is subject to diverse theoretical positions. It has been viewed as manipulative communication (Gunderson, 1984), interpersonal problem solving (Linehan *et al.*, 1987), emotion regulation (Linehan, 1993a), cathartic emotional release (Gardner & Cowdry, 1985), an outcome of intrapsychic conflicts and transference phenomena (Kernberg, 1987), and a result of biochemical dysfunctions (Traskman-Bendz, Asberg, & Schalling, 1986). Whatever the etiology and function, suicidal and parasuicidal behaviors are primary treatment targets in the treatment of BPD by either psychotherapy or pharmacotherapy (Kernberg *et al.*, 1989; Liebowitz, 1987; Linehan, 1993a).

Other features of BPD that have undergone substantial empirical investigation include neurological dysfunctions (Andrulonis, Glueck, Stroebel, & Vogel, 1982), cognitive deficits (O'Leary, Brouwers, Gardner, & Cowdry, 1991), psychotic symptoms (Silk, Lohr, Westen, & Goodrich, 1989; Zanarini, Gunderson, & Frankenburg, 1990), sexual behavior (Zubenko, George, Soloff, & Schulz, 1987), alcoholism (Nace, Saxon, & Shore, 1983; Jonsdottir-Baldursson, & Horvath, 1987), and substance abuse (Dulit *et al.*, 1990; Malow, West, Williams, & Sutker, 1989). In light of the empirical data so far, BPD seems to include a mishmash of behavioral, physiological, and environmental characteristics even beyond its stringent DSM-III criteria, and the interrelationship of all of these factors paints a complicated picture that makes diagnosing, understanding, and treating this disorder difficult.

Prevalence and Epidemiology

Borderline personality disorder is one of the most common personality disorder diagnoses, although official prevalence rates are subject to fluctuations depending on the criteria used, settings, and diagnostic procedures (Widiger & Frances, 1989). In the general population, the prevalence of BPD has been estimated to range from 1.6% to 4% when using strictly defined DSM-III criteria, although Kernberg (as reported in Gunderson and Elliott, 1985), who uses a much broader definition of BPD, has given estimates as high as 15% in the general population. According to Widiger and Frances (1989), in clinical samples prevalence ranges from 8% to 63% depending on the setting. In their review of the literature, they estimate that approximately 11% of psychiatric outpatients and 19% of psychiatric inpatients are diagnosed with BPD. Furthermore, they also estimate that 23% of inpatients who are not schizophrenic or mentally retarded, and who do not have an organic mental disorder, meet criteria for BPD; in addition, they also estimate that 33% of outpatients and 63% of inpatients with a personality disorder meet criteria for BPD. These high prevalence rates among inpatients and outpatients suggest that BPD greatly impacts all areas of the mental health field.

In terms of gender and ethnic distribution, Widiger and Frances (1989) report that 74% of BPD patients in 38 studies were women, although there is some question as to gender bias in the diagnosis of BPD (Widiger & Spitzer, 1991). A few studies have reported a lower proportion of blacks with BPD, although it has been suggested that racial bias may prohibit black borderline patients from receiving adequate mental health treatment in comparison to receiving correctional treatment (Akhtar, Byrne, & Doghramji, 1986; Castaneda & Franco, 1985). Castaneda and Franco reported no differences in prevalence rates between Hispanics and whites, although they noted that more male Hispanics were diagnosed with BPD (47%) than white or black males (27% and 20%, respectively).

Etiological and Developmental Factors

Many developmental factors have been implicated in the etiology of BPD, particularly factors in the familial environment. Many researchers believe that BPD has its roots in early childhood development, and recent research evidence indicates that the borderline diagnosis can be adequately applied to adolescents (Ludolph *et al.*, 1990). However, there is some suggestion that normal adolescent behavior can be misconstrued as borderline behavior. In their retrospective study, Ludolph and colleagues (1990) reported many disruptive parenting variables that predicted a later BPD diagnosis in their adolescent population compared to normals. These variables included an early and recurrent history of disrupted attachments, maternal neglect, maternal rejection, grossly inappropriate parental behavior, a higher number of parental surrogates, and physical and/or sexual abuse. Several other retrospective studies have reported similar problematic factors in parental care as self-reported by BPD patients, including parental neglect (Gunderson, Kerr, & Englund, 1980), inadequate parental bonding (Paris & Frank, 1989), and parental rigidity and borderline behavior (Feldman & Guttman, 1984). In a long-term follow-up study, Paris, Nowlis, and Brown (1988) also reported that disruptive parental relationships, particularly with the mother, was predictive of poor overall global outcome and higher depression over a mean interval of 15 years for a group of 191 borderlines.

Several studies of first-degree relatives of borderline patients have also been reported. Overall, this familial research has indicated that borderline families have higher rates of depression and antisocial personality disorder (Schulz *et al.*, 1989), alcoholism (Loranger & Tulis, 1985), and borderline personality disorder (Links, Steiner, & Huxley, 1988; Loranger, Oldham, & Tulis, 1982) than other psychiatric control groups and the general population. Studies necessary to demonstrate a genetic basis for the disorder, however, have not been conducted.

In addition to disruptive parental behaviors and a high prevalence of familial disorders in BPD probands, there is also some research evidence that implicates neurological and biochemical factors in the etiology of BPD. In a recent study by Andrulonis and colleagues (1982), 38% of 91 BPD patients had some type of neuropsychiatric or organic abnormality which was believed to play an etiological role in the development of the disorder. In another study, 16 BPD outpatients had significantly more impairments on memory tests and visual perceptual tests than normal controls, which could not be attributed to nonneurological factors (O'Leary *et al.*, 1991). In addition, other researchers have reported that BPD patients had significantly more EEG dysrhythmias than depressed control patients, which seems to indicate another form of neurological impairment (Cowdry, Pickar, & Davies, 1985; Snyder & Pitts, 1984). However, all of these findings have recently been challenged in a study by Cornelius and colleagues (1989) which did not find a consistent pattern of abnormalities in neuropsychological testing or higher rates of EEG dysrhythmias in a group of 45 BPD patients compared to depressed and schizophrenic controls. Finally, research on biochemical factors in the etiology of BPD has been sparse. A few studies have indicated that serotonergic dysfunctions may play a role in increased suicidal, impulsive, and aggressive behaviors in BPD patients, although it is unclear whether these biochemical dysfunctions are an antecedent or consequence of the disorder (Coccaro *et al.*, 1989; Traskman-Bendz, Asberg, & Schalling, 1986).

Linehan (1993a) and others (Snyder & Pitts, 1985) have called attention to the temperamental characteristics of borderline individuals. Such characteristics appear to have a genetic basis in the normal population, and, thus, an argument can be made that at least some aspects of BPD may be genetically influenced (Chess & Thomas, 1986; Thomas & Chess, 1985). Taken together, findings on environmental, biological, and temperamental characteristics of borderline individuals suggest a biosocial etiology. Either a diathesis-stress or transactional model (Linehan, 1993; Scarr & McCartney, 1983) may be the best fit here.

Theoretical Conceptualization and Treatment of BPD

Psychodynamic Approaches

From the very beginning, borderline personality disorder has had its conceptual and treatment roots in psychoanalytic theory. In fact in 1938, A. Stern, a prominent psychiatrist, coined the term "borderline" to describe a group of patients who were "too ill for classical psychoanalysis" (Stone, 1980). Thereafter, many psychodynamic clinicians have diverged on the conceptualization and treatment of borderline patients (for a more complete review see Alder, 1989).

Of these theorists, Kernberg's object relations approach to borderline personality organization (of which BPD is a specialized subgroup) has provided a comprehensive approach to understanding the development and subsequent treatment of this disorder (Kernberg, 1975, 1984; Kernberg *et al.*, 1989). Kernberg points to a combination of early constitutional and environmental factors that lead to the development of BPD during the first few years of life. He postulates that infants with intrinsic excessively aggressive drives who are subsequently frustrated by inadequate parenting styles may develop borderline pathology. During ego development, these infants encounter more negative experiences than positive, which in turn cause them to internalize aggression. Thereafter, these internalized negative experiences are represented in negative object relations constructs, including self-representations, object representations, and a concurrent negative affective state that links the two. Since these negative representations are threatening to the overall internal psychic structure, these individuals are distanced from the positive self-object representations through primitive defense mechanisms such as regression and splitting. Overall, this entire psychic process leads to a borderline individual with primary process thinking, identity disturbances, low anxiety tolerance, and high impulsivity. In Kernberg's expressive psychotherapy for borderline patients, the therapist's task is to expose and resolve intrapsychic conflict via the use of interpretations, the maintenance of technical neutrality, and the use of transference analysis. The duration of therapy is expected to last several years, with primary foci on suicidal behaviors and therapy-interfering behaviors.

Other prominent psychodynamic theorists who have formulated approaches to borderline personality include Masterson (1976, 1981) and Rinsley (1982), who believe that the borderline individual has problems with separation and individuation due to conflicts with early pathological maternal attachment. Masterson's and Rinsley's treatment approaches emphasize the importance of the transference relationship as a model and testing ground for the borderline individual to resolve these separation–individuation issues. Thus, the therapist becomes a surrogate "mother" with whom the patient can repeat early attachment experiences and form a more healthy perspective on separation and individuation.

Adler and Buie (Adler, 1985; Adler & Buie, 1979; Buie & Adler, 1982) also emphasize problems with separation in borderline patients. These theorists believe that borderline individuals have an extreme intolerance for being alone, and when they do find themselves alone, their insufficient coping responses lead them to have irrational fears of abandonment. Fears of separation occur mainly because borderline individuals lack the capacity to count upon their own strengths and resources during periods of separation. Consequently, when alone, borderline individuals experience extreme anger and resentment due to the stress of separation and being alone, which interferes with their ability to remember important and stable people in their lives. These emotional responses lead to extreme displays of behavior, including unbridled dependency behaviors and impulsive, self-damaging behaviors. According to Adler and Buie, treatment should focus on the feelings of aloneness, abandonment, and rage until healthy separation responses are learned.

Gunderson's (1984) approach to the borderline individual involves a multilevel conceptualization of patient functioning with concomitant treatment strategies. The first level of treatment is concerned with the patient's inherent need for support and reassurance at the start of therapy and the development of an intimate and stable therapeutic relationship. At the second level, the therapist needs to work through the transference relationship, including any aggressive and manipulative behaviors that develop as a result of therapeutic frustration of the patient. At this level, treatment strategies include interpretations, confrontations, and limit setting. At the third level, the borderline patient experiences feelings of aloneness and self-hatred, which results in panic behavior. Consequently, the patient may engage in impulsive behaviors or experience brief psychotic episodes to relieve these feelings of panic. The therapist works through separation and individuation issues to resolve these crises.

Marziali and Munroe-Blum (1987; Munroe-Blum & Marziali, 1987) have developed a psychodynamic, time-limited, group therapy ("relationship management psychotherapy" [RMP]) for borderline patients. In RMP, the therapist's role is to help the client express internalized conflicts around self-attributes that can be interpreted or disconfirmed in a group therapy setting. The group format of RMP helps diffuse abstruse and potentially destructive projections patients may make by minimizing the intensity of transference and countertransference reactions across patients and cotherapists. The therapist often engages patients individually without necessarily provoking group interaction. Therapist interpretations often are facilitated better in a group format in contrast to individual psychodynamic therapy. Mutual patient support is also accomplished when altruistic patient behaviors are made in response to externalized negative projections, self-concepts, and beliefs other group members may voice. RMP is different than traditional psychodynamic group therapy since it includes an orientation phase to treatment and allows the therapist to be accessible outside of the group format.

Interpersonal Approaches

The interpersonal model is a relatively new approach to conceptualizing and treating personality disorders (McLemore & Brokaw, 1987; Pincus & Wiggins, 1990). The basic premise of this approach is that all intrapsychic and behavioral events are in relationship to other people, and thus personality disorders are just dysfunctional interpersonal behavior. One of the most important interpersonal approaches has been developed by Lorna Benjamin (1974, 1979), whose coding scheme, "structural analysis of social behavior" (SASB), can be used to measure and validate interpersonal and intrapsychic behavior along the dimensions of interdependence, affiliation, and "self" and "other" foci. A SASB analysis consisting of interpersonal and intrapsychic descriptors can be reliably applied to the DSM-III-R criteria for BPD and is thereby useful in describing current interpersonal patterns of behavior in BPD patients and for planning subsequent treatment interventions (Benjamin, in press).

Cognitive-Behavioral Approaches

Behavioral and cognitive-behavioral theorists have been among the last to apply their theories to conceptualizing and treating personality disorders, primarily because behaviorists have often questioned the validity of psychiatric diagnoses and have strong biases in interpreting personality as a changing, environmentally influenced (rather than consistent) phenomena (Turner & Turkat, 1988). Interestingly, cognitive-behaviorists, like their psychoanalytic colleagues, have begun to attend to the influence of personality disorders on the effectiveness of their treatments at approximately the same developmental point in their discipline, the third decade (Linehan, 1993a). In both cases, attention to personality disorders follows widespread acceptance of their respective treatment perspectives.

Among these theorists, Turner (1984; Turner & Hersen, 1981) has proposed an array of behavioral and cognitive interventions for treatment of BPD. Turner's approach emphasizes an information-processing model and reinforced maladaptive schemata over time to understand the development and maintenance of learned borderline behavior. In treatment of BPD, Turner advocates certain cognitive-behavioral components in his treatment plan, including social anxiety reduction group therapy, social skills training, anxiety management training, contingency management, and cognitive-restructuring therapy.

A more strictly behavioral approach to the personality disorders has been the case formulation approach advocated by Turkat (1990; Turkat & Maisto, 1985). Each patient is evaluated individually on a case-by-case basis, and an appropriate behavioral treatment plan is then rendered. In this method, the formulation of each case can be defined by three hypotheses along the dimensions of behavioral patterns: (1) how do the problems presented by the patient relate to each other, (2) what is the etiology of these problems, and (3) what predictions can be made about the patient's behavior in the future. Using this formulation approach over several

BPD patients, Turkat (1990) has proposed that a deficiency in problem-solving abilities is a core feature of BPD. Thus, Turkat recommends several behavioral interventions for treating BPD, including basic problem-solving training, concept formation training, categorization management, and information-processing speed management.

Linehan (1987a, 1987b, 1993a,b) has developed a comprehensive cognitive-behavioral therapy, "dialectical behavior therapy," for the treatment of chronically parasuicidal BPD patients. Linehan uses a biosocial theory to conceptualize BPD, where the constitutional basis of the disorder is one of high emotional reactivity and dysregulation. She proposes that borderline behavioral patterns are a result of the transaction between the emotionally vulnerable child and an environment that invalidates expressions of private experience, particularly emotional expressions (Linehan, 1993; Linehan & Koerner, 1993). In addition, she proposes three bipolar behavioral patterns of BPD that are both a function of and maintained by this core emotional dysregulation within invalidating environments. These behavioral patterns can be thought of along a biosocial axis and include (1) emotional vulnerability versus self-invalidation, (2) active passivity versus apparent competency, and (3) unrelenting crises versus inhibited grieving. From a theoretical stance, those patterns above the axis (emotional vulnerability, active passivity, unrelenting crises) are originally most heavily influenced by biological factors associated with emotion regulation. Those patterns below the axis (invalidation, apparent competency, inhibited grieving) are most heavily influenced by invalidating social responses, both developmentally and presently, to emotional expressiveness. The importance of these patterns is that they interfere with effective treatment and adaptive change.

Linehan's dialectical behavior therapy (DBT) (1993a,b) involves simultaneous individual psychotherapy and behavioral skills training, usually accomplished in group treatment. The group format is psychoeducational, stressing acquisition of behavioral skills such as interpersonal effectiveness, emotion regulation, distress tolerance, mindfulness meditation practices, and self-management. In individual DBT, treatment targets are hierarchically arranged as follows: (1) suicidal and parasuicidal behaviors, (2) behaviors interfering with the conduct of therapy, (3) quality-of-life interfering behaviors, (4) behavioral skills acquisition (as instructed in the group format), (5) posttraumatic stress, (6) respect for self, and (7) individual goals the patient brings to therapy. Essentially, the first goal of DBT individual therapy is to block behaviors in the first three target areas and replace them with behavioral skills in the fourth target area. Thereafter, goals are to uncover and reduce effects of childhood sexual, physical, and emotional trauma (target 5) and then teach individuals how to trust and validate themselves (target 6). DBT is a blend of interventions focusing on acceptance (e.g., validation, reciprocal communication strategies) and on change (e.g., problem solving, skills training, management, cognitive modification strategies). Although primarily a cognitive-behavioral therapy, DBT is based on a dialectical philosophy and employs a range of interventions which Linehan describes as dialectical strategies.

Cognitive Approaches

Cognitive therapy has only recently been applied to the personality disorders (e.g., Murray, 1988; Padesky, 1986; Pretzer & Fleming, 1989; Young, 1990; Young

& Swift, 1988), and more specifically to borderline personality disorder (e.g., Beck & Freeman, 1990; Glat, 1988a, 1988b; Katz & Levendusky, 1990; Millon, 1987). As with these cognitive approaches to other disorders, the basic premise is that personality disorders are a result of dysfunctional cognitive schemata. Schemata are constructs used for organizing and interpreting the environment. Dysfunctional schemata cause individuals to perceive, interpret, and evaluate environmental situations and themselves in an erroneous manner, thus contributing to the behavioral patterns of the disorder in question (Murray, 1988).

Beck and Freeman's (1990) approach to BPD is to challenge dysfunctional thinking patterns. They are particularly concerned with addressing the borderline patient's basic assumptions and errors in thinking ("cognitive distortions"). Beck and Freeman believe the borderline individual holds three basic cognitive assumptions that influence both behavior and emotional responses. They are as follows: "The world is dangerous and malevolent," "I am powerless and vulnerable," and "I am inherently unacceptable." They also believe that the borderline's dichotomous thinking (a cognitive distortion where situations are perceived and interpreted in extremes) plays a crucial role in the development and perpetuation of crises and conflicts. Thus, the combination of both these negative basic assumptions and all-or-none thinking leads to much of the typical borderline behavior. Beck and Freeman advocate a treatment plan that fosters an intense therapeutic alliance, reduces dichotomous thinking, addresses basic assumptions, and works on impulse and emotional control.

Similarly, Young (1990; Young & Swift, 1988) has developed "schema-focused cognitive therapy" to treat personality disorders. According to Young, people who develop enduring, stable, and dysfunctional patterns of thinking ("maladaptive schemas") during childhood may develop a personality disorder in adulthood. The early maladaptive schemata that characterize BPD in childhood include fears of abandonment and loss, unlovability, dependence, lack of individuation, mistrust, poor self-discipline, fear of losing emotional control, excessive guilt, and emotional deprivation. Thus, in schema-focused cognitive therapy, methods for evaluating and modifying these maladaptive schemata are the primary focus of therapy.

Millon (1987) provides a slightly different cognitive-behavioral view to conceptualizing BPD. He proposes a social learning theory which combines biological, psychological, and sociological factors in explaining BPD. Millon postulates that the borderline has an unclear identity and a vacillating sense of self, which becomes the crux of the disorder. This identity crisis leads to inconsistent and poor coping responses, poor impulse control, and extreme dependency needs.

Psychopharmacological Approaches

The psychopharmacological approach to BPD emphasizes the biological nature of the disorder, along with any comorbid diagnoses that complicate the disorder. The typical pharmacological approach to BPD has been to assess and treat the disorder along many affective, cognitive, and behavioral dimensions that have previously shown response to drug therapies (Cowdry, 1987; Stone, 1989a). Because there is no drug treatment of choice for BPD and there is high variability of symptoms among BPD patients, various pharmacological regimens are instigated, including treatment for psychotic thinking, behavioral dyscontrol, and affective lability, including anxiety and depression. This approach of limiting treatment to specific target areas, rather than simultaneously treating the broad array of behaviors associated with the disorder as a whole, has met with limited success. Consequently, pharmacological approaches are typically used in conjunction with some form of psychosocial therapy to form a comprehensive treatment package.

Treatment Research on BPD

Like other Axis II disorders, empirically based treatment research on BPD has been lacking, and the development of systematic treatment manuals for BPD has only recently been promulgated (Hurt & Clarkin, 1990). Some recent controlled studies, however, may provide some insight into the treatment of BPD. In a controlled study of short-term psychodynamic therapy ("brief adaptational psychotherapy") with individuals diagnosed with personality disorders other than BPD, Pollack and colleagues (1990) found some treatment success in terms of reductions in target complaints and improved global social adjustment compared to a wait-list control group; further improvement was achieved in the psychotherapy group on target complains 1–5 years after termination of therapy. Using a cognitive-behavioral problem-solving approach, Salkovskis, Atha, and Storer (1990) reported reductions in depression, hopelessness, suicidal ideation, and target problems in a group of repeated suicide attempters compared to a treatment-as-usual control condition. Although Salkovskis *et al.* did not report diagnoses for patients in their study, repeated parasuicides is one of the most prevalent criteria for BPD, and thus, this type of approach may be amenable to parasuicidal borderline patients.

The actual treatment process of all personality disorders is rife with problems, including selecting a proper therapeutic modality, getting the patient into treatment, the long length of treatment, high attrition rates, and vague criteria for successful outcomes (Liebowitz, Stone, & Turkat, 1986). This is particularly true for BPD. The high prevalence rates of BPD, in conjunction with high treatment failure rates with these patients, has put considerable strain on the mental health field with no immediate solution in sight. Simply put, there is no treatment of choice for BPD. Furthermore, although many therapeutic modalities are regularly applied in treating BPD, the efficacy of these treatments has generally not undergone stringent treatment outcome research. As with treatment, research with borderline individuals can be extraordinarily taxing. Difficulties getting subjects to come to assessment sessions and to complete difficult assessment protocols, lack of standardized assessment procedures (or even moderate agreement on what should be measured), problems training therapists in long-term therapy regimes, and difficulties maintaining adherence to treatment protocols in the face of life-threatening crises are just a sample of the problems the investigator must overcome. It is little wonder that treatment researchers are wary of treading into this area.

Case Study Designs

Although idiosyncratic, individual treatment case histories for BPD (e.g., Chessick, 1982; Glantz, 1981) have often been reported in the literature, Turner (1989) has reported an elaborate and well-assessed case study design with four (two male and two female) BPD patients using a bio-cognitive-behavioral treatment program. The study was divided into six time periods: (1) a baseline period of 2 weeks, (2) a medication-only period lasting 2 weeks, (3) an evocative flooding phase to inoculate patients against emotional instability and anxiety for 2 weeks, (4) a 4-week period using both covert rehearsal strategies to improve emotion control and self-image and cognitive therapy aimed at modifying cognitive distortions, (5) 4 weeks of cognitive therapy aimed at improving interpersonal skills, and (6) a maintenance therapy period of 9 months consisting of skills training and problem solving. Pharmacotherapy (alprazolam) was given over the first 6 months of treatment. All four of the patients were actively engaging in suicidal and parasuicidal behaviors prior to treatment. The primary treatment goals were to reduce parasuicidal behaviors, micropsychotic experiences, and number of psychiatric hospitalizations. All four patients were seen by the same therapist, a third-year psychiatric resident who had been trained in these techniques.

Patients were assessed weekly for weeks 1 through 7, and thereafter at weeks 10, 11, 14, and follow-up. During the baseline period and during each week of treatment, patients were asked to self-report their most problematic behaviors or cognitive states, and these were used as outcome measures. The Hamilton Rating Scales for Anxiety and Depression were also administered by an independent assessor. Reductions in self-reported frequency of the most problematic cognitions and behaviors occurred with each aspect of the treatment plan, except the flooding phase. Turner (1989) also reported gradual reductions in anxiety and depression which could be attributed to the alprazolam treatment. At 12 months, all patients were still in maintenance therapy, and three patients had maintained their treatment gains, including reduced suicidal behavior. At the 2-year follow-up period, two of the patients were still in therapy; two of the four patients had maintained their treatment gains, while one patient had severely relapsed.

There are several problems with Turner's (1989) case study design. The lack of a control group, the small number of subjects, the use of only one therapist, the lack of independent and blind assessment, and the lack of randomization in ordering treatment components contribute to the pitfalls of this case study design. Although this study was not a controlled single-subjects design, it is an interesting preliminary pilot study with this population. Turner's results suggest that a multimodality treatment package may be effective in treating BPD.

Treatment Comparisons with Nonspecific Effects

Due to the lack of controlled treatment research for BPD, there is insufficient data to report any nonspecific treatment effects in outcome studies. Consequently, the few controlled studies that have reported treatment gains should be interpreted with caution.

Interorientation Comparisons

To our knowledge, there have been no interorientation treatment studies conducted on BPD. Although Linehan and colleagues (1991) used a treatment-as-usual naturalistic control condition in their study (see below) that allowed control subjects to receive a variety of therapeutic modalities, the limited number of subjects in this control condition, in conjunction with the variety of therapies received by control subjects, does not give sufficient power for adequate orientation comparisons.

Controlled Clinical Trials

Linehan *et al.* (1991) recently conducted a randomized clinical trial to evaluate the efficacy of an outpatient cognitive-behavioral therapy—dialectical behavior therapy (DBT)—for the treatment of chronically parasuicidal women meeting criteria for BPD. The treatment included both a weekly behavioral skills training group therapy component, along with weekly individual therapy sessions that lasted for 1 year (described previously). The control condition was a treatment-as-usual condition (TAU), where subjects were referred to available treatment resources in the community. After initial screening, 24 subjects were assigned to the DBT condition and 23 subjects to the control condition. All subjects were women who met criteria for BPD and had had at least two incidents of parasuicide in the last 5 years, with one incident within 8 weeks prior to referral to the study. Subjects in the DBT condition consented to taper off psychotropic medications; however, failure to do so was not justified as an adequate reason to terminate them from the study, but instead the problem was addressed in therapy as a treatment issue.

All subjects were assessed at pretreatment and at 4, 8, and 12 months using measures of parasuicide, types and duration of medical and psychiatric treatment, and self-report measures of anger, depression, hopelessness, suicide ideation, and reasons for living. There were no pretreatment differences between conditions on any of these measures. After 1 year of treatment, results indicated that at most assessment points, and over the entire year, subjects assigned to DBT had significantly fewer incidences of parasuicide, less medically severe parasuicides, and fewer inpatient psychiatric days than subjects assigned to TAU. Subjects receiving DBT had significantly less anger and better scores on measures of global social adjustment, employment, household duties, financial adjustment, interpersonal relationships with friends, overall work performance, anxious rumination, emotion regulation, interpersonal problem-solving, and the GAS compared to TAU subjects at post-treatment (Linehan, Tutek, Heard, Armstrong, 1993). However, there were no between-group differences on measures of depression, hopelessness, suicide ideation, or reasons for living, although scores on all four measures improved over the year for subjects in both conditions. These results were maintained when subjects in DBT were compared to just those TAU subjects who were in stable individual psychotherapy during the entire year. This comparison is important since it suggests that the efficacy of DBT is not due simply to a nonspecific relationship effect common to all psychotherapies.

In addition, subjects assigned to DBT had a significantly lower attrition rate over the year (16.7%) compared to all subjects assigned to TAU, as well as to only those subjects who began psychotherapy with a new therapist at the beginning of the treatment year (50%). The ability of DBT to keep patients in active therapy is an extremely significant finding for this population. In a study by Waldinger and Gunderson (1984) with 78 BPD patients, only one-half of these patients continued beyond 6 months of therapy, a rate which appears typical of patients in psychodynamic therapies (H.W. Koenigsberg, personal communication, 1991). These treatment results are promising, and despite the small number of subjects, the high statistical significance of results indicates a powerful effect for treatment, at least in terms of parasuicide reduction, retention rates, and decreased hospitalizations. However, there is some question of the generalizability of these results to less severe BPD patients and to male BPD patients.

In terms of treatment follow-up, Linehan *et al.* (in press) located 37 subjects for 18-month interviews and 35 for 24-month interviews. Many were unwilling to complete the entire assessment battery but were willing to do an abbreviated interview covering essential outcome data. Treatment gains in DBT were maintained the entire period and superiority of DBT over TAU was maintained at the 18-month point but not at the 24-month point. At 18 months, significantly fewer DBT subjects (11%) than controls (63%) reported at least one parasuicide, and DBT subjects reported fewer parasuicides and less anger. At the 24-month point, there were no between-group differences in parasuicide, and the sample size was too small to examine questionnaire data. This loss of DBT superiority at 24 months, was not due to loss of treatment gains in the DBT subjects. Rather, it can be accounted for by improvement in some TAU subjects, the inability of the two most severe TAU subjects to be interviewed due to psychiatric disability, and less power due to smaller sample size.

Linehan *et al.* (1992) also analyzed data pertaining to the group skills training component of DBT (DBT-GST). Eleven subjects were assigned to DBT-GST, and 8 were assigned to a no-DBT-GST control condition. All subjects *already had individual, continuing therapy* in the community and were referred for group skills training by their individual therapist. Other than their therapy status, there were no significant differences between subjects in this study and those in the original outcome study described above. The results suggested that DBT-GST has little if anything to recommend it as an additive treatment to ongoing individual (non-DBT) psychotherapy. There were no significant between-group differences on any variable, nor did effect sizes suggest that the absence of results was due to the small sample size.

In addition, all subjects in stable, individual psychotherapy other than individual DBT were compared to subjects receiving stable, standard DBT (both group and individual therapy). Subjects getting standard DBT did better in all target areas. Subjects in stable, individual TAU, whether or not they received DBT-GST, did no better (or worse) than TAU subjects in the original outcome study. These results do not necessarily indicate that DBT-GST is ineffective or unimportant when offered within the standard DBT format. Nor is it clear whether DBT-GST would be effective if offered alone, without concomitant non-DBT individual psychotherapy. In standard DBT, the skills training conducted in groups is integrated within individual DBT. This integration of both types of treatment may be critical to the success of standard DBT. Furthermore, there is one factor that may have detracted from effectiveness of adding DBT-GST to stable, non-DBT community psychotherapy. The combination of non-DBT individual therapy with skills training DBT might create a conflict for the patient that adversely affects outcome.

Overall, DBT appears to be a somewhat effective treatment with chronically parasuicidal borderline women. Although BPD patients are certainly not cured in the 1-year treatment, the significant progress of patients justifies examining the treatment more intensively to ascertain which components of the treatment are most important. Such studies are currently being planned.

In the only other controlled clinical trial with borderline patients to date, Munroe-Blum and Marziali (1987, 1989; Clarkin, Marziali, & Munroe-Blum, 1991) have recently reported preliminary results of a treatment study involving the dynamically oriented group "relationship management psychotherapy" (RMP). One hundred and ten borderline patients were randomly assigned to either RMP or treatment as usual, which consisted of individual dynamic psychotherapy. Preliminary results on behavioral indicators with 52 subjects indicated that at the 6-month follow-up period there were no differences in treatment outcome between groups. However, patients who remained in either group or individual therapy had significantly more improvement than patients who dropped out of therapy. Group therapists also reported greater satisfaction with therapy than individual therapists. The preliminary nature of these results warrants some caution in interpreting the treatment efficacy of RMP versus individual psychodynamic therapy or versus other therapeutic modalities.

Retrospective Studies

Although the studies of Linehan *et al.* (1991, 1992, 1993, in press) and Munroe-Blum *et al.* (1987, 1989) are the only reported controlled clinical trials to date on BPD, numerous naturalistic follow-up studies have been reported in the literature. In general, most of these studies report long-term global functioning of BPD patients after an index psychiatric hospitalization. Although no controlled experimental treatment studies were conducted *per se*, an analysis of these longitudinal data may give some insight to treatment outcome from psychiatric inpatient settings, particularly where psychodynamic forms of treatment are offered. One must interpret these results with caution since many extraneous variables can influence the long-term course of functioning in this population, regardless of treatment gains made during prior psychiatric treatment (for a more complete review of BPD follow-up studies, see Stone, 1989b).

In the Chestnut Lodge follow-up study (McGlashan, 1986), 81 BPD patients were assessed at 2 to 32 years after an average psychiatric hospital stay of 2 years during which they received intensive psychotherapy (3–4 times a week); one-fourth of these patients had received pharmacotherapy. Subjects meeting criteria for schizophrenia and unipolar depression were used as comparison groups. At follow-up, 70 patients were still alive, but only 2 had confirmed suicides. Of these patients, 46% were still receiving some form of psychiatric treatment. In contrast to patients with schizophrenia, BPD patients had fewer rehospitalizations (45% vs. 8%, respectively). Two-thirds of BPD patients were employed full-time, a rate similar to that for depressed patients but much higher than that for schizophrenics. For those BPD patients who became symptomatic again, they frequently manifested substance abuse, impulsive behaviors, and suicide ideation. The typical life course of BPD patients during follow-up showed poor adaptation from age 20 into the early 30s, followed by good overall functioning in the 40s. Some patients suffered another severe decrease in functioning during their late 40s into their early 50s, particularly if they had some significant loss through death, divorce, or rejection. Overall in global functioning, BPD patients were at a much higher level than schizophrenics, but not performing as well as depressives at follow-up. Most of the BPD patients were doing well in occupational functioning, although several patients were still functioning poorly in social and intimate interpersonal relationships. Many BPD patients at follow-up (over 50%) continued using outpatient psychotherapy in spite of their improvements.

In the New York State Psychiatric Institute follow-up study (Stone, Stone, & Hurt, 1987), 205 BPD patients were compared to a schizophrenic control group. The average follow-up interval was 16 years (range 10–23 years). Among the BPD patients, 127 patients had a comorbid affective disorder, while 61 patients could be diagnosed as "pure" BPD. Both BPD patients and schizophrenic patients had similar suicide rates (9% vs. 10.3%, respectively). BPD patients as a whole had good global functioning (mean Global Assessment Scale [GAS] score = 65.6) compared to poor global functioning of schizophrenics (mean GAS score = 39.4). Poorest functioning overall was for the BPD–major affective disorder males, who had the highest suicide rates (18.5%), and the pure BPD males, who had the lowest mean GAS score (55) in the BPD group. The poor function of the BPD males was attributed to the high prevalence of antisocial traits in this subgroup. Overall, 4 out of 10 of the BPD patients were considered to be recovered (GAS scores > 70) at follow-up, while at least three-fourths were considered to be functioning in the "good" range (GAS scores > 60). These results need to be viewed in light of the fact that most of these BPD patients were in a higher socioeconomic status prior to hospitalization, skewed in terms of higher education and intelligence, and preselected prior to admission for amenability to dynamically oriented psychotherapy. Thus, in some aspects, premorbid functioning of these borderline patients was better than most BPD patients.

Paris, Brown, and Nowlis (1987) reported follow-up information on 100 BPD patients a mean of 15 years after psychiatric hospitalization. Using Gunderson's Diagnostic Index for Borderlines (DIB), 75% of the patients were no longer diagnosable as borderline, and all scales of the DIB (social adaptation, impulse-action, affect, psychosis, and interpersonal relations) showed reduction of symptomatic behavior. Using the Health–Sickness Rating Scale as a measure of global outcome, borderline patients were rated as generally functioning well with few or no symptoms, although work histories and social and familial relationships still showed some level of impairment. The suicide rate was 8.5% for 165 locatable subjects. In this study socioeconomic status was highly variable among patients, and education level of patients did not predict outcome.

In a more recent short-term follow-up study, Links, Mitton, and Steiner (1990) assessed 65 BPD patients at 2 years following an index hospitalization. In this sample, 68.8% required continuous treatment for approximately 1 year during the follow-up period. In terms of hospitalization, 60% of the sample were rehospitalized for less than 5% of the follow-up period. In addition, only 20.3% of the sample was working full-time during the follow-up period, yet 82.5% were deemed as socially active. Overall, only 12.3% of the sample were rated as functioning normally over 50% of the time during the follow-up period. Furthermore, 4.6% had suicided during this short period of time. In contrast to the long-term follow-up studies, the short-term outcome for BPD patients after an initial hospitalization appears to be less satisfactory, if not mediocre.

Many of these follow-up studies should be interpreted with caution. Lifetime parasuicidal behavior is still generally high in BPD patients (Gunderson, 1984), and although much of this behavior is without lethal intent, a sizable number of borderlines (5–10%) eventually do die as a consequence of this behavior (Frances, Fyer, & Clarkin, 1986). McGlashan (1983) has reported that the BPD diagnosis is stable over a 15-year follow-up period, and BPD individuals continue to manifest serious psychosocial impairments comparable to schizophrenic individuals at least

5 years after the initiation of treatment (Pope, Jonas, Hudson, Cohen, & Gunderson, 1983). Furthermore, the long-term improvement described by McGlashan may be a function of unusually extensive treatment including more than 3 years of inpatient hospitalization and intensive psychotherapy (Gunderson & Elliott, 1985). Other than these retrospective studies, there are a few other pseudo-empirical studies looking at the efficacy of psychodynamic treatment for borderlines. Waldinger and Gunderson (1984) performed a retrospective study in which 30 therapists were asked to report treatment outcome with 78 patients meeting criteria for BPD or borderline personality organization. Of the patients in the sample, 59% were treated with psychoanalysis, while the rest were treated with "intensive psychotherapy" (whether other dynamic forms of treatment were used in this group is unclear). Those subjects in the psychoanalysis group had significantly more years of previous therapy (3.91 vs. 1.56 years), more years of therapy with this group of therapists (5.06 vs. 3.50 years), less months of psychiatric hospitalization during treatment (0.17 vs. 2.44 months), and more sessions per week (4.02 vs. 2.53 sessions) than the intensive psychotherapy group. Patients in both groups were judged to have equal levels of impairment prior to treatment. Patients in psychoanalysis were significantly less likely to terminate therapy precipitously than the intensive psychotherapy group, but they were just as likely to terminate therapy against their therapist's advice.

In sum, therapists had rated psychoanalytic patients more improved in areas of better object relations and sense of self compared to the intensive psychotherapy group; there were no between-group differences on improvement ratings for ego functioning and behavior. Furthermore, experience levels of therapist had no effect on outcome. The authors note the many methodological problems with this retrospective study, including the generalizability of their results and the credibility of self-report data by the participating therapists. However, this is one of the few attempts in the psychoanalytic literature to quantify and measure change in the analytic treatment of BPD.

In addition, Koenigsberg *et al.* (1985) have developed an instrument, the Therapist Verbal Intervention Inventory, to measure therapeutic techniques in process research of Kernberg's expressive psychotherapy with borderlines. They achieved sufficient reliability on this instrument over a number of therapist variables after training psychiatric residents to use it. Although this is not a treatment study *per se*, this research is an important step toward measuring treatment adherence for this type of therapy and perhaps a valuable move toward doing more extensive psychodynamic outcome research.

Psychopharmacology

In contrast to psychosocial interventions, several placebo-controlled pharmacological studies have been performed on BPD populations. However, as reported by Soloff (1989), many methodological problems are inherent in the pharmacological study and treatment of BPD, including high comorbidity rates with other Axis I and II disorders, the heterogeneity of BPD symptoms, the "state versus trait" phenomena of borderline behavioral patterns, and a lack of a coherent etiology for BPD. Nevertheless, many research studies have focused on treating three separate areas of borderline behavioral patterns: affective dysregulation patterns, schizotypal (psychotic) patterns, and impulsive behavioral patterns.

Several types of drugs have been studied in BPD populations, including neuroleptics (Cowdry & Gardner, 1988; Goldberg *et al.*, 1986; Soloff *et al.*, 1989), antidepressants (Cowdry & Gardner, 1988; Montgomery, Roy, & Montgomery, 1983; Soloff *et al.*, 1989), minor tranquilizers (Faltus, 1984; Gardner & Cowdry, 1986), anticonvulsant medications (Cowdry & Gardner, 1988), and lithium carbonate (Links, Steiner, Boiago, & Irwin, 1990).

Two well-designed pharmacotherapy studies of BPD have been reported by Cowdry and Gardner (1988) and Soloff and colleagues (1989). Cowdry and Gardner employed a double-blind, crossover trial of placebo, alprazolam (a minor tranquilizer), carbamazepine (an anticonvulsant medication), trifluoperazine (a neuroleptic), and tranylcypromine (an antidepressant) on 16 female BPD patients. Each trial was designed to last 6 weeks. Physicians rated improvement on structured interviews. Overall, physicians rated patients as significantly improved compared to placebo while on trials of tranylcypromine and carbamazepine, while patients rated themselves as significantly improved only on tranylcypromine trials. Patients who received full trials of trifluoperazine showed some improvement. Patients who received full trials of carbamazepine had a decrease in behavioral dyscontrol, while those receiving full trials of alprazolam had increased episodes of serious behavioral dyscontrol.

Soloff and colleagues (1989) employed a randomized, double-blind trial of placebo, amitriptyline (an antidepressant), and haloperidol (a neuroleptic) on 90 BPD patients over a 5-week period. In comparison to placebo, haloperidol produced significant improvement on measures of global functioning, depression, hostility, schizotypal symptoms, and impulsive behavior. Amitriptyline showed significant effects on measures of depression compared to placebo.

Overall, it appears that most of the drug studies with BPD have reported at least moderate improvements in areas of psychosocial functioning (for an excellent review, see Gardner and Cowdry, 1989). Consequently, properly administered pharmacotherapy seems to be a useful adjunct to psychotherapy in treatment of BPD. However, some prudence must be exercised when administering pharmacotherapy to BPD patients; therapists should be particularly aware about compliance issues, contraindicated effects, drug abuse, and the potential for drug misuse in suicide attempts.

Summary and Conclusions

Overall, BPD is one of the most widely researched psychiatric disorders, and by far the most widely researched personality disorder. Although numerous research articles have been done on the epidemiology, etiology, diagnosis, and behavioral patterns of BPD, there are only a handful of studies looking at treatment outcome for BPD (and only two stringently controlled clinical trials of BPD that we know of). Due to the paucity of research in this area, it is difficult to make any strong conclusions about efficacious treatment modalities.

Although significant treatment gains have been reported by the two studies using cognitive-behavioral approaches in the treatment of BPD (Linehan *et al.*, 1991; Turner, 1989) and in the study using a cognitive-behavioral approach for parasuicide (Salkovskis *et al.*, 1990), it would be imprudent to assume this type of approach is the treatment of choice for BPD. However, in light of these results, cognitive-behavioral approaches are the only treatment modalities for BPD that have been shown to be somewhat efficacious through empirical research to date. The efficacy of insight-oriented approaches for BPD still needs to be thoroughly investigated through more controlled clinical trials, especially since recent research indicates that short-term dynamic therapies are less effective overall to alternative therapeutic approaches (particularly cognitive-behavioral approaches) in the treatment of various disorders (Svartberg & Stiles, 1991).

In addition, the limitations of these studies must also be evaluated. All of these studies had few numbers of subjects and have yet to be replicated, indicating the potential for hasty conclusions about effective treatment modalities. Furthermore, several pharmacotherapy studies have also shown beneficial effects in treating BPD with certain classes of drugs, although they too suffer from some of the same methodological flaws and generalizability problems. Consequently, there is a strong need in this area to do more controlled treatment outcome studies. There is a particular need for interorientation comparisons, especially since some researchers are postulating unequivocal similarities between seemingly opposite treatment modalities (e.g., Swenson, 1989; Westen, 1991). Without this important research, we can only continue to speculate about the most effective treatments for BPD.

References

Adler, G. (1985). *Borderline psychopathology and its treatment.* New York: Jason Aronson.

Adler, G. (1989). Psychodynamic therapies in borderline personality disorder. In A. Tasman, R. E. Hales, A. J. Frances (Eds.), *American psychiatric press review of psychiatry: Volume 8* (pp. 48–64). Washington, DC: American Psychiatric Press.

Adler, G., & Buie, D. H. (1979). Aloneness and borderline psychopathology: The possible relevance to child development issues. *International Journal of Psychoanalysis, 60,* 83–96.

Akhtar, S., Byrne, J., & Doghramji, K. (1986). The demographic profile of borderline personality disorder. *Journal of Clinical Psychiatry, 47,* 196–198.

American Psychiatric Association. (1980). *Diagnostic and statistical manual of mental disorders* (3rd ed.). Washington, DC: American Psychiatric Association.

American Psychiatric Association. (1987). *Diagnostic and statistical manual of mental disorders* (3rd ed.-revised). Washington, DC: American Psychiatric Association.

Andrulonis, P. A., Glueck, B. C., Stroebel, C. F., & Vogel, N. G. (1982). Borderline personality subcategories. *The Journal of Nervous and Mental Disease, 170,* 670–679.

Beck, A. T., & Freeman, A. (1990). *Cognitive therapy of personality disorders.* New York: Guilford Press.

Benjamin, L. S. (1974). Structural analysis of social behavior. *Psychological Review, 81,* 392–425.

Benjamin, L. S. (1979). Structural analysis of differentiation failure. *Psychiatry, 42,* 1–23.

Benjamin, L. S. (in press). *Interpersonal diagnosis and treatment of personality disorders.* New York: Guilford Press.

Bryer, J. B., Nelson, B. A., Miller, J. B., & Krol, P. A. (1987). Childhood sexual and physical abuse as factors in adult psychiatric illness. *American Journal of Psychiatry, 144,* 1426–1430.

Buie, D. H., & Adler, G. (1982). The definitive treatment of borderline personality. *International Journal of Psychoanalytic Psychotherapy, 9,* 51–87.

Castaneda, R., & Franco, H. (1985). Sex and ethnic distribution of borderline personality disorder in an inpatient sample. *American Journal of Psychiatry, 142,* 1202–1203.

Chess, S., & Thomas, A. (Eds.). (1986). *Temperament in clinical practice.* New York: Guilford Press.

Chessick, R. D. (1982). Intensive psychotherapy of a borderline patient. *Archives of General Psychiatry, 39,* 413–419.

Clarkin, J. F., Marziali, E., & Munroe-Blum, H. (1991). Group and family treatments for borderline personality disorder. *Hospital and Community Psychiatry, 42,* 1038–1043.

Clarkin, J. F., Widiger, T. A., Frances, A. J., Hurt, S. W., & Gilmore, M. (1983). Prototypic typology and the borderline personality disorder. *Journal of Abnormal Psychology, 92,* 263–275.

Coccaro, E. F., Siever, L. J., Klar, H. M., Maurer, G., Cochrane, K., Cooper, T. B., Mohs, R. C., & Davis, K. L. (1989). Serotonergic studies in patients with affective and personality disorders. *Archives of General Psychiatry, 46*, 587–599.

Cornelius, J. R., Soloff, P. H., George, A. W. A., Schulz, S. C., Tarter, R., Brenner, R. P., & Schulz, P. M. (1989). An evaluation of the significance of selected neuropsychiatric abnormalities in the etiology of borderline personality disorder. *Journal of Personality Disorders, 3*, 19–25.

Cowdry, R. W. (1987). Psychopharmacology of borderline personality disorder: A review. *Journal of Clinical Psychiatry, 48*(Suppl. 8), 15–22.

Cowdry, R. W., & Gardner, D. L. (1988). Pharmacotherapy of borderline personality disorder: Alprazolam, carbamazepine, trifluoperazine, and tranylcypromine. *Archives of General Psychiatry, 45*, 111–119.

Cowdry, R. W., Pickar, D., & Davies, R. (1985). Symptoms and EEG findings in the borderline syndrome. *International Journal of Psychiatry and Medicine, 15*, 201–211.

Dulit, R. A., Fyer, M. R., Haas, G. L., Sullivan, T., & Frances, A. J. (1990). Substance use in borderline personality disorder. *American Journal of Psychiatry, 147*, 1002–1007.

Faltus, F. (1984). The positive effect of alprazolam in the treatment of three patients with borderline personality disorder. *American Journal of Psychiatry, 141*, 802–803.

Feldman, R. B., & Guttman, H. A. (1984). Families of borderline patients: Literal-minded parents, borderline parents, and parental protectiveness. *American Journal of Psychiatry, 141*, 1392–1396.

Finkelhor, D. (1979). *Sexually victimized children*. New York: Free Press.

Frances, A., Fyer, M., & Clarkin, J. F. (1986). Personality and suicide. *Annals of the New York Academy of Sciences, 487*, 281–293.

Fyer, M. R., Frances, A. J., Sullivan, T., Hurt, S. W., & Clarkin, J. (1988). Comorbidity of borderline personality disorder. *Archives of General Psychiatry, 45*, 348–352.

Gardner, D. L., & Cowdry, R. W. (1985). Suicidal and parasuicidal behavior in borderline personality disorder. *Psychiatric Clinics of North America, 8*, 389–403.

Gardner, D. L., & Cowdry, R. W. (1986). Alprazolam-induced dyscontrol in borderline personality disorder. *American Journal of Psychiatry, 143*, 519–522.

Gardner, D. L., & Cowdry, R. W. (1989). Pharmacotherapy of borderline personality disorder: A review. *Psychopharmacology Bulletin, 25*, 515–523.

Gardner, D. L., Leibenluft, E., O'Leary, K. M., & Cowdry, R. W. (1991). Self-ratings of anger and hostility in borderline personality disorder. *The Journal of Nervous and Mental Disease, 179*, 157–161.

Glantz, K. (1981). The use of a relaxation exercise in the treatment of borderline personality organization. *Psychotherapy: Theory, Research, and Practice, 18*, 379–385.

Glat, M. (1988a, February). Borderline syndrome: Cognitive and behavioral treatment for adolescents. Part I—theory. *Carrier Foundation Letter #131*, pp. 1–3.

Glat, M. (1988b, March). Borderline syndrome: Cognitive and behavioral treatment for adolescents. Part II—treatment and practice. *Carrier Foundation Letter #132*, pp. 1–3.

Goldberg, S. C., Schulz, S. C., Schulz, P. M., Resnick, R. J., Hamer, R. M., & Friedel, R. O. (1986). Borderline and schizotypal personality disorders treated with low-dose thiothixene vs placebo. *Archives of General Psychiatry, 43*, 680–686.

Gunderson, J. G. (1984). *Borderline personality disorder*. Washington, DC: American Psychiatric Press.

Gunderson, J. G., & Elliott, G. R. (1985). The interface between borderline personality disorder and affective disorder. *American Journal of Psychiatry, 142*, 277–288.

Gunderson, J. G., Kerr, J., Englund, D. W. (1980). The families of borderlines: A comparative study. *Archives of General Psychiatry, 37*, 27–33.

Herman, J. L. (1986). Histories of violence in an outpatient population. *American Journal of Orthopsychiatry, 56*, 137–141.

Herman, J. L., Perry, J. C., & van der Kolk, B. A. (1989). Childhood trauma in borderline personality disorder. *American Journal of Psychiatry, 146*, 490–495.

Hurt, S. W., & Clarkin, J. F. (1990). Borderline personality disorder: Prototypic typology and the development of treatment manuals. *Psychiatric Annals, 20*, 13–18.

Jonsdottir-Baldursson, T., & Horvath, P. (1987). Borderline personality-disordered alcoholics in Iceland: Descriptions on demographic, clinical, and MMPI variables. *Journal of Consulting and Clinical Psychology, 55*, 738–741.

Katz, S. E., & Levendusky, P. G. (1990). Cognitive-behavioral approaches to treating borderline and self-mutilating patients. *Bulletin of the Menninger Clinic, 54*, 398–408.

Kernberg, O. F. (1975). *Borderline conditions and pathological narcissism*. New York: Jason Aronson.

Kernberg, O. F. (1984). *Severe personality disorders*. New Haven, CT: Yale University Press.

Kernberg, O. F. (1987). A psychodynamic approach. *Journal of Personality Disorders, 1*, 344–346.

Kernberg, O. F., Selzer, M. A., Koenigsberg, H. W., Carr, A. C., & Appelbaum, A. H. (1989). *Psychodynamic psychotherapy of borderline patients*. New York: Basic Books.

Koenigsberg, H. W., Kernberg, O. F., Haas, G., Lotterman, A., Rockland, L., & Selzer, M. (1985). Development of a scale for measuring techniques in the psychotherapy of borderline patients. *The Journal of Nervous and Mental Disease, 173*, 424–431.

Kroll, J. (1988). *The challenge of the borderline patient*. New York: Norton.

Liebenluft, E., Gardner, D. L., & Cowdry, R. W. (1987). The inner experience of the borderline self-mutilator. *Journal of Personality Disorders, 1*, 317–324.

Liebowitz, M. R. (1987). A medication approach. *Journal of Personality Disorders, 1*, 325–327.

Liebowitz, M. R., Stone, M. H., & Turkat, I. D. (1986). Treatment of personality disorders. In A. J. Frances & R. E. Hales (Eds.), *American psychiatric association annual review: Volume 5* (pp. 356–393). Washington, DC: American Psychiatric Press.

Linehan, M. M. (1987a). Dialectical behavior therapy: A cognitive behavioral approach to parasuicide. *Journal of Personality Disorders, 1*, 328–333.

Linehan, M. M. (1987b). Dialectical behavior therapy for borderline personality disorder. *Bulletin of the Menninger Clinic, 51*, 261–276.

Linehan, M. M. (1993a). *Cognitive-behavioral treatment of borderline personality disorder.*. New York: Guilford Press.

Linehan, M. M. (1993b). *The skills training manual for treatment of borderline personality disorder*. New York: Guilford Press.

Linehan, M. M., Armstrong, H. E., Suarez, A., Allmon, D., & Heard, H. L. (1991). Cognitive-behavioral treatment of chronically parasuicidal borderline patients. *Archives of General Psychiatry, 48*, 1060–1064.

Linehan, M. M., Camper, P., Chiles, J. A., Strosahl, K., & Shearin, E. (1987). Interpersonal problem solving and parasuicide. *Cognitive Therapy and Research, 11*, 1–12.

Linehan, M. M., Heard, H. L., & Armstrong, H. E. (1992). *Standard dialectical behavior therapy compared to individual psychotherapy in the community for chronically parasuicidal borderline patients*. Unpublished manuscript.

Linehan, M. M., Heard, H. L., & Armstrong, H. E. (in press). Naturalistic follow-up of a behavioral treatment for chronically parasuicidal borderline patients. *Archives of General Psychiatry*.

Linehan, M. M., & Koerner, K. (1993). Behavioral theory of borderline personality disorder. In J. Paris (Ed.), *Borderline psychopathology: Etiology and treatment* (pp. 103–131). Washington, DC: American Psychiatric Association.

Linehan, M. M., Tutek, D. A., Heard, H. L., & Armstrong, H. E. (1993). *Cognitive behavioral treatment for chronically parasuicidal borderline patients: Effects on social behaviors*. Manuscript submitted for publication.

Links, P. S., Mitton, J. E., & Steiner, M. (1990). Predicting outcome for borderline personality disorder. *Comprehensive Psychiatry, 31*, 490–498.

Links, P. S., Steiner, M., Boiago, I., & Irwin, D. (1990). Lithium therapy for borderline patients: Preliminary findings. *Journal of Personality Disorders, 4*, 173–181.

Links, P. S., Steiner, M., & Huxley, G. (1988). The occurrence of borderline personality disorder in the families of borderline patients. *Journal of Personality Disorders, 2*, 14–20.

Loranger, A. W., Oldham, J. M., & Tulis, E. H. (1982). Familial transmission of DSM-III borderline personality disorder. *Archives of General Psychiatry, 39*, 795–799.

Loranger, A. W., & Tulis, E. H. (1985). Family history of alcoholism in borderline personality disorder. *Archives of General Psychiatry, 42*, 153–157.

Ludolph, P. S., Westen, D., Misle, B., Jackson, A., Wixom, J., & Wiss, F. C. (1990). The borderline diagnosis in adolescents: Symptoms and developmental history. *American Journal of Psychiatry, 147*, 470–476.

Malow, R. M., West, J. A., Williams, J. L., & Sutker, P. B. (1989). Personality disorders classification and symptoms in cocaine and opioid addicts. *Journal of Consulting and Clinical Psychology, 57*, 765–767.

Manos, N., Vasilopoulou, E., & Sotiriou, M. (1987). DSM-III diagnosed borderline personality disorder and depression. *Journal of Personality Disorders, 1*, 263–268.

Marziali, E., Hamilton, J., Sadavoy, S., Book, H., Sadavoy, J., & Silver, D. (1984). Analysis of emotional states during the hospital treatment of a borderline patient. *Canadian Journal of Psychiatry, 29*, 347–349.

Marziali, E. A., & Munroe-Blum, H. (1987). A group approach: The management of projective identification in group treatment of self-destructive borderline patients. *Journal of Personality Disorders, 1*, 340–343.

Masterson, J. (1976). *Psychotherapy of the borderline adult.* New York: Brunner/Mazel.

Masterson, J. (1981). *The narcissistic and borderline disorders.* New York: Brunner/Mazel.

McGlashan, T. H. (1983). The borderline syndrome, II: Is it a variant of schizophrenia or affective disorder? *Archives of General Psychiatry, 40*, 1319–1323.

McGlashan, T. H. (1986). The Chestnut Lodge follow-up study. III. Long-term outcome of borderline personalities. *Archives of General Psychiatry, 43*, 20–30.

McGlashan, T. H. (1987). Testing DSM-III symptom criteria for schizotypal and borderline personality disorders. *Archives of General Psychiatry, 44*, 143–148.

McGlashan, T. H., & Heinssen, R. K. (1989). Narcissistic, antisocial, and noncomorbid subgroups of borderline disorder. *Psychiatric Clinics of North America, 12*, 653–670.

McLemore, C. W., & Brokaw, D. W. (1987). Personality disorders as dysfunctional interpersonal behavior. *Journal of Personality Disorders, 1*, 270–285.

Millon, T. (1987). On the genesis and prevalence of the borderline personality disorder: A social learning thesis. *Journal of Personality Disorders, 1*, 354–372.

Modestin, J. (1987). Quality of interpersonal relationships: The most characteristic DSM-III BPD criterion. *Comprehensive Psychiatry, 28*, 397–402.

Morey, L. (1988). Personality disorders under DSM-III and DSM-III-R: An examination of convergence, coverage, and internal consistency. *American Journal of Psychiatry, 145*, 573–577.

Munroe-Blum, H., & Marziali, E. (1987). *Randomized clinical trial of relationship management time-limited group treatment of borderline personality disorder.* Unpublished manuscript, Ontario Mental Health Foundation, Hamilton, Ontario.

Munroe-Blum, H., & Marziali, E. (1989). *Continuation of a randomized control trial of group treatment for borderline personality disorder.* Unpublished manuscript, Canadian Department of Health and Human Services, Hamilton, Ontario.

Murray, E. J. (1988). Personality disorders: A cognitive view. *Journal of Personality Disorders, 2*, 37–43.

Nace, E. P., Saxon, J. J., & Shore, N. (1983). A comparison of borderline and nonborderline alcoholic patients. *Archives of General Psychiatry, 40*, 54–56.

Ogata, S. N., Silk, K. R., Goodrich, S., Lohr, N. E., & Westen, D. (1989). *Childhood abuse and clinical symptoms in borderline patients.* Unpublished manuscript.

O'Leary, K. M., Brouwers, P., Gardner, D. L., & Cowdry, R. W. (1991). Neuropsychological testing of patients with borderline personality disorder. *American Journal of Psychiatry, 148*, 106–111.

Padesky, C. A. (1986, September). *Personality disorders: Cognitive therapy into the 90's.* Paper presented at the meeting of the International Conference on Cognitive Psychotherapy, Umea, Sweden.

Paris, J., Brown, R., & Nowlis, D. (1987). Long-term follow-up of borderline patients in a general hospital. *Comprehensive Psychiatry, 28*, 530–535.

Paris, J., & Frank, H. (1989). Perceptions of parental bonding in borderline patients. *American Journal of Psychiatry, 146*, 1498–1499.

Paris, J., Nowlis, D., & Brown, R. (1988). Developmental factors in the outcome of borderline personality disorder. *Comprehensive Psychiatry, 29*, 147–150.

Perry, J. C., Herman, J. L., van der Kolk, B. A., & Hoke, L. A. (1990). Psychotherapy and psychological trauma in borderline personality disorder. *Psychiatric Annals, 20*, 33–43.

Perry, J. C., & Klerman, G. L. (1980). Clinical features of the borderline personality disorder. *American Journal of Psychiatry, 137*, 165–173.

Pincus, A. L., & Wiggins, J. S. (1990). Interpersonal problems and conceptions of personality disorders. *Journal of Personality Disorders, 4*, 342–352.

Pollack, J., Winston, A., McCullough, L., Flegenheimer, W., & Winston, B. (1990). Efficacy of brief adaptational psychotherapy. *Journal of Personality Disorders, 4*, 244–250.

Pope, H. G., Jonas, J. M., Hudson, J. L., Cohen, B., & Gunderson, J. F. (1983). The validity of DSM-III borderline personality disorder. *Archives of General Psychiatry, 40*, 23–30.

Pretzer, J., & Fleming, B. (1989). Cognitive-behavioral treatment of personality disorders. *Behavior Therapist, 12*, 105–109.

Raczek, S. W., True, P. K., & Friend, R. C. (1989). Suicidal behavior and personality traits. *Journal of Personality Disorders, 3*, 345–351.

Rinsley, D. (1982). *Borderline and other self disorders.* New York: Jason Aronson.

Rosenberger, P. H., & Miller, G. A. (1989). Comparing borderline definitions: DSM-III borderline and schizotypal personality disorders. *Journal of Abnormal Psychology, 98,* 161–169.

Salkovskis, P. M., Atha, C., & Storer, D. (1990). Cognitive-behavioral problem solving in the treatment of patients who repeatedly attempt suicide: A controlled trial. *British Journal of Psychiatry, 157,* 871–876.

Scarr, S., & McCartney, K. (1983). How people make their own environments: A theory of genotype-environmental effects. *Child Development, 54,* 424–435.

Schulz, P. M., Soloff, P. H., Kelly, T., Morgenstern, M., Di Franco, R., & Schulz, S. C. (1989). A family history study of borderline subtypes. *Journal of Personality Disorders, 3,* 217–229.

Serban, G., Conte, H. R., & Plutchik, R. (1987). Borderline and schizotypal personality disorders: Mutually exclusive or overlapping? *Journal of Personality Assessment, 51,* 15–22.

Shearer, S. L., Peters, C. P., Quaytman, M. S., & Ogden, R. L. (1990). Frequency and correlates of childhood sexual and physical abuse histories in adult female borderline inpatients. *American Journal of Psychiatry, 147,* 214–216.

Silk, K. R., Lohr, N. E., Westen, D., & Goodrich, S. (1989). Psychosis in borderline patients with depression. *Journal of Personality Disorders, 3,* 92–100.

Snyder, S., & Pitts, W. M. (1984). Electroencephalography of DSM-III borderline personality disorder. *Acta Psychiatrica Scandinavica, 69,* 129.

Snyder, S., & Pitts, W. M. (1985). Characterizing anger in the DSM-III borderline personality disorder. *Acta Psychiatrica Scandinavica, 72,* 464–469.

Soloff, P. H. (1989). Psychopharmacologic therapies in borderline personality disorder. In A. Tasman, R. E. Hales, & A. J. Frances (Eds.), *American psychiatric press review of psychiatry: Volume 8* (pp. 65–83). Washington, DC: American Psychiatric Press.

Soloff, P. H., George, A., Nathan, R. S., Schulz, P. M., Cornelius, J. R., Herring, J., & Perel, J. M. (1989). Amitriptyline versus haloperidol in borderlines: Final outcomes and predictors of response. *Journal of Clinical Psychopharmacology, 9,* 238–246.

Stone, M. H. (1980). Borderline conditions: Early definitions and interrelationships. In M. H. Stone (Ed.), *The borderline syndrome* (pp. 1–43). New York: McGraw-Hill.

Stone, M. H. (1981). Borderline syndromes: A consideration of subtypes and an overview, directions for research. *Psychiatric Clinics of North America, 4,* 3–13.

Stone, M. H. (1989a). The role of pharmacotherapy in the treatment of patients with borderline personality disorder. *Psychopharmacology Bulletin, 25,* 564–571.

Stone, M. H. (1989b). The course of borderline personality disorder. In A. Tasman, R. E. Hales, & A. J. Frances (Eds.), *American psychiatric press review of psychiatry: Volume 8* (pp. 103–122). Washington, DC: American Psychiatric Press.

Stone, M. H., Stone, D. K., & Hurt, S. W. (1987). Natural history of borderline patients treated by intensive hospitalization. *Psychiatric Clinics of North America, 10,* 185–206.

Svartberg, M., & Stiles, T. C. (1991). Comparative effects of short-term psychodynamic psychotherapy: A meta-analysis. *Journal of Consulting and Clinical Psychology, 59,* 704–714.

Swenson, C. (1989). Kernberg and Linehan: Two approaches to the borderline patient. *Journal of Personality Disorders, 3,* 26–35.

Thomas, A., & Chess, S. (1985). The behavioral study of temperament. In J. Strelau, F. H. Farley, & A. Gale (Eds.), *The biological bases of personality and behavior* (pp. 213–235). Washington, DC: Hemisphere.

Traskman-Bendz, L., Asberg, M., & Schalling, D. (1986). Serotonergic function and suicidal behavior in personality disorders. In J. J. Mann & M. Stanley (Eds.), *Annals of the New York Academy of Sciences: Vol. 487. Psychobiology of suicidal behaviors* (pp. 168–174). New York: The New York Academy of Sciences.

Turkat, I. D. (1990). *The personality disorders: A psychological approach to clinical management.* New York: Pergamon Press.

Turkat, I. D., & Maisto, S. A. (1985). Personality disorders: Application of the experimental method to the formulation and modification of personality disorders. In D. H. Barlow (Ed.), *Clinical handbook of psychological disorders* (pp. 502–570). New York: Guilford Press.

Turner, R. M. (1984, November). *Assessment and treatment of borderline personality disorders.* Paper presented at the meeting of the Association for Advancement of Behavior Therapy, Philadelphia, PA.

Turner, R. M. (1989). Case study evaluations of a bio-cognitive-behavioral approach for the treatment of borderline personality disorder. *Behavior Therapy, 20,* 477–489.

Turner, S. M., & Hersen, M. (1981). Disorders of social behavior: A behavioral approach to personality disorders. In S. M. Turner, K. S. Calhoun, & H. E. Adams (Eds.), *Handbook of clinical behavior therapy* (pp. 103–123). New York: Wiley.

Turner, S. M., & Turkat, I. D. (1988). Behavior therapy and the personality disorders. *Journal of Personality Disorders, 2,* 342–349.

Wagner, A. W., & Linehan, M. M. (in press). Relationship between childhood sexual abuse and topography of parasuicide among women with borderline personality disorder. *Journal of Personality Disorders.*

Waldinger, R. J., & Gunderson, J. G. (1984). Completed psychotherapies with borderline patients. *American Journal of Psychotherapy, 38,* 190–202.

Westen, D. (1991). Cognitive-behavioral interventions in the psychoanalytic psychotherapy of borderline personality disorders. *Clinical Psychology Review, 11,* 211–230.

Westen, D., Ludolph, P., Misle, B., Ruffins, S., & Block, J. (1990). Physical and sexual abuse in adolescent girls with borderline personality disorder. *American Journal of Orthopsychiatry, 60,* 55–66.

Widiger, T. A., & Frances, A. J. (1989). Epidemiology, diagnosis, and comorbidity of borderline personality disorder. In A. Tasman, R. E. Hales, & A. J. Frances (Eds.), *American psychiatric press review of psychiatry: Volume 8* (pp. 8–24). Washington, DC: American Psychiatric Press.

Widiger, T. A., & Spitzer, R. L. (1991). Sex bias in the diagnosis of personality disorders: Conceptual and methodological issues. *Clinical Psychology Review, 11,* 1–22.

Young, J. E. (1990). *Cognitive Therapy for Personality Disorders: A Schema-Focused Approach.* Sarasota, Florida: Professional Resource Exchange, Inc.

Young, J., & Swift, W. (1988). Schema-focused cognitive therapy for personality disorders: Part I. *International Cognitive Therapy Newsletter, 4,* 13–14.

Zanarini, M. C., Gunderson, J. G., & Frankenburg, F. R. (1990). Cognitive features of borderline personality disorder. *American Journal of Psychiatry, 147,* 57–63.

Zimmerman, M., Pfohl, B., Coryell, W., Stangl, D., & Corenthal, C. (1988). Diagnosing personality disorder in depressed patients: A comparison of patient and informant interviews. *Archives of General Psychiatry, 45,* 733–737.

Zubenko, G. S., George, A. W., Soloff, P. H., & Schulz, P. (1987). Sexual practices among patients with borderline personality disorder. *American Journal of Psychiatry, 144,* 748–752.

16

Strategies for the Treatment of Alcoholism

John P. Allen and Margaret E. Mattson

Introduction and Background

Alcoholism is an exceedingly common and serious problem in our society. State-of-the-art estimation procedures place the number of alcohol-dependent persons in the United States at approximately 9 million with an additional 6 million persons diagnosable as nondependent alcohol abusers. Alcohol abuse and alcohol dependence are most prevalent among younger males. For both genders these problems tend to decrease with age (Williams, Grant, Harford, & Noble, 1989).

The financial burden to this country resulting from misuse of alcohol is not definitively known, despite employment of methodologically sophisticated data collection and econometric techniques. Different lines of research, however, conservatively estimate that the cost, including attendant health care expenses, losses due to diminished productivity, and premature death, is $100 billion per year (National Institute on Alcohol Abuse and Alcoholism, 1991).

Beyond the specific problems to which abuse and/or dependence on alcohol contribute, including a panoply of adverse legal, family, employment, and social consequences, heavy consumption of alcohol is associated with several serious medical problems, especially alcoholic hepatitis and cirrhosis (Grant, Dufour, Harford, 1988) pancreatitis (Korsten, 1989), organic brain syndrome (Berman, 1990), cancers of head and neck (Lieber, Garro, Leo, & Warner, 1986), and fetal alcohol syndrome. It has been estimated that there were approximately 100,000 alcohol-related deaths in the United States in 1980 (Ravenholt, 1984).

So, too, the large-scale Epidemiologic Catchment Area survey (Regier *et al.*, 1984) conducted with household samples in five cities in the United States revealed high rates of lifetime co-occurrence of alcoholism and several other psychiatric diagnoses, in particular, antisocial personality, drug abuse and dependence, hypomania, schizophrenia, and a variety of neurotic diagnoses (Helzer & Pryzbeck,

John P. Allen and **Margaret E. Mattson** • National Institute on Alcohol Abuse and Alcoholism, Rockville, Maryland 20857.

Handbook of Effective Psychotherapy, edited by Thomas R. Giles. Plenum Press, New York, 1993.

1987). In fact, 44% of male alcoholics and 65% of female alcoholics were reported to have at some time in their lives met the criteria for a diagnosis for at least one of the twelve psychiatric conditions surveyed. While many possible reasons have been offered for the disproportionate co-occurrence of these conditions with alcoholism (and their simultaneous existence may well be particularly high in alcoholism treatment settings), it remains generally unclear how their presence or successful resolution might relate to choice of intervention or outcome for alcoholism treatment. A range of issues on comorbidity and alcoholism are succinctly summarized in an issue of *Alcohol Alert* (National Institute on Alcohol Abuse and Alcoholism, 1991).

Many definitions for alcoholism are implied in common parlance. Researchers, treatment personnel, and third-party treatment reimbursers, however, typically confine the term "alcoholism" to conditions which satisfy the criteria for alcohol dependence as specified by DSM-III-R. The conceptualization of alcohol dependence as a distinct clinical syndrome has been most clearly articulated by Edwards and Gross (1976). This definition posits seven key characteristics which distinguish the alcohol dependence syndrome from related conditions such as heavy drinking and alcohol abuse:

- Narrowing of the drinking repertoire
- Salience of drink-seeking behavior
- Increased tolerance to alcohol
- Repeated withdrawal symptoms
- Relief or avoidance of withdrawal symptoms by further drinking
- Subjective awareness of the compulsion to drink
- Reinstatement of the syndrome after abstinence

Although serious questions have been raised on the utility of the construct of the alcohol dependence syndrome (Caetano, 1985), this concept continues to dominate the fields of alcoholism research and treatment practice.

Extensive research has been performed on the etiology of alcoholism and its possible subtypes. Limitations of space, however, prohibit review of this body of literature here. Nevertheless, we believe that the research strongly supports certain important conclusions. Most importantly, it appears that a diversity of conditions are included under the rubric of "alcoholism," despite certain common features such as decreased tolerance for ethanol, persistence of drinking even in light of the individual's awareness of the adverse consequences of drinking on his or her welfare, and frequent relapses following periods of freely chosen and motivated periods of abstinence or diminished consumption. Evidence from many lines of research argues strongly for at least two distinct types of alcohol dependence. One type begins early, seems to have a clear component of genetic vulnerability, is especially common among males, is closely associated with acting-out behaviors, and has a rather negative treatment prognosis. The second type differs on each of these dimensions. Cluster analyses and Q-type factor analyses of personality inventories and drinking measures with alcoholics also strongly suggest that alcoholism is not a unitary phenomenon (Babor & Dolinski, 1988).

Although over 40 types of alcoholism interventions have been identified (Holder, Longabaugh, Miller, & Rubonis, 1991), traditional treatment in the United States generally conforms to the "Minnesota Model," a multimodal treatment strategy including Alcoholics Anonymous, lectures on the nature of alcoholism, group and individual counseling, and intervention with family members and employers to avoid "enabling" drinking by the alcoholics (Cook, 1988). Traditional individual and group psychotherapy approaches have been employed in alcoholism treatment. These interventions seem to assume that alcoholism is a manifestation of unconscious conflicts or other emotional problems and that insight into the nature of these difficulties should result in decreased consumption. With the exception of behaviorally focused techniques and treatment strategies which include the spouse in the psychotherapy sessions, these interventions have not generally been demonstrated as effective. For example, in a recent review of alcoholism treatment research, only 5 of 31 controlled studies on counseling or traditional group or individual psychotherapy showed positive effects for these approaches (Holder *et al.*, 1991).

This chapter will address three more recently developed strategies that have been shown to have promise in the treatment of alcoholism: the community reinforcement approach, social skills training, and patient–treatment matching.

In addition to these methods, we will briefly mention some encouraging work in the area of pharmacotherapy for alcoholism.

The first two interventions were chosen for discussion because of a growing body of research on their effectiveness with alcohol-dependent patients (Holder *et al.*, 1991), and, in fact, no controlled trials were located which failed to demonstrate their benefits. We have also chosen to discuss differential effects of various interventions as a function of patient characteristics (patient–treatment matching) since research in this area is also quite positive and suggests a different, but possibly complementary, strategy for effectively intervening with alcoholics. Our decision to include pharmacotherapies in the report was based both on some exciting preliminary data on the topic and on our desire to suggest future benefits of formal, but nonpsychotherapeutic, adjuncts to the treatment process. Nevertheless, since the major emphasis in this chapter is on psychotherapeutic interventions, the discussion on pharmacotherapy will be brief.

In presenting results of the various studies, we will focus on the effectiveness of the intervention on reducing drinking itself. Nevertheless, several of the investigations also present findings on other types of outcome, such as improvement in employment, social and psychological status, and other indices of life functioning, and we will note these. All of the studies reviewed employed a controlled experimental design, either random assignment to conditions or some type of equating of subjects on pretreatment variables. Nonetheless, we will comment on what we consider substantive deficiencies in the design or in the conclusions reached. Although we have restricted our inclusion of studies to those which involve alcohol-dependent, as opposed to alcohol-abusing, subjects, we will describe the nature of the subject population in considerable detail, since such information establishes "comfortable" limits of generalizability on the effectiveness of the intervention with other alcoholic groups.

Community Reinforcement Approach

The community reinforcement approach (CRA) to alcoholism treatment should not be viewed as a single interventional approach. Rather, it is a family of techniques, the specific ones of which are selected according to the needs of a particular patient. CRA may thus be described as a "menu-driven" treatment strategy. Contemporary "full" CRA consists of the following elements:

- Disulfiram (Antabuse®) with a rather complex set of procedures to enhance compliance
- Marital counseling
- A "job club" to help clients find work which does not present high-risk drinking situations (effectiveness of the "Job-Finding Club" on reducing unemployment and obtaining higher salaries was evaluated by Azrin, Flores, & Kaplan, 1975)
- Training in skills to cope with urges to drink
- Counseling on constructive leisure-time activities
- Training in techniques to resist social pressures to drink

These CRA components are described in detail by Sisson and Azrin (1989). The rationale for most of the CRA techniques derives from operant conditioning theory, which argues that drinking will be deterred if reinforcers for not drinking (such as more pleasant interaction with the spouse and more rewarding work experiences) are maximized, frequent, varied in nature, and closely contiguous to and contingent upon not drinking (Hunt & Azrin, 1973). CRA may be performed in groups or individually and with inpatients or outpatients. In addition to the counselor, spouses, "buddies," and employers typically play key roles in the treatment.

The original research on CRA (Hunt & Azrin, 1973) involved patients admitted to a state hospital for treatment of alcoholism. Patients were rural males diagnosed as alcoholics and evidencing alcohol withdrawal symptoms. Individuals with serious medical problems that precluded employment were excluded from sample consideration. Eight cases were selected and matched individually with eight other patients on employment history, family stability, age, educational level, and previous drinking history. On the basis of a coin flip, patients from each pair were randomly assigned to CRA with standard treatment or to the standard treatment alone. The standard treatment consisted of about 25 hour-long educational lectures and films on Alcoholics Anonymous and on the extent and nature of behavioral, sexual, and physical problems suffered by alcoholics.

The usual duration of treatment is not noted in the report, but the report does state that CRA patients were discharged as soon as they acquired a job that they stated was satisfactory for them. Following treatment, at least the CRA patients were visited once or twice a week for the first month by a counselor.

Six-month follow-up results of the project were quite positive. CRA-treated patients differed significantly on all outcome measures from their peers who had received the standard treatment regime alone. They spent only 14% of their time drinking versus 79% of the control group. They were employed 95% of the time, whereas the control group was employed 38% of the time. They were away from their families or "synthetic families" created by the trial only 16% of the time versus 36% of the time for the other group. Finally, they were institutionalized posttreatment only 2% of the time versus 27% of the time for the control group. Interestingly, the report also includes plots of monthly posttreatment status on each dependent variable. These graphs generally suggest little decay of treatment effect for either group as time passed, with the exception that the control group showed a slight temporal U shape on the time-away-from-home dimension. While not emphasized, the report also shows that the mean monthly income of the CRA group was almost twice that of the control group and that CRA patients engaged in social activities more than three times as frequently as those in the other group.

Azrin (1976) conducted a second study on CRA by adding a "buddy," a recovering alcoholic similar to the patient but with at least a year of sobriety. The buddy was to meet regularly with the patient to discuss practical techniques to maintain sobriety. Also added was an elaborated disulfiram compliance program, including pairing the taking of the drug with some well-established habit and spouse monitoring of the disulfiram administration. Behavioral rehearsal of techniques to handle high-risk drinking situations and daily inventories to monitor marital satisfaction by both spouses were also added in the second CRA trial. Treatment was done in small patient groups with spouses rather than individually as had been the case in the initial trial. Finally, written contracts for all the major CRA procedures seem to have played a significant role in the intervention.

Selection criteria were as before with the further restriction that the patients be between 20 to 60 years of age and reside within an hour's drive to the hospital. Matching was done on the basis of job satisfaction, job stability, family stability, social life, and drinking history. Again, patients were assigned to CRA or to traditional treatment alone according to a flip of a coin. Blind 6-month follow-up of the clients was also conducted as before.

Results were again quite supportive of CRA. Posttreatment drinking days were reduced to 2% for CRA patients but only to 55% for the control group. Unemployment time declined to 20% for the experimental group, although it was 56% for the traditional treatment group. Time away from the family was 7% for the CRA group, yet 67% for the control group. No time for the CRA patients was spent in posttreatment institutionalization. Forty-five percent of the control group's days were, however, spent in institutions following treatment. All outcome measures differed at $p < .005$.

Of interest, this study also revealed that the three different CRA counselors were approximately equal in effectiveness. A 2-year follow-up of the patients showed that the CRA-treated group was abstinent for 90% of the four 6-month follow-up periods. The author also notes that the augmented CRA procedures reduced the total amount of counseling time to 30 hours. (In the original study, 50 hours had been spent in CRA counseling.) It is, however, unclear if this reduction was in counselor time or patient time. (It will be recalled that the first study involved individual counseling and the second employed group sessions.)

Three additional studies have been conducted to assess the contribution of specific components of CRA. Mallams, Godley, Hall, and Meyers (1982) directed their attention to the nondrinking social club. Subjects for the project were 40 outpatient alcoholics receiving treatment in a rural alcoholism program. Exclusionary criteria were age over 65, severe psychiatric, cognitive, or physical problem, and residence in an institution. Subjects were randomly assigned to a control group, which received written and verbal descriptions of the club, or to the experimental group, which received these instructions plus an average of 10 sessions of encouragement by the counselor to attend the club following the session, letters advertising forthcoming events, transportation to the club when needed, membership cards and materials, counseling to resolve problems in attending such as needs for child care, encouragement from club members for attendance, and attempts to ascertain and provide recreational activities desired by the client. The club was described as a self-governing club for alcoholics, their families, and nonalcoholic guests. It met Saturday evenings from 7 p.m. to midnight and included a range of recreational activities such as table games, dancing, pool, ping-pong, and potluck suppers. Alcohol was not available, and clients were denied admission or continued stay if they arrived intoxicated or if they drank while in attendance.

Follow-up was conducted at 3 months postintake and consisted of a standardized questionnaire dealing with drinking behaviors over the last 30 days of the preceding 3 months. Days of institutionalization and attendance at the social club were also monitored. Not surprisingly, the experimental group attended the social club significantly more frequently than did the control group. Interestingly, however, the experimental subjects attended the club only 2.47 times on average.

Quantity–frequency indices of alcohol consumption were significantly different and revealed a major decline in posttreatment drinking for the experimental group and minimal improvement for the control group. Similarly, the groups differed significantly on the global indices of physical and behavioral problems related to drinking and time spent in situations in which drinking is common. The groups did not differ in institutionalization levels subsequent to treatment.

In discussing the results, the researchers not only opine about the benefits of the nondrinking social club as a means of occupying high-risk time (Saturday night) in a way incompatible with drinking but also about the possible benefits of the club in promoting and reinforcing social skills without the presence of alcohol. They further observe that the social club provided the entire family reinforcement for nondrinking behaviors.

Sisson and Azrin (1986) evaluated CRA-based counseling of family members of alcoholics. Subjects were 12 women with a male family member (usually a spouse) whom they reported was "alcoholic" in terms of loss of control of drinking and physical withdrawal when not drinking. All subjects reported verbal abuse from the alcoholic and six also reported physical abuse. A coin flip determined assignment of the subject to a traditional program involving education on the disease concept of alcoholism, supportive counseling, catharsis, and referral to Al-Anon or assignment to the experimental condition consisting of "awareness of problem training" (completion of an inventory and discussion of possible problems caused to the client by the alcoholic's drinking); training in how to motivate the alcoholic to enter treatment and, once admitted, to take disulfiram; instruction on how to reinforce the alcoholic for not drinking and how to communicate effectively with him; advice on how to schedule activities for the alcoholic in which heavy drinking was unlikely; encouragement to the client to seek outside activities so that she would be less dependent on the alcoholic; instruction on techniques to use while the alcoholic was drinking to diminish his alcohol consumption; training to withhold reinforcers if he was intoxicated; instruction on avoidance of "enabling" drinking such as making excuses for others for his condition; and training on how to recognize and escape situations in which she felt at physical risk from the alcoholic.

Results revealed than none of the alcoholic family members of control subjects entered treatment. All but one of those of experimental subjects did so. Analysis of 3-month follow-up data also showed that alcoholic family members of clients in the experimental group were intoxicated on fewer days, consumed less ethanol per drinking occasion, and took disulfiram more frequently than did those of clients in the traditional program, although it is unclear to what extent these benefits may be ascribed fully to the family member's treatment rather than to the treatment that the alcoholic entered. Nevertheless, post hoc comparisons among those alcoholics who entered treatment revealed that, while the number of drinking days declined in the 30-day period before the alcoholic himself entered treatment, the number of drinking days decreased significantly more after he entered treatment. Little change in drinking days or intoxication days per month or average alcohol consumption per drinking episode was found among the alcoholics whose family member was treated in the traditional program.

Azrin, Sisson, Meyers, and Godley (1982) contrasted the value of the disulfiram assurance component of CRA to traditional treatment including disulfiram as well as to full CRA with the disulfiram assurance component. Subjects were outpatients in a rural community alcoholism program. All clients were considered as potential subjects if they were willing and medically able to take disulfiram, had lived in the local area for at least 6 months, and were not psychotic or dependent on a drug other than alcohol. Of the subjects, 83% were male, 67% were married or cohabitating, and 46% were employed. The mean age and education were 33.9 and 11.2 years, respectively. Average ethanol consumption per drinking day was 8.8 ounces, and subjects reported drinking on an average of 21.1 days per month.

All subjects were encouraged to take disulfiram, and the usual dosage was 250 mg. They were also all scheduled for five weekly sessions and monthly sessions thereafter. All were given educational materials on alcoholism. They were taught to record improvements in drinking, job performance, arrests, family status, and institutionalization on a monthly calendar. These self-reports were brought to treatment sessions. The record was also reviewed by someone close to the patient who would be aware of the information recorded. Counselors visited the client's home or workplace.

Clients were randomized to one of three interventions at the second session:

1. Traditional treatment with no special disulfiram assurance procedures. Sessions included films on alcoholism, discussion of the course of alcoholism, sympathetic listening to problems, and encouragement of total abstinence.
2. Traditional treatment with disulfiram assurance including observation of disulfiram administration; instruction on when and where to take the drug and that it should be done in the presence of a significant other; role play and instruction with the client and significant other on taking disulfiram when either one did not want it used or was uncooperative.
3. Full CRA as needed by the client and including the above two interventions and deep muscle relaxation training.

Overall results were obtained on seven outcome measures 6 months following admission to treatment. The three groups did not differ on days unemployed, days institutionalized, or days absent from home. They did, however, differ significantly on number of days on which disulfiram was taken, number of drinking days, and number of days intoxicated. They also differed on mean amount of ethanol consumed per drinking occasion, with the mean ounces of alcohol drunk being 4.1, 1.7, and .7 for the traditional, disulfiram assurance, and full CRA interventions, respectively. Visual inspection of results on the four outcome measures revealing significant effects suggests that CRA yielded better results than disulfiram assurance only and that disulfiram assurance did better than traditional treatment alone. However, it seems that post hoc t tests were not performed on the data, which would have more definitively indicated the incremental effectiveness of full CRA over disulfiram assurance only and these two interventions over the traditional program.

This study is also important because it suggested a thought-provoking patient–treatment interaction on the four follow-up measures showing significant improvements. The interaction effect between marital status (single versus married) and the three treatment conditions was significant and seemed to indicate that married patients did as well with disulfiram assurance only as with full CRA, but that single patients gained more if they received full CRA than if they simply received disulfiram compliance treatment. However, again no post hoc t-test results were reported.

As suggested in the studies summarized above, CRA appears to offer considerable potential as a time-limited, practical, effective treatment for alcoholism. Additional research, however, needs to be done since the data base remains quite small. It would be of particular interest to determine the effectiveness of CRA with alcoholics suffering collateral psychiatric or drug dependence problems. Unlike most alcoholism interventions, CRA seems especially geared to alcoholics with serious adjustment problems such as unemployment, marital strife, and deficits in social functioning. It would be of interest to assess its effectiveness also with clients who do not suffer such clear liabilities.

While as yet there is not much research on CRA, it is impressive that "dismantling" studies have already been undertaken to evaluate the relative impact of its various components. Beyond these, it seems important to assess the role of the nonformal intervention aspects of CRA, such as the high level of involvement by the spouse, the "buddy," and the employer in treatment; the high degree of optimism and activity of the counselor; the prominent role of self-monitoring by the patient; the use of behavior-change contracts; and the motivational value of selecting particular interventions based on perceived client needs.

Social Skills Training

Complex relationships exist between social skills deficits and drinking problems (Monti, Abrams, Kadden, & Cooney, 1989), and it has been hypothesized that deficiencies in certain social skills may make it difficult for alcoholics and problem drinkers to appropriately and effectively resist interpersonal pressures to drink. So too, deficiencies in social skills may cause personal unhappiness or disappointment, and drinking may be engaged in to dissipate these dysphoric feelings.

Social skills training involves employment of didactic instruction, modeling of appropriate responses, coaching, role play, and feedback on performance of social skills. Social skills training represents a subclass of coping skills strategy, which, in addition to training patients in more effective interpersonal skills, assists them in techniques to monitor and modify mood, solve problems more effectively, and change dysfunctional personal habits.

It seems that the first controlled trial of social skills training as a treatment for alcoholism was conducted by Chaney, O'Leary, and Marlatt (1978). Subjects for the investigation were male VA inpatients with a primary diagnosis of alcoholism but who were not actively psychotic or suffering severe organic impairment. The mean age of subjects was 45.6 years and the modal social class was lower middle class. Prior to the trial, patients had been detoxified and received 2 weeks of standard training including group therapy, therapeutic community group sessions, and alcohol education. Further, they had verbally committed themselves to a rather demanding level of ongoing VA care. Of the 70 patients eligible to participate, 56 did so, although 16 dropped out before or after randomization to treatment. Dropout did not seem related to the treatment condition to which patients were assigned. Dropouts were not followed. Subjects were randomly assigned to three conditions:

1. *Skills-training group.* These subjects were taught general problem-solving and assertion skills in small groups of three to five patients each. They were then presented problematic situations and asked to generate possible responses to them. Therapists discussed the likely consequences of these responses and suggested alternatives. For interpersonal situations, one of the therapists role-played the response and the other reacted. For intrapersonal responses, a therapist "thought aloud," defining the problem, considering alternative responses, deciding on a solution, and planning the response. Following these demonstrations, subjects decided on responses, role-played them, and received feedback from the group on likely consequences of the response. Two examples from each of the four most frequently cited classes of high-risk relapse situations discovered in previous research by Marlatt and Gordon (1978) were chosen for the exercises. Subjects also chose one or two situations to practice which they believed might be particularly problematic for them following hospital discharge.
2. *Discussion group.* Subjects in this condition discussed the same eight situations as in the skill-training condition. However, rather than engaging in active practice and receiving instruction on how to appropriately respond to the situation, they were urged to explore and discuss their feelings and motivations.
3. *Control group.* Subjects assigned to this condition received the same amount of treatment as those in the two experimental conditions but participated only in the regular treatment program.

All subjects were discharged following the eight treatment sessions and entered into the standard weekly aftercare group sessions.

Results for drinking variables are reported for 1, 3, 6, and 12 months following day-care discharge. Discharge and 3-month performance were reported on the Situational Competency Test (SCT) (Chaney, 1989), a measure of adequacy of responses to 16 situations similar to those involved in the training of experimental groups. The discussion group and control group did not differ in performance on the SCT at treatment exit. The skills-training group, however, had a longer mean duration of response than the other two groups. The difference diminished at subsequent retest. At treatment exit the three groups differed on the amount of detail they offered in how they would respond to the SCT stimuli with the skills group doing best, followed by the control group and with the discussion group scoring most poorly. The skills group continued to score significantly higher than the discussion group at 3-month follow-up.

The discussion and control groups did not differ on the drinking measures at the follow-up periods and, hence, they were combined into a single group for comparison with the skills-training group. At 1-year follow-up, subjects in the experimental group were significantly improved compared to those in the combined control group in number of days intoxicated (one-sixth as many), average alcohol consumption per day (one-fourth as much), and average length of drinking episode (one-eighth as long). The groups did not differ on days hospitalized, days abstinent, days of controlled drinking, or days employed. Subsequent analyses related latency of response on the SCT to the positive drinking outcomes.

Jones, Kanfer, and Lanyon (1982) performed a partial replication of the Chaney, O'Leary, and Marlatt (1978) study synopsized above. Major differences in their methodology included a higher socioeconomic and more socially stable cohort of patients, reduced intensity of the three conditions, slightly modified interventions, and use of different assessment instruments.

While also having a primary diagnosis of alcoholism, the Jones, Kanfer, and Lanyon subjects were in a private inpatient alcoholism treatment program, had to have attended at least five of six treatment sessions, ultimately had to have received a "regular" discharge from the inpatient facility in order to be included in the study, were primarily middle class, were more often currently married, and were more likely to be employed.

The three treatment conditions were largely comparable to those of the earlier study. The social skills group and the discussion groups participated in six biweekly 90 min small-group sessions. These treatments began 1 week after entry into the inpatient program. The same training manuals were used as in the original study. The authors do, however, note that the discussion group in their study probably focused on patients' emotional reactions to high-risk relapse situation descriptions more than was the case in the previous project.

Rather than use the SCT as a dependent measure, the authors employed their own Adaptive Skills Battery (ASB) (Jones & Lanyon, 1981). The ASB presents potential relapse-related situations to subjects via audiotape. Responses were scored on a 3-point scale of expressed coping skills by a rater blind to treatment condition.

Follow-up testing on the ASB was conducted at discharge and self-report drinking measures were obtained at the 1-year follow-up. The groups did not differ on the ASB score at discharge. Long-term results of the interventions were seriously flawed due to a follow-up rate of slightly fewer than half the patients. The authors report a statistical trend toward significant differences on a composite drinking variable. Step-down univariate analyses of covariance suggested that the skills-training group and the discussion group did not differ on total alcohol consumption or days drinking posttreatment but that both groups did better on these outcome measures than the control group.

The authors ascribe their weaker results than those of Chaney *et al.* to possible differences in subject selection. It may be that their patients were higher functioning and, hence, may not have required concrete practice in the skills. Also influential may have been changes in procedures for the discussion group and diminished intensity of treatment for the two experimental groups. It is also, of course, possible that the subjects available for follow-up differed as a function of treatment condition.

Oei and Jackson (1980) conducted a project both to evaluate the benefits of social skills training and to determine if differences in effects resulted from the training being conducted according to an individual or a group format. Subjects for the study were men and women admitted for inpatient treatment of chronic alcohol dependence. The mean age was 33.5 years. Interestingly, average alcohol consumption was reported in dollars spent per week. Little other information on patient characteristics was reported.

Patients were matched on age, number of previous admissions for alcoholism treatment, alcohol consumption, and scores on an assertion and social skills inventory. The matching procedure and bounds on the pairing variables for what constituted a match were not described.

Subjects were assigned to four treatment conditions of identical frequency and duration:

1. Group social skills training involved 12 sessions of 2 hours per day conducted over a 3-week period. The therapy sessions involved training in six basic interpersonal skills. Sessions included instruction on the skill, demonstration of the skill by the therapists, and role play of two situations in which the skill could be employed. These performances were videotaped and replayed to patients with feedback provided by clients and therapists. Patients were also encouraged to practice the skills on their own between sessions.
2. Individual social skills training was conducted by the same therapists who offered the group variant of the approach. The same instruction was also given on the skills. Videotapes of the performances by the subjects in the group social skills training condition were then shown for the remainder of the session. As in the previous condition patients were encouraged to practice the skills between sessions.
3. Group traditional supportive therapy involved encouraging patients to "mentally explore themselves" with the therapists' assistance. Clients themselves raised topics of concern, often of a general, practical nature, such as marital or monetary problems.
4. Individual traditional supportive therapy seems identical to the group-format approach except that patients were treated on a one-to-one basis.

Baseline, discharge, and 3-, 6-, and 12-month postdischarge data were collected on six measures, one of which assessed self-reported alcohol intake. A main effect for alcohol consumption was found, favoring the social skills strategy across the follow-up periods. No differences were found between strategies as a function of individual versus group format.

Nurses' ratings of assertiveness across time also favored the social skills training approach. Again, no difference was found between the individual and group approaches. Nevertheless, the group format of social skills training led to more rapid improvement during and after treatment on measures of social avoidance and fear of negative evaluation from others. The group format of traditional treatment was also more successful than the individual format on these dependent measures. Subjects treated by the social skills approach improved more than those treated in the traditional approach on the assertion skills inventory and on a quantitatively scored, disguised-intent behavioral interview conducted by a psychologist blind to treatment condition. Results on the assertion inventory also favored group over individual social skills training.

It is difficult to determine if the differences between the individual and group formats in social skills training were related to the group versus individual format itself or to other differences, such as a single therapist being involved in the individual format, the individual approach failing to include active practice, or possible difficulties of patients in individual sessions in adequately identifying with the videotaped performances since they involved different patients.

It is also difficult to fully determine if the benefits of the social skills training were due to the content of the sessions themselves or if there were simply no incremental benefits of increasing traditional supportive techniques which both groups had likely received in the treatment program. To eliminate the possibility of a potential "ceiling effect" in the benefits available from traditional treatment, it would have probably been necessary to conduct the research outside of the context of a traditional inpatient treatment setting. This concern, of course, is not limited to the current investigation. It applies to most research evaluating a new type of intervention within the context of traditional treatment.

A very tightly controlled trial in social skills training was conducted by Eriksen, Bjornstad, and Gotestam (1986) in Norway. Subjects for the investigation were inpatients who had already been in alcoholism treatment for at least 8 weeks, employed or eligible for employment, and diagnosed as alcohol dependent according to criteria of DSM-III. Additionally, entry criteria for the unit from which research subjects were selected included voluntary admission to the facility and absence of psychosis, retardation, or serious other drug addiction. (The authors note that one of the social skills subjects was eventually discovered to be an opiate addict but was not subsequently dropped from the study.)

Patients were randomly assigned to social skills training or to the control group, except that a married couple was assigned to each of the conditions based on randomization of the first member. Groups differed only on age, with the social skills group having a higher mean than the control group. (Secondary analyses, however, showed that age was negatively associated with treatment outcome in the control group.) A review of patient preintervention characteristics suggests that the control group, if anything, had more positive prognostic indicators, although a multivariate contrast of groups on the pretreatment characteristics combined was not reported.

Control group therapy involved discussion of attitudes and feelings toward drinking, alcohol consequences, reasons for drinking, and techniques to stop drinking.

The social skills training was conducted in two small-group sessions for eight weekly 90-min sessions. Mean attendance was 6.4 sessions. The control group also was divided into two small groups and received eight weekly 90-min sessions in which a range of alcohol topics were discussed. Mean attendance was 6.7 sessions. The social skills training model of Chaney *et al.* (1978) discussed above was employed.

Following the research interventions, patients were reassigned to standard discussion group aftercare sessions. All patients had also previously received the traditional treatment program involving occupational, academic, and physical rehabilitation training and personal counseling.

Beginning at discharge, clients completed biweekly self-report questionnaires on drinking, sleeping at home, and taking disulfiram. Compliance was 100% for 23 of the 24 subjects. One patient (assigned to social skills) returned no reports and was unreachable. For most analyses maximally negative scores were imputed for this subject. Primary and secondary significant others were also asked to submit collateral reports, and all but three did so. Correlations between self-reports and reports of primary significant others ranged from .91 to 1.00.

Independent one-tailed *t* tests on 1-year posttreatment means for total alcohol consumption, days drinking, days employed, length of abstinence, admissions to subsequent alcohol or other treatment, and nights slept at home all strongly favored the social skills group. For example, the social skills group averaged 6.5 drinks per week, 77% sober days, 2 days of drinking per week, and 51.6 days to relapse, whereas comparable figures for the control group were 10.5, 32%, 5 days, and 8.3 days, respectively. The social skills group also did far better on employment, working 77% of the possible work days versus 45% for the control group. While formal trend analyses were not performed, biweekly figures suggested little change in treatment effect for either group during the postdischarge year.

Research has also been directed toward specifically evaluating assertion training, one of the key components of social skills training. The earliest investigation of this seems to be by Freedberg and Johnston (1981), who evaluated possible advantages of enhancing a 3-week residential alcoholism treatment program with assertion training. Ninety percent of the subjects in the study had been compelled to enter treatment by their employers under threat of job loss.

Four consecutive treatment cohorts consisting of a total of 56 subjects, of whom 54 were male, entered the program with assertion training. The group receiving no assertion training also consisted of four treatment cohorts and was also almost entirely male. Subjects for this study differed from those of most other projects assessing the benefits of social skills training with alcoholics in that they were older (mid-40s) and all were employed and earning at least moderate salaries. No discussion was offered on other potentially important subject variables, such as how diagnostic criteria for alcoholism were satisfied, severity of dependence on alcohol, number of previous treatments, and pretreatment alcohol consumption. Also, the cohort nature of subject selection constituted at least a slight statistical confound since it is impossible to determine if the nature of the treatment population varied across time, and, unfortunately, statistical tests of possible experimental group–control group differences were not reported.

The assertion training group received approximately 70 hours of supervised traditional treatment and six 2½ to 3-hour sessions of assertion training. The control group received between 80 and 90 hours of traditional treatment. Regrettably, traditional treatment modules are not described, and the discussion of assertion training is limited to noting that it involved role play and behavioral rehearsal with video, peer, and therapist feedback after each role-playing situation, and practice continued until all other group participants agreed that the behavior was satisfactory. Subjects were also encouraged to practice assertive responses between sessions with an assigned partner. It is unclear if the practiced vignettes involved specific high-risk drinking situations or were of a more general nature.

Data were collected at program admission and discharge as well as at 3, 6, and 12 months postdischarge. While the assertion training group appeared to fare better with regard to drinking, the summary measure of drinking was quite complex and included judgments by therapists, who were not blind to treatment condition and who may well have been unintentionally biased. More objective data were collected on employment status. At 12-month follow-up, 80.4% of the assertion group were employed as contrasted with 68.8% of the control group. The groups also differed on three self-report scales dealing with assertion skills.

Unfortunately, statistical analyses were limited to chi-squares, rather than an overall multivariate analysis of variance with repeated measures and subsequent step-down analyses. On the positive side, this investigation had a very high follow-up rate in both conditions.

Ferrell and Galassi (1981) contrasted human relations training with assertion training in chronic alcoholic inpatients in a public facility. The average length of self-reported problem drinking was 14.5 years. Most importantly, subject selection was limited to patients who scored below the 40th percentile on the Adult Self-Expression Scale (ASES) (Gay, Hollandsworth, & Galassi, 1975), a measure of assertion skill. Patients were matched as closely as possible on scores from this measure, age, gender, marital status, race, and education and assigned to either assertion training or human relations training groups. Regardless of condition, subjects received 2 hours of therapy per day for 10 consecutive days. Posttests were conducted 1 day after the intervention and 6 weeks later. Drinking behavior was reassessed at 2 years and included corroboration by next of kin, records, and outside counselor reports.

Assertion training involved bibliotherapy, discussion, modeling, behavioral rehearsal, coaching, feedback, and homework assignments designed to teach the patient to more effectively express feelings and refuse unreasonable requests. (It is unclear from the report if the refusal behavior training included drink refusal skill training.)

The human relations training involved verbal and nonverbal exercises intended to help patients become more aware of themselves, how they were perceived by others, and how to communicate feelings more clearly.

Both interventions were conducted in a group format, and both groups received milieu therapy in addition to the specific assigned treatment condition. Patients given assertion training scored higher on several measures of assertion at the conclusion of treatment and on another index at 6-week follow-up. While the two groups did not differ on the total ASES score at the conclusion of treatment, the assertion training group did score significantly higher by the 6-week follow-up. So too, they scored lower on trait anxiety at this point.

Data on sobriety were reported for 6, 12, and 24 months postdischarge. Rates of sobriety for the assertion training group were 62.5%, 37.5%, and 25% for the successive follow-up periods. For the human relations condition, comparable rates were 33.3%, 11.1%, and 0%, respectively. The investigators reported that the assertion group maintained sobriety significantly longer than the human relations group and noted that for both groups the 6 month rates compared quite favorably with previously published data for the same facility when only milieu therapy was used.

Research has also been conducted on cognitive restructuring, an alcoholism treatment in its own right as well as a common component of social skills training for alcoholism. Cognitive restructuring involves techniques to rectify maladaptive perceptions and assumptions about situations. The theoretical underpinnings of cognitive restructuring as a behavioral-change modality highlight the potential role of anxiety in inhibiting the application of appropriate social skills currently in the individual's behavioral repertoire. To determine if the long-term benefits of social skills training might be enhanced by combining cognitive restructuring with it, Jackson and Oei (1978) evaluated the effectiveness of social skills training with and without a secondary component of cognitive restructuring.

Subjects for the project were inpatients in a public alcohol dependence treatment facility. They were matched for age, amount spent per week for alcohol, number of previous alcohol treatment admissions, and scores on a personality inventory. The subjects were assigned to one of three experimental conditions: social skills group training; cognitive-restructuring group training, involving discussion of the social and assertive skills covered in the first experimental condition without direct training in the skills; and traditional therapy consisting of supportive, general discussions with the group therapists. All therapies consisted of 12 two-hour sessions.

A repeated-measures two-way analysis of variance contrasting results on the three conditions for pretreatment, discharge, and 3 months postdischarge measures showed both experimental conditions as more effective than traditional treatment on several dependent variables and cognitive restructuring as more effective than the other two approaches. The dependent measures were Eysenck Personality Questionnaire (EPQ) scales, a behavioral assertion scale, the Social Interaction Scale, a behavioral interview (unexplained), nurses' ratings (unexplained), and alcohol intake.

While this study revealed a rather consistent pattern of positive results, unfortunately, the measures are little described and means on the scales are not provided. Also, it is disconcerting that the actual procedures included in the three strategies are not described. Finally, it is surprising that the follow-up period was so brief, considering the investigators' stated belief that the major benefit of cognitive restructuring is in producing "long-term" skill increments.

Many of these deficiencies were resolved by a subsequent investigation by the same research team (Oei & Jackson, 1982). Patients were from the same facility as in the previous project. Subject selection was, however, limited to those who scored in the mild to severe range on a scale of assertiveness. Patients were matched on age, ethanol consumption during the last 7 drinking days, number of previous treatment admissions, number of years of drinking problems, and the assertiveness scale score and assigned to one of four treatment conditions. Self-reports of alcohol consumption were verified by an outside corroborator. The four conditions were as follows:

1. *Social skills training.* This intervention appears identical to the group format of social skills training involved in the Oei and Jackson (1980) study cited above.
2. *Cognitive restructuring.* The six social skills covered in the social skills training were discussed by patients and therapists without direct training on appropriate responses. Discussions focused on patients' opinions regarding effective and ineffective behavioral and attitudinal options and techniques to change them. Rational persuasion techniques were employed to assist patients in modifying false assumptions about the situation.
3. *Combined social skills training and cognitive restructuring.* In this integrated approach patients were given social skills training after they indicated acceptance of the cognitive-restructuring rationale.
4. *Traditional treatment.* This intervention also appears identical to the group traditional supportive treatment included in Oei and Jackson (1982).

All treatments were conducted with groups of eight patients each in 12 two-hour sessions over a 3-week period.

Results were reported contrasting the four groups on a series of measures taken at treatment entry, discharge, and 3, 6, and 12 months postdischarge. Findings revealed that the patients in the three experimental conditions did better across time than those in the traditional treatment group on the social interaction, assertion measures, and the neuroticism, psychoticism, and extraversion scales of the EPQ.

All three of the experimental condition therapies resulted in much lower weekly alcohol consumption over the year following treatment. The combined cognitive-restructuring–social skills training approach and the approach using cognitive restructuring alone also yielded significantly better results than social skills training without cognitive restructuring in reducing alcohol intake.

An extremely well-controlled, well-documented project contrasting communication skills training with (CSTF) and without (CST) significant others and cognitive-behavioral mood management (CBMMT), including cognitive restructuring, was conducted by Monti *et al.* (1990). (This investigation will be discussed in further detail in the "Patient–Treatment Matching" section of this chapter since it evaluated interaction effects in addition to main effects of treatment.)

Subjects were male inpatients receiving treatment in a 28-day Minnesota Model-based Veterans Administration program. The subject sample was characterized as having a primary diagnosis of alcohol dependence, unusually high daily alcohol consumption (averaging 11.6 drinks per day while in a noncontrolled environment), and rather low social stability in terms of employment and marital status.

Subjects were assigned by cohorts to one of three interventions: communication skills training with active practice and emphasis on high-risk drinking situations; the same training but with the closest significant other participating; and cognitive behavioral mood management training, consisting of relaxation training, training in avoidance of or response-substitution for high-risk drinking situations, and training in cognitive restructuring to cope with drinking urges and negative mood states. Each of the interventions were 4 weeks in length and involved 12 hours.

The 6-month follow-up rate was only 77%, but the groups did not differ on attrition in terms of pretreatment drinking variables, demographics, or role-play skills.

All groups appeared to show marked pre–post treatment differences on almost all drinking variables. CSTF and CST groups did better than CBMMT in reducing their alcohol consumption per actual drinking day and did not differ from each other. Number of drinks per drinking day posttreatment were 7.35, 9.61, and 18.40 for the three groups, respectively.

Results of the studies cited above reveal that social skills training is consistently more effective than "traditional" forms of alcoholism treatment on posttreatment drinking and on a range of psychological and social functioning dimensions. Assertion training, a component of social skills training, also appears to be rather effective in its own right. It also seems that cognitive restructuring augments the effectiveness of social skills training and that cognitive restructuring, even without direct training in social skills, yields very positive benefits. Some evidence exists that social skills training when performed in a group context is more efficient and effective than when it is offered on a one-to-one basis. The beneficial results of social skills training seem most pronounced for patients who score low in general assertion and social skills. Future research should assess possible benefits of these approaches with patients who do not clearly evidence such liabilities. It would also be of interest to evaluate the benefits of cognitive restructuring and social skills training in those specific situations indicated by individual patients as presenting particularly high-risk drinking stimuli for them. Finally, it would be worthwhile to evaluate the relative benefits of general interpersonal skills training as opposed to training in social skills directly proximal to drinking situations.

Patient–Treatment Matching

As researchers more fully understand the heterogeneous nature of alcoholism, it has become increasingly clear that no single rehabilitation approach can be expected to prove equally effective for all alcohol-dependent patients. The goal of patient–treatment matching research is to develop valid and practical guidelines for assigning patients to treatment regimens particularly suited to their needs. Although this seems an obvious direction for alcoholism research and one which certainly is not new in the field, only recently have efforts been made to systematically develop, test, and disseminate matching paradigms for the treatment of alcoholism. This section will first briefly discuss types of matching and application of matching models in clinical settings and then summarize examples of recent research on matching.

"Matching" most commonly refers to interactions of patient characteristics with particular types of treatment. Four classes of patient variables that may serve as potential matching variables may be distinguished: demographics; psychopathology; alcohol-specific factors such as attitudes or behaviors; and social and psychological characteristics such as social support, conceptual level, and neuropsychological functioning. An example of a match involving an interaction between treatment and alcohol-specific behavior is the work of Annis and Davis (1989). They found that individuals able to identify high-risk drinking situations derived more benefit from specific, focused relapse prevention than from traditional counseling. However, drinkers with a more "generalized" drinking response (i.e., absence of a distinct set of situations prompting drinking) did equally as well with both treatments. Another study (Azrin *et al.*, 1982) involving a demographic patient matching variable found that marital status interacted with choice of treatment in a disulfiram program with either traditional assurance or a multifaceted program that featured behavioral, social, and vocational components. Single men did much better with the multifaceted intervention than the disulfiram assurance program, whereas for married men both the less intense and the more intense programs were equally effective.

Although most of recent matching research has focused on patient–treatment interactions, matching can refer to other types of treatment interactions. For example, "self-matching" might be employed by the patient, rather than treatment assignment based on formal assessment-based algorithms. The "cafeteria approach" (Ewing, 1977) offers patients a menu of treatment options, with varying degrees of advice from the clinician. The efficacy of such client-directed matching has yet to be fully evaluated, although it incorporates the important element of imparting a sense of partnership and participation that may be important for compliance, motivation, and retention in treatment.

Another approach to matching stems from the suspected influence of therapist characteristics on successful outcome that may in some cases be so powerful that they may exceed formal intervention effects. Considerable information on patient–therapist matches in the general area of psychotherapy is available (Luborsky & McLellan, 1981), and hopefully these findings will be tested and extended into the alcoholism treatment domain in the future.

Turning now to application of matching models in the clinical setting, three variants of patient–treatment matching effects can be distinguished, each having very different interpretations for clinical decision making: overall treatment effects, generalized predictors of outcome, and "true matching" (or interactions between patient characteristics and treatment modality).

Panel A of Figure 16.1 depicts the overall treatment effects for two therapies. There is a linear relationship between patient characteristic "A" and improvement in both of the treatments under consideration. However, despite the small but consistent effect of characteristic "A," the overall strength of effect of treatment 1 is so much greater than treatment 2 that it appears to be the treatment of choice, regardless of any considerations related to factor "A." In this example, the main effect is so large that interactions (at least with characteristic A) are not of practical clinical significance.

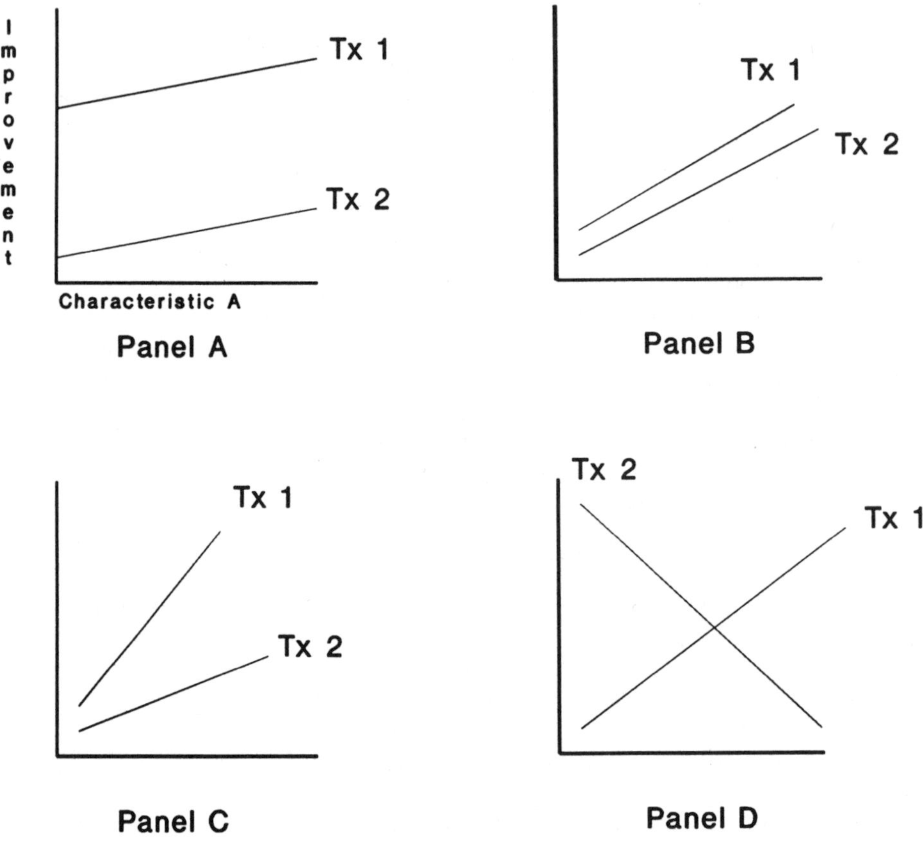

Figure 16.1. Variants of patient–treatment "matching" effects. See text for explanation. (Adapted from Mattson & Allen, 1991.)

Panel B of Figure 16.1 presents a different situation. Here, as levels of patient characteristic "A" increase, there is a marked and linear improvement on outcome. For example, the more socially stable the patient, the better his or her outcome in treatment. In this case, the effect of "A" upon improvement holds true for both treatments 1 and 2. In addition, the similarity in slopes and intercepts of the two lines suggests that both treatments are nearly equally effective, in contrast to panel 1. Thus, if faced with a choice between treatment 1 or treatment 2, both appear equally advantageous, and the clinician's decision would not be influenced by the patient's level of "A." Characteristic "A" is thus a generalized predictor of outcome, and, at least for treatments 1 and 2, it does not behave as a matching variable—that is, it does not interact with treatment type.

Panels C and D depict examples of true patient–treatment matching. In panel C, at very low levels of "A," both treatment 1 and treatment 2 seem equally, but modestly, effective. However, as the level of "A" increases, it becomes more apparent that treatment 1 offers meaningful benefits over treatment 2. Thus, although the response to both treatments is influenced to a degree by "A," treatment 1 seems differentially sensitive to the presence of this factor. Thus, if faced with a choice between the two treatments, the clinician might decide to offer either one for those low in "A," but should prescribe treatment 1 over treatment 2 for those with higher levels of "A."

Another type of matching effect is shown in panel D. In panel C, the choice of treatment was governed by the fact that patients "do better" with 1 than with 2 for higher levels of "A." In panel D, however, the two treatments have opposite effects, depending upon the level of characteristic present. As levels of "A" increase, outcome with treatment 1 is enhanced; however, the opposite occurs with treatment 2. Hence, in our hypothetical treatment choice, the levels of "A" should be a major factor in choosing the most appropriate treatment. For low levels of "A," treatment 2 is suggested and treatment 1 is contraindicated. For high levels of "A," treatment 1 is to be preferred and treatment 2 is contraindicated.

The patient–treatment matching literature is varied in both the nature of the matches examined and the type and rigor of the methodology used. Although the overall consensus from the literature by groups such as the Institute of Medicine (1990) is that matching may represent one of the most promising approaches to improving treatment outcome rates for alcoholism treatment, uniformity in research methodology is still at an early stage. Therefore, caution must be exercised in interpreting and comparing matching reports.

While the reports of matching studies are suggestive, caution must also be observed before results are incorporated into treatment programs. Few replication studies have yet been done. Thus, particular matches, although convincing in one report, have not been evaluated with other populations and by other investigators. Another shortcoming in the field of alcoholism research in general and patient treatment research in particular is cross-study variability in outcome measures (both primary measures of drinking and secondary measures of quality-of-life functioning). Variations in selection of measures, follow-up periods, criteria for improvement, psychometric properties of assessment instruments, relevance of both the primary and secondary measures chosen to the goals of the particular treatment under study, and efforts to assure validity of self-report render making meta-analyses, or even simple comparisons, difficult.

In addition to the experimental literature, there is a rather substantial body of information on conceptual and theoretical issues, and unique complexities inherent in the design and analysis of interaction studies (Finney & Moos, 1986; Glaser, 1980; Institute of Medicine, 1990; Marlatt, 1988; Miller, 1989; Miller & Hester, 1986). The reader is encouraged to consult these sources for a broad perspective.

Several examples of studies published in the 1980s and 1990s that satisfy basic criteria for a controlled clinical investigation will be summarized below, with emphasis upon the methodology employed and the nature of the matches discovered.

Kadden, Cooney, Getter, and Litt (1989) hypothesized that patients with higher levels of sociopathy, psychopathy, and neuropsychological impairment would do better with coping skills therapy than with interactional therapy. Conversely, those with lower levels on these characteristics were predicted to experience more favorable outcomes with interactional therapy than with cognitive skills training.

One hundred male and female patients who had completed a 21-day inpatient program were randomly assigned to one of these two treatments. Patients met DSM-III criteria for alcohol dependence or abuse. Assessment methods included the Psychiatric Severity subscale composite score of the Addiction Severity Index to gauge psychopathology; the California Psychological Inventory Socialization Scale to measure sociopathy; and the WAIS-R Digit Symbol subtest, Wisconsin Card Sorting Test, Trail-Making Test, Four-Word Short-Term Memory Test, and the face–name paired associates test to assess neuropsychological functioning. The Time-Line Follow-Back method of Sobell was used to assess drinking within 55 days of completion of the 26-week interventions.

The hypotheses were largely confirmed: Coping skills training was indeed more effective for subjects higher in sociopathy or psychopathology, and interactional therapy was more effective for those lower in sociopathy and, on one of three outcome measures, for subjects lower in psychopathology. Results, however, based on neuropsychological status were less consistent, with only one out of six analyses revealing a matching effect.

The Kadden *et al.* study is a significant example of current matching research for several reasons. The clinical trial methodology employed was highly rigorous, the treatment conditions were distinct and well documented, and the hypotheses were derived from a sound theoretical basis. In addition, the investigators conducted a second follow-up 2 years later to examine the durability of the matching effects (Cooney, Kadden, Litt, & Getter, 1991). Survival analysis of 24-month data showed that relapses (defined as the first heavy drinking, i.e., more than 3 ounces of ethanol) occurred significantly later for high-psychopathology patients who had received coping skills therapy and for low-psychopathology patients who had received interactional therapy. Likewise, relapse rates were lower for high-sociopathy subjects treated with coping skills and for low-sociopathology who had been given interactional therapy. Cognitively impaired patients had better outcomes in interactional therapy and worse outcomes in coping skills therapy. Those without cognitive impairment did equally well with either intervention.

In another example of matching research, Rohsenow *et al.* (1991) employed the social skills training techniques described in the previous section. The patient population consisted of 52 of the subjects from the original subject pool (Monti *et al.*, 1990). As noted earlier, patients were randomized to one of three experimental conditions: (1) communication skills training group (CSTG), (2) communication skills training group with a family member or close friend participating (CSTF), or (3) cognitive-behavioral mood management training group (CBMMT).

Alcohol-related anxiety was rated from responses to alcohol-specific role-play tapes. The Alcohol Dependence Scale was used to measure severity of alcohol dependence symptoms and the Irrational Beliefs Test assessed dysfunctional beliefs associated with negative mood and trait anxiety. Drinking in the 6 months prior to treatment and for the 6 months posttreatment was measured by the Time-Line Follow-Back procedure. The dependent measures were average number of standardized drinks per day and proportion of days abstinent.

The two communication skill modalities were combined into a single group (CST) for analysis purposes since they did not differ on effectiveness for any of the drinking variables. Overall, CST appeared to be equally effective regardless of pretreatment coping skill, anxiety in high-risk alcohol role-play situations, alcohol dependence, marital status, or education. CBMMT, however, was less successful in reducing drinking rate among alcoholics with lower education and more anxiety and urge to drink in high-risk role plays at pretreatment. CST subjects did equally well regardless of their pretreatment anxiety level, whereas subjects high in anxiety drank more in the CBMMT condition than in the CST.

A second interaction effect related to the urge-to-drink variable was observed. Subjects in CST again did equally well regardless of pretreatment urge-to-drink level. Patients high in urge to drink responded less favorably in CBMMT than did those low in urge to drink.

Litt, Babor, DelBoca, Kadden, and Cooney (1992) conducted a unique matching trial in which the patient variable was not a single characteristic, but rather a typology of characteristics. Using cluster-analytic techniques, they distinguished two groups of alcoholics; (1) a "high-risk/high-severity" group suffering early onset of problem drinking, more familial alcohol problems, greater dependence and higher levels of sociopathy and (2) a "low-risk/low-severity" group. The project was designed to determine whether matches existed between these opposite constellations of characteristics and two distinctly different therapies: coping skills therapy and interactional therapy.

Subjects in the study were 70 men recruited from a 21-day inpatient alcoholism treatment program. Eligibility criteria included DSM-III diagnosis of abuse or dependence and completion of the inpatient program. Excluded were those having current opioid dependence, severe organic brain syndrome, current thought disorder, reading or transportation impediments, or need for further hospitalization. Group therapy was employed for both interventions, consisting of twenty-six 90-min weekly sessions. The coping skills training included lectures, behavioral rehearsal, and homework practice exercises. The interactional therapy was focused on exploring the participants relationships with one another emphasizing immediate feelings and issues within the group.

The specific hypothesis, which was confirmed by the experiment, was that the high-risk/high-severity group would do better with coping skills than with interactional treatment. The opposite interaction was postulated, and also borne out empirically, with the low-risk/low-severity group.

The disulfiram trial reported by Fuller *et al.* in 1986 is unique in that it is among the scant handful of cooperative multicenter trials in the alcoholism field. Post hoc analyses revealed that older men who had abused alcohol longer, who were more socially stable, and who were more compliant tended to benefit more from disulfiram than did those who varied on these characteristics. (It will be recalled that the "full" CRA disulfiram contrast project reported above also found that married clients did as well with the disulfiram assurance intervention only as with "full" CRA.)

In 1989, Dorus and colleagues replicated, on a much larger scale, earlier work of Merry, Reynolds, Bailey, and Coppen (1976) on the effects of lithium in reducing drinking in depressed and nondepressed alcoholics. The earlier work had reported that, although the entire group showed little difference between placebo and lithium, the depressed group did much better with lithium than did the nondepressed group. The outcome measure was number of days incapacitated by alcohol. However, no beneficial effect of lithium was observed by Dorus *et al.* for either the depressed or nondepressed patients on a wider variety of outcome measures: abstinence, alcohol-related hospitalizations, and average number of days of drinking per 4-week period. Likewise, survival analysis revealed no significant difference in time to fifth and tenth days of drinking. The subjects were 457 men free from antisocial personality disorder and major psychiatric illnesses other than nonpsychotic depression and being treated in a VA inpatient alcoholism treatment facility.

The Dorus *et al.* study had sufficient power and a better rate of follow-up than is often the case in these types of studies, although as in other studies with this population, compliance to the medication regimen was lower than desired. It is surprising that Dorus *et al.* did not also include a group of hypomanic patients, since lithium is believed to be particularly beneficial with them.

In 1990, Longabaugh, Beattie, Noel, Stout, and Malloy reported results of a study examining a patient–treatment match in which the patient matching variable was moderated by another characteristic. They attempted first to determine whether the relationship between alcohol involvement and alcohol-specific social support (i.e., degree to which significant others stimulate or reinforce alcohol consumption) is influenced by the degree to which the patient values such support. Second, the project examined whether there was a match between involvement–support variables and type of intervention (relationally focused treatment, which involved significant others from the patient's environment, and individually focused therapy, which teaches cognitive behavioral techniques to motivate the patient to choose more adaptive behaviors that will reduce alcohol involvement and improve psychological functioning).

Two hundred and twenty-nine patients were randomized into either individual or relationally focused outpatient treatments and followed for 12 months. The population was drawn from a private psychiatric hospital. Eighty one percent were alcohol dependent according to DSM-III-R criteria, 29% had a current non-substance-related Axis I diagnosis, and 47% had a diagnosis of abuse or dependence on a substance other than alcohol. The average number of standard drinks per day in the preceding 90 days was 9.3. Patients were interviewed monthly by telephone and in person every 6 months with the Time-Line Follow-Back method.

Results indicated that alcohol involvement after treatment was a function of posttreatment alcohol-specific support for high "investors," but not for low "investors." Relative to treatment matching effects, the study showed that for high investors, support was an important determinant of outcome in relational therapy. That is, low support led to poor outcome and high support led to improved outcome. However, low investors were unaffected by levels of support, and high investors in individually focused therapy were likewise unaffected by level of support.

This study identified an important element of social investment as it relates to alcoholism treatment and suggested that provision of support is useful for those who place considerable value on it. Further, treatment is best delivered in a relationally oriented treatment milieu. Expending resources on provision of support either to those who do not value it or to those not receiving concomitant relational therapy does not appear fruitful.

A drawback of the study was that only the 107 subjects with complete follow-up data were included in the analyses. In addition, there appeared to be slightly more attrition in the individually focused treatment than in the relational condition. Importantly, however, the analysis group and the total group appeared quite similar on major prognostic indicators such as ethanol dependence, current Axis I diagnoses, marital status, employment, prior experience with social learning treatments, and gender.

Given the potential of the matching approach to enhance the effectiveness of treatment assignment decisions, the National Institute of Alcohol Abuse and Alcoholism has recently undertaken a multicenter cooperative clinical trial to assess patient–treatment interactions. The investigation includes sufficient numbers of cases and patient diversity to allow testing of a range of matches. Project MATCH consists of nine clinical research units and a data coordinating center. Two separate, but parallel, studies are being conducted, one with clients recruited at five outpatient settings, the second at four sites with patients receiving aftercare following an episode of standard residential treatment. Hypotheses being tested and research designs are nearly identical. Patients are being randomly assigned to one of three alcoholism treatment approaches: twelve-step approach incorporating principles of Alcoholics Anonymous, cognitive-behavioral therapy, or motivational enhancement therapy. Assessment at baseline and at sequential follow-ups over 15 months includes extensive information on a wide array of patient characteristics to explore interaction effects. The size of the data base will permit exploratory analyses as well as testing of *a priori* matching hypotheses.

Pharmacotherapy

The dual observation that 5-hydroxyindoleacetic acid, a metabolite of the neurotransmitter serotonin, is elevated in alcoholics in withdrawal (Ballenger, Goodwin, Major, & Brown, 1979) and that after 4 weeks of abstinence declines to levels *below* nonalcoholic controls has led some researchers to posit that serotonin uptake inhibitors might attenuate alcohol consumption. Various investigations of pharmacological agents which inhibit serotonin re-uptake (reviewed by Litten & Allen, 1991) suggest that these substances, in fact, reduce alcohol consumption in animals as well as in human social drinkers and alcoholics. Suppression of alcohol intake in humans has been consistent, though not dramatic, and differs somewhat across individuals, and the various serotonin re-uptake inhibitors differ in their specific benefits. Some reduce alcohol intake per drinking occasion. Others increase the number of abstinence days. While the serotonin re-uptake inhibitors are best known for their antidepressant effects, their effects on alcohol consumption do not seem to derive primarily from this property, although the possibility remains that the decreased drinking effect may be related to general curbing of appetitive behaviors (Litten & Allen, 1991). An interesting secondary benefit of the serotonin re-uptake inhibitors seems to be some improvement in learning and memory (Weingartner, Buchsbaum, & Linnoila, 1983), and this might enhance the patient's responsiveness to psychosocial interventions.

Another line of research suggests that opioid antagonists may diminish alcohol consumption (although, interestingly, quite different rationales have been proposed for their mode of action in this regard). Investigation of opioid antagonists with alcoholics is in very early stages. Volpicelli and his colleagues (1990) found that naltrexone reduced the number of drinking days, the frequency and duration of relapse, and the craving for alcohol in chronic alcoholics. O'Malley *et al.* (1992) largely confirmed these findings. O'Malley, Jaffe, Schottenfeld, and Rounsaville (1991) further reported that the effectiveness of two forms of psychosocial therapy was enhanced by collateral use of naltrexone.

Conclusion

Sufficient research on social skills training and the community reinforcement approach has now been conducted to demonstrate their effectiveness in alcoholism treatment. So too, the patient–treatment matching literature lends considerable support to the concept of matching as beneficial, although insufficient research has yet been performed to demonstrate which types of matching will ultimately prove most advantageous. Pharmacotherapies to diminish drinking urges may ultimately prove useful adjuncts to treatment, but this research is in even earlier stages.

Key questions remain about each of these four approaches. Research on social skills therapy with identifies the relative benefits of general training on interpersonal skills versus training specifically on skills related to drinking is needed. So too, it is important to show whether patients deficient in social skills, be they general or alcohol-specific, profit more from the training than do those who are not low in interpersonal skills.

Future CRA research might focus on developing algorithms for choosing which specific CRA components are most effective for which type of patients. In a sense, such research might be termed patient–treatment matching within CRA.

The prospects of patient–treatment matching seem particularly intriguing but, as we have noted, investigations in this field have to date involved so much variability in follow-up periods, outcome measures, sample description, and description of interventions that it is difficult to contrast the relative impact of various types of matches.

Most treatment efficacy research on social skills training, CRA, and patient–treatment matching has been conducted in the context of or following closely after traditional, generally Minnesota Model, treatment programs. Dismantling research is needed which evaluates the effectiveness of these techniques independent of standard alcoholism treatment.

Efforts to develop pharmacotherapeutic adjuncts are so early that we would urge that primary emphasis be placed on conducting more exploratory research and research on the wider range of agents that animal research has suggested might be useful in curbing ethanol consumption. Such studies should, however, attempt to discover the mechanisms of effectiveness of the medication and which alcohol-related phenomena—craving, drinking per occasion, time to resumption of drinking following treatment, alcohol consequences, and so forth—are affected.

Finally, we believe that ultimately research on effective interventions and patient–treatment matching strategies will prove complementary. In light of the fact that an array of alcoholism interventions exist, it is probably prudent to consider as potential treatments for matching effects those which have demonstrated meaningful main effects in alcoholism treatment.

Many questions remain on effective techniques for alcoholism treatment. Nevertheless, important research strides are being made, and the prospects for ultimately enhancing outcomes for alcoholism patients are quite favorable. As more is learned about drug agents which can effectively curb drinking, patient–treatment matching trials can be conducted with interventions that combine pharmacotherapies with behavioral interventions.

We believe that the research findings reviewed above offer important implications for the practice of alcoholism treatment. Sufficient research has been done on CRA to merit its incorporation in treatment programs, especially those dealing with patients suffering employment problems, lacking social reinforcements which do not focus on drinking, or deficient in general social stability. The literature has become quite extensive and strongly supportive of social skills training as an alcoholism intervention. Training in general interpersonal skills such as assertion training and expression of emotions and training in specific alcohol-related social skills such as drink-referral training have proven to be useful adjuncts to alcoholism treatment. Such training has been shown to be particularly helpful with alcoholics overtly deficient in these skills, but it may also be useful for those who have more subtle interpersonal deficits. There appears to be no reason why CRA and social skills training cannot be employed in consort with alcoholic patients.

Research on patient–treatment matching and medications to suppress drinking is at earlier stages. We would not yet argue for their matter-of-course inclusion in alcoholism treatment programs. We would urge treatment providers to remain conversant on such research since initial findings are quite promising. The matching research conducted to date does seem to suggest the value of tailoring treatment programs to specific patient needs rather than offering an intensive, time-consuming standard regime to all patients.

We do not have data on the extent to which the techniques described in this review are currently being employed in alcoholism treatment settings. It is our impression that unfortunately their use has been largely restricted to formal research programs. It is our hope, however, that as research findings are better disseminated to the treatment community that this state of affairs will improve.

ACKNOWLEDGMENTS. The authors gratefully acknowledge the contributions of Dr. William Miller and Dr. Scott Tonigan in the conceptualization of several key issues in this chapter and appreciate their advice and support.

References

Annis, H. M., & Davis, C. S. (1989). Relapse prevention. In R. K. Hester & W. R. Miller (Eds.), *Handbook of alcoholism treatment approaches* (pp. 170–182). New York: Pergamon Press.

Azrin, N. H. (1976). Improvements in the community-reinforcement approach to alcoholism. *Behaviour Research and Therapy, 14,* 339–348.

Azrin, N. H., Flores, T., & Kaplan, S. J. (1975). Job-finding club: A group-assisted program for obtaining employment. *Behaviour Research and Therapy, 13*, 17–27.

Azrin, N. H., Sisson, R. W., Meyers, R., & Godley, M. (1982). Alcoholism treatment by disulfiram and community reinforcement therapy. *Journal of Behavior Therapy and Experimental Psychiatry, 13*, 105–112.

Babor, T. F., & Dolinsky, Z. S. (1988). Alcoholic typologies: Historical evolution and empirical evaluation of some common classification schemes. In R. M. Rose & J. E. Barrett (Eds.), *Alcoholism: Origins and outcome* (pp. 245–266). New York: Raven Press.

Ballenger, J., Goodwin, F., Major, L., & Brown, G. (1972). Alcohol and central serotonin metabolism in man. *Archives of General Psychiatry, 36*, 224–227.

Berman, M. O. (1990). Severe brain dysfunction. *Alcohol Health and Research World, 14*, 120–129.

Caetano, R. (1985). Two versions of dependence: DSM-III and alcohol dependence syndrome. *Drug and Alcohol Dependence, 15*, 81–103.

Chaney, E. (1989). Social skills and training. In R. K. Hester & W. R. Miller (Eds.), *Handbook of alcoholism treatment approaches* (pp. 206–221). New York: Pergamon Press.

Chaney, E. F., O'Leary, M. R., & Marlatt, G. A. (1978). Skill training with alcoholics. *Journal of Consulting and Clinical Psychology, 46*, 1092–1104.

Cook, C. C. H. (1988). The Minnesota Model in the management of drug and alcohol dependency: Miracle, method or myth? Part I. The philosophy and the programme. *British Journal of Addiction, 83*, 625–634.

Cooney, N. L., Kadden, R. M., Litt, M. D., & Getter, H. (1991). Matching alcoholics to coping skills or interactional therapies: Two year follow-up results. *Journal of Consulting and Clinical Psychology, 59*, 598–601.

Dorus, W., Ostrow, D. G., Anton, R., Cushman, P., Collins, J. F., Schaefer, M., Charles, H. L., Desai, P., Hayashida, M., Malkerneker, U., Willenbring, M., Fiscella, R., & Sather, M. R. (1989). Lithium treatment of depressed and nondepressed alcoholics. *Journal of the American Medical Association, 262*, 1646–1652.

Edwards, G., & Gross, M. M. (1976). Alcohol dependence: Provisional description of a clinical syndrome. *British Medical Journal, 1*, 1058–1061.

Eriksen, L., Bjornstad, S., & Gotestam, K. G. (1986). Social skills training in groups for alcoholics: One-year treatment outcome for groups and individuals. *Addictive Behaviors, 11*, 309–329.

Ewing, J. A. (1977). Matching therapy and patients: The cafeteria plan. *British Journal of Addiction, 72*, 13–19.

Ferrell, W. L., & Galassi, J. P. (1981). Assertion training and human relations training in the treatment of alcoholism. *The International Journal of Addictions, 16*, 959–968.

Finney, J., & Moss, R. (1986). Matching patients with treatments: Conceptual and methodological issues. *Journal of Studies on Alcohol, 47*, 122–134.

Freedberg, E. J., & Johnston, W. E. (1981). Effects of assertion training within the context of a multi-modal alcoholism treatment program for employed alcoholics. *Psychological Reports, 48*, 379–386.

Fuller, R. K., Branchey, L., Brightwell, D. R., Derman, R. M., Emrick, C. D., Iber, F. L., James, K. E., Lacoursiere, R. B., Lee, K. K., Lowenstam, I., Maany, I., Neiderhiser, D., Nocks, J. J., & Shaw, S. (1986). Disulfiram treatment of alcoholism: A Veterans Administration cooperative study. *Journal of the American Medical Association, 256*, 1449–1455.

Gay, M. L., Hollandsworth, J. G., & Galassi, J. P. (1975). An assertiveness inventory for adults. *Journal of Counseling Psychology, 22*, 340–344.

Glaser, F. B. (1980). Anybody got a match: Treatment research and the matching hypothesis. In G. Edwards & M. Grant, *Alcoholism treatment in transition* (pp. 178–196). Baltimore, MD: University Park Press.

Grant, B. F., Dufour, M. C., & Harford, T. L. (1988). Epidemiology of alcoholic liver disease. *Seminars in Liver Disease, 8*(1), 12–25.

Helzer, J. E., & Pryzbeck, T. R. (1987). The co-occurrence of alcoholism and other psychiatric disorders in the general population and its impact on treatment. *Journal of Studies on Alcohol, 49*, 219–224.

Holder, H. D., Longabaugh, R., Miller, W. R., & Rubonis, A. V. (1991). The cost effectiveness of treatment for alcohol problems: A first approximation. *Journal of Studies on Alcohol, 52*, 517–540.

Hunt, G. M., & Azrin, N. H. (1973). A community-reinforcement approach to alcoholism. *Behaviour Research and Therapy, 11*, 91–104.

Institute of Medicine. (1990). *Broadening the base of treatment for alcohol problems*. Washington DC: National Academy Press.

Jackson, P., & Oei, T. P. S. (1978). Social skills training and cognitive restructuring with alcoholics. *Drug and Alcohol Dependence, 3*, 369–374.

Jones, S. L., Kanfer, R., & Lanyon, R. I. (1982). Skill training with alcoholics. *Addictive Behaviors, 7*, 285–290.

Jones, S., & Lanyon, R. (1981). Relationship between adaptive skills and sustained improvement following alcoholism treatment. *Journal of Studies on Alcohol, 42*, 521–525.

Kadden, R. M., Cooney, N. L., Getter, H., & Litt, M. D. (1989). Matching alcoholics to coping skills or interactional therapies: Posttreatment results. *Journal of Consulting and Clinical Psychology, 57*, 698–704.

Korsten, M. A. (1989). Alcoholism and pancreatitis: Does nutrition play a role? *Alcohol Health and Research World, 13*, 229–231.

Lieber, C. S., Garro, A. J., Leo, M. A., & Warner, T. M. (1986). Mechanisms for the interrelationship between alcohol and cancer. *Alcohol Health and Research World, 10*(3), 10–17.

Litt, M. D., Babor, T. F., DelBoca, F. K., Kadden, R. M., & Cooney, N. L. (1992). Types of alcoholics: III. Application of an empirically-derived typology to treatment matching. *Archives of General Psychiatry, 49*, 609–614.

Litten, R. A., & Allen, J. P. (1991). Pharmacotherapies for alcoholism: Promising agents and clinical issues. *Alcoholism: Clinical and Experimental Research, 15*, 620–633.

Longabaugh, R., Beattie, M., Noel, N., Stout, R., & Malloy, P. (1990, August). *Matching alcoholic patients to relationally focused treatments*. Paper presented at the annual convention of the American Psychological Association, Boston, MA.

Luborsky, L., & McLellan, A. T. (1981). Optimal matching of patients with types of psychotherapy: What is known and some designs for knowing more. In E. Gottheil, A. McLellan, & K. A. Druley (Eds.), *Matching patients needs & treatment methods in alcoholism and drug abuse* (pp. 51–71). Springfield, IL: Thomas.

Mallams, J. H., Godley, M. D., Hall, G. M., & Meyers, R. J. (1982). A social-system approach to resocializing alcoholics in the community. *Journal of Studies on Alcohol, 43*, 1115–1123.

Marlatt, G. A. (1988). Matching clients to treatment: Treatment models and stages of change. In D. M. Donovan & G. A. Marlatt (Eds.), *Assessment of addictive behaviors* (pp. 474–483). New York: Guilford Press.

Marlatt, G. A., & Gordon, J. R. (1980). Determinants of relapse: Implications for the maintenance of behavior change. In P. Davidson & S. Davidson (Eds.), *Behavioral medicine* (pp. 410–452). New York: Brunner-Mazel.

Mattson, M. E., & Allen, J. P. (1991). Research on matching alcoholic patients to treatments: Findings, issues, and implications. *Journal of Addictive Diseases, 11*(2), 33–49.

Merry, J., Reynolds, C. M., Bailey, J., & Coppen, A. (1976). Prophylactic treatment of alcoholism by lithium carbonate. *Lancet, 2*, 481–487.

Miller, W. R. (1989). Matching individuals with interventions. In R. K. Hester & W. R. Miller (Eds.), *Handbook of alcoholism treatment approaches* (pp. 261–272). New York: Pergamon Press.

Miller, W. R., & Hester, R. K. (1986). Matching problem drinkers with optimal treatments. In W. R. Miller & N. Heather (Eds.), *Treating addictive behaviors: Processes of change* (pp. 175–203). New York: Pergamon Press.

Monti, P. M., Abrams, D. B., Binkoff, J. A., Zwick, W. R., Liepman, M. R., Nirenberg, T. D., & Rohsenow, D. J. (1990). Communication skills training, communication skills training with family and cognitive behavioral mood management training for alcoholics. *Journal of Studies on Alcohol, 51*, 263–270.

Monti, P. M., Abrams, D. B., Kadden, R. M., & Cooney, N. L. (1989). *Treating alcohol dependence*. New York: Guilford Press.

National Institute on Alcohol Abuse and Alcoholism. (1991). Estimating the economic cost of alcohol abuse. *Alcohol Alert.*

National Institute on Alcohol Abuse and Alcoholism. (1991). Alcoholism and reoccurring disorders. *Alcohol Alert, 14*.

Oei, T. P. S., & Jackson, P. R. (1982). Social skills and cognitive behavioral approaches to the treatment of problem drinking. *Journal of Studies on Alcohol, 43*, 532–547.

Oei, T. P. S., & Jackson, P. (1980). Long-term effects of group and individual social skills training with alcoholics. *Addictive Behaviors, 5*, 129–136.

O'Malley, S., Jaffe, A., Chang, G., Witte, G., Schottenfeld, R., & Rounsaville, B. (1992). Naltrexone in the treatment of alcohol dependence: Preliminary findings. In C. Naranjo and E. Sellers (Eds.), *Novel pharmacological interventions for alcoholism* (pp. 148–160). New York: Springer-Verlag.

O'Malley, S., Jaffe, A., Schottenfeld, R., & Rounsaville, B. (1991). Naltrexone and coping skills therapy in the treatment of alcohol dependence. *Alcoholism: Clinical and Experimental Research, 15,* 382.

Ravenholt, R. T. (1984). Addiction mortality in the United States, 1980: Tobacco, alcohol, and other substances. *Population and Development Review, 10,* 697–724.

Regier, D. A., Myers, J. K., Kramer, M., Robins, L. N., Beager, D. G., Hough, R. L., Eaton, W. W., & Locke, B. Z. (1984). The NIMH Epidemiologic Catchment Area program: Historical context, major objectives, and study population characteristics. *Archives of General Psychiatry, 41,* 934–941.

Rohsenow, D. J., Monti, P. M., Binkoff, J. A., Liepman, M. R., Nirenberg, T. D., & Abrams, D. B. (1991). Patient–treatment matching for alcoholic men in communication skills versus cognitive-behavioral mood management training. *Addictive Behaviors, 16,* 63–69.

Sisson, R. W., & Azrin, N. H. (1986). Family-member involvement to initiate and promote treatment of problem drinkers. *Journal of Behavior Therapy and Experimental Psychiatry, 17,* 15–21.

Sisson, R. W., & Azrin, N. H. (1989). The Community Reinforcement Approach. In R. K. Hester & W. R. Miller (Eds.), *Handbook of alcoholism treatment approaches* (pp. 242–258). New York: Pergamon Press.

Volpicelli, J., O'Brien, C., Alterman, A., & Hayashida, M. (1990). Naltrexone and the treatment of alcohol-dependence: Initial observations. In L. Reid (Ed.), *Opioids, bulimia and alcohol abuse and alcoholism* (pp. 195–214). New York: Springer-Verlag.

Weingartner, H., Buchsbaum, M., & Linnoila, M. (1983). Zimelidine effects on memory impairments produced by ethanol. *Life Sciences, 33,* 2159–2163.

Williams, G. D., Grant, B. F., Harford, T. C., & Noble, J. (1989). Epidemiologic Bulletin no. 23: Population projections using DSM-III criteria. *Alcohol Health and Research World, 13,* 366–370.

III

CRITICAL COMMENTARY

17

Beyond Effectiveness

Uses of Consumer-Oriented Criteria in Defining Treatment Success

Gene Pekarik

Since the rise of behavioral and cognitive-behavioral treatments in the late 1960s and early 1970s, the mental health field has become increasingly empirically oriented, relying on experimentally designed outcome studies to demonstrate impact relative to no treatment and among alternative treatments. This empirical orientation to assessing therapy has had a multitude of benefits, including enhancement of psychotherapy's credibility (and associated increased service provision and insurance coverage), identification of the most effective treatments, clear descriptions of therapy procedures and associated dissemination of the most effective treatments, and increased efforts to refine treatments and improve their impact.

These accomplishments are all very important and have contributed greatly to the vitality of the psychotherapy field. Basic outcome research is so important that it is tempting to equate treatment outcome with treatment *utility*. These are quite distinct issues, however. Outcome is a necessary but insufficient criterion for treatment utility. For treatment to be truly useful it must be *used* by those in need. This means that clients in need must elect to *enter* treatment, *comply* with treatment, and *remain* in treatment till its completion. Variables such as treatment duration, cost, cost-effectiveness, and reimbursability determine these client decisions to enter and remain in treatment, yet they are rarely manipulated in psychotherapy research.

It is the thesis of this chapter that pragmatic and humanitarian concerns dictate that researchers broaden the application of their outcome technology to address such consumer and public policy-relevant issues. This need to do so is increased by evidence that psychotherapy has low utility as just defined: Later it will be documented that less than one-fourth of those with mental disorders receive professional mental health treatment, half of clients drop out of treatment, and half of both public clinic and private clients terminate by their fourth visit.

Gene Pekarik • Department of Psychology, Washburn University, Topeka, Kansas 66621.

Handbook of Effective Psychotherapy, edited by Thomas R. Giles. Plenum Press, New York, 1993.

Recent scientific and market forces that encourage therapists to deliver the most effective and efficient treatments provide a unique opportunity for the field to make great advances in the consumer-oriented aspects of treatment; these same forces, however, threaten to curtail mental health benefits subsidized by insurance plans and public mental health programs. The outcome for consumers and the mental health profession greatly depends on how we respond to these forces.

The Current Climate: Forces Affecting Psychotherapy Delivery

The 1990s find the mental health profession in the midst of clashing forces. Psychotherapy currently benefits from unprecedented credibility, third-party reimbursement, demonstrated effectiveness (e.g., Giles, Chapter 20, this volume; Shapiro & Shapiro, 1982; Weisz, Weiss, Alicke, & Klotz, 1987), and the potential for "cost-offset" effects by reducing medical service use (Jones & Vischi, 1979; Mumford, Schlesinger, Glass, Patrick, & Cuerden, 1984). Advances are being made toward the identification of the most effective treatments for each disorder (Davison & Neale, 1990). On the one hand, such accomplishments make mental health treatment and associated professions stronger and better than ever. On the other hand, the increased access to and utilization of mental health services is costly, being the third most expensive category of all disorders treated in the United States (Kiesler & Morton, 1988). Mental health care has been part of the escalating cost of all health care and increasingly will be subjected to the same kinds of cost containment strategies applied in general health care, for example, risk shifting, risk capitation, and the use of managed mental health. Policies such as severely limiting the number of outpatient hours reimbursed by third-party payers and tying inpatient stay to a prospective payment system based on diagnosis-related groups impose constraints on treatment duration that most mental health professionals and their treatments do not accommodate well and have so far resisted (Kiesler & Morton, 1988). As mental health treatment has become more accessible through third-party payment, it also has become severely curtailed with respect to duration and the total amount available for each case treated due to cost-containment policies of third-party payers.

Ironically, the cost-containment policies of third-party payers have forced mental health professionals to address—and redress—certain long-standing weaknesses in the mental health field. In general, these pertain to the consumer issues referred to earlier; in particular, they pertain to the mental health field's historic ignoring of clients' expressed needs, preferences, and high dropout rates, a general unconcern with cost-effectiveness, and a failure to respect clients' moral autonomy regarding treatment choices. (These criticisms apply to almost all approaches to psychotherapy.) These of course are very serious accusations. The documentation of their existence along with the proposal of possible solutions to them make up the bulk of the rest of this chapter.

These allegations of consumer neglect and insensitivity are made more serious by the fact that psychotherapy has certain inherent liabilities even under the best of circumstances. First, while there has been increased support for the overall effectiveness of psychotherapy in recent years, it is far from a sure remedy for all disorders and problems. Second, and more important, psychotherapy as designed is very costly to the consumer in terms of time, effort, and money—only very disabling or life-threatening physical disorders entail the same high costs. This combination of high cost and generally moderate benefit makes the cost-effectiveness ratio of psychotherapy quite poor relative to other health care. To illustrate this point consider the cost-effectiveness of the following common treatments:

1. A common filling for dental caries costs about $45.00 ($22.50 with typical 50% insurance reimbursement), requires about 30 min duration, and a very high percentage of the time results in a total cure of the problem.
2. "Root canal" work is usually perceived as a relatively extensive and invasive intervention. It usually requires three visits of about 45 min each, costs about $300 ($150 with 50% insurance coverage), and a very high percentage of the time it also results in total cure of the disorder.
3. An eye examination and eyeglasses for common nearsightedness secured from an optometrist costs about $200 and requires one or two office visits of about 30 min each. Most corrections with eyeglasses yield close to 20/20 (excellent) vision.
4. Conditions prompting visits to physicians are extremely variable. The five principal reasons for visits to general and family practitioners are general medical examinations, throat symptoms, blood pressure tests, coughs, and head colds (Silver, 1985). The average person has between two and one-half (National Center for Health Statistics [NCHS], 1988) and four and one-half (Silver, 1985) physician visits per year for all conditions, each of which lasts about 15 min and costs about $35 (NCHS). About one-third of visits do not result in a subsequent planned appointment (NCHS, 1988). Typically, about 80% of this is reimbursed by health insurance, requiring out-of-pocket payment of about $30 total per year without a deductible or about $125 for policies with a common $200 deductible.

Treatments (1) through (4) above represent the experience of the typical citizen with the U.S. health care system: one to two visits per problem episode, each lasting 15 to 30 min, with a total out of pocket payment less than $200; more severe conditions, such as the root canal treatment, entail a sequence of two to four visits and somewhat greater cost. Often treatments result in rapid and total cessation of intense pain or dysfunction.

5. Psychotherapy of depression requires about 12 to 20 one-hour visits using the most acclaimed treatments, Beck-style cognitive-behavioral treatment (Hollon, Shelton, & Loosen, 1991) and interpersonal psychotherapy of depression (Cornes, 1990). Considerable out-of-session treatment assignments are added to the 16 hours of in-session treatment. Total cost for 16 sessions would be about $1,200 (at a conservative $75 per hour). Typical insurance coverage (100% coverage for first $100, 80% of next $100, and 50% of next $1,640) would result in the client paying about $520 out of pocket. The same treatment with an also common 50% copayment after a $200 deductible would result in about $700 of charges. A strong majority of clients benefit from treatment, but about 25% to 50% relapse within one year (Hollon *et al.*, 1991).
6. While there is no single typical psychotherapy client, Corsini (1991) attempted to depict several representative treatment approaches to a normal

person with minor though persistent problems. The modal *recommended* treatment was 20 (sessions) hours (as documented later, this is the modal duration for most empirically oriented treatment programs described in the outcome literature). Using the figures presented under (5), the total cost would be $1,500 with an out-of-pocket payment of about $650. The overall effect of psychotherapy is that about 80% of those treated are better off than untreated people with similar conditions (Shapiro & Shapiro, 1982).

I am not arguing that general health care is comparable or even analogous to mental health care, but that the professional treatment expectations of most people are shaped by their experience with general health care. There is a dramatic contrast with mental health care prescriptions: one to a few 15–30 min visits, high success, and low cost versus 15 to 20 visits, medium success, and medium to high cost.

When similar conditions of relatively high cost and moderate benefit occur in general health care there is a high rate of noncompliance (Dunbar & Agras, 1980). It is not surprising then that high rates of noncompliance as indicated by a 50% dropout rate (Baekeland & Lundwall, 1975; Wierzbicki & Pekarik, 1991) are found in psychotherapy. Under these high cost–moderate benefit circumstances, compliance (continuance) could only be reasonably expected if therapists worked hard to take client desires into consideration. While all treatment approaches put a premium on thorough understanding of the client, therapists (of all orientations) *typically* pursue a course of treatment at variance with client preferences for treatment length, goals, and content. The evidence for this will be reviewed later in this chapter. These problems have occurred in a historical context of considerable consumer neglect in the mental health field. Because of the influence of this historical context, a brief review of the recent history of the mental health field's responsiveness to consumers follows.

Recent History of the Mental Health Field's Responsiveness to Consumers

Until relatively recently, mental health care for the average emotionally disturbed citizen has not been very available or very good. Before the Community Mental Health Centers Act of 1963, most emotionally disturbed individuals had little access to outpatient mental health treatment. In 1961, the Joint Commission on Mental Illness and Health concluded that outpatient and inpatient mental health services in the United States were woefully inadequate. Other studies from that era also found that services and professionals were unavailable and that the general public made little use of mental health treatment when emotionally upset (Albee, 1959; Gurin, Veroff, & Feld, 1960). Kiesler and Morton (1988) report that the 1950s per capita number of psychiatrists and psychologists was only one-tenth current levels, while even now less than one-fourth of those with a mental disorder currently receive treatment by a mental health professional (Shapiro *et al.*, 1984).

Before the mid-1960s, the professional treatment most accessible to the general public was inpatient state hospital treatment. A large number resorted to this option. In 1955, the average daily census of public mental hospitals was about

600,000 persons, who had an average length of stay of 5 years (Bloom, 1984). The average daily cost per client was $4.50, compared to $27.00 per day for general hospital care (Bloom, 1984). The Joint Commission (1961) concluded that treatment there was woefully inadequate.

Even those lucky enough to afford and gain access to outpatient psychotherapy received a suspect treatment. Following Freud's preference for case studies rather than aggregated data in the study of psychotherapy, psychotherapists widely neglected to systematically assess the impact of their work. Probably the most famous of the early assessments of psychotherapy outcome was Eysenck's 1952 indictment of the field which suggested that even those who could afford treatment need not bother because of its ineffectiveness. Even though some later interpretations of the same data concluded that Eysenck overstated his case against psychotherapy (e.g., Bergin & Lambert, 1978) the poverty of relevant data itself indicates consumer neglect. For years after Eysenck's 1952 publication, the mental health establishment did little to create new data in response to his conclusions—most rejoinders were criticisms of Eysenck's analysis rather than presentation of new data (Garfield, 1980). This dearth of outcome research did not improve until alternatives to psychodynamic treatment emerged in the 1950s and 1960s, notably Rogers' client-centered group and then, more vigorously, the behaviorists and cognitive-behaviorists.

Much of psychotherapy's consumer neglect can be traced to its early history. Freud's therapy did not begin as a response to consumer demand, but as an intellectual inquiry and treatment of an esoteric but especially interesting disorder, hysteria. This orientation to the treatment of mental disorders remained throughout his career. As late as 1919, about 30 years after he began treating hysterics, Freud (1919/1963, p. 88) acknowledged that psychoanalysis "is still directed principally to the cure of this [hysteria] affliction." This focus on the analytically interesting disorders (rather than those most prevalent) continued through the modern era.[1] Inspection of the content of analytically oriented texts reveals continued emphasis on hysterias, paranoia, and obsessions (e.g., Langs, 1975; Murphy, 1965; Strecker, 1952; Sullivan, 1956), all relatively rare disorders (Myers *et al.*, 1984). This was all in addition to the aforementioned aversion to aggregated data, reliance on the case study for treatment evaluation, and analytic concept of resistance making the client's stated treatment goals an object of skepticism. The combined impact of these influences was to make treatment more suited to therapists' interests than to client-consumers' needs.

As already noted, the behavioral/cognitive-behavioral ascendance provided many benefits to consumers, including the option of a treatment that was heralded for both effectiveness and efficiency (Wilson, 1981). Here, too, however, there were technical shortcomings that did not bode well for consumers. An emphasis on analogue studies of subclinical problems has been acknowledged as a shortcoming of the early outcome literature generated by this group (Emmelkamp, 1986; Hollon & Beck, 1986; Shapiro & Shapiro, 1982). In addition, early treatment

[1]Traditional psychodynamic approaches to treatment continue to emphasize treatment that is the least accessible (long-term), have a fascination with esoteric and rare disorders, deem most influential and prestigious those practitioners who do intensive long-term treatment with a very few clients (Bloom, 1984), and screen cases to fit the treatment method rather than adapt the method to the client or problem (Garfield, 1986).

models emphasized such trivial conditions as simple phobias as their targets. Thankfully, this has changed in recent years with increased outcome research on clients who have serious (diagnosable) disorders (Emmelkamp, 1986; Giles, Chapter 20, this volume; Kendall & Lipman, 1991; Morris & Kratochwill, 1983). As with outcome research in general, however, most research has not been conducted in standard practice settings with actual clinic populations (Emmelkamp, 1986; Hollon & Beck, 1986). Of more relevance to this chapter is the fact that even the behavioral/cognitive-behavioral approach to treatment duration and scope is far different from the average client's treatment preferences. Given the extreme treatment duration of the psychodynamic competition (consider the Menninger Foundation outcome study that averaged 289 to 835 hours of treatment per client!; Kernberg *et al.*, 1972), the behaviorists/cognitive-behaviorists could be *relatively* efficient and consumer-oriented while still prescribing quite lengthy treatment.

Other current influences also impede responsiveness to consumers. In different ways, the exigencies of public and private practice management run counter to consumer benefit. Public clinics have few incentives to do quality work. After a brief flirtation with assessing treatment quality via outcome studies in the late 1970s, public clinics have reverted to their previous reliance on reviews of utilization and chart completeness as evaluation measures. As Lachenmeyer (1980) points out, public mental health programs are maintained by contingencies independent of service quality. Their chronic underfunding relative to need creates an excess of service demand regardless of the quality of the treatment provided, removing incentives for quality work.

Private practitioners publish almost no assessment of their work, but at least they have financial incentives for keeping clients satisfied. This is partly offset, unfortunately, by the clear financial incentive to be inefficient, that is, to keep clients in treatment as long as possible. There are virtually no practical incentives but plenty of disincentives to make treatment efficient in all outpatient settings (Budman & Gurman, 1988; Giles, Chapter 20, this volume).

In summary, psychotherapy is a treatment that is especially prone to noncompliance and discontinuance due to its inherent high cost and moderate benefit. Until quite recently, consumer needs were little considered in treatment content or delivery systems. Since the entry of the federal government into the provision of services and the influence of empirically oriented treatments in the 1960s, services have improved: They have become more accessible, effective, and efficient. These improvements, however, are relative to a very poor baseline of performance and have been hampered by the history and traditions of the field and lack of practical incentives to do quality work in typical practice settings.

Psychotherapy has always been designed and primarily intended only for that subgroup of clients who accept the psychotherapy subculture's value for therapeutic and technical perfectionism (Budman & Gurman, 1988), that is, those willing to persist through a course of medium to long treatment, often aimed at basic or general functioning. It appears that most therapists fail to realize that only a minority of clients who request (and need) help want or attend even moderately lengthy treatment. The next section is devoted to demonstrating this allegation and argues that we should provide treatment to the majority of clients who "aren't buying" therapy as offered but who need help, that is, resetting priorities to help the majority who seek help rather than the minority who complete "textbook" prescribed treatment.

Client versus Therapist Preferences Regarding Treatment Length, Content, and Goals

Treatment Length

Clients clearly expect treatment to last only a short time. Pretherapy surveys of clients find that over 70% expect treatment to consist of 10 visits or less, and about half expect five or fewer visits (Garfield & Wolpin, 1963; Pekarik, 1991a; Pekarik & Wierzbicki, 1986). Clients at a managed mental health care setting expected even briefer treatment: 88% expected five or fewer visits (Pekarik, 1991b). In a study that distinguished expectations from preferences, McGreevy (1987) found that 62% of college undergraduates expected psychotherapy to be 10 or fewer visits, but 79% preferred it to be that short.

Therapists have a clear preference and expectation for treatment to be considerably longer than clients. Therapy textbooks provide information on such duration prescriptions. Treatment directed at personality reorganization is considered to require years (Garfield, 1980), with one report identifying an average of 835 hours of treatment (Kernberg *et al.*, 1972). This admittedly represents the extreme high end of treatment duration. Duration expectation and prescription is more commonly in the 20- to 50-visit range. Lambert, Shapiro, and Bergin (1986) represent the psychotherapy establishment with their reference to improvement after 26 sessions as an effect "that occurs in a relatively short period of time" (p. 162). Of mainstream delivery of behavior therapy, Wilson (1981) acknowledged that "therapy lasting from 25 to 50 sessions is commonplace" (p. 141) and then cited one clinic where treatment averages 50 sessions. Behaviorally oriented practitioners clearly perceive their treatment as of moderate length rather than very short. Norcross and Wogan's (1983) survey of members of the Association for the Advancement of Behavior Therapy found that only about a fourth of their clients were estimated to terminate in less than 3 months of treatment. These references are representative of commonly accepted views of the length of standard contemporary psychotherapies. Further indication of treatment duration prescriptions can be found in therapy technique texts. Corsini's (1991) book is representative; in it, prescribed durations for a fictitious case example are: person-centered—19 sessions, rational emotive therapy—21 sessions, behavior therapy—32 sessions, eclectic—20 sessions. It is important to note that the case example is of a *normal* person with minor though persistent problems.

An additional source of duration prescription can be found in recently published outcome studies. A recent edition of the *Journal of Consulting and Clinical Psychology* (February, 1991) with special sections on outcome research is representative: All outcome reports addressed treatment of a single disorder (e.g., agoraphobia, hyperactivity, depression), and the great majority of treatments were for 15 to 25 sessions.

In order to identify mainstream contemporary prescriptions of empirically oriented brief treatment, recently published texts on brief therapy were consulted. These identify the lower limits of treatment duration prescribed by experts. The following duration prescriptions were found for these popular brief therapies: multimodal therapy—20 to 30 sessions (Lazarus & Fay, 1990); brief behavioral marital therapy—20 sessions of 60 to 90 min each (Whishman & Jacobson, 1990); brief sex therapy—8 to 25 sessions (Beck, 1990); cognitive therapy (Beck-style treatment of anxiety or depression)—20 sessions (Moretti, Feldman, & Shaw, 1990); and brief behavior therapy—generally 15 to 20 sessions (Wilson, 1981). With very few exceptions, brief therapy associated with the other schools of therapy also recommend 10 to 20 sessions when duration is specified (Budman & Gurman, 1981; Wells & Giannetti, 1990; Zeig & Gilligan, 1990). Of mainstream approaches, only crisis intervention—not regarded as sufficient treatment of mental disorders (Aguilera & Messick, 1982; Slaikeu, 1984)—is generally prescribed for less than 10 sessions.

In one of the very few surveys of practitioners, Pekarik and Finney-Owen (1987) asked community mental health center therapists to indicate the length of treatment they preferred for most clients. Of 165 therapists, 30% selected 21 or more sessions and an additional 43% selected 11 to 20 sessions; overall, about three-quarters of the therapists selected 11 or more sessions.

It is clear from the foregoing analysis that clients expect and prefer a treatment course that is considerably briefer than that preferred by psychotherapists, even when compared to most brief therapists and practitioners in public clinics.

Treatment Content and Goals

Not surprisingly, clients' expectations and preferences for treatment content and goals are compatible with their ideas on treatment length; that is, they have modest, pragmatic aspirations for both treatment length and goals. Studies generally find that clients expect a high level of direct advice, concrete problem definition, problem solving, and therapist activity (e.g., Benbenishty & Schul, 1987; Hornstra, Lubin, Lewis, & Willis, 1972; Llewelyn, 1988; Overall & Aronson, 1962). Therapists prefer less of the treatment characteristics just identified than clients do; therapists prefer more extensive treatment and more insight and feeling expression (Benbenishty & Schul, 1987; Hornstra *et al.*, 1972; Llewelyn, 1988). Overall and Aronson (1962) found that clients' expectations regarding treatment directiveness usually were not met. When clients and therapists were asked their treatment preference, clients preferred problem-oriented treatment and therapists preferred treatment oriented toward personality change (Pekarik, 1985b; Pekarik & Wierzbicki, 1986).

Research on treatment dropouts also suggests that many clients have modest, problem-focused treatment goals. Baekeland and Lundwall's (1975) dropout literature review concluded that many clients attend therapy until acute crises subside, then terminate. This suggests that clients seek crisis relief as a primary treatment goal. Surveys of dropouts consistently find that perceived improvement is one of the most common reasons given for dropping out (Acosta, 1980; Garfield, 1963; Pekarik, 1983b, in press b). Pekarik (1983b, 1992b) found that the dropouts who cited problem improvement as a dropout reason did, as a group, improve significantly based on intake and follow-up symptom inventory scores. These findings are consistent with the broader medical treatment literature which consistently finds symptom abatement as one of the primary reasons for treatment noncompliance (Dunbar & Agras, 1980).

Further evidence of therapists' preference for more ambitious treatment is found in the extensive literature devoted to preparing clients for psychotherapy (reviewed by Heitler, 1976); the preparation usually consists of correction of clients' expectation for immediate, direct help and indoctrination into the therapy subculture's ethic of longer treatment and ambitious goals.

Actual Treatment Attendance Patterns

In the real world of both public clinic and private practice settings, treatment is typically very brief. This very brief treatment is sometimes by design but often by default, due to premature termination.

The mean number of sessions attended by community mental health center (CMHC) outpatients is about five (National Institute of Mental Health [NIMH], 1981). This finding was based on a survey of the universe of all federally funded CMHCs. Incredibly, this often-cited statistic is an exaggeration of the actual treatment duration since it is distorted (skewed) by the few clients who attend very high numbers of sessions. The median is a more appropriate measure: It is about three and a half sessions (NIMH, 1979; Rosenstein & Milazzo-Sayre, 1981). Rosenstein and Milazzo-Sayre's (1981) report, based on a sample of over 1,500 clinics, found that 63% of clients terminated before their fifth session, 75% terminated before the seventh session, and 86% terminated before the eleventh session! The great majority of early terminators have the same sorts of disorders (Rosenstein & Milazzo-Sayre, 1981) and problem severity (Pekarik, 1983a, 1992a) as outpatients in general.

Private-setting treatment duration is longer than public setting but still extremely brief. Taube, Burns, and Kessler (1984) reported a mean number of private practice sessions of about twelve and a median of about four and a half. The modal number of sessions in both public and private clinic samples was one. About 44% of the private practice clients terminated before the fourth session and about 64% before the tenth. Other surveys of private practices also have found that less than half their clients attend 10 to 15 sessions (Knesper, Pagnucco, & Wheeler, 1985; Koss, 1979).

The foregoing studies are typical of reports of treatment duration in public and private settings. It is most likely that they, if anything, are overestimates of current treatment duration, since the recent policy of third-party payers is to increasingly restrict the number of reimbursable outpatient sessions (Kiesler & Morton, 1988). In any case, more recent reports of treatment in standard practice settings (e.g., Weisz & Weiss, 1989) indicate continued very brief treatment.

In summary, it is clear that treatment in standard practice public and private settings ends up being far briefer (for the great majority of clients) than the typical prescriptions and preferences of almost all therapists; this holds for standard therapy, behavioral and cognitive-behavioral therapy, and even most brief therapies. The great majority of clients do not receive anywhere near the "dose" of treatment widely assumed necessary and for which treatment is designed. To review: Only about 14% of public clinic clients and 36% of private clients attend even brief therapy's minimum prescription of 10 visits, much less the 20-visit minimum of more commonly prescribed treatment. To put this another way, mainstream therapies are designed to serve only a small minority of the clients who seek assistance. What happens to the "untreated" majority? This is addressed next.

Premature Termination

Rates. Considering the steep attrition curve from outpatient psychotherapy, it is not surprising that a large percentage of cases are considered premature terminations by therapists. Reviews of dropout research generally find that about 50% of clients are considered dropouts (Baekeland & Lundwall, 1975; Wierzbicki & Pekarik, 1991). A report from the universe of federally funded CMHCs found similarly high dropout rates (NIMH, 1981).

Virtually nothing is known about private practice dropout rates, unfortunately. The best estimate is that they parallel the findings of attrition in public versus private settings; that is, dropout rates are probably lower in private settings but, given the great disparity between prescribed and actual treatment duration, a significant percentage of private clients probably drop out of treatment also.

Effects. Although hundreds of archival studies have addressed the dropout problem, very few have addressed that most salient aspect of dropouts, their treatment outcome. Garfield (1986) fairly recently concluded that "detailed evaluations of the outcome of early terminators have not been made" (p. 232). Until very recently, dropouts were not even routinely identified or their outcome reported in outcome research. This failure to address the posttreatment functioning of dropouts is part of what we can now see is a pattern: the neglect of those clients who fail to conform to the professions' stereotyped prescription for treatment duration. It is almost as if therapists are unaware that dropouts and early terminators exist when it comes to prescribing, devising, and evaluating outcome of treatment.

In real-world clinic and practice settings, the outcome for dropouts plays an important, though generally unacknowledged, role in the assessment of psychotherapy's effectiveness. Since dropouts' outcome is rarely evaluated, it is safe to say that conclusions about psychotherapy's effectiveness are really only conclusions about its effectiveness with that portion of clients who complete treatment. This becomes a very meaningful issue when the normal dropout rate is about 50%, as it is in standard practice settings. The result is that we really do not know the true (overall) impact of psychotherapy. Actually, this very issue plays a prominent role in the history of psychotherapy outcome research. In his landmark 1952 study, it was Eysenck's decision to categorize dropouts as failures that led to his conclusion that therapy was ineffective (Bergin & Lambert, 1978).

Contrary to the common assumption that all dropouts are treatment failures (Garfield, 1986), the few studies that have reported the posttreatment adjustment of dropouts consistently find that clients who drop out early in treatment have very poor outcome, while those who drop out later have better outcome, in some cases similar to treatment completers (Pekarik, 1986). A substantial minority—about one-third—of dropouts claim to terminate due to problem abatement (Acosta, 1980; Garfield, 1963; Pekarik, 1983b, 1992b). When outcome measures have been available, these studies find that clients' claims of improvement are corroborated.

In addition to the treatment outcome consideration, there are administrative, therapist morale, and fiscal problems posed by dropouts (Pekarik, 1985a). Premature termination is also consistently related to lower client satisfaction with treatment (Lebow, 1982).

Causes. Research on the cause of dropout is also a good place to look for the cause of high early attrition. (It should be noted that these are not identical issues, however; it is common to find low-session completers and high-session dropouts; Pekarik, 1985b.)

There is no single simple cause of dropout or early termination. Literature reviews have found virtually no single client or therapist variable that is strongly and consistently related to dropout (Baekeland & Lundwall, 1975; Pekarik, 1985a; Wierzbicki & Pekarik, 1991). Stronger relationships have been found between dropout and more complex therapist–client interactions. For example, Duehn and Proctor (1977), Epperson, Bushway, and Warman (1983), and Pekarik (1988) have all found a two- to fourfold higher dropout rate when therapists have been unable to accurately identify clients' perceptions of their problems. Among studies of early termination, it appears that client expectations regarding treatment length is more highly related to actual length than any single client variable (Pekarik, 1991a; Pekarik & Wierzbicki, 1986). Given the finding that any major discrepancy between treatment expectation and actual treatment content contributes to increased dropout (Horenstein & Houston, 1976), it is highly probable that the discrepancy between client and therapist expectations regarding treatment length, goals, and content cited earlier contributes to dropout rates.

The investigation of noncompliance with medical treatment, an issue very similar to mental health dropout, has found some very clear-cut results which are applicable to the dropout phenomenon. Reviewers of this literature consistently report that aspects of the treatment regimen and symptom abatement are the most important determinants of noncompliance. Specifically, long treatment duration, high treatment cost (in money, discomfort, or inconvenience), treatment complexity, and reduction of symptoms are strongly and consistently associated with noncompliance (Blackwell, 1976; Dunbar & Agras, 1980; Houpt, Orleans, George, & Brodie, 1979). Psychotherapy dropouts also consistently have cited symptom abatement and dislike of the treatment regimen or therapist as two of their top-three dropout reasons; practical problems such as transportation and cost was the third (Acosta, 1980; Garfield, 1963; Pekarik, 1983b, 1992b). Psychotherapy designed for even 10 to 20 visits is high in cost (in money, time, and inconvenience), complex, and results in its greatest impact (symptom abatement) long before its prescribed termination point (Howard *et al.*, 1986). In other words, it has all the right ingredients for noncompliance.

In summary, psychotherapy dropout rates are quite high but entirely understandable given therapy's high cost, long duration, and the discrepancy between prescribed and actual treatment duration. Dropout rates are a major obstacle to the delivery of treatment-as-designed and are associated with fiscal, administrative, and therapist morale problems. Very few studies have addressed treatment outcome for dropouts or ways to reduce dropout rates (Pekarik, 1985a). Of the latter, the major strategy has been to do "pretherapy preparation" of clients, that is, to indoctrinate them in the need to attend treatment as prescribed by therapists. Almost no suggestion is given to *altering the nature of the treatment* that seems to inevitably lead to high dropout rates.

Treatment Efficiency: Brief versus Standard Therapies

There is overwhelming evidence that brief treatment is generally as effective as longer treatment and far more efficient in both outpatient and inpatient settings. Despite this, there is continued prescription of moderate to longer treatment in texts and resistance to brief treatment in practice, especially in its briefest forms. Because cost-effectiveness and efficiency are extremely important consumer issues, an elaborated analysis of the relative benefits of standard and brief therapies and resistance to brief therapies follows. In the reviews that follow, standard and brief therapy are defined in terms of treatment duration, not theoretical orientation.

Outpatient

Outcome for Time-Limited versus Time-Unlimited Treatment. Research bearing on the issue of treatment duration and outcome is complex and addressed by several different literatures. First and foremost are the studies that have experimentally assigned clients to standard (time-unlimited) and brief (time-limited) treatment. The reviews of this literature all reach the same conclusion: There is no reliable difference in the effectiveness of time-limited and time-unlimited treatment (Bloom, 1984; Koss & Butcher, 1986; Gurman & Kniskern, 1978; Luborsky *et al.*, 1975; Miller & Hester, 1986). These studies include investigations of individual, family, and child therapy. The studies include a wide range of visits in their comparison groups; for example, Piper *et al.* (1984) had brief therapy that averaged 22 visits and long therapy that averaged 76 visits, while Edwards *et al.* (1977) randomly assigned clients to either two sessions or a 1-year treatment program. It is impressive that regardless of the client population studied, the duration of brief and long treatment, the theoretical orientation of the brief therapy, or the dependent measures of outcome, the brief treatments fared as well as the longer ones.

Like the general treatment outcome literature, many of the studies that compare brief and long-term treatment have methodological shortcomings; furthermore, they are relatively small in number. For that reason, other research that bears on this issue will be examined.

Comparisons between Brief Treatments. There is a substantial body of research that has compared brief therapy to no therapy and has assessed the relative effectiveness of different types of brief treatments. Studies typically find improved functioning of the briefly treated groups relative to the control groups (Koss & Butcher, 1986). Budman and Gurman (1988) make the cogent point that "virtually every major review of the efficacy of various individual therapies . . . has been an unacknowledged review" (p. 7) of brief therapy since the great majority of studies reviewed have assessed quite brief treatment. They note that the two most widely cited meta-analyses of treatment outcome (Shapiro & Shapiro, 1982, and Smith *et al.*, 1980) reviewed treatments that were very brief—the typical treatment reviewed by Shapiro and Shapiro was only 7 hours. These analyses concluded that the brief treatments analyzed were significantly more effective than no treatment (all used some type of untreated control group). Smith *et al.* (1980) concluded that there were no meaningful differences between the therapies with respect to outcome, while Shapiro and Shapiro (1982) found evidence for superiority of cognitive-behavioral and behavioral approaches.

Treatment Length and Outcome in Long-Term Treatment. The one study that is most often cited as a defense of long-term treatment (Howard *et al.*, 1986), upon critical inspection, actually provides some support for short-term treatment. Howard *et al.* analyzed data from 15 studies of long-term treatment and assessed improvement at each visit. The studies Howard *et al.* review are not representative of standard practice. Nine of the fifteen studies had a median of 10 or more visits, and seven had a median of 15 or more visits; these numbers are far in excess of the CMHC median of three and a half visits (NIMH, 1981) and the private practice median of five (Taube *et al.*, 1984). Therapists were also unrepresentative, in that they all had psychodynamic or "interpersonal" orientations. Settings were also unusual, with 6 of the 15 being university clinics.

The authors present data that shows continued improvement up through the twenty-sixth session. The improvement measures emphasized by the authors are based upon *therapist* ratings, however, and a substantial body of research has shown that therapist-rated measures of improvement are consistently biased in favor of long-term treatment when compared to behavioral measures and psychological tests (Johnson & Gelso, 1980). This, in fact, reveals a typical bias of long-term treatment advocates, namely, that the therapist, rather than the client, should choose treatment goals. Howard *et al.*'s *client-rated* measures of improvement present a different picture—with them the greatest improvement occurs in the first eight visits. The percentage of improved clients increased from 53% at 8 visits to 60% at 26 visits, a very modest increase considering the time invested. This is consistent with Smith *et al.*'s (1980) meta-analyses which found most improvement to occur in the first six to eight sessions.

Several studies have assessed the relationship between treatment length and satisfaction. Reviews of this literature have concluded that treatment length is unrelated to client satisfaction with treatment (Bloom, 1984; Lebow, 1982).

Impact of Brief Therapy on Subsequent Medical Care Utilization. A substantial literature has shown that brief psychotherapy has been associated with subsequent lowered use of medical treatment (Jones & Vischi, 1979; Mumford *et al.*, 1984). Most dramatic in this literature are studies that show reduced medical care after a single psychotherapy visit. Cummings and Follette (1968; Cummings, 1977a, 1977b; Follette & Cummings, 1967) found this to be the case in a series of studies. One of the groups they studied was a group of 80 emotionally upset clients assigned to a single psychotherapy session. They found a dramatic and surprising outcome: That single interview (with no subsequent psychotherapy) was associated with a 60% reduction in medical care use which was maintained over the entire 5-year follow-up period.

In a similar type of study, Rosen and Wiens (1979) found that clients who received only a single evaluation interview had a significant reduction in a wide range of medical care treatment, both outpatient and inpatient. The more recent analyses of studies of this type (e.g., Mumford *et al.*, 1984) find reduced medical care utilization to be primarily inpatient care.

Impact of Very brief (One- to Two-Session) Therapy. Data from diverse sources suggest that very brief (one or two visits) treatment may be effective for at least some outpatients. Edwards *et al.* (1977) randomly assigned alcohol abuse clients to either two conjoint sessions (client and spouse) or treatment options covering a variety of outpatient and inpatient services over a year's time. No significant differences were found between groups on any measure (including objective drinking measures and more subjective adjustment measures) at 1- and 2-year follow-ups. In a series of studies, Miller and his colleagues randomly assigned alcohol abuse clients to either a structured one to two session treatment emphasizing self-directed treatment or longer treatment ranging from six to eighteen visits. No outcome differences were found over the follow-up periods, which ranged from 6 to 24 months (Miller & Hester, 1986). Where employed, no-treatment control groups were less improved than treatment groups.

These impressive studies done by Edwards and Miller and their colleagues were the only ones found in the literature that compared clients assigned to *planned* very brief treatment and longer treatment. A host of other studies suggest that very brief treatment may be effective, however. Bloom (1981) and Talmon (1990) both reported that a very large proportion of clients, about 90%, seen for planned one- or two-session treatment reported improvement at follow-ups ranging from 3 to 12 months, and that most did not seek additional time-unlimited treatment though it was offered. These two reports, unfortunately, rely on simple client report using Likert-type scales; a more thorough assessment of planned single-session therapy is in progress (Hoyt, Rosenbaum, & Talmon, in preparation, cited in Talmon, 1990).

In addition to the foregoing studies of *planned* formal brief therapy, there is evidence that *unplanned* brief treatment (i.e., treatment that is brief by default—dropouts who terminate early in treatment) and informal brief therapy (i.e., a brief course of treatment delivered by a therapist trained in and usually having a preference for longer-term treatment) are often associated with positive treatment outcome. These studies are especially important because of the large percentage of clients in standard practice settings who terminate by default or after "informal" brief therapy (Budman & Gurman, 1988; Garfield, 1986). There are a number of "naturalistic" psychotherapy studies that have assessed the posttreatment adjustment of clients who have attended only a few outpatient sessions. Weisz and Weiss (1989) found that child outpatients who attended a single session with their parents were significantly improved at 6- and 12-month follow-up using a behavior checklist, focal problems identified by parents, and teacher reports as dependent measures. When compared with treatment completers (who averaged 12.4 visits), the single-session groups were as much or more improved, depending on the measure and follow-up period.

Pekarik (1983a) assessed the posttreatment adjustment of very briefly treated adults (one to two sessions) using a symptom checklist at intake and 3-month follow-up. Overall, only a small percentage of early terminators were improved at follow-up. When the early terminators were divided between dropouts and completers, however, it was found that the very briefly treated completers were as improved as the completers who attended three or more sessions. Pekarik (1991) replicated this result with a separate sample of outpatients. Getz *et al.* (1975), Gottschalk *et al.* (1967), Pekarik and Tongier (1993), and Silverman and Beech (1979) all reported that a majority of very briefly treated terminators were improved at follow-up.

All the studies just described employed fairly standard psychotherapy outcome criteria and are uniform in finding that a substantial proportion of very briefly treated clients improved at follow-up. Those studies that employed the most rigorous research methods (Edwards *et al.*, 1977, the Miller studies, and Weisz and Weiss, 1989) found that very brief and longer treatments had equal impact for the client groups examined.

Inpatient

As with outpatient studies, there is a substantial literature on comparisons of both mental health and alcohol inpatient treatments of varying lengths. Two reviews of the mental health literature (Bloom, 1984; Riessman *et al.*, 1977) have concluded that, as with outpatient treatment, short-term inpatient treatment is as effective as long-term treatment. Like the outpatient studies, the lengths of stay vary among studies. The contrasted treatment lengths range from 11 versus 60 days to 90 versus 177 days. Regardless of contrasted length range, the briefer treatments fare as well as the longer ones.

After reviewing the inpatient alcohol literature, Miller and Hester (1986) arrived at virtually the same conclusion: Overall, there is virtually no difference in the impact of programs of varying lengths. Furthermore, in comparisons of 10 studies of random assignment to inpatient versus outpatient care, Miller and Hester found that the outpatient care was superior.

Clients Appropriate for Brief Treatment. In the previous section, several literature reviews, each reviewing many individual studies, were found to reach the same conclusion: No consistent difference has been found between the outcomes for brief and longer treatment. The great majority of the individual studies did not restrict assignment of cases to the briefer treatment; that is, the results reported are generally for the wide range of outpatients and inpatients. Furthermore, there is no reliable evidence that briefer treatment is only effective with certain select subgroups. Koss and Butcher (1986), after investigating this issue, concluded that none of the client characteristics they investigated were found to be related to brief treatment outcome. While future research *may* find that briefer treatments are most appropriate for certain client subgroups, there is no evidence for it at this time. More research is clearly needed on this matter. While some proponents for brief problem-focused treatments recommend selecting only certain clients for such therapy, there are no empirical grounds for such selection.

Brief Therapy Methods. A very wide range of theoretical orientations to brief therapy are encompassed in the studies cited. In some studies a certain school of brief therapy was employed, while in a significant number of others the techniques of brief therapy were not controlled, time was simply limited.

The single characteristic most associated with brief treatment technique is that treatment is highly focused, usually on a single, circumscribed issue; this occurs in virtually all brief treatments (Budman & Gurman, 1988; Koss & Butcher, 1986; Pekarik, 1990). Beyond that, an extremely diverse set of theories of psychopathology and behavior change are associated with brief therapies.

Mental Health Professionals' Reactions to Brief Therapy. The pragmatic incentives created by very recent attempts to contain costs of health and mental health care (Kiesler & Morton, 1988) have caused a tremendous increase in interest in brief therapy, with a proliferation of related texts and seminars. The field is clearly now in a state of transition with respect to brief therapy because of these factors. The current climate of greater acceptance represents a distortion of the earlier "natural" response to brief therapy. That response was generally negative, relegating brief therapy to a "second-class" treatment appropriate for only select cases (Baldwin, 1977; Bloom, 1984; Budman & Gurman, 1988). Bloom (1984) has noted that short-term therapy "flies in the face of a deeply ingrained mental health professional value system . . . [in which] . . . brief treatment is thought of as superficial, longer is equated with better, and the most influential . . . practitioners . . . undertake long-term therapy" (p. 58).

There remains, at best, a strong ambivalence about brief therapy. Those with a stake in more intensive treatments continue to defend them (e.g., Goldfarb, 1991; "Who Needs What," 1991), as do more empirically oriented supporters of longer treatments (e.g., Howard *et al.*, 1986). As noted earlier in this chapter, mainstream therapies and *even purportedly brief therapies typically* have a textbook prescribed duration of around 20 visits, a duration considerably longer than both the average actual length of treatment and the time limits of many of the effective treatments in the brief versus standard therapy outcome comparisons. It is interesting to note that 20 visits is almost exactly the number of visits typically reimbursed by nonmanaged medical insurance coverage (Blue Cross and Blue Shield Association, personal communication, May, 1991). I am not suggesting a conspiracy within the mental health profession, merely that treatment will be affected by pragmatic forces such as reimbursement policies.

Summary and Analysis of Consumer-Issues Literature Review

There are six major findings in the literatures reviewed in this chapter:

1. Clients expect and prefer treatment that is very brief and has modest problem-oriented goals.
2. Therapists prefer and prescribe courses of treatment significantly longer and with more ambitious goals than expected or wanted by clients.
3. In both public and private settings, the majority of clients terminate before the (a) textbook-prescribed duration of standard therapy, (b) therapist preferred duration of therapy, and even (c) text-prescribed duration of most brief therapies. A majority of clients terminate by the fifth visit, before the treatment duration prescribed for virtually all therapies that have been subjected to extensive empirical outcome study. Over one-third of clients in both public and private settings terminate after only one or two visits. These early terminators have the same need for treatment (i.e., the same disorders and severity) as later terminators. Virtually no effort has been put into addressing the needs of these early terminators by designing and evaluating the impact of very brief treatments.
4. About half of psychotherapy clients in public clinic settings drop out of treatment. The rate in private settings is unknown, but suspected to be high. This high rate is to be expected given that psychotherapy has most of the problematic characteristics associated with high noncompliance/dropout rates in general health care: high cost, effort, time, and inconvenience and moderate benefit.
5. Treatment duration appears little related to client satisfaction and treatment outcome, especially from the client's perspective. Planned brief therapy in particular is as effective and satisfying to clients as longer treatment. It also has the benefit of a better fit with clients' expectations regarding treatment duration and goals. In spite of these advantages, the mental health field has failed to enthusiastically embrace brief therapy and devote adequate resources to researching and refining it. This is especially true for therapies designed to last less than five to ten visits.
6. While the lower limit of duration for effective therapy has not been thoroughly researched, there is a distinct possibility that a significant

proportion of clients could benefit from planned very brief treatment (one to three sessions). This prospect has been ignored and unexplored by almost all psychotherapy researchers and authors.

These findings seem to be a clear mandate to reorient research and service delivery toward treatments designed for less than ten visits, perhaps less than five visits. This clearly has not happened. As noted earlier, the shift toward abbreviating treatment has been slow and directed at the high end (10 to 20 visits) of brief therapy. Even this trend would probably not have emerged if it were not for the cost-containment strategies of third-party payers *forcing* treatment abbreviation. This leads us to the question of why the field has been so slow to respond to these unmet client needs, so neglectful of the early terminating majority even when technology exists to treat them effectively. There are probably many factors that contribute to this state of affairs, including the profession's tradition of consumer unresponsiveness. The most parsimonious explanation, however, is that professionals are unaware of the virtual inevitability of massive early attrition in standard practice settings. This lack of awareness is probably due to several factors. Authors of psychotherapy texts pay very little attention to those who terminate early, orienting therapists to the longer-term client from the beginning of their careers. Many researchers have had little need to be concerned about early attrition since many outcome studies have very low attrition rates. This is due to several influences: the subclinical and analogue nature of many published outcome studies (Shapiro & Shapiro, 1982; Weisz *et al.*, 1987); the special circumstances of even clinical sample treatment in published outcome studies (e.g., setting credibility, client self-selection, therapist motivation); and outcome studies' reliance on treatments that are brief, highly structured, and problem oriented, characteristics found to contribute to lower dropout rates (Sledge, Moras, Hartley, & Levine, 1990; Straker, 1968).

There is evidence that practicing clinicians have an exaggerated view of the duration and completeness of treatment. Pekarik and Finney-Owen (1987) found that CMHC therapists estimated the average number of sessions of their clients to be three times greater than their actual number and estimated a dropout rate half of the actual rate. This misperception is probably widespread. Norcross and Wogan's (1983) survey of American Psychological Association Division 29 (Psychotherapy) found that respondents estimated that 89% of clients persisted in therapy 3 or more months. In light of Taube *et al.*'s (1984) and Koss's (1979) findings with private practitioners (cited earlier), this is almost certainly an exaggeration.

The reason for practitioner-exaggerated perception of duration is easy to understand; therapists naturally pay more attention to those clients they spend the most time with. Data generated by Taube *et al.* (1984) is illustrative. They found that while only 17% of psychologists' clients attended 25 or more visits, this group accounted for 65% of their fees (and hence, time) for service; the 25% of clients who attended 10 or more visits accounted for 80% of the charges and time of therapists. This same pattern holds for CMHCs. Based on NIMH (1979) data, only 10% of therapist time is devoted to the 42% of clients who attend one or two visits. The average full-time clinic therapist has only a few openings per week. Most therapist time is spent with longer-term clients they have accumulated even though most clients who seek treatment attend very few visits. This paradoxical situation makes it easy to ignore and be unaware of that majority of clients—early terminators.

In summary, there are many historical and practical reasons why those who work in the mental health field (clinic administrators, practitioners, researchers, text authors, and even reimbursement policymakers) have focused undue attention and resources on that small minority of consumers who receive the "full dosage" of prescribed treatment.

New Directions for a Consumer-Oriented Psychotherapy

Earlier I noted that the literature reviewed in this chapter seems to be a mandate to reorient outcome research and service delivery toward treatments designed for less than ten visits and even less than five visits. In this section, I will advocate precisely such a reorientation as part of a more basic shift toward client-consumers' treatment preferences. I will also describe some steps that can be taken toward this goal.

Regardless of any arguments in favor of standard duration therapy, it is clear that the majority of clients have never wanted nor received such treatment. The disparity between prescribed and actual therapy is so immense that it cannot be attributable to failings of therapists or client characteristics; it must be integral to the therapy process. We may conclude that psychotherapy never was and never will be attended for the duration currently prescribed by texts and desired by therapists. This holds even for the modal contemporary short-term therapies of the 10- to 20-visit range. The client attendance patterns are so consistently, pervasively, and extremely brief that they are virtually inevitable. This presents the field with a choice: We can (1) continue to devote most resources to the development of treatments designed for the small minority who complete a moderate to long treatment and lament (or ignore) the fact that most troubled clients do not want and will not fully use such treatments, or (2) we can adapt therapy to suit that majority who desire modest goals and brief treatment, including those who attend only a few visits. The former option is a dismissal of the suffering of those clients who refuse to buy into the prescribed treatment model. It is the course the field has taken for its first hundred years, justified by concepts such as resistance and low client motivation, and somewhat understandable in light of the factors cited in the preceding section. Given what is known about the impact of brief therapies, it seems indefensible to maintain this course. It seems to me far more ethical to devote our resources to the development of treatments that are usable by the majority of clients and have goals compatible with clients' desires.

In contrast to the prevailing attitude, this approach grants clients the legitimacy of their usually modest treatment goals. It is compatible with the position of medical ethicists which states that the patient has final authority in treatment choices, even when contrary to a physician's recommendations (Jonsen, Siegler, & Winslade, 1986). This holds even when a medical patient is emotionally upset and that upset is thought to affect the client's judgment. Indeed, physicians are clearly cautioned against even subtle interference with client treatment choices:

> Although patients have the legal and moral authority over physician-patient relationship, physicians have enormous power in these relationships. They can shape the course and moral dimensions of medical care by their psychological dominance, specialized knowledge, and technical skills. *The physician's power can . . . destroy the fragile moral autonomy of the patient.* (Jonsen *et al.*, 1986, p. 49; italics added)

In psychotherapy, such unequivocal statements about the legitimacy of client choices are difficult to find (Keith-Spiegel & Koocher, 1985), reflecting the ingrained skepticism regarding client choices and the disparity between client and therapist treatment expectations.

The traditional therapist-oriented approach to treatment will *not* be changed by a grudging acceptance of third-party payers' reimbursement restrictions and associated gradual lowering of prescribed treatment duration and shifts away from inpatient treatment. Significant gains in treatment impact for the universe of treatment needers and requesters (as opposed to high session completers) can only be accomplished by reordering priorities toward consumer preferences, treatment efficiency, and treatment accessibility. This will entail a major shift away from glorification of the ideal long-term "cured" treatment completer as personified by the typical case study and completers of 20 session programs.

Action toward Consumer-Oriented Treatment

Specific actions within each of the domains of professional mental health activity can be taken to achieve the consumer-oriented approach to treatment advocated in this chapter.

Research. The single-disorder outcome and comparative outcome research model is an appropriate way of initially developing and comparing treatments. After treatments have been identified as successful this way, outcome studies should be done using treatment duration as an independent variable in order to assess treatment efficiency (cost-effectiveness). This would entail packaging successful treatments in varying durations and comparing outcomes. It would be a relatively simple variation of the single-disorder comparative outcome design. Practical models are available for cost-effectiveness assessment (e.g., Yates, 1980).

In order to increase generalization to standard practice settings, it is important to also use duration as an independent variable in the assessment of more general treatment strategies. This can be done in university settings where the treatment can be more tightly operationalized (e.g., cognitive-behavioral), applied to a broad spectrum of clinical or subclinical problems (e.g., child behavior problems), then analyzed for duration × problem subgroup interactions.

Much more outcome research needs to be done in standard practice settings. Even clinical samples treated in nonstandard settings are ultimately only analogous to actual therapy delivery because of self-selection of clients and the other peculiarities of research-oriented settings. True treatment utility can only be demonstrated in the settings where the great majority of people receive it. The efficacy of time-limited treatment of moderate duration has been demonstrated sufficiently that random assignment into such a condition (with access to more intensive or longer treatment if wanted by the client and warranted) can now be done without ethical constraint. With proper screening, informed consent, and access to further treatment if warranted, assessment of downward extensions of brief therapy (i.e., very brief—one to three sessions) can also be done. Quasi-experimental assessment of the effect of treatments of differing durations can and should be done, then, in standard practice settings. Recent research in public clinics (e.g., Sledge *et al.*, 1990) and HMOs (e.g., Talmon, 1990) demonstrates the feasibility and utility of such approaches.

An important issue for outcome research in normal practice settings is the outcome assessment for dropouts, a sizable proportion of all those treated. Dropouts and completers should be evaluated with the same methods. Since it has been demonstrated that clients who drop out at different stages of treatment have different outcome (Pekarik, 1986), such assessment should also be part of an overall treatment evaluation.[2] There is evidence that intentional abbreviation of treatments does reduce dropout rates (Pekarik, 1987; Sledge *et al.*, 1990; Straker, 1968).

The goals of the recommended research are to more thoroughly assess efficiency, therapy acceptability, the relationship of duration to outcome, the duration × treatment interactions, and to identify clients appropriate for treatments of varying durations. The unorthodox step of assessing (and designing) treatments of very short durations (a few sessions) should be part of this research.

Adoption of Consumer Criteria in Defining Treatment Success. The foregoing strategy only makes sense if one adopts the consumer's perspective on what is desirable therapeutically: modest and narrow goals, pragmatism, efficiency, and greater reliance on client than therapist assessment. That may mean valuing moderate improvement with a very few sessions more than greater improvement in longer treatment. Many clients probably would rather attend only two sessions and have a 50% reduction in symptoms than eight sessions with 80% reduction. And many more would opt for the briefer duration if the first two sessions were totally reimbursed and the remainder required a 50% copayment. Does this imply that we should design treatments to suit insurance coverage policies? We certainly should if those policies influence treatment attendance (as they do). Clients' modest goal and brief duration preferences exist regardless of insurance reimbursement policies however—the latter only exacerbate this predilection. Rather than lament the lack of motivation of clients (or the tyranny of third-party payers), this consumer-oriented approach *enthusiastically* pursues the same efficient treatment as the client. It celebrates the prospect of giving the client "a good deal," with significant benefit from a small investment rather than greater benefit from a much greater investment in time and money. Clearly this is a reversal of the traditional celebration of the few who go along with the therapist subculture's preference for "deep," "thorough-going," "personality," or "basic" change and denigration of "superficial," "naive" client goals often associated with "resistance" and "dropout."

While the consumer-oriented philosophy described here has never been accepted by the mental health establishment, it is not a new idea. It is very similar to the original ideals of the community mental health movement, with a focus on "least restrictive" treatment and "acceptability, accessibility, and availability" of services for all in need of treatment (Bloom, 1984). This is not to be confused with the traditional treatment that ended up being delivered by CMHCs (Chu, 1974), often characterized as "old wine in new bottles."

Brief Therapy. The psychotherapy movement most compatible with the consumer-oriented philosophy described here is the brief therapy movement,

[2]Many would claim that outcome for dropouts is an inappropriate concept, since treatment has not been fully delivered to them. I disagree with this position because (1) the reality of high (50%) dropout rates makes them an important portion of all treatment efforts, (2) there is evidence that *some* treatment is delivered in very early sessions, with corresponding improvement early in course of treatment, and (3) this sounds too much like blaming the client for the failings of treatment.

including its very brief versions. It has become popular in recent years because of its compatibility with cost-containment strategies which, by all accounts, represent the current and future realities of health and mental health care in the United States (Keisler & Morton, 1988). Brief therapy, then, is perhaps the single most important psychotherapy influence today.

It is ironic and unfortunate that those who have seized the leadership in comparative outcome research—that is, those prolific publishers, the cognitive-behaviorists—have been virtually absent from the brief therapy movement. Scholarly reviews (e.g., Koss & Butcher, 1986), popular texts (e.g., Budman & Gurman, 1988), advocacy for the model (e.g., Bloom, 1984), edited handbooks (e.g., Wells & Giannetti, 1990; Zeig & Gilligan, 1990), professional workshops (e.g., annual conventions of the American Psychological Association) and the specific "brands" or models of brief therapy (e.g., Bellack & Small, 1978; Malan, 1973; Wolberg, 1980) are almost all written by authors with other than cognitive-behavioral orientations, primarily those who have psychodynamic, "interpersonal," and strategic orientations. The most innovative treatments, the very brief therapies (one to two sessions), have been created and advocated primarily by psychodynamically oriented therapists (Bloom, 1981; Hoyt, 1990; Talmon, 1990). While cognitive-behaviorists may consider their therapies to be brief (e.g., Ellis, 1990; Lazarus & Fay, 1990; Wilson, 1981), they rarely align themselves with the brief therapy approach. Koss and Butcher (1986) note that inclusion of behavioral therapies as brief therapy may be questionable. Using the simple criterion of treatment duration, behavioral therapy is at least sometimes not at all brief. Fishman and Lubetkin (1980, reported in Wilson, 1981) claim an average of 50 sessions at their Institute for Behavior Therapy, and Norcross and Wogan's (1983) survey of members of the Association for the Advancement of Behavior Therapy found that about three-quarters of respondents' clients were seen for 3 or more months of primarily once-a-week treatment. Earlier it was shown that treatments from this orientation are typically designed for around 20 sessions, far in excess of the earlier cited actual medians of three and a half to five sessions.

Several authors have attempted to identify the elements common to the varieties of brief therapy. All have emphasized the importance of having a central treatment focus (Budman & Gurman, 1988; Koss & Butcher, 1986; Pekarik, 1990; Reid, 1990) which is defined as a (usually single) problem explicitly acknowledged by the client rather than what the practitioner may see as the "real," underlying problem. By this definition, also, cognitive-behavioral treatment fails to be necessarily brief. While client problems are typically conceptualized as discrete problems in this orientation, multiple problems may be addressed in a course of treatment. And in their own way, cognitive-behaviorists are often taught to address the real, underlying problem (or at least a more general "basic problem") rather than the simpler one explicitly identified by the client. For example, representing a cognitive-behavioral approach, Haaga and Davison (1986) state that social problem-solving training

> seeks to teach a client a *general procedure* to use in solving problems, *as opposed to alleviating* only the client's *most pressing problem*. . . . Clients frequently enter therapy *expecting rapid help in solving a particular problem, not generalized training*. . . . [In social problem-solving training] the client is a student learning a *generally applicable* self-control technique. (p. 261; italics added)

Rather than insist on character change or even "generalized training," the brief therapist accepts that most clients desire specific changes in circumscribed aspects of their lives and, in any case, only attend enough visits to deal with such modest goals. The brief therapist is content to focus on the most pressing problem rather than teach a general procedure because (1) this maximizes the client's cooperation, (2) the client has an ethical right to choose (even modest) treatment goals, (3) there is a much greater chance of achieving more modest goals, and (4) most clients will only stay in treatment long enough to attain modest goals.

In summary, cognitive-behavioral treatment is not necessarily brief therapy. Cognitive-behavioral treatment does not inherently or automatically possess the duration, technical elements, or the philosophy and values of brief therapy (Budman & Gurman, 1988). This does not imply that cognitive-behavioral treatment is incompatible with brief, consumer-oriented treatment. To the contrary, it possesses many technical and value elements amenable to brief therapy, and most approaches to brief therapy have borrowed heavily from cognitive-behavioral technique and strategy. It just seems as though the cognitive-behaviorists have been content to demonstrate their *relative* efficiency and effectiveness compared to traditional psychodynamic approaches and have thus failed to take the initiative to test limits of efficiency within their own orientation. While they earlier invested heavily in criticisms of traditional psychodynamic treatment's inaccessibility, they have failed to acknowledge the inaccessibility of their prescription for 10 or more sessions for the two-thirds to three-quarters of clients who terminate before that criterion. Just as psychoanalysts were content to rely on their traditional way of addressing efficacy (case studies) for decades, the cognitive-behaviorists seem content to rely on their traditional way of addressing efficacy (assessment of 15- to 20-session treatments). Both approaches are valuable as far as they go, but neither goes far enough in exploring treatment utility.

The failure of the cognitive-behavioral group to get fully involved in issues such as efficiency, uses of very brief treatments, and cost-effectiveness assessment in standard service settings is unfortunate. Their empirical orientation combined with therapy techniques highly adaptable to consumer-oriented treatment would greatly facilitate research progress on these issues. Most of the very important research comparing brief and longer treatments has *not* been conducted by researchers whose therapeutic orientations have an empirical assessment tradition; consider the advances that might be made if the research expertise and therapy technology of the cognitive-behaviorists were applied to the efficiency, duration, and other consumer-oriented issues described in this chapter. We might also consider the prospect of declining influence of cognitive-behavioral treatments if their advocates decide to sit out these investigations; witness the recent increased advances (and credibility) of such brief treatments as interpersonal psychotherapy of depression (Klerman, Weissman, Rounsaville, & Chevron, 1984), de Shazer's (1985) family treatment, and Kaiser-Permanente's far flung brief psychodynamic service delivery system. It is indeed ironic that those researchers who have led the field in the search for the most effective treatment under ideal circumstances seem to have conceded to others the search for delivery of the most cost-effective treatments in the real world of standard practice.

Reimbursement and Service Delivery Policy. Mental health program administrators and third-party payers can play especially important roles in making therapy more consumer oriented. Earlier it was noted that there are many disincentives for clinicians to do more efficient treatment. Two of the several identified by Budman and Gurman (1988) and Pekarik (1990) are that it is harder work than standard therapy and requires more paperwork since there is higher client turnover. Some incentives should be provided by clinic administrators to offset these penalties in their settings.

Reimbursement policies are currently reshaping treatment more powerfully than any single influence. The expectations for brief treatment by clients and clinicians and actual shorter treatment duration at managed mental health facilities (Pekarik, 1991b) are evidence of this. If research identifies reasonable cost-effective strategies, these are likely to be incorporated into reimbursement policies; failure to identify reasonable cost-cutting strategies is likely to result in unreasonable ones being imposed and/or mental health benefits being cut (Kiesler & Morton, 1988; Jencks & Goldman, 1987).

Pursuit of cost-effective treatments that are "consumer friendly" as advocated in this chapter presents the opportunity to identify those clients and disorders most (and least) amenable to brief, efficient treatments. Widespread application of designed abbreviated treatments, including very brief one- or two-session treatment to those appropriate, would provide a cost savings that could be applied to client subgroups empirically identified as needing more costly treatment. The alternative is shrinking blanket coverage for all clients, ignoring the clinical needs of specific conditions. The unavailability of reimbursement for longer-term and more intensive (e.g., inpatient) treatment for those conditions that really need it is the fault of us in the mental health profession, not the insurance companies, because we are failing to distinguish problems that can benefit from less costly treatment from those that require costlier ones.

Conclusion

In spite of refinement of psychotherapy technique by empirically oriented outcome researchers, subsidization of mental health treatment by public funds, and widespread third-party reimbursement of mental health treatment, there are major service delivery problems. Three-quarters of those with mental disorders do not receive treatment from mental health professionals. Of those who begin psychotherapeutic treatment, 50% drop out. And the great majority of those treated receive a treatment far briefer than prescribed and deemed optimal by mental health professionals.

The recent introduction of cost-containment strategies in mental health threatens to reduce client access to treatment's intensity and duration but, ironically, also presents the field with the opportunity to improve its service delivery problems: Cost-containment policies may force mental health professionals to develop and deliver the treatments that most consumers have always wanted, that is, brief, very brief, and less intensive treatments. Whether cost containment helps or harms consumers depends on how we professionals respond to this challenge. We have basically two options. The first is the current course and one compatible with traditional consumer unresponsiveness—to whittle away at psychotherapy's current prescribed duration so that it is kept within increasingly restrictive duration, that is, to reduce modal treatment prescriptions from 20 to about 12 or 15 visits. This strategy will be relatively ineffective for containing costs and, more importantly, will fail to meet the treatment needs of most clients. The second option is to be truly creative and consumer responsive by *designing* treatments to meet the *actual* service utilization patterns and preferences of consumers, identifying client problems responsive to treatments of *widely* varying durations and intensities (including single-session therapy and outpatient alternatives to inpatient treatment), calculating the cost-effectiveness of the treatments, and then providing clients with these treatment options. Given the known client preferences for very brief and less intensive treatments, this could result in an increase in both client satisfaction and access to treatment by removing time and cost barriers for the majority of clients who prefer (and will only use) very brief and less intensive treatments.

Reliance on very brief, brief, and outpatient alternatives to inpatient treatment could also result in cost offset and cost containment sufficient to retain longer and more intensive treatments for those empirically shown to benefit from only these costlier treatments. Perhaps the only hope of retaining the costlier treatments is to "buy them" with the savings gained by much wider use of very brief and less intensive treatments. To do this, conditions effectively treated by only long-term treatment must be identified. The key to enlightened cost containment is to provide longer and intensive treatments to only those who both desire and can benefit from them. The net result could be treatment far better for the consumer because of greatly increased efficiency, accessibility, and increased treatment options consistent with client preferences.

There is a far grimmer alternative scenario, unfortunately. We can allow insurance companies to contain costs by treatment made cheaper by (1) applying brief and low intensity treatment to all clients, regardless of needs, and (2) contracting treatment to the lowest bidder, irrespective of demonstrated efficacy. This scenario is the only cost-containment option currently open to third-party payers because we have not investigated the efficiency issues sufficiently. It is up to us to develop other options.

References

Acosta, F. X. (1980). Self-described reasons for premature termination of psychotherapy by Mexican American, Black American, and Anglo-American patients. *Psychological Reports*, *47*, 435–443.

Aguilera, D. C., & Messick, J. M. (1982). *Crisis intervention.* St. Louis: Mosby.

Albee, G. W. (1959). *Mental health manpower trends.* New York: Basic Books.

Baekeland, F., & Lundwall, L. (1975). Dropping out of treatment: A critical review. *Psychological Bulletin*, *82*, 738–783.

Baldwin, B. A. (1977). Crisis intervention in professional practice: Implications for clinical training. *American Journal of Orthopsychiatry*, *47*, 659–670.

Beck, J. G. (1990). Brief psychotherapy for the sexual dysfunctions. In R. A. Wells & V. J. Giannetti (Eds.), *Handbook of brief psychotherapies* (pp. 461–492). New York: Plenum.

Bellak, L., & Small, L. (1978). *Emergency psychotherapy and brief psychotherapy* (2nd ed.). New York: Grune & Stratton.

Benbenishty, R., & Schul, Y. (1987). Client-therapist congruence of expectations over the course of therapy. *British Journal of Clinical Psychology*, *26*, 17–24.

Bergin, A. E., & Lambert, M. J. (1978). The evaluation of therapeutic outcomes. In S. L. Garfield & A. E. Bergin (Eds.), *Handbook of psychotherapy and behavior change* (2nd ed., pp. 139–190). New York: Wiley.

Blackwell; B. (1976). Treatment adherence. *British Journal of Psychiatry*, *129*, 513–531.

Bloom, B. L. (1981). Focused single-session therapy: Initial development and evaluation. In S. H. Budman (Ed.), *Forms of brief therapy* (pp. 167–218). New York: Guilford Press.

Bloom, B. L. (1984). *Community mental health: A general introduction* (2nd ed.). Monterey, CA: Brooks/Cole.

Budman, S. H., & Gurman, A. S. (1988). *Theory and practice of brief therapy*. New York: Guilford Press.

Chu, F. D. (1974). The Nader report: One author's perspective. *American Journal of Psychiatry, 131*, 770–775.

Cornes, C. (1990). Interpersonal psychotherapy of depression. In R. A. Wells & V. J. Giannetti (Eds.), *Handbook of brief psychotherapies* (pp. 261–276). New York: Plenum.

Corsini, R. J. (1991). *Five therapists and one client*. Itasca, IL: Peacock Publishers.

Cummings, N. A. (1977a). The anatomy of psychotherapy under national health insurance. *American Psychologist, 32*, 711–718.

Cummings, N. A. (1977b). Prolonged (ideal) versus short-term (realistic) psychotherapy. *Professional Psychology, 8*, 491–501.

Cummings, N. A., & Follette, W. T. (1968). Psychiatric services and medical utilization in a prepaid health plan setting: Part II. *Medical Care, 6*, 31–41.

Davison, G. C., & Neale, J. M. (1990). *Abnormal psychology* (5th ed.). New York: Wiley.

De Shazer, S. (1985). *Keys to solution in brief therapy*. New York: Norton.

Duehn, W. D., & Proctor, E. K. (1977). Initial client interaction and premature discontinuance in treatment. *American Journal of Orthopsychiatry, 47*, 284–290.

Dunbar, J. M., & Agras, W. S. (1980). Compliance with medical instructions. In J. M. Ferguson & C. B. Taylor (Eds.), *The comprehensive handbook of behavioral medicine* (pp. 115–145). New York: Spectrum.

Edwards, G., Orford, J., Egert, S., Guthrie, S., Hawker, A., Hensman, C., Mitcheson, M., Oppenheimer, E., & Taylor, C. (1977). Alcoholism: A controlled trial of "treatment" and "advice." *Journal of Studies on Alcohol, 38*, 1004–1031.

Ellis, A. (1990). How can psychological treatment aim to be briefer and better? The Rational Emotional approach to brief therapy. In J. K. Zeig & S. G. Gilligan (Eds.), *Brief Therapy* (pp. 291–302). New York: Brunner/Mazel.

Emmelkamp, P. J. (1986). Behavior therapy with adults. In S. L. Garfield & A. E. Bergin (Eds.), *Handbook of psychotherapy and behavior change* (3rd ed., pp. 385–442). New York: Wiley.

Epperson, D. L., Bushway, D. J., & Warman, R. E. (1983). Client self-terminations after one counseling session: Effects of problem recognition, counselor gender, and counselor experience. *Journal of Counseling Psychology, 30*, 307–315.

Eysenck, H. J. (1952). The effects of psychotherapy: An evaluation. *Journal of Consulting Psychology, 16*, 319–324.

Follette, W., & Cummings, N. A. (1967). Psychiatric services and medical utilization in a prepaid health plan setting. *Medical Care, 5*, 25–35.

Freud, S. (1963). Turnings in the way of psychoanalytic therapy. In P. Rieff (Ed.), *The collected papers of Sigmund Freud* (Therapy and technique). New York: Collier Books. (Original work published in 1919)

Garfield, S. L. (1963). A note on patients' reasons for terminating therapy. *Psychological Reports, 13*, 38.

Garfield, S. L. (1980). *Psychotherapy: An eclectic approach*. New York: Wiley.

Garfield, S. L. (1986). Research on client variables in psychotherapy. In S. L. Garfield & A. E. Bergin (Eds.), *Handbook of psychotherapy and behavior change* (3rd ed., pp. 213–256). New York: Wiley.

Garfield, S. L., & Wolpin, M. (1963). Expectations regarding psychotherapy. *Journal of Nervous and Mental Disease, 137*, 353–362.

Getz, W. L., Fujita, B. N., & Allen, D. (1975). The use of paraprofessionals in crisis intervention: Evaluation of an innovative program. *American Journal of Community Psychology, 3*, 135–144.

Goldfarb, R. (1991). Strengthening treatment effectiveness. *Employee Assistance, 3*, 16–35.

Gottschalk, L., Mayerson, P., & Gottlieb, A. (1967). Prediction and evaluation of outcome in an emergency brief therapy clinic. *Journal of Nervous and Mental Disease, 144*, 77–96.

Gurin, G., Veroff, J., & Feld, S. (1960). *Americans view their mental health: A nationwide interview survey*. New York: Basic Books.

Gurman, A. S., & Kniskern, D. P. (1978). Research on marital and family therapy: Progress, perspective and prospect. In S. L. Garfield & A. E. Bergin (Eds.), *Handbook of psychotherapy and behavior change* (2nd ed., pp. 817–902). New York: Wiley.

Haaga, D. A., & Davison, G. C. (1986). Cognitive change methods. In J. H. Kanfer & A. P. Goldstein (Eds.), *Helping people change* (3rd ed., pp. 236–282). New York: Pergamon Press.

Heitler, J. B. (1976). Preparatory techniques in initiating expressive psychotherapy with lower class, unsophisticated patients. *Psychological Bulletin, 83*, 339–352.

Hollen, S., & Beck, A. T. (1986). Research on cognitive therapies. In S. L. Garfield & A. E. Bergin (Eds.), *Handbook of psychotherapy and behavior change* (3rd ed., pp. 443–482). New York: Wiley.

Hollon, S. D., Shelton, R. C., & Loosen, P. T. (1991). Cognitive therapy and pharmacotherapy for depression. *Journal of Consulting and Clinical Psychology, 59*, 88–99.

Horenstein, D., & Houston, B. K. (1976). The expectation-reality discrepancy and premature termination from psychotherapy. *Journal of Clinical Psychology, 32*, 373–378.

Hornstra, R., Lubin, B., Lewis, R. & Willis, B. (1972). Worlds apart: Patients and professionals. *Archives of General Psychiatry, 27*, 553–557.

Houpt, J. L., Orleans, C. S., George, L. K., & Brodie, H. K. (1979). *The importance of mental health services to general health care*. Cambridge, MA: Ballinger.

Howard, K. I., Kopta, S. M., Krause, M. S., & Orlinsky, D. E. (1986). The dose-effect relationship in psychotherapy. *American Psychologist, 41*, 159–164.

Hoyt, M. F. (1990). On time in brief therapy. In R. A. Wells & V. J. Giannetti (Eds.), *Handbook of the brief psychotherapies* (pp. 115–144). New York: Plenum.

Hoyt, M. J., Talmon, M., & Rosenbaum, R. (1991, August). *Single session psychotherapy: Increasing effectiveness and training clinicians*. Workshop presented at the annual convention of the American Psychological Association, New York.

Jencks, S. F., & Goldman, H. H. (1987). Implications of research for psychiatric prospective payment. *Medical Care, 25*(Suppl. 9), 542–551.

Johnson, D. H., & Gelso, C. J. (1980). The effectiveness of time limits in counseling and psychotherapy: A critical review. *The Counseling Psychologist, 9*, 70–83.

Joint Commission on Mental Illness and Health. (1961). *Action for mental health*. New York: Basic Books.

Jones, K. R., & Vischi, R. R. (1979). Impact of alcohol, drug abuse and mental health treatment on medical care utilization: A review of the research literature. *Medical care, 17*(Suppl. 12), 1–82.

Jonson, A. R., Siegler, M., & Winslade, W. J. (1986). *Clinical ethics* (2nd ed.). New York: Macmillan.

Keith-Spiegel, P., & Koocher, G. P. (1985). *Ethics in psychology*. New York: Random House.

Kendall, C. C., & Lipman, A. J. (1991). Psychological and pharmacological therapy: Methods and modes for comparative outcome research. *Journal of Consulting and Clinical Psychology, 59*, 78–87.

Kernberg, O. F., Burstein, E. D., Coyne, L., Appelbaum, A., Horwitz, L., & Voth, H. (1972). Psychotherapy and psychoanalysis: Final report of the Menninger Foundation's psychotherapy research project. *Bulletin of the Menninger Clinic, 36*, 1–276.

Kiesler, C. A., & Morton, T. L. (1988). Psychology and public policy in the "Health Care Revolution." *American Psychologist, 43*, 993–1003.

Klerman, G. L., Weissman, M., Rousauville, B., & Chevron, E. (1984). *Interpersonal psychotherapy of depression*. New York: Basic Books.

Knesper, D. J., Pagnucco, D. J., & Wheeler, J. R. (1985). Similarities and differences across mental health services providers and practice settings in the United States. *American Psychologist, 40*, 1352–1369.

Koss, M. P. (1979). Length of psychotherapy for clients seen in private practice. *Journal of Consulting and Clinical Psychology, 47*, 210–212.

Koss, M. P., & Butcher, J. N. (1986). Research on brief therapy. In S. L. Garfield & A. E. Bergin (Eds.), *Handbook of psychotherapy and behavior change* (3rd ed., pp. 627–670). New York: Wiley.

Lachenmeyer, C. (1980). A complete evaluation design for community mental health programs. In M. S. Gibbs, J. R. Lachenmeyer, & J. Siegal (Eds.), *Community psychology* (pp. 339–361). New York: Gardner.

Lambert, M. J., Shapiro, D. A., & Bergin, A. E. (1986). The effectiveness of psychotherapy. In S. L. Garfield & A. E. Bergin (Eds.), *Handbook of psychotherapy and behavior change* (3rd ed., pp. 157–212). New York: Wiley.

Langs, R. (Ed.). (1975). *International Journal of Psychoanalytic Psychotherapy*, Vol. 4.

Lazarus, A. A., & Fay, A. (1990). Brief psychotherapy: Tautology or oxymoron? In J. K. Zeig & S. G. Gilligan (Eds.), *Brief therapy* (pp. 36–54). New York: Brunner/Mazel.

Lebow, J. L. (1982). Consumer satisfaction with mental health treatment. *Psychological Bulletin, 91*, 244–259.

Llewelyn, S. P. (1988). Psychological therapy as viewed by clients and therapists. *British Journal of Clinical Psychology, 27*, 223–237.

Luborsky, L., Singer, B., & Luborsky, L. (1975). Comparative studies of psychotherapies. *Archives of General Psychiatry, 32*, 995–1008.

Malan, D. H. (1973). *A study of brief psychotherapy*. New York: Plenum.

McGreevy, M. K. (1987). *A survey of psychotherapy expectations and preferences of university students*. Unpublished Master's thesis, Washburn University, Topeka, KS.

Miller, W. R., & Hester, R. K. (1986). Inpatient alcoholism treatment: Who benefits? *American Psychologist, 41*, 794–805.

Moretti, M. W., Feldman, L. A., & Shaw, J. (1990). Cognitive therapy: Current issues in theory and practice. In R. A. Wells & V. J. Giannetti (Eds.), *Handbook of brief psychotherapies* (pp. 217–238). New York: Plenum.

Morris, R.J., & Kratochwill, T. R. (1983). *The practice of child therapy*. New York: Pergamon Press.

Mumford, E., Schlesinger, H. J., Glass, G. V., Patrick, C., & Cuerdon, T. (1984). A new look at evidence about reduced cost of medical utilization following mental health treatment. *American Journal of Psychiatry, 141*, 1145–1158.

Murphy, W. F. (1965). *The tactics of psychotherapy*. New York: International Universities Press.

Myers, J. K., Weissman, M. M., Tischler, G. L., Holzer, C. E., Leaf, P. J., Orvaschel, H., Anthony, J. C., Boyd, J. H., Burke, J. D., Kramer, M., & Stoltzman, R. (1984). Six month prevalence of psychiatric disorders in three communities. *Archives of General Psychiatry, 41*, 959–967.

National Center for Health Statistics. (1988). *The national ambulatory medical care survey* (Series 13, No. 93, DHHS Publication No. PHS 88-1754). Washington, DC: U.S. Government Printing Office.

National Institute of Mental Health. (1979). Report of the work group on health insurance, 1974. In C. Windle (Ed.), *Reporting program evaluations: Two sample community mental health center annual reports*. Rockville, MD: U.S. Department of Health, Education and Welfare.

National Institute of Mental Health. (1981). *Provisional data on federally funded community mental health centers, 1978–79*. Report prepared by the Survey and Reports Branch, Division of Biometry and Epidemiology. Washington, DC: U.S. Government Printing Office.

Norcross, J. C., & Wogan, M. (1983). American psychotherapists of diverse persuasions. Characteristics, theories, practices, and clients. *Professional Psychology: Research and Practice, 14*, 529–539.

Overall, W. C., & Aronson, H. (1962). Expectations of psychotherapy in lower socioeconomic class patients. *American Journal of Orthopsychiatry, 32*, 271–272.

Pekarik, G. (1983a). Follow-up adjustment of outpatient dropouts. *American Journal of Orthopsychiatry, 53*, 501–511.

Pekarik, G. (1983b). Improvement in clients who have given different reasons for dropping out of treatment. *Journal of Clinical Psychology, 39*, 909–913.

Pekarik, G. (1985a). Coping with dropouts. *Professional Psychology: Research and Practice, 16*, 114–123.

Pekarik, G. (1985b). The effects of employing different termination classification criteria in dropout research. *Psychotherapy, 22*, 86–91.

Pekarik, G. (1986). The use of treatment termination status and duration patterns as an indicator of treatment effectiveness. *Evaluation and Program Planning, 9*, 25–30.

Pekarik, G. (1987). The effect of treatment duration on continuance in a behavioral weight loss program. *Addictive Behaviors, 12*, 381–384.

Pekarik, G., (1988). The relationship of counselor identification of client problem description to continuance in a behavioral weight loss program. *Journal of Counseling Psychology, 35*, 66–70.

Pekarik, G. (1990, January). *Rationale for consumer-oriented treatment strategies*. Invited address at the annual executive director's meeting of the Metropolitan Clinics of Counseling (CIGNA Corp.), Phoenix, AZ.

Pekarik, G. (1991a). Relationship of expected and actual treatment duration for child and adult clients. *Journal of Child Clinical Psychology, 20*, 121–125.

Pekarik, G. (1991b). *Treatment impact at a managed mental health care clinic*. Unpublished manuscript. Metropolitan Clinics of Counseling, Topeka, KS.

Pekarik, G. (1992a). Posttreatment adjustment of clients who drop out early vs. late in treatment. *Journal of Clinical Psychology, 48*, 379–388.

Pekarik, G. (1992b). Relationship of clients' reasons for dropping out of treatment to outcome and satisfaction. *Journal of Clinical Psychology, 48*, 91–98.

Pekarik, G., & Finney-Owen, K. (1987). Psychotherapists' attitudes and beliefs relevant to client dropout. *Community Mental Health Journal, 23*, 120–130.

Pekarik, G., & Tongier, P. (1993, April). *Variables associated with successful and unsuccessful early termination from psychotherapy*. Presented at the Annual Meeting of the Midwestern Psychological Association, Chicago, IL.

Pekarik, G., & Wierzbicki, M. (1986). The relationship between expected and actual psychotherapy duration. *Psychotherapy, 23*, 532–534.

Piper, W. E., Debbane, E. G., Bienvenu, J. P., & Garant, J. (1984). A comparative study of four forms of psychotherapy. *Journal of Consulting and Clinical Psychology, 52*, 268–279.

Reid, W. J. (1990). An interpretive model for short-term treatment. In R. A. Wells & V. J. Giannetti (Eds.), *Handbook of brief psychotherapies* (pp. 55–78). New York: Plenum.

Riessman, C. K., Rabkin, J. G., & Struening, E. L. (1977). Brief versus standard psychiatric hospitalization: A critical review of the literature. *Community Mental Health Review, 2*, 2–10.

Rosen, J. C., & Wiens, A. N. (1979). Changes in medical problems and use of medical services following psychological intervention. *American Psychologist, 34*, 420–431.

Rosenstein, M. J., & Milazzo-Sayre, L. J. (1981). *Characteristics of admissions to selected mental health facilities 1975*. (DHHS Publication No. ADM 831005). Washington, DC: U.S. Government Printing Office.

Shapiro, D. A., & Shapiro, D. (1982). Meta-analysis of comparative therapy outcome studies: A replication and refinement. *Psychological Bulletin, 92*, 581–604.

Shapiro, S., Skinner, E. A., Kessler, L. G., Von Korff, M., German, P. S., Tischler, G. L., Leaf, P. J., Benham, L., Cottler, L., & Regier, D. A. (1984). Utilization of health and mental health services: Three epidemiologic catchment area sites. *Archives of General Psychiatry, 41*, 971–978.

Silver, A. P. (1985). *The universal health care almanac 1984–1985*. Phoenix, AZ: R-C Publication.

Silverman, W. H., & Beech, R. P. (1979). Are dropouts, dropouts? *Journal of Community Psychology, 7*, 236–242.

Slaikeu, K. A. (1984). *Crisis intervention*. Boston: Allyn and Bacon.

Sledge, W. H., Moras, K., Hartley, D., & Levine, M. (1990). Effects of time-limited psychotherapy on patient dropout rates. *American Journal of Psychiatry, 147*, 1341–1348.

Smith, M. L., Glass, G. V., & Miller, T. I. (1980). *The benefits of psychotherapy*. Baltimore: The Johns Hopkins University Press.

Straker, M. (1968). Brief psychotherapy in an outpatient clinic: Evolution and evaluation. *American Journal of Psychiatry, 24*, 1219–1226.

Strecker, E. A. (1952). *Basic psychiatry*. New York: Random House.

Sullivan, H. S. (1956). *Clinical studies in psychiatry*. New York: Norton.

Talmon, M. (1990). *Single-session therapy*. New York: Jossey-Bass.

Taube, C. A., Burns, B. J., & Kessler, L. (1984). Patients of psychiatrists and psychologists in office-based practice: 1980. *American Psychologist, 39*, 1435–1437.

Weisz, J. R., & Weiss, B. (1989). Assessing the effects of clinic-based psychotherapy with children and adolescents. *Journal of Consulting and Clinical Psychology, 57*, 741–746.

Weisz, J. R., Weiss, B., Alicke, M., & Klotz, M. L. (1987). Effectiveness of psychotherapy with children and adolescents: A meta-analysis for clinicians. *Journal of Consulting and Clinical Psychology, 55*, 542–549.

Wells, R. A., & Giannetti, V. J. (Eds.). (1990). *Handbook of brief psychotherapies*. New York: Plenum.

Whishman, M. A., & Jacobson, N. S. (1990). Brief behavioral marital therapy. In R. A. Wells & V. J. Giannetti (Eds.), *Handbook of brief psychotherapies* (pp. 325–350). New York: Plenum.

Who needs what? (1991, February). *Employee Assistance*, pp. 24–26.

Wierzbicki, M., & Pekarik, G. (in press). A meta-analysis of psychotherapy dropout. *Professional Psychology: Research and Practice*.

Wilson, G. T. (1981). Behavior therapy as a short-term therapeutic approach. In S. H. Budman (Ed.), *Forms of brief therapy* (pp. 131–166). New York: Guilford Press.

Wolberg, L. R. (1980). *Handbook of short-term psychotherapy*. New York: Thieme-Stratton.

Yates, B. T. (1980). *Improving effectiveness and reducing costs in mental health*. Springfield, IL: Thomas.

Zeig, J. K., & Gilligan, S. G. (1990). *Brief therapy*. New York: Brunner/Mazel.

18

Dynamic Cognitive-Behavior Therapy

Ralph M. Turner

Cognitive-behavior therapy is at a critical juncture in its development. It is in the midst of a second cognitive revolution (Mahoney, 1991). Cognitive psychology no longer views the mind as a collection of static self-statements and passive schemata. The mind is a dynamic, constructive process. Cognitive processing affects how information is stored and retrieved. Cognitive processing also influences what information is perceived and attended to in the first place. Cognitive psychology's tenets of tacit, or unconscious, mental processing and a feed-forward mechanism have opened the portal for dynamic theorizing in cognitive-behavior therapy (Turner, 1989; 1993a,b).

While the cognitive revolution in behavior therapy practice has created abundant commotion, there has occurred a hushed cognitive revolution within psychoanalytically oriented psychotherapy. Psychoanalytic thinkers such as Bowlby (1988), Luborsky (1984), Luborsky and Crits-Christoph (1990), and Horowitz (1987; 1988a,b) have constructed cognitive revisions of the psychoanalytic model. Many aspects of these cognitive psychoanalytic models are consistent with findings in modern cognitive psychology. As such, they are compatible with the neoclassical model of cognitive-behavior therapy. In fact, the cognitive psychoanalytic models have solved some problems that have proved daunting to cognitive-behavior theorists, such as developing methods to specify individuals' tacit cognitive schemata.

This chapter's purpose is to describe the development of a model of cognitive-behavior therapy which incorporates reliable and valid components from cognitive-psychodynamic psychotherapy. This model is called Dynamic Cognitive-Behavior Therapy. In developing this model I will, first, review the assumptions of classical cognitive-behavior therapy and neoclassical cognitive-behavior therapy. Next, I will review the recent advances in psychoanalytically oriented psychotherapy and detail

---

Ralph M. Turner • Center for Research on Adolescents and Families, Temple University, and Department of Psychiatry, Temple University School of Medicine, Philadelphia, Pennsylvania 19140.
Preparation of this chapter was facilitated by NIDA grant 1P50DA7697-01.

Handbook of Effective Psychotherapy, edited by Thomas R. Giles. Plenum Press, New York, 1993.

the strategies which appear most promising for integration into a dynamic, cognitive-behavior therapy framework. Finally, I will conclude the chapter with a description of the dynamic cognitive-behavior therapy model.

Cognitive-Behavior Therapy: A Review of the Classical and Neoclassical Models

Cognitive-behavior therapy provides a fitting basis for the development of an integrative psychotherapy model. Its origins are in cognitive psychotherapy (Beck, 1970; Ellis, 1962; Meichenbaum, 1977), social learning theory (Bandura, 1977a, 1977b, 1985), and behavior therapy (Lazarus, 1976). Interestingly, several of the founders of cognitive therapy were originally psychoanalytically oriented practitioners (i.e., Beck, Ellis, and Meichenbaum).

Mahoney (1977) and Kendall and Bemis (1984) have described cognitive-behavior therapy as a hybrid, or integrative, form of psychotherapy. Cognitive-behavioral therapy is best thought of as an amalgam of empirically established techniques and procedures drawn from both cognitive and behavioral research. Due to cognitive-behavior therapy's close ties to basic research, it is constantly expanding. So, in practice it is difficult to specify the exact procedures that are cognitive-behavior therapy. However, rather than being a flaw, this elasticity and permeability results in a model of treatment that is dynamic and robust.

The Basic Assumptions of Cognitive-Behavior Therapy

Despite the wide variety of approaches to cognitive-behavior therapy, eight basic assumptions characterize this therapeutic orientation.

The basic premise of cognitive therapy is that our cognitive processes causally affect our behavior and emotions. This does not mean that the direction of causality is always from cognition to behavior and emotions. A recursive and reciprocal set of causal influences exists among the domains of cognition, behavior, and affect. However, what the pioneers in cognitive therapy did bring into focus for the first time is that our cognitive processes do impel our behavior and emotions in critically important ways.

A second assumption is that learning is a critical factor in psychopathology ontogenesis and the development of psychosocial treatments. Learning is more than Pavlovian and operant conditioning, however. The majority of human learning is cognitively mediated. Cognitive science, not classical animal learning theory, is the basis for the cognitive-behavioral approach.

A related assumption is that people's cognitive representations of themselves and the world, rather than the phenomenon of the actual environment, influence their reactions. These representations occur at both conscious and unconscious levels of awareness.

Cognition is an active process. People do not simply take in the world around them. They actively seek information and mentally construct it. Consequently, people often see what they want to see, hear what they are prepared to hear, and negate or circumvent information out of keeping with their expectations.

Understanding cognitive systems is essential for understanding psychopathology. Cognitive processes such as attitude formation, expectancies, causal attributions, conscious and unconscious self-statements, and expected scripts and roles for self and others are central to psychological functioning and emotional well-being or illness.

It is also assumed that reliable and valid findings in the cognitive, biological, and behavioral sciences are applicable for incorporation into the cognitive-behavioral perspective. So, cognitive-behavioral theory and practice need to accommodate advances in cognitive psychology research.

The task of the cognitive-behavioral clinician is to act as a diagnostician, educator, and technical consultant to the client. The therapist works with the client to design learning experiences aimed at lessening the symptoms of mental illness. Cognitive-behavior therapy is a collaborative relationship between the therapist and the client. The goal is to teach clients enough knowledge and skills to be their own cognitive-behavior therapist.

Taken together, these seven assumptions provide a broad-based platform for integrative thinking about psychotherapy. This is the primary reason cognitive-behavior therapy is the best starting point for the development of an integrative psychotherapy model.

The Framework of Classical Cognitive-Behavior Therapy

There are several models of cognitive-behavior therapy. The model developed by Beck (1967; 1976; Rush, Shaw, & Emery, 1979) is the most studied and commonly used version.

Beck and his colleagues (Beck *et al.*, 1979) focus on three interrelated concepts in explaining the cognitive theory of the genesis and maintenance of emotional disorders. These concepts are the cognitive triad, cognitive distortions, and the schemata which undergird them.

The cognitive triad reflects the three domains of attributions individuals have to contend with to be emotionally stable. The first domain is the self; a person can feel either positive or negative about his or her own self. The second domain is the individual's experience of the world; he or she can feel helpless or vigorous about his or her experience of the world. The third domain of the cognitive triad represents the individual's expectations for the future; he or she can feel pessimistic or optimistic. Clients are assessed regarding their status in each of these domains. Any given client might show negativistic thinking in one domain only, two of the areas, or in all three. The function of the cognitive-triad conceptualization is to permit the clinician to focus quickly on the domain or domains in which the client has problems with negativistic thinking.

Cognitive distortions are the common and habitual ways that persons pervert environmental information. The distortions are typically the central focus of therapy. Common cognitive distortions include dichotomous thinking, overgeneralization, biasing judgments, emotional reasoning, "should" statements, catastrophizing, disqualifying the positive, and personalization, to name several. Freeman (1990) provides a more detailed catalog of cognitive distortions. The cognitive distortions are pivotal in maintaining depressive and anxious states of mind. The principal task of therapy is to educate clients about who they are and how they function.

Beck has adopted Piaget's (1926) concept of the *schema* as a third pivotal element in his model. Schemata are cognitive structures that propagate both the cognitive triad and the distortions. Schemata develop during our earliest experiences with the world, and they store global generalizations about our self-worth and hope for the future. Cognitive therapy strives to illuminate the individual's schemata, or core beliefs, and change them. Altering the deeply ingrained schemata is essential and key for long-term therapeutic success.

The Neoclassical Cognitive-Behavioral Therapy Framework

If any one factor defines the distinction between classical cognitive-behavior therapy and the neoclassical model, it is the neoclassical model's stricter adherence to the principles of cognitive psychology.

Classical cognitive-behavior therapy did not derive its basis from cognitive psychology. Cognitive therapy was developed from observations that patients often engage in negativistic thinking patterns. The use of the term *cognitive* did not define an approach as much as it delineated distinctions. Primarily, cognitive therapy was demarcated as nonbehavioral and nonpsychodynamic. The aim of the early founders of the cognitive therapy movement was to develop a talk therapy that did not rely on psychodynamic theory. With time, the discrimination against behavior therapy-based interventions ceased. This resulted in the amalgam—cognitive-behavior therapy.

Neoclassical cognitive behavior therapy is more formally tethered to cognitive psychology (Mahoney, 1985, 1991). Empirical findings and theoretical perspectives on the structure of semantic memory, the characteristics of natural categories, schema theory, metacognition, concept formation, decision making, and problem solving play a central role in the neoclassical cognitive therapy model. There is not space in this chapter to review the significance of all of these topics. However, I will pursue several themes that are particularly relevant to the discussion of integrating aspects of the psychodynamic approach within the cognitive-behavioral model.

Mahoney (1985, 1991), after reviewing the cognitive psychology literature, has championed the distinction between explicit (i.e., conscious) and tacit (i.e., unconscious) cognition. According to Mahoney, much cognitive processing occurs at the tacit level. It is automatic, overarching, and out of our day-to-day awareness. The tacit level consists of the rules and strategies that guide and direct information processing. It reflects basic assumptions, premises, and world hypotheses that act on the information available to us. Thus, cognitive-behavior therapists now consider tacit, or unconscious, processes in their work with clients.

Integrally linked with the notion of tacit mental mechanisms is the feed-forward mechanism. Working from recent findings in cognitive psychology, Mahoney stipulates that humans actively seek information and meaning structures by mentally creating a significant proportion of the environmental information they take in. This process is akin to a mixture of the mechanisms of projection and transference in psychoanalytic theory. Humans project and transfer meaning schemata onto their experiences. This dramatically influences how and what they perceive of environmental events.

These phenomena have long been of interest to psychodynamically oriented researchers and clinicians (Turner, 1988, 1992, 1993a). Luborsky (1984) and Horowitz (1989) have developed measurement techniques designed to assess tacit interpersonal schemata and their feed-forward affects. The assessment procedure development by Luborsky (1984) is called core conflictual relationship theme analysis. Horowitz (1988a, 1988b, 1989) has produced a complementary approach called role-relationship model analysis. Both models assume distortions in the individual's tacit and feed-forward cognitive strategies that cause emotional disorders.

The approach to cognitive-behavior therapy described in this chapter integrates both psychodynamic assessment techniques to clarify clients' tacit and feed-forward cognitive processes (Turner 1983; 1988; 1989; 1993a,b). Thus, in addition to the usual cognitive and behavioral assumptions, the current approach emphasizes the role of unconscious and active mental processing in human functioning. For these reasons I refer to this model as dynamic cognitive-behavior therapy (D-CBT).

The D-CBT approach stresses the significance of interpersonal relationships in human functioning. Change comes about through interpersonal interaction. The therapeutic relationship is the primary vehicle through which treatment works. Other factors such as performance of homework and education are critical for successful treatment, but the relationship provides the laboratory for assessing and modifying cognitive distortions.

A detailed description of the D-CBT approach will be provided in the final portion of this chapter.

"Copiously Cognitive" Psychodynamic Psychotherapy

Luborsky, Crits-Christoph, Mintz, and Auerbach (1988) defined psychoanalytically oriented psychotherapy's primary mechanism of change as "copiously cognitive." The authors were referring to the fact that psychoanalytically oriented psychotherapy works by modifying persons' cognitive schemata concerning interpersonal relations. These interpersonal schemata are stored in both tacit and explicit cognitive structures which guide and direct individuals' behavior, affect, and related cognitions.

However, Luborsky *et al.*'s (1988) colorful description reflects a more general orientation in psychodynamic thinking. Bowlby's (1940, 1980, 1982, 1988) biologically based concept of attachment and bonding hinges heavily on cognitive psychological theorizing. Bowlby's proposal asserts that persons' early experiences with the family of origin (particularly the mother) generate durable schemata about interpersonal relationships. Individuals' sense of self-security, self-efficacy, and relational security are formed in their nuclear families. This information is stored in long-term memory as tacit schemata. These tacit schemata guide and direct much of a person's life-long interpersonal behavior, affect, thinking, and global mental health status.

Horowitz (1988a, 1988b, 1989) has taken Bowlby's cognitive view farther by reconceptualizing psychoanalytic theory in cognitive terms. According to Horowitz, interpersonal schemata are dynamic cognitive structures. They do not simply contain true and false beliefs about interpersonal interactions. These schemata contain projected roles for the self and others, predesigned scripts for self and others across a wide variety of potential interactions, and expectancies about synchrony and conflict between self and others. The schemata contain information about conflict within the self about one's wishes and needs. Importantly, interpersonal schemata are nested in superordinate schemata networks related to one's multifaceted experience of self. Finally, these intricate networks of interpersonal schemata have motivational properties. Horowitz calls these interpersonal schemata role-relationship models. He has developed a cognitive assessment procedure that maps individuals' tacit cognitive organization of interpersonal relations.

In keeping with his cognitive reevaluation of psychodynamic theory, Horowitz has also conceptualized the defense mechanisms as control processes involved with information processing. Their function is to modulate the speed of information processing as well as accentuate or dampen attention to specific information.

Luborsky's work has provided a solid empirical foundation for several key psychoanalytic concepts. Foremost among his contributions, Luborsky has operationalized the construct of transference. The principle of transference states that patients will respond to the therapist in predictable ways based upon their learned, interpersonal schemata. In point of fact, the principle of transference asserts that individuals carry a mental template of learned expectancies for interpersonal relations into all interpersonal episodes. The transference in relation to the therapist is just a special case of transference. The core conflictual relationship theme assessment procedure devised by Luborsky provides a reliable and valid method of illuminating the tacit, interpersonal schema called the transference.

My interest in the utility and quality of psychodynamically oriented treatment procedures is not predicated only on the fact that the prominent theorists have attended to developments in cognitive psychology. More importantly, these theorists and researchers have developed research programs which have clearly delineated the reliable and valid components of the psychodynamically oriented treatment model. It is to these issues that I now turn my attention.

The Fundamentals of Modern Psychodynamic Psychotherapy

The Role of the Therapist

The classical psychoanalytic treatment model specified that the therapist interact minimally with the patient—the therapist was to be a blank screen. A patient would eventually project his or her problems onto the therapist, and at that point the therapist would have an understanding of the patient's conflicts and interpret them for the patient. Over a lengthy period patients would begin to understand their conflicts and eventually resolve them. The therapist was not an active participant in the process; therefore, treatment was prescribed in years.

The role of the therapist changed dramatically, however, with the advent of the short-term dynamic treatment model. During the last three decades in Britain (Balint, Ornstein, & Balint, 1972; Malan, 1963, 1976) and the United States (Davenloo, 1979, 1980; Mann, 1973; Sifneos, 1972, 1979), psychodynamic theorists developed robust short-term treatment models. The time-limited treatment movement changed the therapist's role from passive participant to active teacher. First, the clinician teaches patients about how psychodynamics work. Then the therapist teaches patients about their personal psychodynamic structure, the nature of their focal conflicts, and how these conflicts interfere with their interpersonal relationships. The short-term model assumes patients need to learn cognitive skills (the psychodynamic world view) to solve their problems and live more effectively. The assumption that the therapist is an active teacher is identical to the view of the role of the therapist in classical and neoclassical cognitive-behavior therapy.

The Centrality of the Helping Alliance

Both theoretically and empirically, the helping alliance is a paramount curative factor in psychodynamic psychotherapy. The helping alliance (Luborsky, 1976) has also been called "the therapeutic alliance" (Zetzel, 1958) and the working alliance (Greenson, 1965). The construct of the helping alliance attempts to capture the extent to which patients experience the relationship with the therapist as helpful in achieving their goals.

Luborsky, Crits-Christoph, Mintz, and Auerbach (1988) define two subtypes of the helping alliance. The first class of alliance captures patients' experience of the therapist as supportive and helpful. The second class of the helping alliance describes patients' perception that the therapist is working with them in a joint struggle to overcome their problems. However, research reported by Luborsky *et al.* (1988) indicates the two types of alliance overlap 82% in the eyes of patients. Thus, in practice patients appear to experience one principal factor of the helping relationship.

This factor is critical for the success of psychotherapy, however. Luborsky *et al.* (1988) report that 25% of outcome variance in the Penn Psychotherapy Project was accounted for by the quality of the therapeutic alliance. This estimate is consistent with other studies on the impact of the therapeutic alliance on outcome (Hartley & Strupp, 1983; Horowitz, Marmar, Weiss, DeWitt, & Rosenbaum, 1984; Marziali, Marmar, & Krupnick, 1981). It is also consistent with similar work conducted on cognitive-behavior therapy (e.g., Turner & Ascher, 1982).

What are the implications for the practice of cognitive-behavior therapy from this research? The answer is that the therapeutic alliance should be given a high priority in both research and practice. Although behavior therapists have often suggested that the quality of the relationship is important in treatment outcome, no treatment manuals explicitly define tactics to enhance it. Dynamic cognitive-behavior therapy does emphasize the central curative role of the therapeutic relationship and incorporates tactics to strengthen it.

Cognitive Schemata for Interpersonal Relations

The most important curative factor in psychodynamically oriented psychotherapy is the accurate interpretation of transference. Luborsky *et al.* (1988) report that accurate attention to transference interpretation accounts for 25% of the successful outcome of treatment.

Transference refers to the process of interacting with others on the basis of cognitive maps of similar relationships in one's past. Individuals learn to view interpersonal situations as prototypes of interpersonal situations in their family of origin. From our earliest days of life we develop expectations, role definitions, and behavioral and affective action patterns based on the culture of the family environment.

This complex interpersonal information is stored in schemata, most of which are out of awareness. These schemata form a network of beliefs and expectations about ourselves and others that operate implicitly on any new interpersonal information. In fact, they exercise anticipatory control over our thoughts, behaviors, and affects in social situations. These social situations include interactions with significant others outside the family of origin and the therapeutic relationship.

Unfortunately, our cognitive maps of interpersonal situations are sometimes in error. They can be in error because adult goals are often different from the typical goals of children. They can also be wrong because the people we are now dealing with have characteristics very different from those of our family members.

Yet, we continue to carry forth tacit constructions of interpersonal life based upon these early templates. Why? There are two principal reasons. First, because of the necessity of the child to bond with his or her parents for survival purposes, the early schemata are highly reinforced. Second, because the schemata are learned during the earliest phases of life, they form the foundation on which all other learning is built. The early schemata serve as the scaffolding for the development of subsequent interpersonal schemata. Since a large proportion of our interpersonal schemata are developed during the preverbal period, we are not aware of their impact upon our day-to-day thinking. They are tacit knowledge.

That such tacit cognitive schemata exist and direct behavior, affect, and overt cognition is verified by research in cognitive psychology (Matlin, 1989). In fact, the phenomenon is so robust it influences our visual perception and recall of furnishings in a university professor's office. In their well-controlled study, Brewer and Treyens (1981) demonstrated that subjects would recall having seen objects typical of a university professor's office, such as books, even when such typical objects were not present in the office. In addition, subjects did not recall objects out of keeping with an office setting, such as a wine bottle or picnic basket. Schema theory argues that humans selectively attend to environmental stimuli based on their previously held schemata about a particular situation. Cognition is profoundly affected by the heuristic "when overwhelmed with stimuli, encode mainly the stimuli consistent with the schema" (Matlin, 1989, p. 288). Transference schemata operate on the same principle.

The principal cognitive agenda for psychodynamically oriented psychotherapy is to generate for patients an understanding of interpersonal schemata that form their transference. This is accomplished by the therapist achieving an understanding of patients' schemata in two domains and interpreting (i.e., teaching) this understanding for patients. The first domain is called the triangle of insight. The second domain is termed the impulse-defense triad.

The *triangle of insight* defines the territory of transference reactions. There are three main spheres of interaction corresponding to the three points of a triangle. The first is the nuclear family, where our cognitive maps of interpersonal relations are formed. The second sphere of operation is with significant others in our daily life, such as schoolmates, co-workers, lovers, and our children. The third area delineated is the relationship with the therapist. It is because transference patterns, or cognitive maps, operate in the therapy session that the therapist can gain an understanding of them and teach patients about their structure and function.

The *impulse-defense triad* consists of three components: motivational constructs, beliefs, and emotional and behavioral reactions. The first component consists of wishes, aims, or needs persons possess in relation to significant others that may be developmentally appropriate or inappropriate. For instance, it is fitting for a 10-year-old to depend on his or her parents for nurturance and life direction. It is not developmentally appropriate for healthy adults to need total life direction and nurturance from significant others.

The second component of the impulse-defense triad is the beliefs individuals hold about the probability that significant others will fulfill their needs and wishes. This component represents persons' expectancies about others' responses to them. The negation of an individual's needs may be reality based because of a rejecting other. The lack of need gratification may also be based on erroneous beliefs about the other's predicted response, which blocks the person from making a clear request for need gratification. It is this component that often contains erroneous schemata based on early experiences.

The third component specifies the emotional and behavioral reactions of individuals to having their needs and wishes ignored or denied by significant others. The first aspect of the reaction is the experience of anxiety, depression, or both. The second aspect of the response is behavioral. There are three potential paths the behavioral expression can take. The first is the development of overt psychiatric symptoms such as panic attacks or disruptive interpersonal behavior. The alternative is for the person to engage in a compromise solution such as avoidance behavior and alcohol or drug abuse. Of course, these two paths describe the maladaptive solution to reducing anxiety and depression.

A third path involves solving the interpersonal problem. This involves tolerating the anxiety and depression until individuals can clarify their needs and wishes and achieve an adaptive solution which satisfies their need. However, as schema theory predicts, their cognitive maps cause individuals to ignore new solutions and push them toward known, quick solutions for reducing dysphoria. Consequently, they remain caught in the impulse-defense triad. In addition, the interpersonal schemata are so powerful and controlling that persons never question their veracity. They think "this is the way we and other people are and this is just the way the world is." Importantly, research on both cognitive therapy and psychodynamically oriented psychotherapy has shown that these maladaptive schemata can be modified.

Despite the critical role of understanding patients' transference schemata, it is only recently that reliable and valid methods of assessing these schemata have been developed. The two most promising procedures are Luborsky's (1984) core conflictual relationship theme method and Horowitz's (1988a,b) role-relationship model analysis.

The core conflictual relationship them (CCRT) method is an assessment system for reliably drawing inferences about relationship patterns from relationship narratives. The relationship narratives consist of the parts of sessions in which patients either spontaneously, or at the request of the therapist, present episodes about their interpersonal relationships. Luborsky refers to these stories as relationship episodes. A minimum of 10 relationship episodes is a desirable number with which to provide a basis for deriving the CCRT. The steps in the CCRT method were chosen because they represent a kind of formalization of the inference process used by clinicians in adducing transference patterns. Within each relationship episode, the CCRT judge makes inferences about types of: (1) wishes, needs and intentions, (2) responses from others, and (3) responses from the self. Then, to be sure the inferences are being made at the most appropriate level, the same judge goes through the process a second time and modifies the inferences. The final CCRT is an assemblage of the most frequent types of wishes and responses across all the relationship episodes. The CCRT method is described in detail in Luborsky (1974) and Luborsky and Crits-Christoph (1990).

A series of studies by Luborsky and his colleagues have examined the reliability for interjudge agreement on identifying relationship episodes and the core theme (Crits-Christoph *et al.*, 1988; Levine & Luborsky, 1981; Luborsky & Crits-Christoph, 1990). The pooled-judge intraclass correlation is .68 for judges' ability to identify relationship episodes from the transcript. The reliability of judges' agreement on the components of the CCRT is reflected in weighted kappa values of .61 to .70. These reliability estimates are very good, and they argue that the CCRT method can be used reliably to assess transference schema.

Luborsky *et al.* (1988) have established impressive validity data for the CCRT method. First, the degree of congruence between the CCRT pattern and the content of interpretations has been shown to significantly correlate with the outcomes of psychotherapy (multiple r = .49 to .54). Second, changes in the pervasiveness of CCRT themes have been shown to significantly correlate with the outcome of psychotherapy (r = .32 to .54). Studies are currently underway to further evaluate the validity of the CCRT method. However, these initial reports indicate that the CCRT method is both a reliable and valid measure of tacit relationship schemata.

Horowitz (1988a, 1989) has developed a complementary method for assessing transference schemata. Horowitz's system is called the Role-Relationship Model analysis. A *role-relationship model* portrays a schema of self in interaction with another person. An individual's inner view of an interpersonal situation is typically organized simultaneously by several schemata. Thus, each schemata is thought to possess tacit cognitive views of self. For each of these self-schemata there are different configurations of the wish, response-from-other, and response-from self sequences.

The role-relationship model analysis provides a method for describing a person's multiple self-schemata (Horowitz, 1987). The method also maps three distinct types of conflict: (1) conflict between one's wishes or needs and one's actions, (2) conflict between different solutions for the specific relationship problem, and (3) conflict between divergent views of self.

Horowitz's conceptual model for intrapsychic conflict about relationships contains predictions about the nature of self and other representations and the scripts for interpersonal transactions between self and other. These person schemata are assumed to function unconsciously and simultaneously in the construction of mental working models of actual interpersonal situations. The working models are assumed to guide the individuals behavior, thought, and affect during the real-world experience.

A single role-relationship model is a format that contains a conceptual position for seven different elements. These consist of (1) the self-schema, (2) the schema of the other person, and the aims, acts, or emotional expressions scripted as stemming from each toward the other. These scripted elements are (3) the anticipated action or expressed emotion of self (often a wish), (4) the responses of the other, (5) the reactions of self to the response of the other, (6) the self-estimation of these reactions, and (7) the other's expected self-estimation of these reactions. According to Horowitz (1988) it is often sufficient to use the first five of these several elements in constructing a role-relationship model from observation of recurrent interpersonal patterns.

Three separate types of interpersonal relations conflict can be interpreted using the role-relationship model format. The first level of conflict is between the wish to act or express emotion and the fear of the consequences in terms of responses of others and ensuing reactions of the self.

The second level of conflict is between different intrapsychic views of the same interpersonal situation. This level describes the conflict between two or more role-relationship models as alternative schemata for organizing experience and action. These different role-relationship models offer the self alternative solutions for the immediate interpersonal conflict.

The third level of conflict is between different types of self-schemata. A set of weak self-schemata might organize a group of potential solutions, and that cluster of schemata might conflict with a cluster of schemata organized by a strong self-concept. Similarly, there might be conflicts between passive and active, masculine and feminine, good and bad, intact or damaged sets of self-schemata. This method provides a complex, but cognitively accurate, view of the levels of dynamic interaction at the tacit level. The reader is referred to Horowitz (1988a) for a more in-depth discussion of the method.

Role-relationship model analysis refers to a format rather than in instrument, such as a rating scale. One of its strengths is its idiographic nature. However, for psychometric research this presents limitations. Consequently, reliability studies have not focused on consensual agreement. However, reliability analyses have been conducted on ratings made by two teams of configural analysts. The results, which indicate a good sense of consensual agreement (.63), can be obtained by using the team approach (Horowitz, 1989).

Reliability studies have also been completed using the multiple role-relationship models to describe recurrent maladaptive interpersonal patterns of relationships between difficult psychotherapy patients and their therapists. The average intraclass correlation of the pooled judges was .74 (Horowitz, Rosenbaum, & Wilner, 1988).

Transference schemata, or tacit interpersonal schemata, are as critical to the cognitive-behavior therapist as they are to the psychoanalytically oriented therapist. What the CCRT and role-relationship model methods add to the cognitive-behavioral approach is the inclusion of dynamic properties to the cognitive interpersonal schemata. In addition, they add the capacity to extract tactic schemata which are out of patients' awareness. Thus, by incorporating them into the cognitive-behavior therapy model we can now derive the tactic foundation of individuals' irrational beliefs.

The Role of Attachment Theory in Modern Psychodynamic Practice

In the earliest model of psychoanalytic theory, Freud (1912) postulated that individual motivation was determined by biological need gratification. For Freud this amounted to sexual gratification. Other psychodynamic theorist such as Adler and Sullivan argued that social factors, not biological, were the key organizing phenomena. There has been much controversy over this issue within the psychoanalytic school (Rychlak, 1981).

However, beginning in 1940, John Bowlby initiated a theoretical perspective and line of research which integrated the biological and social views. Following the lead of ethology researchers, Bowlby hypothesized that the unitary instinct in the human organism, at the time of birth, is the propensity to make strong emotional bonds to parents (or parent substitutes). Bowlby (1973, 1980, 1982, 1988) assumes that emotionally significant bonds between individuals have basic survival value. Infants cannot survive on their own. The nurturance of parental figures is required. In addition, the quality of the emotional bond between children and their parents determines the offsprings' potential personality strength and emotional stability. A significant strength of Bowlby's theoretical perspective is that it is firmly rooted in biology. Ethologists such as Lorenz (1935) have shown that attachment and bonding phenomena occur in a wide range of mammalian and avian species and that these phenomena are integrally related to survival of species.

Bowlby (1988, p. 162) specifies four principal propositions of his theory:

a. that emotionally significant bonds between individuals have basic survival functions and therefore a primary status;
b. that they can be understood by postulating cybernetic systems, situated within the central nervous system of each partner, which have the effect of maintaining proximity or ready accessibility of each partner to the other;
c. that in order for the system to operate efficiently each partner builds in his mind working models of self and other, and of patterns of interaction that have developed between them;
d. that present knowledge requires that a theory of developmental pathways should replace theories that invoke specific phases of development in which it is postulated a person may become fixated and/or to which he may regress.

Four important conclusions can be drawn from these propositions. First, the modern psychodynamic view does away with psychosexual stages of development and the notions of fixation and regression. This rids the model of much that has been found objectionable by cognitive-behavior therapists. Second, individuals' histories of attachment with their parents can provide important information about their difficulties in interpersonal relations as adults. Third, Bowlby's perspective provides a biological and motivational basis for the development of tacit and implicit cognitive schemata of role-relationship models. Fourth, it suggests that during therapy the therapist must form an attachment bond with the patient. Thus, it provides a basic science rational for the critical importance of the helping alliance in therapeutic outcome. From Bowlby's perspective, the helping alliance, or the quality of the therapeutic relationship, is not a nonspecific factor in therapy outcome. Rather, the relationship is a core, essential ingredient for human interaction, as it is in all of the rest of life.

The Efficacy of Psychodynamic Psychotherapy

We have now reviewed the essential elements of modern, cognitively oriented psychodynamic psychotherapy. Since this book is dedicated to discussing effective psychotherapy methods, we must address the efficacy of the short-term psychoanalytically oriented approach. I do not intend to review the literature on efficacy since Luborsky *et al.* (1988) have provided an extensive review. However, I will underscore some of the conclusions Luborsky *et al.* (1988) have drawn about the efficacy of psychodynamically oriented psychotherapy.

In study after study the results indicate that around 68% of patients, with markedly different psychiatric disorders, are very much improved. Across 10 studies with similar protocols, using true psychiatric outpatients, the effect sizes, or benefit estimates, have ranged from .51 to 2.72. This efficacy rate has occurred even under conditions of low helping alliance ratings and inadequacy of interpretations. Thus, it probably represents a lower boundary for the success of the approach.

Second, very few patients finish therapy worse off than when they started. No more than approximately 10% of patients show deterioration at termination. For those patients who do worsen, it is possible that their illness trajectory was actually dampened, or mitigated, by treatment.

Interestingly, patients who make large gains in resolving their presenting symptoms show improved physical health. In addition, patients tend to maintain their gains following the end of treatment. There is a small posttreatment decrease in level of functioning by 1-year follow-up for most patients. However, most gains are maintained. The extent of loss during the year appears to be parallel to the typical forgetting phenomenon associated with any learning situation.

The factors predictive of successful psychodynamic treatment are the quality of the therapeutic alliance, the development of an accurate conceptualization of the patient's core conflict, vigorous interpretation of the core conflict for the patient, adequate caring attitude on the therapist's part, adequate intelligence and psychological mindedness on the patient's part, and the severity of the patient's illness at pretreatment. Some of these factors are under the therapist's control, while, of course, others are not. It is clear to me, however, that there are significant strengths to the psychodynamic treatment model.

My belief is that by adding the strengths of the psychoanalytically oriented approach with the potency of the cognitive-behavioral techniques a model of treatment can be developed that achieves higher posttreatment success rates and more durable long-term gains.

Summary

Modern psychodynamically oriented psychotherapy's foundation rests on attachment theory (Bowlby, 1988) and cognitive psychology (Horowitz, 1988a,b). Freud's contribution has diminished. However, his insight concerning the role of transference phenomena remains a seminal cornerstone of theory and treatment. Recent empirical research on schema theory in cognitive psychology has verified the critical function tacit mental models play in behavioral and cognitive regulation (Matlin, 1989).

The role of the therapist is active teacher. The therapist-teacher focuses on developing and enhancing the helping alliance to promote the acquisition of therapeutic goals. Once the helping alliance is established, numerous and accurate interpretations teach patients about their cognitive maps of interpersonal relations. Finally, the therapist uses patients' in-session transference episodes to teach patients how to modify their interpersonal cognitive schemata, behavior, and emotions.

Psychoanalytically oriented psychotherapy is reasonably effective for the treatment of anxiety and depression related to interpersonal problems. The average success rate is 68%. The quality of the helping alliance accounts for 25% of this success; the application of accurate interpretations concerning core conflictual relationship themes accounts for another 25% of the outcome of treatment.

The changes in the psychodynamic model make it much more compatible with the cognitive-behavioral approach. Both models place an emphasis on cognition and learning. Recent psychodynamically oriented advances in assessing tacit interpersonal schemata provide cognitive-behavior therapists with the tools to take them beyond working with static self-statements. In addition, the therapeutic relationship can serve as a basis for enhancing treatment effectiveness and an arena for generating change. This integration can occur without perturbing the fundamental assumptions of neoclassical cognitive-behavior therapy.

The Dynamic Cognitive-Behavior Therapy Model

Dynamic cognitive-behavior therapy (D-CBT) is based on the principles of neoclassical cognitive-behavior therapy, cognitive psychology, and developmental psychodynamics as developed by Mahoney (1991), Matlin (1989), Bowlby (1988), Horowitz (1988a,b), Luborsky (1974), Luborsky *et al.* (1988), and Luborsky & Crits-Christoph (1990). Therapists conceptualize their cases from a dynamic cognitive point of view. The therapist assesses clients' tacit, dynamic cognitive structure with regard to interpersonal relationships, faulty cognitive information processing, emotional disregulation, and behavioral adaptation.

D-CBT is based on the assumptions of neoclassical cognitive-behavior therapy defined earlier in this chapter. The model adapts three assumptions from the psychodynamic approach. First, a stress is placed on the power of the therapeutic alliance to affect the outcome of treatment. Second, investigation of patients' attachment bonds with parental figures is considered important in understanding their current interpersonal relationship problems and cognitive distortions. Third, an accent is placed on elucidating and modifying patients' tacit working models of relationships as well as their overt cognitions.

The D-CBT treatment plan has five phases. The early phase consists of assessment and establishing a treatment contract. In addition, the therapist provides the client with an overview of the treatment process. During the initial session the clinician needs to get a clear description of the client's problems. The clinician should perform a formal diagnostic evaluation if the problems are symptomatic of a psychiatric disorder. Depending on the patient's circumstances, a mental status exam might be necessary.

Typically, the clinician will get some type of psychometric information on the client's symptom status. For instance, if the client is depressed, the Beck Depression Inventory (Beck, Ward, Mendelson, Mock, & Erbaugh, 1961) should be administered. In the case of obsessive–compulsive disorder or panic disorder, for instance, the client is asked to self-record the frequency, severity, and environmental conditions surrounding the daily occurrence of symptoms. Virtually any reliable and valid psychometric assessment device can be used for assessment. In addition, the clinician needs to provide the client with an overview of the therapy approach.

Although the D-CBT is short term, therapists do not always set a definitive termination date. However, having a fixed endpoint provides a focus for the therapeutic work.

An important task of the first session is for the clinician to check the capacity of the patient to develop a sound working relationship with the clinician. The simplest means to accomplish this is to ask clients, at the close of the first session, if they feel comfortable working with the therapist.

Assessment occurs over the first several sessions. The therapist's goal is to form a cohesive conceptualization of the case. The conceptualization includes specifications about the genesis of the problem, the types of schemata and distortions involved, and a prescription for treatment.

The early-middle phase of treatment is designed to enable the therapist to clarify patients' tacit working models of role relationships and their core conflictual relationship themes. During this phase, patients are invited, and helped, to tell the therapist stories about their interpersonal life history. Exploration of interpersonal life history events are made in the context of the parental relationships, immediate family relationships, and significant relationships at school, work, and with friends. This exploration provides a format for the therapist to understand patients' dynamic cognitive structure and promotes a strengthening of the therapeutic alliance. The formal analysis of the tacit working models of role relationships and conflict schemata is based on transcripts derived from audiotapes of these sessions. Utilizing the techniques of Luborsky (1984), Luborsky and Crits-Christoph (1990), and Horowitz (1988a,b), the therapist and the supervision group review the tapes and map out patients' interpersonal schemata.

The middle phase of treatment begins an intensive cognitive therapy program. Patients are taught to understand and self-monitor their tacit and overt cognitions. Cognitive tactics such as guided discovery, testing idiosyncratic meanings, reattribution, examining options and alternatives, self-instruction, and labeling of cognitive distortions are utilized. In addition, the therapist educates patients about the wishes and needs that all humans have in the context of significant interpersonal relationships. An understandable linkage is made between the patients' wishes and needs, emotional reactions, and behavior.

The late-middle phase of treatment is focused on enhancing the client's skills in self-management. Behavioral intervention tactics, such as systematic desensitization, flooding, problem-solving training, social skills training, and assertiveness training, are applied during this phase of treatment. Behavioral intervention is not viewed as just a way to modify behavior. Rather, the D-CBT approach views these techniques as powerful tools to modify emotional and tacit cognitive schema.

Also, if it is warranted, cognitive-behavioral family therapy or cognitive-behavioral couples therapy is instituted during the late-middle phase. Time is also devoted to teaching patients meditation techniques in order to facilitate enhanced self-control. Finally, imagery and role rehearsal are utilized to reinforce the newly learned skills.

The final phase of therapy is focused upon termination issues and relapse prevention. The termination phase is viewed as the period when the learning and gains made in therapy are consolidated.

The D-CBT session typically lasts from 45 to 60 min. The therapist starts by asking the client to provide an overview of the previous weeks events. The clinician's job is to help the client relate the recent experiences to the focus of treatment. Since homework is integral to this approach, the clinician next reviews the previous homework assignment with the client. The therapist ties these reports into the central focus of treatment and sets up a problem focus for the current session. The session problem focus serves as the basis for interpretation of core conflictual relationship themes and the targeting of cognitive and behavioral interventions during the session. The next homework assignment is based on the session focus. In closing the session the clinician briefly reviews the material discussed during the hour and links the session to the overall context of the therapeutic process.

Evidence for the efficacy of the D-CBT approach consists of multiple-baseline studies and two single-case evaluations. Turner (1989) demonstrated the treatment was effective in reducing symptoms associated with borderline personality disorder. Two case studies by Turner (1993a,b) indicated that D-CBT was effective in reducing drug and alcohol abuse with adolescents. More recently a controlled trial comparing D-CBT to a treatment-as-usual control group has been completed. The subjects were 22 patients treated for symptoms associated with borderline personality disorder. The data are currently being analyzed from this project.

Also, a controlled clinical outcome study sponsored by the National Institute on Drug Abuse is underway at Temple University. This study is contrasting D-CBT with multidimensional family therapy and a community treatment control group. The experimental comparison will run for 5 years. Adolescents, aged 12 through 17, with drug-use problems are targeted for treatment in the study. At the end of that time we will have a clearer understanding of the effectiveness rate for D-CBT as well as a better understanding of its effective components.

A final note about the nature of D-CBT will be helpful for the reader. D-CBT is an integrative blend of psychodynamic, cognitive, and behavioral therapy procedures into a cohesive framework. The clinician needs to be careful to note those points at which the model is discontinuous with assumptions associated with any of the three models in their pure practice.

Unlike behavior therapy, the D-CBT model does assume there is a tacit level of information processing which affects and guides day-to-day explicit information processing. Unlike psychodynamically oriented models, D-CBT does not assume that the tacit level is a burning cauldron of fixations and psychologically dangerous material; nor does the D-CBT model assume that insight about the full workings of the tacit level is sufficient for therapeutic change. Change at both the tacit and overt levels of cognitive processing requires understanding plus emotional and behavioral change. However, unlike classical cognitive therapy models, the D-CBT model does not assume that the simple substitution of positive cognitions for maladaptive, explicit cognitions provides a basis for durable personal self-regulation.

The D-CBT model does assume that tacit working models of role relationships, scenario schemata, and self-schemata are critical influences upon overt cognition, emotion, and behavior. It is assumed that these schemata are developed during attachment and bonding experiences. It is also assumed that these tacit schemata provide the soil from which explicit, automatic cognitions grow and influence overt behavior and emotional regulation. Emotion and its personal meanings are influenced by both the tacit and explicit levels of cognition, as well as by behavior. Behavior consolidates the personal system and provides a window for understanding the self-system and reorganizing it.

D-CBT attempts to bring the relevant components of a person's tacit processes into awareness. It accomplishes this goal through the process of education in the context of a safe, secure environment. D-CBT emphasizes education in cognitive, emotional, and behavioral coping strategies in support of one's development of an integrated sense of self.

References

Balint, M., Ornstein, P. H., & Balint, E. (1972). *Focal psychotherapy.* Philadelphia: Lippincott.

Bandura, A. (1977a). Self-efficacy: Towards a unifying theory of behavior change. *Psychological Review, 84,* 191–215.

Bandura, A. (1977b). *Social learning theory.* Englewood Cliffs, NJ: Prentice-Hall.

Bandura, A. (1985). Model of causality in social learning theory. In M. Mahoney & A. Freeman (Eds.), *Cognition and psychotherapy* (pp. 81–100). New York: Plenum.

Beck, A. T. (1967). *Depression: Clinical, experimental, and theoretical aspects.* New York: Hoeber.

Beck, A. T. (1970). Cognitive therapy: Nature and relation to behavior therapy. *Behavior Therapy, 1,* 184–200.

Beck, A. T. (1976). *Cognitive therapy and the emotional disorders.* New York: International Universities Press.

Beck, A. T., Rush, A. J., Shaw, B. F., & Emery, G. (1979). *Cognitive therapy of depression.* New York: Guilford Press.

Beck, A. T., Ward, C. H., Mendelson, M., Mock, J. E., & Erbaugh, J. K. (1961). An inventory for measuring depression. *Archives of General Psychiatry, 4,* 561–571.

Bowlby, J. (1940). The influence of early environment in the development of neurosis and neurotic character. *International Journal of Psycho-Analysis, 21,* 154–178.

Bowlby, J. (1973). *Attachment and Loss, Vol. 2. Separation: Anxiety and anger.* Harmondsworth: Penguin.

Bowlby, J. (1980). *Attachment and Loss, Vol. 3. Loss: Sadness and depression.* Harmondsworth: Penguin.

Bowlby, J. (1982). *Attachment and Loss, Vol. 1. Attachment* (2nd ed.). Harmondsworth: Penguin.

Bowlby, J. (1988). *A secure base.* New York: Basic Books.

Brewer, W. F., & Treyens, J. C. (1981). Role of schemata in memory for places. *Cognitive Psychology, 13,* 207–230.

Crits-Christoph, P., Luborsky, L., Dahl, L., Popp, C., Melon, J., & Mark, D. (1988). Clinicians can agree in assessing relationship patterns in psychotherapy: The core conflictual relationship method. *Archives of General Psychiatry, 45,* 1001–1004.

Davenloo, H. (1979). Technique of short-term psychotherapy. *Psychiatric Clinics of North America, 2,* 11–12.

Davenloo, H. (1980). *Short-term dynamic therapy, Vol. 1.* New York: Jason Aronson.

Ellis, A. (1962). *Reason and emotion in psychotherapy.* New York: Lyle Stuart.

Freeman, A. (1990). Cognitive therapy. In A. S. Bellack & M. Hersen (Eds.), *Handbook of comparative treatments for adult disorders* (pp. 64–87). New York: Wiley.

Freud, S. (1912). The dynamics of transference. In J. Strachey (Ed.), *The standard edition of the complete psychological works of Sigmund Freud* (Vol. 12, pp. 99–108). London: Hogarth Press.

Greenson, R. (1965). The working alliance and transference neurosis. *Psychoanalytic Quarterly, 34,* 158–181.

Hartley, D., & Strupp, H. (1983). The therapeutic alliance: Its relationship to outcome in brief psychotherapy. In J. Masling (Ed.), *Empirical studies of psychoanalytic theory* (Vol. 1). Hillsdale, NJ: Erlbaum.

Horowitz, M. J. (1987). *States of mind* (2nd ed.). New York: Plenum.

Horowitz, M. J. (1988a). *Introduction to psychodynamics: A new synthesis.* New York: Basic Books.

Horowitz, M. J. (1988b). *Psychodynamics and cognition.* Chicago: University of Chicago Press.

Horowitz, M. J. (1989). Relationship schema formulation: Role relationship models and intrapsychic conflict. *Psychiatry, 52,* 260–274.

Horowitz, M. J., Marmer, C., Weiss, D. S., DeWitt, K. N., & Rosenbaum, R. (1984). Brief psychotherapy and grief reactions: The relationship of process to outcome. *Archives of General Psychiatry, 41,* 438–448.

Horowitz, M. J., Rosenbaum, R., & Wilner, N. (1988). Role relationship dilemmas: A potential new process variable. *Psychotherapy, 25,* 241–248.

Kendall, P. C., & Bemis, K. M. (1984). Cognitive-behavioral interventions: Principles and procedures. In N. S. Endler & J. M. Hunt (Eds.), *Personality and the behavioral disorders* (2nd ed., pp. 1069–1109). New York: Wiley.

Lazarus, A. (1976). *Multimodal behavior therapy*. New York: Springer.

Levine, F. J., & Luborsky, L. (1981). The core conflictual relationship theme method: A demonstration of reliable clinical inferences by the method of mismatched cases. In S. Tutman, C. Kayne, & M. Zimmerman (Eds.), *Object and self: A developmental approach* (pp. 501–526). New York: International Universities Press.

Lorenz, K. Z. (1935). Der kumpan in der umvelt des vogels. In C. H. Schiller (Ed.) *Instinctive Behaviour*. New York: International Universities Press.

Luborsky, L. (1976). Helping alliances in psychotherapy: The groundwork for a study of their relationship to outcome. In J. L. Claghorn (Ed.), *Successful psychotherapy* (pp. 92–116). New York: Brunner/Mazel.

Luborsky, L. (1984). *Principles of psychoanalytic psychotherapy: A manual for supportive-expressive treatment*. New York: Basic Books.

Luborsky, L., & Crits-Christoph, P. (1990). *Understanding transference*. New York: Basic Books.

Luborsky, L., Crits-Christoph, P., Mintz, J., & Auerbach, A. (1988). *Who will benefit from psychotherapy? Predicting therapeutic outcomes*. New York: Basic Books.

Mahoney, M. J. (1977). Reflections on the cognitive-learning trend in psychotherapy. *American Psychologist, 32*, 5–13.

Mahoney, M. J. (1985). Psychotherapy and human change processes. In M. J. Mahoney & A. Freeman (Eds.), *Cognition and psychotherapy* (pp. 3–48). New York: Plenum.

Mahoney, M. J. (1991). *Human change processes: The scientific foundations of psychotherapy*. New York: Basic Books.

Malan, D. H. (1963). *A study of brief psychotherapy*. New York: Plenum.

Malan, D. H. (1976). *Toward the validation of dynamic psychotherapy*. New York: Plenum.

Mann, J. (1973). *Time-limited psychotherapy*. Cambridge, MA: Harvard University Press.

Marziali, E., Marmar, C., & Krupnick, J. (1981). Therapeutic alliance scales: Their development and relationship to psychotherapy outcome. *American Journal of Psychiatry, 138*, 361–364.

Matlin, M. M. (1989). *Cognition* (2nd ed.). Orlando: Holt, Rinehart & Winston.

Meichenbaum, D. (1977). *Cognitive behavior modification*. New York: Plenum.

Piaget, J. (1926). *The language and thought of the child*. New York: Harcourt, Brace.

Rychlak, J. F. (1981). *Introduction to personality and psychotherapy* (2nd ed.). Boston: Houghton Mifflin.

Sifneos, P. E. (1972). *Short-term psychotherapy and emotional crisis*. Cambridge, MA: Harvard University Press.

Sifneos, P. E. (1979). *Short-term psychotherapy: Evaluation and technique*. New York: Plenum.

Turner, R. M. (1983). Cognitive-behavior therapy with borderline patients. *Carrier Foundation Letter, 88*, 1–4.

Turner, R. M. (1988). The cognitive-behavioral approach to the treatment of borderline personality disorders. *International Journal of Partial Hospitalization, 5*, 279–289.

Turner, R. M. (1989). Case study evaluation of a bio-cognitive-behavioral approach for the treatment of borderline personality disorder. *Behavior Therapy, 20*, 477–489.

Turner, R. M. (1992). Launching cognitive-behavior therapy. In S. Budman, M. Hoyt, & S. Friedman (Eds.), *The first session of brief therapy* (pp. 135–154). New York: Guilford Press.

Turner, R. M. (1993a). Cognitive therapy for the borderline patient: Cogito ergo sum. In A. Freeman & F. Datillio (Eds.), *Cognitive therapy casebook* (pp. 215–222). New York: Guilford Press.

Turner, R. M. (1993b). The utility of psychodynamic techniques in the practice of cognitive-behavior therapy. *Journal of Integrative and Eclectic Psychotherapy*, 230–253.

Turner, R. M., & Ascher, L. M. (1982). Therapist factor in the treatment of insomnia. *Behaviour Research and Therapy, 20*, 33–40.

Zetzel, E. (1958). Therapeutic alliance in the analysis of hysteria. In E. Zetzel (Ed.), *The capacity for emotional growth* (pp. 182–196). London: Hogarth Press.

19

"Are Some Psychotherapies More Equivalent Than Others?"

Robert Elliott, William B. Stiles, and David A. Shapiro

Introduction

We found reading, reflecting on, and discussing a sample of the material in this book to be challenging, informative, and stimulating. Thus, we welcome this opportunity to update and continue our earlier analysis (Stiles, Shapiro, & Elliott, 1986) of the debate over the equivalence or nonequivalence of different psychotherapies.

In this chapter we begin by reviewing the position taken in our earlier paper (Stiles *et al.*, 1986). We then review and evaluate the key tasks and relevant themes in a sample of chapters in this book. Next, we attempt to clarify the key issues involved in the debate and to suggest how it might be more productively carried forward. We hope these clarifications will facilitate the process of appraising the strengths and limitations of the literature reviewed and the recommendations contained in this volume. Finally, we address a set of pressing broader philosophical, ethical, and professional issues raised by this review volume. Throughout, our primary tasks are to enhance mutual understanding between researchers and clinicians of different theoretical persuasions and to strengthen and broaden the data base from which future, more complete theoretical conclusions and treatment recommendations can be made.

Robert Elliott • Department of Psychology, University of Toledo, Toledo, Ohio 43606. **William B. Stiles** • Department of Psychology, Miami University, Oxford, Ohio 45056. **David A. Shapiro** • MRC/ESRC Social and Applied Psychology Unit, University of Sheffield, Sheffield S10 2TN, England.

Handbook of Effective Psychotherapy, edited by Thomas R. Giles. Plenum Press, New York, 1993.

Review of Our Earlier Position

In our earlier paper (Stiles *et al.*, 1986), we began by stating a troubling paradox: the fact that "a substantial body of evidence and opinion points to the conclusion that the outcomes of different psychotherapies with clinical populations are equivalent" (p. 166), in spite of clearly documented differences in the content and techniques used in those therapies. Our purpose was to organize, describe, and show how psychotherapy researchers' attempts to address this paradox have driven the field for the past 40 years:

> The paradox . . . challenges some cherished beliefs of practitioners and underlines our comparative ignorance as to the mechanisms whereby psychotherapies achieve their effects. Researchers have attempted to resolve the paradox by demonstrating differential outcomes (thus overturning the Dodo's verdict), by identifying a common core of therapeutic process (thus disputing the relevance of the technical diversity), or by reconceptualizing the issues. (p. 175)

A prime goal of our 1986 article was to consider how the field might progress more productively. Thus, our key recommendation was that the entire field of psychotherapy research would benefit greatly from greater specificity or precision, in the form of more fine-grained questions, methods, and answers. In our analysis, this call for "a closer look" took a variety of forms, including treatment manualization, dismantling studies, description of client and therapist in-session behaviors, behavioral and weekly measures of outcome, Paul's (1967) specificity or matrix paradigm, and the study of important change events in therapy. Our advocacy of specificity was also evident in the somewhat critical stance we took toward "equivalent mechanism" explanations of outcome equivalence; we argued that general factors such as client expectancy and therapeutic alliance were too abstract to be clinically useful and needed to be analyzed in more precise terms.

In their introductory chapter to this book, Giles, Neims, and Prial (Chapter 2) oversimplify our 1986 position by including it in an "equivalency literature . . . which argues that all therapies yield essentially similar results." In fact, the title of our article, "Are all psychotherapies equivalent?" was in quotation marks. This was intended to convey our somewhat ironic intent, which was to examine the meaning of this question for psychotherapy researchers. It was never our intention to decide this issue within the confines of a single article. As it is usually stated, the equivalence position is a logically flawed, overly simplistic endorsement of the null hypothesis. While our stance in this chapter is again an ironic one, critical of sweeping conclusions on either side, we will also offer constructive suggestions for deciding specific issues of equivalence or nonequivalence.

Summary and Assessment of Main Tasks and Themes of This Book

In our view, this volume employs two rather different strategies to dissolve the equivalence paradox, both of them attacking the assertion of outcome equivalence. The first strategy, *general outcome nonequivalence* is found most clearly in Giles *et al.*'s chapter, in which the authors marshall an impressive range and quantity of information in order to prove that "prescriptive" therapies are generally superior to "traditional" therapies. The second strategy is a version of what we (Stiles *et al.*, 1986) referred to as the *matrix paradigm*, which argues that it is possible to show nonequivalence of treatments for specific disorders. This latter strategy is the main task of the review chapters we read. Thus, the main thrust of the book is to continue in the tradition of important previous works on matching treatments to clients and disorders (especially Beutler & Clarkin, 1990; Goldstein & Stein, 1976). In other words, important clinical disorders are each presented, and the relevant outcome literature is reviewed, providing the basis for treatment recommendations, wherever possible.

In order to form our evaluation of the success with which these two strategies have been carried out, we requested and were able to study, in addition to the keynote chapter (Giles, Niems, & Prial), eight review chapters (covering alcohol abuse, borderline personality disorder, developmental disability, nocturnal enuresis, major depressive disorder, obsessive–compulsive disorder, posttraumatic stress disorder, and schizophrenia).

Because of the need to summarize the diversity of data and opinion reviewed in these chapters, we carried out an analysis of the major relevant themes which we found to cut across these reviews. This analysis is presented in Table 19.1. While these are certainly not the only themes present in these chapters, we think that our statement of them will help to illustrate and focus the discussion.

To begin with, it is clear that all but one of these reviewers (Tutek & Linehan, Chapter 15) have concluded (with varying degrees of certainty) that, in the treatment of the specific disorders under review, certain cognitive/behavioral treatments are more effective than other therapies, which they usually define as "traditional," "conventional," "treatment as usual" or "psychodynamic/humanistic."

However, what is more striking is the degree of concern shown by these reviewers with the limitations of the existing treatments. Furthermore, all of the reviewers urged adoption of one or both of two complementary solutions to these limitations. First, almost all reviewers advocated greater consideration of contextual factors in selecting and designing treatments, especially client individual differences in diagnostic subgrouping (Blake *et al.*, Chapter 9), prognostic factors (Steketee & Lam, Chapter 11), and situational factors (Lutzker, Chapter 4). Second, almost all argued that improved outcomes would be obtained if more complex, flexible treatments were adopted, including multimodal treatment packages (Allen & Mattson, Chapter 16), individualized or case formulation approaches (Persons, Chapter 13), relationship or emotional treatment components (Tutek & Linehan, Chapter 15), or long-term treatments (Mueser & Glynn, Chapter 14). Thus, to our ears, these authors seemed less interested in proving the superiority of cognitive/behavioral treatments and more concerned with the limitations of these treatments and how their efficacy can be improved.

A final general theme which we note here is a general dissatisfaction with the research data base on which the comparative effectiveness statements were made, leading six of the reviewers to remark on the dearth of research on psychodynamic, humanistic, and/or supportive treatments. Some of the reviewers (e.g., Kaplan & Busner, Chapter 6) interpret this absence of data as evidence for the ineffectiveness of the alternative treatments, but at least three (e.g., Persons, Chapter 13) advocate further research on these treatments. The nonequivalence verdict returned by at least some of these reviewers is thus a tentative one, based on "best available data," but by no means definitive.

Table 19.1. Analysis of Relevant Themes in Nine Selected Review Articles in This Book

I. Treatment Issues

- A. Differential treatment recommendations
  1. None possible: BPD
  2. Cross-study variability makes it difficult to recommend one treatment over others: Alc
  3. Differential effectiveness of cognitive/behavioral assumed but not explicitly stated: OC
  4. Cognitive/behavioral claimed better than nonbehavioral treatments: Intro, Alc, DD, En, MDD, PTSD, Sc
     - a. Other approaches ignored; superiority of CB taken for granted: DD
     - b. Redefining effective treatments as behavioral/cognitive/prescriptive: Intro, DD, Sc (i.e., family therapy)
     - c. Lack of data is taken to indicate ineffectiveness: Intro, Alc, DD, En
- B. Limitations of existing treatments
  1. Attrition/dropout rates are a problem: BPD, En, MDD, PTSD
  2. Treatment failure is a problem: BPD, En, MDD, PTSD
  3. Relapse, failure to maintain treatment gains is a problem: Alc, En, MDD, PTSD, Sc
  4. Results of present research literature may not generalize well to practice situations: MDD, PTSD
  5. Current treatments show limited range of effects, don't generalize to untreated symptoms, have too narrow a range of effect: OC, PTSD
  6. Current treatments haven't been tried with entire range of disorder: PTSD
- C. Treatment contextualization
  1. Individual differences are important for outcome and call for different treatments: Alc, BPD, MDD, OC, PTSD
     - a. Clients within diagnostic group are heterogeneous, have a variety of different problems: Alc, BPD, MDD, PTSD
     - b. Comorbidity (other concurrent diagnoses) is an important complicating factor: BPD, PTSD
     - c. Client individual differences (prognostic factors) affect outcome: Alc, OC, PTSD
     - d. Client individual differences interact with treatment to produce different outcomes: Alc (research evidence presented), PTSD (claimed likely)
  2. Situational context calls for different treatments: DD
  3. Therapist effects are important: Alc
- D. More complex, flexible treatments advocated
  1. Multimodal treatments are important in dealing with disorder; treatment package approach: Alc, BPD, DD, OC, Sc
     - a. Limited range of modalities recommended: En, OC
     - b. Broad range of modalities recommended: Alc, BPD, DD, Sc
  2. Case formulation approach or individualized treatment is advocated as useful: Alc, BPD, MDD
  3. Relationship/emotional treatment components are important: Alc, BPD
  4. Long-term treatment (1+ yr) is called for: BPD, Sc
     - a. Necessity of long-term treatment can be inferred: DD

II. Methodological and Philosophy of Science Issues

- A. Present research base is inadequate; more is needed
  1. There is an inadequate base of research on psychodynamic, humanistic, or supportive treatments: Intro, BPD, DD, En, MDD, OC, PTSD
     - a. More research is needed: BPD, MDD, PTSD
  2. Need to study treatments as they are employed in practice settings: MDD, PTSD
- B. View of nonspecific or placebo control groups
  1. Use emphasized or advocated as definitive of good therapy outcome design: Intro, BPD, MDD, OC, En
  2. Described as not necessary or helpful or reinterpreted to include no-treatment controls: Sc, En, PTSD
- C. View of case study and uncontrolled group research
  1. Controlled single-case designs are informative: Intro, BPD, DD, En, MDD, OC, PTSD

(*continued*)

Table 19.1. Analysis of Relevant Themes in Nine Selected Review Articles in This Book (*continued*)

2. Traditional case study (and uncontrolled group) research contains useful information: PTSD
3. Case study and uncontrolled group research ignored or devalued: Alc, Sc

D. Other
1. "Empirical" used in narrow positivistic sense: Intro, BPD, DD, En
2. Specific studies producing contrary results are singled out for criticism in order to discredit them: PTSD, Sc

Note. Intro = Giles *et al.*, Ch. 2; Alc = alcohol abuse (Allen & Mattson, Ch. 16); BPD = borderline personality disorder (Tutek & Linehan, Ch. 15); DD = developmental disabilities (Lutzker, Ch. 4); En = nocturnal enuresis (Kaplan & Busner, Ch. 6); MDD = major depressive disorder (Persons, Ch. 13); OC = obsessive–compulsive disorder (Steketee & Lam, Ch. 11); PTSD = posttraumatic stress disorder (Blake *et al.*, Ch. 9); Sc = schizophrenia (Mueser & Glynn, Ch. 14).

What, then, is our assessment of the project of this book, viewed from the perspective of our earlier analysis of attempts to resolve the equivalence paradox? In our view, the reviews we have seen are more successful in making recommendations about which therapies have been shown to be effective than they are in making comparative judgments about the superiority of one treatment over another. In all eight reviews available to us, we were struck by how little research there is within each disorder which directly compared the authors' favored cognitive or behavioral treatments to other well-specified treatments. Time and again, the comparative treatment studies reviewed ended up as horse races between a Thoroughbred racehorse and a nondescript nag: one well-defined cognitive or behavioral treatment against a vaguely psychodynamic "treatment-as-usual" condition.

Perhaps that is why Giles *et al.* take the general nonequivalence strategy in their introductory chapter, which is to argue that there never was a paradox, that the claim of general equivalence between major treatment categories is an error reflecting the bias of nonbehavioral reviewers. If this argument were to succeed, it would greatly simplify the task of figuring out which therapies work best with which disorders, since it would rule most of the possible treatments out of court from this point on! Researchers could then carry on studying the most effective blends of cognitive and behavioral components (e.g., Steketee & Lam).

However, our view is that Giles *et al.* have not yet convincingly demonstrated that, however they are relabeled, the class of cognitive/behavioral therapies shows a clear, clinically significant advantage over the class of psychodynamic/experiential therapies. We base this conclusion on a series of conceptual, statistical, and methodological arguments. More importantly, we take issue with the whole enterprise of addressing the equivalence question in such a broad, nonspecific manner.

On the other hand, we support the reviewers' repeated emphasis on the need for continued specification of outcome in terms of domain (e.g., classes of symptoms, social adjustment, generalization to nontargeted domains) and modes of effect (attrition from treatment, posttreatment outcome, maintenance of gain or relapse prevention, efficiency/rapidity of treatment). Such distinctions also serve as convincing illustrations of the complexity of psychotherapy process and outcome.

Key Issues Raised by the Equivalence Debate

In this part of our chapter, we will put forward the position that the important, continuing search for specific effective treatments is not well served by broad and invidious comparisons such as "prescriptive" versus "traditional" therapies. In support of this point, we will offer a series of arguments and suggestions for moving the field beyond this debate into more productive avenues.

Problems with the Prescriptive versus Traditional Therapy Distinction

Central to Giles *et al.*'s analysis of the therapy outcome literature is the division of treatments into two groups, which they label "prescriptive" (or "directive") and "traditional." As shown in Table 19.2, Giles *et al.* have modified the traditional verbal versus behavioral dichotomy (e.g., Smith, Glass, & Miller, 1980) to suit their purposes. Thus, prescriptive therapies are brief and present focused, address specific symptoms, and are empirically based, directive, and collaborative, while traditional therapies are the opposite. It is our contention that the continued division of therapies into "sheep" and "goats" categories is a gross oversimplification and is no longer productive.

There are several problems with this two-category model of therapy types. First, there is the logical problem that defining prescriptive therapies as empirically based means that *any* therapy for which there is efficacy data can be included, thus making a tautology out of the claim that prescriptive therapies are more effective. Second, the distinction reinforces a stereotype about nonbehavioral treatments, characterizing them in terms applicable really only to a caricature of traditional psychoanalysis. This dichotomy is too limiting to describe the current scene and was never really accurate of psychodynamic therapy, which does have an empirical (but not experimental) basis and which does attempt to foster a collaborative client–therapist relationship (see Luborsky, 1984).

More importantly, there are many therapies which cut across traditional and prescriptive categories. These include various focused, time-limited dynamic therapies (see Svartberg & Stiles, 1991, for a meta-analysis). Research on short-term focused experiential therapies is now also emerging (e.g., Beutler *et al.*, 1991; Elliott *et al.*, 1990; Greenberg & Webster, 1982). A number of these short-term nonbehavioral therapies have been designed for use with a particular disorder, such as bereavement reactions (Horowitz *et al.*, 1984) or depression (Beutler *et al.*, 1991). Furthermore, some of the new treatments resemble behavioral or cognitive therapies in their problem focus, making use of specific, experimentally re-

Table 19.2. The Two Major Types of Therapy according to Giles, Neims, and Prial

Feature	Traditional	Prescriptive
Length	Long	Brief
Temporal focus	Historical	Present
Goals	General personality change	Specific symptoms
Empirical base	No	Yes
Techniques	Interpretation, reflection, confrontation, catharsis-induction, support	Advisement, information
Collaborative	No	Yes

searched techniques to help clients resolve specific emotional problems such as internal conflict or puzzling personal reactions (Greenberg, Rice, & Elliott, 1993; Rice & Greenberg, 1984), but without giving instruction or prescribing solutions to clients' problems. Finally, virtually all therapies see themselves as entering into a collaborative relationship with clients.

The distinction is fuzzy on the prescriptive side as well. For example, Smith *et al.* (1980) classified cognitive therapies such as rational emotive therapy as verbal (vs. behavioral) treatments (cognitive therapies have since been "adopted" into the prescriptive "family"). More recently, Beck and others (see Tutek & Linehan, Chapter 15, this volume) have begun to use cognitive/behavioral therapies with personality disorders, necessitating considerably longer treatments (i.e., on the order of a year). Behavioral and cognitive therapists have become interested in emotional-change processes such as helping clients to become more aware of and acceptant of feelings (Afari, Hayes, Wilson, McCurry, & Taylor, 1991). Also, cognitive therapy has been combined with traditional Christian beliefs in order to treat depression in religious individuals (see Propst, Ostrom, Watkins, Dean, & Mashburn, 1992).

Finally, the field is beginning to see the emergence of integrated treatments which combine educative-behavioral elements with exploratory-insight-oriented elements (e.g., Tutek & Linehan, Chapter 15, this volume; Norcross, 1986). It is clear that the prescriptive versus traditional therapy distinction is overly restrictive and unlikely to foster the development of new, potentially effective treatments.

In fact, two-category models (no matter what form they take) are too simplistic to properly classify therapies. At present there is no coherent theoretical or procedural basis for grounding such categories. Attempts to dichotomize therapies always yield problematic examples that do not fit the proposed categories.

The cause of this fuzziness is a radical underfactoring of the domain of therapies. Therapies differ in important ways on a number of underlying dimensions. For example, Smith *et al.* (1980) report, but do not utilize, a multidimensional-scaling analysis which resulted in a three-dimensional model, with dimensions corresponding roughly to (1) action versus verbal-analytic mode of operation, (2) fantasy versus reality focus, and (3) nondirective versus directive client–therapist relationship. Any two-category model is thus an attempt to collapse these and other distinctions onto a single dimension, resulting in the many exceptions listed above. In short, there is probably as much (and perhaps more) within-group variance in the prescriptive and traditional headings as there is between them. Such oversimplifications are no longer warranted and do not serve to advance our knowledge about psychotherapy.

A close reading of Giles *et al.*'s chapter, as well as other information (personal communication, Dec. 9, 1991), leads us to suspect that the real distinction underlying their traditional versus prescriptive dichotomy is not substantive but methodological: the degree of explicitness or specification of a treatment (e.g., manualization). In other words, we agree that for research purposes it may be useful to distinguish between "specified" and "unspecified" treatments, whether these be psychodynamic or behavioral. *Specified* treatments are those which are guided by a single, explicit treatment model, whether it be behavioral, psychodynamic, or humanistic, and often targeted on a specific disorder; *unspecified* treatments consist of "treatment as usual," "mixed behavioral and cognitive treatments" (e.g., Sloane, Staples, Cristol, Yorkston, & Whipple, 1975), or "generic or nonspecific counseling." This does not mean that nothing specific is being done, only that the researcher is not in a position to be specific about it. This degree of ignorance seriously undermines the clarity and validity of researchers' efforts.

It is our view that "unspecified treatment conditions" should be studied only when there are strong practical or theoretical reasons for doing so, and that results should not be generalized between unspecified and specified treatments, even if they are both of the same general type (e.g., "cognitive therapy"). In most cases, knowing that a specified treatment does better than an unspecified one is not a particularly informative finding.

Logic of Argument in the Equivalence Debate

Several aspects of the logic used by Giles *et al.* as well as some (but not all) of the other reviewers bear explication. Some of these forms of reasoning appear to us to be sound, while others do not:

1. *The claim of universal or blanket equivalence ("All have won") can be demolished by counterexamples.* Giles *et al.* argue this quite effectively. We seriously doubt that any psychotherapy researcher (or clinician) ever seriously believed in universal equivalence, but it is still useful to show that claims of universal equivalence are absurd. At the same time, counterexamples also provide an effective means for demolishing universal claims of superiority of one type of therapy other another.
2. *It is possible to prove the general superiority of directive therapies by citing numerous examples of studies which found such superiority.* We disagree with this form of reasoning. Examples are not an adequate basis for making general knowledge claims; citing numerous examples doesn't "prove" anything. Proving that nonequivalence (or equivalence) occurs is not the same as showing nonequivalence (or equivalence) is the rule in psychotherapy. Given the wide study-to-study variations in outcome that are characteristic of the field, general knowledge claims, that is, claims about what is *generally* or probabilistically true, must be made on the basis of reasonably inclusive and systematic sampling and systematic combination of the available evidence (e.g., meta-analysis or self-critical, balanced narrative reviewing).
3. *The absence of data may be taken as evidence for lack of effectiveness and used as the basis for negative recommendations against treatments.* That lack of evidence is the same as negative evidence, that is, evidence for the relative inefficacy of the treatment, appears to be the underlying logic used in several of the reviews in this book (e.g., Kaplan & Busner, Chapter 6; see also Table 19.1). When faced with a total or nearly total absence of data, however, it seems more logical to us to conclude that we simply do not yet know whether the unstudied treatment is effective or not.

In their chapter, Giles *et al.* present a tour de force of evidence for the nonequivalence position, combining the previous two arguments: They hold that the numerous examples of the superiority of directive over traditional therapies, coupled with the near absence of examples of the opposite form of nonequivalence, proves the superiority of directive therapies. To this end, they cite single-case experimental designs, "attention-placebo" studies, meta-analytic studies, and comparative treatment studies. For this strategy to work, however, each of these sets of evidence (1) must be truly relevant (apply in a logical fashion to the issue of nonequivalence), (2) must be reasonably valid (not confounded with other factors such as allegiance effects), (3) must be accurately cited and summarized, and (4) must be substantial enough to be clinically meaningful. We will expand upon these issues in later sections.

The Need for Greater Specificity in Therapy Research

As we noted earlier, the central theme of our 1986 paper was the turn toward greater specificity. Although this trend took many different forms, all can be characterized as attempts to identify the contexts under which a treatment is effective. However, 6 years later we find that researchers and reviewers are still overlooking most important sources of variation in outcome; the lack of specificity in primary and meta-analytic research on psychotherapy seems to us to be a continuing problem.

The importance of greater specificity is dictated by the complexity inherent in psychotherapy process and outcome (Elliott & Anderson, in press). This complexity is evident both within and between studies. First, within studies, most treatments show wide variations across clients in treatment outcomes. These variations, especially clients who drop out, get worse, do not change enough, or later relapse, are of great interest to clinicians and researchers interested in understanding the application of a particular treatment to a particular disorder, and, as noted earlier, the reviewers in this volume are no exception. Who are these clients, and how do they differ from the clear "treatment successes"?

Complexity and the consequent need for greater specificity are also apparent at the study level, and can be readily seen in the large variations in effect size found in most meta-analyses. For example, in Smith *et al.* (1980), the overall effect size for the 1,761 effects reviewed was .85 *sd*, but the standard deviation of these effects was 1.25 *sd*, suggesting more variation than consistency: furthermore, in their analyses, means and standard deviations for effect sizes were consistently of the same order of magnitude, no matter how the data were broken down (e.g., type and modality of therapy, client disorder, researcher allegiance), For example in Svartberg and Stiles's (1991) meta-analysis of comparative outcome research with short-term dynamic treatments, the cited advantage of cognitive-behavioral treatments in the treatment of depression reflects the impact of a single study (Gallagher & Thompson, 1982)!

The consistent presence of these large variations within and between studies of the same particular type of therapy points to the importance of contextual factors in determining therapy outcome. Two main sources of these variations will be discussed briefly in this section; a third, researcher allegiance, will be taken up later.

Client Individual Differences. One of the most common themes we found in the review chapters was what we called "treatment contextualization" (see Table 19.1). This refers to reviewers' concerns about nonmanipulated client and situational factors strongly influencing outcome. Clients within particular treatments vary widely in their outcomes, even when they have been selected for diagnostic homogeneity. Some of this inherent heterogeneity can be attributed to comorbidity, the widespread presence of concomitant DSM-III-R Axis I or II disorders. Furthermore, clients with a given diagnosis often present very different clinical patterns (e.g., poor coping skills, negative self-statements, loss issues; Persons, Chapter 13, this volume). These client variations typically result in variations in how and to what degree the treatment is implemented with each client. Along this line, several reviewers underlined the traditional wisdom of strengthening treatments through individualized case formulation (e.g., Allen & Mattson, Chapter 16; Persons, Chapter 13).

Beyond differences in client symptom pattern, other differences in client ideology or coping style may interact systematically with type of treatment. For example, Beutler *et al.* (1991), Shoham-Solomon and Hannah (1991) and others have reported an interaction between client reactance (resistance to influence) and type of treatment. Clients higher in reactance tend to do better in nondirective or paradoxical treatments, while more compliant clients do better in more directive behavioral or cognitive treatments. In this volume, Allen and Mattson's delineation of types of patient–treatment matching effects provides a useful clarification. However, there are many pitfalls in traditional matching research (Snow, 1991), including poor statistical power and failure to replicate.

Therapist Effects. After a number of years of relative neglect, therapist effects have once again captured the attention of therapy researchers (see Crits-Christoph *et al.*, 1991; Lambert, 1989). In a recent meta-analysis, Crits-Christoph *et al.* (1991) found that therapists accounted for an average of about 9% of the variance in 27 separate treatment groups, with very large variations between studies (0–49%); they also found that therapist effects were larger in nonmanualized treatments and in those conducted by less experienced therapists. As a result, Crits-Christoph and Mintz (1991) warn that many treatment effects in the literature may be due to therapist effects instead.

Examining the effects of treatments or client or therapist variables independently of one another is unlikely to be productive. Because different therapies make different demands of clients (Bordin, 1979) and therapists, the interplay between these three factors needs to be studied. A standard strategy for investigating the interplay would be an exploratory or hypothesis-testing investigation of a particular treatment used to treat a particular problem (e.g., Beutler *et al.*, 1991). By contrast, more intensive, discovery-oriented case studies of treatment failures and successes may prove to be a productive strategy, as in Ross's (1981) deviant case analysis or Strupp's (1980) case comparison method. We support the efforts in this direction evidenced in a number of the reviews and predict that these efforts will ultimately prove more clinically useful than interorientation comparative studies.

Shadish and Sweeney (1991) further argue that moderating and mediating situational and methodological variables must be incorporated in any meta-analyses of the relationship between treatment orientation and outcome. It is implausible to suggest that any single variable, such as treatment orientation, is solely responsible for all variation in outcome. In meta-analysis, multivariate model testing is required to produce useful information about when, where, and how therapy works.

Placebo Control Groups and the Need to Be Specific about Nonspecific Effects

A "nonspecific" or "placebo" control cannot be defined except within a particular therapeutic approach (Kazdin, 1991b); that is, it has no general or universal meaning but varies in meaning from one treatment model to another. Your placebo is my active ingredient. That means that if you and I subscribe to different treatment models, we will consistently misunderstand each other if we talk about "placebos" and "nonspecific factors."

In addition, the concepts of placebo and nonspecific factors have numerous conceptual and practical problems (Butler & Strupp, 1986; Lambert, Shapiro, & Bergin, 1986; Parloff, 1986; Wilkins, 1986). In particular, because "placebo effects" in drug research are identified with "psychological effects," the term cannot be translated into psychological discourse without losing its original denotation. In psychology, "placebo effect" has come to refer to some subclass of psychological effect. However, understanding is not advanced without specifying the particular effect, whether it be empathic listening, non-problem-focused group discussion, a credible-sounding rationale, and so on. Once the so-called placebo effect has been specified, there is no longer any point in referring to it as a nonspecific effect.

In addition, the very word *placebo* is pejorative in meaning. When the "placebo" or "nonspecific control" label is applied to, say, client-centered therapy, it is offensive to practitioners within that tradition who regard what they do as built on specific, research-based factors. In the language of the psychotherapy integration movement (Norcross, 1986), these words are "x-rated"; they impair communication across orientations and cause more trouble than they are worth.

An example of this can be found in Giles *et al.*'s chapter, in which they equate traditional therapies with "attention/placebo/nonspecific" factors. Doing this has great rhetorical value: First, it allows them to attach the negative connotations of the word *placebo* to a collection of therapies which they don't like. Second, it then allows them to make the claim that single-case research studies which demonstrate effects in relation to baseline phases provide evidence for the "comparative superiority" of behavioral treatments (T. Giles, personal communication, December 9, 1991). Third, it allows them to claim the generally accepted superiority of specified treatments over so-called placebo controls as further evidence for the comparative effectiveness of behavioral treatments over traditional therapies. In other words, equating nonspecific factors with traditional therapy allows the authors to marshall large sets of additional evidence in support of their case.

Their argument, however, is misleading, because the so-called traditional therapies in fact comprise a wide variety of specific factors; empathy, credibility, transference interpretation, and support have all clear behavioral and experiential referents and are just as specific as systematic desensitization and thought stopping! The claim that traditional therapies consist of nothing but placebo or nonspecific factors is tautological, since nonspecific factors are defined as what goes on in traditional therapies. Single-case and nonspecific control group designs provide useful information about the efficacy and effective ingredients in particular treatments, but they bear little if any evidence for the comparative superiority of prescriptive over traditional therapies.

It also seems clear that the "placebo" label has been applied carelessly in the past, as when Giles *et al.* conflate paraprofessional helping with placebo conditions, citing Strupp and Hadley (1979) as evidence for the equivalence of traditional and placebo therapies.

In an attempt to move the debate ahead, Lambert *et al.* (1986) prefer to speak of "common factors"; however, we find even that to be conceptually sloppy. Instead, in light of the confusions and invidious comparisons engendered, we suggest that the time has come to retire the terms *attention placebo* and *nonspecific factors* from the working vocabularies of psychotherapy researchers. "Placebo" should be restricted to its original context, that is, "pill placebo." "Nonspecific factors," such as empathic listening, reassurance and support, nonproblem-focused group discussion and contact, bibliotherapy/self-help, relaxation training, credible-sounding rationale, and so on, should be specified and studied.

Investigator and Reviewer Allegiance Effects

Investigator Allegiance. Researcher and reviewer allegiance effects still present the most plausible explanation for broad behavioral versus nonbehavioral treatment differences obtained in the literature, or at least cannot be ruled out on the basis of the available evidence. The investigator allegiance problem arises from the following facts:

1. The majority of investigators (in contrast to the majority of practicing clinicians) hold allegiance to behavioral/cognitive treatments.
2. As Giles *et al.* (Chapter 2, this volume) and others have noted, the balance of evidence from controlled comparisons of the kind reported and reviewed in mainstream psychology journals favors behavioral/cognitive treatments.
3. Investigator allegiance to a treatment is often correlated with reports of beneficial outcomes of that treatment, particularly when the investigator has a behavioral orientation (Shadish & Sweeney, 1991).
4. Statistical control for either investigator allegiance or measurement factors associated with allegiance (e.g., reactivity) abolishes the superiority of behavioral/cognitive methods.

To elaborate, in three comparative meta-analytic reviews of the effects of different psychotherapies, researchers' theoretical allegiance (inferred from their reports' introductions or the authors' other writings) has been found to predict the direction and size of the treatment effects obtained (Berman, Miller, & Massman, 1985; Robinson, Berman, & Neimeyer, 1990; Smith *et al.*, 1980).

For example, Robinson *et al.* (1990) reviewed studies of treatment for unipolar depression. They found that two raters' highly reliable judgments of investigators' differential allegiance to one of the compared treatments correlated .58 with the difference in treatment effect size across 30 studies directly comparing different treatments. That is, "therapies that were preferred by the investigator tended to achieve better results than the less favored therapies with which they were compared" (p. 35). A reanalysis using ratings of investigators' previous writings to predict present study effects, carried out to check the possibility that the allegiance shown in the introductions had been influenced by the studies' results, yielded a similar correlation, .51. Taking this a step further, Robinson *et al.* (1990) found that when the effect of researcher allegiance was statistically partialed out, "there remained no evidence for the relative superiority of any one type of therapy" (p. 36).

Two earlier analyses of researcher allegiance effects also turned up statistically significant allegiance effects, but of wildly divergent sizes. On the one hand, a recalculation of the data given in Smith *et al.* (1980) yields a correlation coefficient of only .12 (statistically significant because of the large *n*). On the other hand, Berman *et al.* (1985) also assessed investigator allegiance in their analysis of 15 studies comparing cognitive therapy with systematic desensitization for treatment of a variety of conditions (mainly anxiety disorders). Translating their results into terms comparable with the other two studies yields a very large correlation of .86 (74% of the variance). Obviously the three values cited here are so divergent that averaging them would be misleading. Shadish and Sweeney's (1991) finding that researchers with a behavioral orientation show stronger allegiance effects may help to explain the differences between these three studies.

There are three rival interpretations for these allegiance data: real difference, data bias, and sensitivity/selection bias. The first is that the differences in effectiveness are real, and the differences in allegiance are essentially a consequence of differential effectiveness. Investigators are rational and form their allegiances in the light of the evidence.

A second interpretation is that the apparent superiority of behavioral and cognitive methods is an artifact of investigator's allegiances, to be understood in terms of mediating experimenter effects. Using the formulation of Shadish and Sweeney (1991), methodological factors associated with allegiance may mediate the relationship between treatment orientation and outcome; such mediator variables have hitherto been ignored by meta-analysts.

In their illustrative meta-analysis of marital and family interventions, Shadish and Sweeney (1991) found that mediators of the relationship between behavioral orientation and effect size included treatment standardization and implementation, use of a behavioral dependent measure, and publication status (journal vs. dissertation). Instead of indexing actual treatment differences, the nonequivalence effects cited by Giles *et al.* may in fact be a measure of the behavioral researchers' methodological preferences, especially the use of behavioral dependent measures and manualized and more fully implemented treatments. The resulting problem is one of construct validity, the meaning of the obtained treatment differences (Cook & Campbell, 1979).

A third interpretation is that allegiance motivates researchers to design, carry out, and analyze their studies in such a way as to maximize sensitivity to the effects of the favored therapy. In Shadish and Sweeney's (1991) terms, the apparent superiority of cognitive-behavioral treatments may reflect the operation of moderator variables. For example, behavioral methods were particularly effective in university settings, and particularly ineffective with nonreactive measures. The degree of specificity of outcome measurement was strongly related to effectiveness for behavioral treatments, but not for nonbehavioral treatments. In other words, the obtained interorientation treatment differences are real within the context of the research, but they may not generalize to actual practice situations, having been subtly "selected" from the range and variety of possible effects which might be obtained in such research. Thus, allegiance effects are a problem of external validity.

We suspect that the choice between these three explanations cannot be made on available evidence; in fact, all three may contribute to the relationship between allegiance and outcome. As we see it, investigator allegiance is both powerful and subtle. Thus, we do not suggest that investigators are consciously fudging or misrepresenting their data. On the other hand, designing, implementing, and measuring comparisons of psychotherapies requires hundreds of decisions that can be influenced by an investigator's conceptions of what constitutes each treatment and how its effects may be best realized and measured.

One example is in the selection of measures. Psychotherapeutic approaches carry different ideas about what is an appropriate target for an intervention and consequently how one should assess it. Behavioral approaches tend to see treatment as focused on specific, easily observable behaviors, and to use target symptom measures that assess changes in these behaviors (Shadish & Sweeney, 1991). Such measures tend to produce very large effects, lend themselves to what is called in educational circles as "teaching to the test" (narrowly organizing an intervention around the change measure), and are vulnerable to treatment sensitization effects (Cook & Campbell, 1979) or reactivity effects (Smith *et al.*, 1980).

Psychodynamic treatments, by contrast, tend to see treatment as focused on broad intrapsychic structures that cannot be assessed directly and to favor general life adjustment or personality measures (see Blake *et al.*, Chapter 9, this volume). Such measures tend to produce smaller effect sizes (Smith *et al.*, 1980).

Another example is in the construction of comparison groups. Investigators with an allegiance to one treatment may be likely to design and conduct comparison treatments in ways that are suboptimal from the viewpoint of advocates. This need not be an intentional downgrading. The very fact that an investigator has an allegiance in the first place suggested that in his or her understanding, the competitors are inferior. Comparison groups in allegiance-guided treatment research are like the disfavored stepchild of folklore who is resented and resentful (resentfully demoralized?). Advocates of the favored treatment are likely to have a view of it that is not just more positive, but also more fully implemented, subtle, differentiated, and problem focused, so when they put it into practice it is in fact likely to be more effective than the "step-therapy."

In the few studies where investigators do not have any marked differential allegiance (e.g., Shapiro, Barkham, Hardy, & Morrison, 1990; Shapiro & Firth, 1987; Sloane *et al.*, 1975) or where each treatment is conducted by its own advocates (e.g., Elkin *et al.*, 1989), results tend to show equivalent effectiveness. Perhaps these investigators owe allegiance to equivalent outcomes!

Reviewer Allegiance. A plausible extension of the investigator allegiance effect is the reviewer allegiance effect. Reviewers, like investigators, are faced with many decisions regarding what to include in a review and how to evaluate, summarize, and present evidence, with concomitant opportunities for values to manifest themselves. If there is such an effect, the editor and authors of this book must be considered as candidates.

As he notes, the editor was trained in, has made numerous public commitments to, and has a professional and administrative stake in directive treatments. Most of the chapter reviewers also have training and previous research experience in behavioral or cognitive approaches. Finally, we, too, bear a set of allegiances, best summed up as a commitment to psychotherapy pluralism/integration and research-based understanding of the change processes involved in psychotherapy.

In our review of the subset of chapters in this book, we found numerous examples of reviewer allegiance effects, some of which we have described in previous sections. For example, Blake *et al.* (Chapter 9), in their review of post-traumatic stress disorder research, casually lumped Horowitz *et al.*'s (1984) specific short-term dynamic treatment with less effective conventional or unspecified treatments. We also noted instances in which reviewers went to great pains to single out and discredit studies which went contrary to their theoretical orientation (e.g., Mueser and Glynn's critique (Chapter 14) of Karon and VandenBos, 1972). Giles *et al.* argued almost entirely by selection of favorable examples, citing studies as favorable to behavioral or cognitive approaches on the basis of a single variable (e.g., Shapiro & Firth, 1987) and dismissing or ignoring ties or treatment effects opposite to their theoretical preference (e.g., the better showing of interpersonal therapy with more depressed clients in Elkin *et al.*, 1989; Giles, personal communication, December 8, 1991). Finally, large areas of research on nonbehavioral treatments were dismissed out of hand in the reviews. Virtually all reviewers ignored the evidence of effectiveness provided by nonbehavioral uncontrolled group and case study research, while a number cited behavioral single-case studies in a favorable manner (e.g., Persons, Chapter 13). Sadly, such exercise of double standards has a long history in our field (see Shapiro & Shapiro, 1977).

We suspect that the definitive word on the role of researcher and reviewer allegiance effects cannot be made on the basis of the available evidence. Partialing out allegiance over the narrow range that is sampled in a literature largely devoid of studies whose authors' allegiance is to dynamic and experiential therapies cannot tell us what the results would look like, were there similar numbers of authors holding allegiance to all the methods under comparison. In the absence of such true deconfounding of allegiance and treatment method, the adherents of behavioral and cognitive methods can simply assert that their allegiance is based on the evidence. Only by removing the manifest bias in the literature can the comparative outcome question be advanced.

While we certainly see the need for more research by adherents of nonbehavioral methods, we would like to suggest more powerful strategies for working with allegiance problems. One possibility is a much greater use of collaborative, "blended family" research in which behavioral/cognitive researchers and researchers of other traditions work together to design and carry out studies whose methods and results will be acceptable to both parties. Another possibility is incorporating a "dialectical" reviewing process in future disorder-based treatment reviews, with reviewers of at least two different theoretical persuasions asked to carry out parallel reviews of treatment outcome literatures and to comment on each other's reviews.

Refining the Concepts of Equivalence and Nonequivalence

It has become increasingly clear that the key concepts in the equivalence debate, "equivalence" and "nonequivalence," stand in need of considerable refinement. What does it mean to say that two treatments are equally effective? What does it mean to say that one treatment is more effective that the other? It is our view that the resulting lack of conceptual clarity is partly to blame for the widely diverging interpretations of the same therapy outcome literature and that more precise definitions are essential for further progress in this field.

As noted earlier, the equivalence position is a null hypothesis. Meehl (1978, 1990) has forcefully pointed out that it is very unlikely that the difference between any two treatments on any variable is exactly zero; finding a significant difference between any two treatments on any variable is simply a matter of conducting a sufficiently powerful test (e.g., a large enough *n*).

From a logical point of view, it might be more valid to assert that *no* therapies were equivalent. That is, each therapy case is unique in terms of a variety of factors. These include the precise pattern of client presenting problems, client and therapist background and personal characteristics, actual implementation of the treatment, as well as its effects across problems and time. In fact, this is just a restatement of Paul's (1967) specificity "litany."

We are thus under no illusion about the fact that virtually all specific no-difference results in the therapy literature, whether they be individual primary research studies or meta-analyses, may be simply artifacts of small sample size (Kazdin & Bass, 1989)! *All* types of treatments used to treat a specific disorder can be shown to differ in their effectiveness, given enough time and resources to collect the data.

The important question then becomes whether actual differences between treatments are large enough to be *clinically* significant, since neither researchers nor practicing therapists wish to waste their time dealing with trivial effects. Jacobson, Follette, and Revensdorf (1984), Nietzel, Russell, Hemmings, and Gretter (1987), and others have proposed specific statistical criteria for evaluating the clinical significance of the effects of particular treatments. These criteria can be extended to comparisons between treatments, but a more straightforward approach may be that of equivalency testing.

Rogers, Howard, and Vessey (in press), building in part on earlier work by Cook and Campbell (1979) and others, present a fascinating set of methods for "proving the null hypothesis." This approach, known as "equivalency testing," was developed by biostatisticians for evaluating the equivalence of experimental drugs. These methods have great relevance for evaluating claims regarding the equivalence or nonequivalence of different therapies:

> . . . this procedure is used to determine whether two groups are sufficiently near each other to be considered equivalent. Equivalency testing is appropriate when the investigator is able to specify a small, non-zero difference between two treatments that would serve to define an "equivalence interval" around a difference of zero (e.g., +/−10%). Any difference small enough to fall within that equivalence interval would be considered clinically and/or practically unimportant. (Rogers *et al.*, in press, p. 5).

Using the now-familiar metric of effect size, Rogers *et al.* (in press) go on to suggest Cohen's (1988) "+/−.2 *sd*" definition of a small effect size as one reasonable for their equivalency boundary, for "the minimum value considered to be substantively important" (p. 7).

Rogers *et al.* then use this approach to reanalyze Robinson *et al.*'s (1990) meta-analysis of therapies of depression (values controlled for researcher allegiance). They argue that if the obtained effect size can be shown to be significantly smaller than +/−.2 *sd*, then the difference is too small to be clinically important, and a verdict of equivalency should be returned. In their reanalysis, they found that the four comparisons Robinson *et al.* carried out between psychotherapy (including both "general verbal" and cognitive-behavioral treatments) and drug treatments all met the criteria for equivalence. However, they found that comparisons between "verbal" and cognitive and behavioral therapies were equivocal; that is, there was so much variability in the data that neither equivalence nor nonequivalence could be inferred.

Finally, Rogers *et al.* note that with a large enough sample it is perfectly possible for two treatments to be *both* significantly different and significantly equivalent, that is, trivially different. In fact, they note that instead of two different verdicts in the redefined equivalence–nonequivalence debate, there are four (p. 28):

- *Different*: statistically different but not statistically equivalent
- *Equivalent*: statistically equivalent but not statistically different
- *Trivially different*: both statistically different and statistically equivalent
- *Equivocal*: neither statistically equivalent nor statistically different

It is worth noting that Rogers *et al.*'s effect size lower limit of .2 *sd* may be unreasonably small, in that one could readily argue that social science research in general and psychotherapy research in particular should be concerned with effects which are at least "medium" in size. In fact, as Cohen (1988) notes, an effect size of .2 accounts for only about 1% of the variance and involves an 85% overlap in distributions between the two groups. If psychotherapy research is an applied field, then surely we want to concern ourselves with larger effects than that! Thus, we suggest that the lower limit for substantive equivalence be set at an effect size of .4, which accounts for about 4% of the variance and involves a 73% overlap in distributions. (An alternative would be to adopt a "medium" effect size of .5, which involves an effect still only accounting for roughly 6% of the variance and a 67% overlap in distributions. However, .4 *sd* offers a reasonable compromise.)

Applying our revised criterion to Robinson *et al.*'s (1990) results, the allegiance-controlled comparison between "general verbal therapy" and cognitive, behavioral, and cognitive-behavioral treatments would remain equivocal, while the three directive therapies would meet the statistical equivalency criterion at the .05 probability level, as would the drug–cognitive therapy comparison. These treatments could then be said to be more equivalent than the general verbal therapies studied.

Suggested Criteria for Substantive Nonequivalence. In quantitative terms, what evidence would satisfy us that the outcomes of two treatment methods for a given disorder meaningfully differ from one another ("substantive nonequivalence")? Substantive nonequivalence has to be dependable in statistical terms, but also of sufficient magnitude to be relevant to practical decisions, such as the design of treatment services, the training of therapists, and treatment recommendations for individual clients. Since no single study is a sufficient basis for inferring substantive nonequivalence, the criterion must be a meta-analytic one. We would thus require an average effect size over a sufficient number and quality of independent studies that (1) is statistically reliable (i.e., allows rejection of the statistical null hypothesis), (2) fails an equivalency test (i.e., mean difference between treatments not statistically significantly less than .4 sd), and (3) yields absolute differences in mean posttreatment values sufficient for reliable clinical change (Jacobson *et al.*, 1984); (4) nonequivalence must be obtained even in the presence of controls for allegiance effects (either through the study design or statistical).

Recommended Criteria for Substantive Equivalence. What evidence would indicate that two treatment methods are meaningfully equal in effectiveness ("substantive equivalence")? Strict criteria must be employed here as well, including the following: (1) There would have to be a meta-analytic average effect size over a sample of studies large enough to be statistically significantly less than the proposed difference of .4 *sd*; (2) average differences between treatments on mean posttreatment values would have to be trivially small from a practical point of view (less than the reliable clinical change range—e.g., 5 points on the BDI); (3) controls for investigator allegiance should also be implemented in the meta-analysis. Note that this definition of substantive equivalence would encompass Rogers and colleagues' (in press) "trivially different" verdict (mean difference between treatments significantly greater than zero and less than .4 *sd*).

At the present time we expect that these two sets of criteria would yield equivocal (i.e., neither equivalent nor nonequivalent) verdicts on most disorder-specific comparisons. In other words, in most cases, too little is known to justify either an equivalence or a nonequivalence verdict. Nevertheless, although they may sound stringent, we believe these criteria to be capable of demonstrating nonequivalence and equivalence in well-developed areas of comparative therapy research, and certainly to show nonequivalence between a well-developed treatment and a category of "unspecified treatments" (although such a comparison would be of greater methodological than substantive interest).

Broader Issues in the Equivalence Debate

As we have read selected chapters from this book and thought about and discussed the various technical and methodological issues raised by the equivalence debate, we have repeatedly encountered a set of broader issues involving the epistemology, ethics, and professional aspects of psychotherapy research, an enterprise to which we have each devoted most of our professional lives. We are aware that some of these issues are not usually raised in this debate, but we have come to see that it would be a mistake not to make them explicit.

Epistemology and Psychotherapy Research

Epistemology is the area of philosophy which is devoted to understanding the nature and sources of knowledge (e.g., Hamlyn, 1970). No science can proceed without an agreed-upon epistemological position, although the degree to which that position is made explicit may vary from discipline to discipline, and from time to time over the development of a given discipline. Epistemological assumptions are most often articulated and debated at times of uncertainty and change.

Over the years, psychotherapy researchers have adopted and refined an epistemological position in the form of a set of procedures for developing knowledge claims and evaluating their truth. This "received view" includes the traditional principles of measurement, experimental design, and data summarization and inference. These procedures have been very helpful in establishing the identity and credibility of psychotherapy research and for establishing the general efficacy of psychotherapy, but they have sometimes had a limiting effect on what could be studied, how it could be studied, and, ultimately, what kinds of knowledge could be obtained.

This is as true for the reviewers in this volume as it is within the mainstream of psychological research more generally. Guided by a correspondence theory of truth (see Hamlyn, 1970), cognitive/behavioral researchers have largely abandoned historical or nonexperimental case study methods, as is clear from the reviews we looked at. Collection of verbal data and open, thematic procedures of data analysis have also been ignored in favor of quantitative behavioral observation or psychometrically constructed questionnaires. Clients' experiences of what helped them in therapy have been regarded as suspect compared to experimental manipulation of treatment conditions.

Over the past 10 years, however, many psychological, educational, and medical researchers have become dissatisfied with the limitations of these ways of defining and developing knowledge (for a survey, see Lincoln, 1989). Some, such as Lincoln and Guba (1990), have called for an abandonment of the traditional methods of experimentation and quantification; others have simply proposed methodological pluralism, a broadening of the range of methods and subject matter (e.g., Patton, 1990; Polkinghorne, 1983).

Our purpose here is certainly not to advocate for one approach to research over another. For example, in our experience, advocates of the new research paradigm are often long on rhetoric and "positivism-bashing" and short on concrete, practical demonstrations of alternatives. Instead, we are pointing out that issues about how we do our science have been opened up and need to be addressed by those involved with psychotherapy research.

Let us take as an example, the chapter on posttraumatic stress disorder (PTSD) by Blake *et al.* (Chapter 9, this volume). In our view, this is a thoughtful, well-written, reasonably balanced review. It shows that there is now good evidence that behavioral treatments, particularly systematic desensitization and flooding, can significantly reduce certain symptoms of PTSD, especially those involving hyperarousal and anxiety.

Nevertheless, the clear impression left by the review is that there has been little research of any sort on nonbehavioral treatments of PTSD. As one important facet of this, all of the cited case reports are behaviorally oriented, in spite of the fact that there is a substantial body of psychoanalytic and other psychodynamic case reports on survivors of war, the Nazi Holocaust, child abuse, natural disasters, and other traumas (for some examples of psychoanalytic successes, see Lindy *et al.*, 1988). Along the same line, several reviewers (e.g., Kaplan & Busner, Chapter 6, this volume) make references to excluding studies which do not include control groups; given the context of normative information provided by existing research, such exclusions are now arbitrary and unnecessary.

The central point here is that qualitative and case study methods are just as "empirical" as received-view methods, in the ordinary, original sense of utilizing practical experience. These alternative methods have standards, which, while different, are not necessarily less rigorous than the traditional methods (e.g., Lather, 1986; Lincoln & Guba, 1990; Mishler, 1990; Stiles, in press; Sullivan, 1984).

Unlike some radical critics, we do not see the value in abandoning traditional research and standards; instead, we are advocating a thoughtful consideration of the range of methods and standards. As we see it, this requires two kinds of effort:

first, an examination of the assumptions and truth criteria in both traditional and emerging research genres (e.g., Stiles, in press); second, a clearer articulation of the relationships between research questions and research methods, and the relative place of both qualitative-narrative and quantitative-experimental research methods.

Ethics, Clinical Practice, and Psychotherapy Research

As Lincoln and Guba (1985) and others (e.g., Rappoport, 1977) have pointed out, most of us have been trained in the received view of science as a value-free enterprise. In the process of preparing this chapter, however, the moral and ethical overtones of psychotherapy research and the equivalence debate have been brought firmly home to us (see Imber *et al.*, 1986, for a discussion of other ethical issues in psychotherapy research).

Giles (personal communication, December 9, 1991) has pointed out that there is a real ethical danger in inflicting second-rate or inferior care on large numbers of suffering individuals when clearly more effective treatments are available. There is an additional danger in making public pronouncements which might discourage practicing therapists from learning about or taking seriously data which show that a particular treatment is more effective than some other treatment.

We find it surprising to be considered responsible for indirectly causing harm to clients by supporting lax standards of care. As we noted earlier, our interest was not in advocating equivalence but in understanding the issues raised by it and encouraging better, more specific research, for the ultimate benefit of clients. Nevertheless, this experience has helped us to clarify a complementary set of ethical issues. Harking back to our discussion of epistemological issues, what knowledge claims do we see as justified by the current state of psychotherapy research? More concretely, what should researchers say to therapists? What should clinicians say when asked to recommend a treatment for a given disorder?

First, it seems quite reasonable to say to practicing therapists and potential clients that specific empirically tested treatments X and Y appear to be effective for disorder A in a majority of cases. This knowledge claim can be made for a number of treatments for most disorders, but it cannot by any means be made about any or all treatments.

Second, on the basis of our current state of knowledge, it is also reasonable to recommend against alternatives such as no treatment, staying on a waiting list for an extended period of time, or taking part in an apparently irrelevant treatment such as a discussion group (i.e., a so-called placebo therapy). The effectiveness of many specified treatments against these alternatives is well established.

Third, if, on the other hand, we, like Persons (Chapter 13, this volume) were asked to recommend between specific time-limited cognitive, interpersonal, psychodynamic, or experiential therapy or tricyclic antidepressant treatments for clinical depression, what would be the most ethical thing to do? If this were a multiple-choice question, we might offer the following alternatives for consideration:

a. Recommend the tricyclics strongly because they are faster, equally effective, and less expensive than the psychotherapies.

b. Recommend cognitive therapy or tricyclics strongly and warn the client or therapist to avoid the other treatments because there is less research showing their effectiveness.
c. Recommend them all and tell the person that it is a matter of personal taste and seeing what works for the individual client.
d. Recommend cognitive, interpersonal, and pharmacological therapies moderately because there is a body of literature on each, and tell the person that not much is known about the effectiveness of psychodynamic and experiential treatments.
e. Evaluate the person's style, ideology, and previous treatment history and then make one or two recommendations to the person, explaining your reasoning and the state of knowledge about each.

While we realize that different readers will view these alternatives in different ways, we are troubled by the ethics of making strong recommendations between treatments for which there exist at least some positive efficacy. Our point is that, for depression, there is not yet an adequate scientific basis for strong, precise differential treatment recommendations. It is not at all clear to us that such recommendations would substantially increase the probability of success for particular clients.

At the same time, making strong blanket recommendations may also be ethically questionable because of the large variation in outcome for all existing treatments of depression, and because of the danger of raising unrealistic expectations. Knowing how important therapist effects are, we might do better to recommend a therapist we know to be generally good with depressed clients, regardless of the brand of therapy he or she does. Or we might quickly gain the impression that the pattern of symptoms presented by this potential client would best be treated in, say, cognitive therapy, and recommend on that basis (see Persons, Chapter 13, this volume). Blanket treatment recommendations also pose the ethical danger of depriving clients of a treatment which they might find to be particularly effective, or subjecting them to treatments which "go against the grain" or which they have previously tried unsuccessfully.

Professional Issues: Using Our Differences More Productively

Differences between Treatment Orientations. One of our main concerns in writing this chapter is what we see as a set of continuing dysfunctional relationships. We have been most occupied with the adversarial relationship between those (almost always of a behavioral or cognitive persuasion) who take a strong nonequivalence interpretation of the results of comparative outcome research, and those (usually researchers of a psychodynamic or humanistic persuasion) who support an equivalence position.

While such adversarial relationships have their value during early or "school" phases of scientific development, and may help get all the issues out on the table in a process of interorientation dialogue, they can also become counterproductive. Such continuing conflicts tend to force all parties into polarized, exaggerated, rigid, and defensive scientific and professional positions, positions which neither facilitate the accumulation of knowledge nor serve our clients well. Furthermore, there are now forums (e.g., *Journal of Psychotherapy Integration*) which make it possible for researchers from different theoretical orientations to discuss their differences in an open, self-reflective manner.

Differences between Researchers and Therapists. The other dysfunctional relationship has been well documented in the literature (e..g, Barlow, Hayes, & Nelson, 1984; Kazdin, 1991a; Morrow-Bradley & Elliott, 1986). As in every problematic relationship, there are two sides to the rift between researchers and practicing therapists. On the one hand, researchers blame therapists for not utilizing research findings and for being biased, irresponsible, or antiscientific. We caught hints of this attitude in some of the chapters we reviewed (e.g., Kaplan & Busner, Chapter 6, this volume). On the other hand, therapists blame researchers for not researching the treatments or populations therapists work with (Kazdin, 1991a; Morrow-Bradley & Elliott, 1986) and for being "scientistic," boring, and irrelevant.

Such mutual blaming sounds to us like a bad marriage in which there is a history of mutual hurt and injury, and it raises the question of whether any accommodation is possible. One possibility is to recognize and accept the fact that researchers and therapists live in different realities and they should therefore stop trying to change each other.

If researchers are not happy with this course of action, they might begin by trying to understand the resistance to therapist utilization of research findings and what if any positive incentives exist for narrowing the gap. Trainees and practitioners may resist research findings because they believe that research is not a search for understanding but a procedure for justifying theoretical allegiances. We touched on another resistance earlier when we described differences between the styles and criteria of research favored by adherents of differing therapeutic orientations.

Thus, one way to reaffirm the favored scientist-practitioner model of clinical training would be to broaden our vision of science to include both traditional experimental or received-view research *and* qualitative methods, critical inquiry, and narrative forms of explanation, as a means of training practitioners who do research and researchers who practice. Incentives to integrate research and practice may come only from persuading researchers that they will be better researchers if they make use of their clinical skills and from helping therapists to see how they may become better therapists if they become more involved in research.

Summary

To sum up our analysis of central issues raised by the reviews in this volume: We suggest that the prescriptive versus traditional therapy distinction is not a useful one, and we argue that the debate about which treatments are *generally* more effective for all disorders should be replaced by a series of smaller-scale discussions about the specific effects of specific treatments on specific types of clients.

To this end, we have suggested the need for continued disorder- or problem-focused treatment outcome research, coupled with more intensive investigation of client and therapist individual differences and in-therapy processes aimed at identifying how and when change occurs, in order to improve treatments. Furthermore, we agree with several of the reviewers (e.g., Blake *et al.*, Chapter 9, this volume) in recommending research on a broader range of treatments more representative of actual treatment practice, with the added suggestion that this research be carried out in collaboration with adherents of these treatments. In addition, where appropriate, we advocate the use of a set of specific criteria based on biometric equivalency tests for determining whether two treatments are equivalent or nonequivalent.

Finally, we tried to explicate some of the underlying issues in the controversy, including how we go about developing knowledge about the effectiveness of different psychotherapies, the practical and ethical implications of the existing body of psychotherapy research, and the nature of the professional–scientific relationships researchers of different therapeutic orientations have with each other and with practicing therapists.

ACKNOWLEDGMENTS. We thank Tom Giles, Les Greenberg, David P. Knight, and Margaret O'Dougherty Wright for very helpful discussions of the issues dealt with in this chapter.

References

Afari, N., Hayes, S. C., Wilson, K., McCurry, S. M., & Taylor, N. (1991, July). *Acceptance and commitment therapy as a treatment for emotional avoidance in agoraphobics*. Paper presented at the meeting of the Society for Psychotherapy Research, Lyon, France.

Barlow, D. H., Hayes, S. C., & Nelson, R. O. (Eds.). (1984). *The scientist practitioner: Research and accountability in clinical and educational settings*. New York: Pergamon Press.

Berman, J., Miller, R. C., & Massman, P. J. (1985). Cognitive therapy versus systematic desensitization: Is one treatment superior? *Psychological Bulletin, 97*, 451–461.

Beutler, L. E., & Clarkin, J. F. (1990). *Systematic treatment selection: Toward targeted therapeutic interventions*. New York: Brunner/Mazel.

Beutler, L. E., Engle, D., Mohr, D., Daldrup, R. J., Began, J., Meredith, K., & Merry, W. (1991). Predictors of differential response to cognitive, experiential, and self-directed psychotherapeutic procedures. *Journal of Consulting and Clinical Psychology, 59*, 333–340.

Bordin, E. S. (1979). The generalizability of the psychoanalytic concept of working alliance. *Psychotherapy: Theory, Research and Practice, 16*, 252–260.

Butler, S. F., & Strupp, H. H. (1986). Specific and nonspecific factors in psychotherapy: A problematic paradigm for psychotherapy research. *Psychotherapy, 23*, 30–40.

Cohen, J. (1988). *Statistical power analysis for the behavioral sciences* (2nd ed.). Hillsdale, NJ: Erlbaum.

Cook, T. D., & Campbell, D. T. (1979). *Quasi-experimentation: Design and analysis issues for field settings*. Chicago: Rand McNally.

Crits-Christoph, P., Baranackie, K., Kurcias, J. S., Beck, A. T., Carroll, K., Perry, K., Luborsky, L., McLellan, A. T., Woody, G. E., Thompson, L., Gallagher, D., & Zitrin, C. (1991). Meta-analysis of therapist effects in psychotherapy outcome studies. *Psychotherapy, 1*, 81–91.

Crits-Christoph, P., & Mintz, J. (1991). Implications of therapist effects for the design and analysis of comparative studies of psychotherapies. *Journal of Consulting and Clinical Psychology, 59*, 20–26.

Elkin, I., Shea, T., Watkins, J. T., Imber, S. D., Sotsky, S. M., Collins, J. F., Glass, D. R., Pilkonis, P. A., Leber, W. R., Docherty, J. P., Fiester, S. J., Parloff, M. B. (1989). National Institute of Mental Health Treatment of Depression Collaborative Research Program: General effectiveness of treatments. *Archives of General Psychiatry, 46*, 971–982.

Elliott, R., & Anderson, C. (in press). Simplicity and complexity in psychotherapy research. In R. L. Russell (Ed.), *Psychotherapy research: Assessing and redirecting the tradition*. Plenum.

Elliott, R., Clark, C., Wexler, M., Kemeny, V., Brinkerhoff, J., & Mack, C. (1990). The impact of experiential therapy on depression: Initial results. In G. Lietaer, J. Rombauts, & R. Van Balen (Eds.), *Client-centered and experiential psychotherapy towards the nineties* (pp. 549–577). Leuven, Belgium: Leuven University Press.

Gallagher, D. E., & Thompson. L. W. (1982). Treatment of major depressive disorder in older adult outpatients with brief psychotherapies. *Psychotherapy: Theory, Research and Practice, 19*, 482–490.

Goldstein, A. P., & Stein, N. (1976). *Prescriptive psychotherapies*. New York: Pergamon Press.

Greenberg, L. S., Rice, L. N., & Elliott, R. (1993). *Facilitating emotional change: The moment-by-moment process*. New York: Guilford Press.

Greenberg, L. S., & Webster, M. (1982). Resolving decisional conflict by means of two-chair dialogue: Relating process to outcome. *Journal of Counseling Psychology, 29*, 468–477.

Hamlyn, D. W. (1970). *The theory of knowledge*. Garden City, NY: Anchor Books.

Horowitz, M. J., Weiss, D. S., Kaltreider, N., Krupnick, J., Marmar, C., Wilner, N., & DeWitt, K. (1984). Reactions to the death of a parent: Results from patients and field subjects. *Journal of Nervous and Mental Disease, 172*, 383–392.

Imber, S. D., Glanz, L. M., Elkin, I., Sotsky, S. M., Boyer, J. L., & Leber, W. R. (1986). Ethical issues in psychotherapy research: Problems in a collaborative clinical trials study. *American Psychologist, 41*, 137–146.

Jacobson, N. S., Follette, W. C., & Revenstorf, D. (1984). Psychotherapy outcome research: Methods for reporting variability and evaluating clinical significance. *Behavior Therapy, 15*, 336–352.

Karon, B. P., & VandenBos, G. R. (1972). The consequences of psychotherapy for schizophrenic patients. *Psychotherapy: Theory, Research & Practice, 9*, 111–119.

Kazdin, A. E. (1991a). Effectiveness of psychotherapy with children and adolescents. *Journal of Consulting and Clinical Psychology, 59*, 785–798.

Kazdin, A. E. (1991b). *Research design in clinical psychology* (2nd ed.). Elmsford, NY: Pergamon Press.

Kazdin, A. E., & Bass, D. (1989). Power to detect differences between alternative treatments in comparative psychotherapy outcome research. *Journal of Consulting and Clinical Psychology, 57*, 138–147.

Lambert, M. J. (1989). The individual therapist's contribution to psychotherapy process and outcome. *Clinical Psychology Review, 9*, 469–486.

Lambert, M. J., Shapiro, D. A., & Bergin, A. E. (1986). The effectiveness of psychotherapy. In S. L. Garfield & A. E. Bergin (Eds.), *Handbook of psychotherapy and behavior change* (3rd ed., pp. 157–211). New York: Wiley.

Lather, P. (1986). Issues of validity in openly ideological research: Between a rock and soft place. *Interchange, 17*, 63–84.

Lincoln, Y. (1989). Trouble in the land: The paradigm revolution in the academic disciplines. *Higher education: Handbook of theory and research, 5*, 57–133.

Lincoln, Y., & Guba, E. G. (1985). *Naturalistic inquiry*. Beverly Hills, CA: Sage.

Lincoln, Y. S., & Guba, E. G. (1990). Judging the quality of case study reports. *Qualitative Studies in Education, 3*, 53–59.

Lindy, J. D., with Green, B. L., Grace, M. C., MacLeod, J. A., & Spitz, L. (1988). *Vietnam: A casebook*. New York: Brunner/Mazel.

Luborsky, L. (1984). *Principles of psychoanalytic psychotherapy: A manual for supportive-expressive treatment*. New York: Basic Books.

Meehl, P. E. (1978). Theoretical risks and tabular asterisks: Sir Karl, Sir Ronald, and the slow progress of soft psychology. *Journal of Consulting and Clinical Psychology, 46*, 806–834.

Meehl, P. E. (1990). Appraising and amending theories: The strategy of Lakatosian defense and two principles that warrant it. *Psychological Inquiry, 1*, 108–141.

Mishler, E. G. (1990). Validation in inquiry guided research: The role of exemplars in narrative studies. *Harvard Educational Review, 60*, 415–442.

Morrow-Bradley, C., & Elliott, R. (1986). The utilization of psychotherapy research by practicing psychotherapists. *American Psychologist, 41*, 188–197.

Nietzel, M. T., Russell, R. L., Hemmings, K. A., & Gretter, M. L. (1987). Clinical significance of psychotherapy for unipolar depression: A meta-analytic approach to social comparison. *Journal of Consulting and Clinical Psychology, 55*, 156–160.

Norcross, J. C. (Ed.). (1986). *Handbook of eclectic psychotherapy*. New York: Brunner/Mazel.

Parloff, M. B. (1986). Placebo controls in psychotherapy research: A sine qua non or a placebo for research problems? *Journal of Consulting and Clinical Psychology, 54*, 79–87.

Patton, M. Q. (1990). *Qualitative evaluation and research methods* (2nd ed.). Beverly Hills, CA: Sage.

Paul, G. L. (1967). Strategy of outcome research in psychotherapy. *Journal of Consulting Psychology, 31*, 109–118.

Polkinghorne, D. (1983). *Methodology for the human sciences*. Albany, NY: SUNY Press.

Propst, L. R., Ostrom, R., Watkins, P., Dean, T., & Mashburn, D. (1992). Comparative efficacy of religious and nonreligious cognitive-behavioral therapy for the treatment of clinical depression in religious individuals. *Journal of Consulting and Clinical Psychology, 60*, 94–103.

Rappoport, J. (1977). *Community psychology: Values, research and action*. New York: Holt, Rinehart & Winston.

Rice, L. N., & Greenberg, L. (Eds.). (1984). *Patterns of change*. New York: Guilford Press.

Robinson, L. A., Berman, J. S., & Neimeyer, R. A. (1990). Psychotherapy for the treatment of depression: A comprehensive review of controlled outcome research. *Psychological Bulletin, 108*, 30–49.

Rogers, J. L., Howard, K. I., & Vessey, J. T. (in press). Using significance tests to evaluate equivalence between two experimental groups. *Psychological Bulletin.*

Ross, A. O. (1981). Of rigor and relevance. *Professional Psychology, 12*, 319–327.

Shadish, W. R., Jr., & Sweeney, R. B. (1991). Mediators and moderators in meta-analysis: There's a reason we don't let dodo birds tell us which psychotherapists should have prizes. *Journal of Consulting and Clinical Psychology, 59*, 883–893.

Shapiro, D. A., Barkham, M., Hardy, G. E., & Morrison, L. A. (1990). The Second Sheffield Psychotherapy Project: Rationale, design and preliminary outcome data. *British Journal of Medical Psychology, 63*, 97–108.

Shapiro, D. A., & Firth, J. (1987). Prescriptive vs. exploratory psychotherapy: Outcomes of the Sheffield psychotherapy project. *British Journal of Psychiatry, 151*, 790–799.

Shapiro, D. A., & Shapiro, D. (1977). The "double standard" in the evaluation of psychotherapies. *Bulletin of the British Psychological Society, 30*, 209–210.

Shoham-Solomon, V., & Hannah, M. T. (1991). Treatment interaction in the study of differential change processes. *Journal of Consulting and Clinical Psychology, 59*, 217–232.

Sloane, R. B., Staples, F. R., Cristol, A. H., Yorkston, N. J., & Whipple, K. (1975). *Psychotherapy versus behavior therapy*. Cambridge: Harvard University Press.

Smith, M. L., Glass, G. V., & Miller, T. I. (1980). *The benefits of psychotherapy*. Baltimore: The Johns Hopkins University Press.

Snow, R. E. (1991). Aptitude-treatment interaction as a framework for research on individual differences in psychotherapy. *Journal of Consulting and Clinical Psychology, 59*, 205–216.

Stiles, W. B. (in press). Quality control in qualitative research. *Clinical Psychology Review.*

Stiles, W. B., Shapiro, D. A., & Elliott, R. (1986). "Are all psychotherapies equivalent?" *American Psychologist, 41*, 165–180.

Strupp, H. H. (1980). Success and failure in time-limited psychotherapy. *Archives of General Psychiatry, 37*, 595–603.

Strupp, H. H., & Hadley, S. W. (1979). Specific versus nonspecific factors in psychotherapy: A controlled study of outcome. *Archives of General Psychiatry, 36*, 1125–1136.

Sullivan, E. V. (1984). *A critical psychology: Interpretation of the personal world*. New York: Plenum.

Svartberg, M., & Stiles, T. C. (1991). Comparative effects of short-term psychodynamic psychotherapy: A meta-analysis. *Journal of Consulting and Clinical Psychology, 59*, 704–714.

Wilkins, W. (1986). Placebo problems in psychotherapy research. *American Psychologist, 41*, 551–556.

20

Consumer Advocacy and Effective Psychotherapy

The Managed Care Alternative

Thomas R. Giles

It may be anticipated that psychoanalysts will disregard these findings as blissfully as they have in the past disregarded other criticisms of their theories and methods.
Wolpe, 1959, p. 233

Failure to provide exposure with response prevention for obsessive–compulsive disorder is unethical.
E. Foa (personal communication, cited from Meredith and Milby, 1980)

But a more serious development is the realization that many clinicians are not even influenced by clinical research findings, resorting instead to a trial-and-error eclectism in their clinical practice.
Barlow, 1981, p. 147

One of the sad realities of alcohol treatment has been the sometimes shocking gap between research and practice. The most commonly used and accepted treatment approaches have little or no empirical support. The use of certain methods has persisted long after their ineffectiveness or even harmfulness has been demonstrated. Other more promising approaches have been developed through research over the past 20 years, yet many of these suffer general disuse. If our success in treating problem drinkers has been less than heroic, perhaps in part this has been due to this chasm between empirical evidence and clinical application.
Miller, 1982, p. 15

. . . and, despite the absence of any evidence supporting the efficacy of the approach, 75% of 196 therapist members of the American Association for Marriage and Family Therapy, when surveyed, choose individual psychotherapy or family therapy over behavioral conditioning as the treatment of choice for bedwetting.
Kaplan and Busner, Chapter 6, this volume

Thomas R. Giles • Associates in Managed Care, Denver, Colorado 80231.

Handbook of Effective Psychotherapy, edited by Thomas R. Giles. Plenum Press, New York, 1993.

The tenacity with which these theories were kept alive in the analytic community . . . despite the fact that their therapeutic application did not improve the patient's condition, reflects the strength of an ideological structure disregarding clinical facts.

American Psychiatric Association, 1989, p. 511

It remains striking . . . that the vast majority of patients admitted to private psychiatric hospitals have no opportunity even to be considered for any behavior therapy.

Dickerson, 1989, p. 158

As of 1986, several hundred different psychotherapies had been developed (Garfield, 1989) despite insufficient empirical support for the bulk of this proliferation. This disparity between research and practice might have been more alarming to professionals had it not been for the mitigating influence of the equivalence of therapies hypothesis (Giles, 1983). According to this point of view (see Chapter 2, this volume), all treatments, due to common inclusion of nonspecific elements, yield the same results regardless of the particulars of client or therapist variables, disorders, manners of implementation, or additive combinations of therapeutic techniques.

Although this hypothesis makes palatable the startling profusion of techniques, other, less suitable consequences result. These were summarized in Wilson and Rachman's (1983) commentary on the initial findings of meta-analysis:

> The reassurance that can be derived from the claimed benefits of psychotherapy may prove to be less sweet than expected; . . . For example, there was no relation between therapeutic effect size and duration of treatment, experience of the therapist, diagnosis of the client, or form of therapy (group vs. individual). Where did these results leave the elaborate theories, the rigorous selection of suitable patients, the extended courses of treatment, the lengthy and demanding training of therapists, the prestigious and well-endowed training institutes, the emphasis placed upon experience and expertise, the honors accorded to the experts, and the patients? (pp. 62–63)

Much of the available data suggest that Wilson and Rachman's warnings *per se* present only minor concern. The reviews in this handbook, for example, indicate that the equivalence of therapies hypothesis is invalid and that certain techniques indeed provide an influence relevant to the outcome of care. Professional surveys (e.g., Garfield and Kurtz, 1976; Norcross, Prochaska, and Gallagher, 1989; Smith, 1982), however, indicate that only a minority of psychotherapists use empirical results to guide their practices. Most therapists are eclectics (e.g., Garfield, 1989). Dynamic intervention remains the primary training orientation for psychiatric residents (Wolpe, 1990), and it is rare to observe a graduate school curriculum in which the insight-oriented schools suffer irrepresentation (cf. Giles, 1990a).

A disturbing implication of these findings is that therapies with greatest proven efficacy are not implemented by the majority, or perhaps even a significant minority, of practitioners. This may be due in part to orientations. When a therapist chooses a particular approach, it is not often relinquished in the face of contravening data (Garfield, 1980). Furthermore, the problems of implementation of a new treatment approach apparently are more difficult than previously realized. Backer, Liberman, and Kuehnel (1986), for example, delineated several worrisome limitations of traditional dissemination methods (such as general articles and conferences) relative to interpersonal contact, outside consultation, organizational support, "championship" by agency staff, and adaptability of the innovation.

Motivational factors have also seemed to provide significant contributorship to the utilization problem; that is, until recently the great majority of provider claims were paid on a fee-for-service basis by indemnity insurance carriers. This reimbursement system has been instrumental to the cost explosion of health care in the United States (Giles, 1993; Kiesler & Morton, 1988), encouraging practitioners to provide services which are comparatively lengthy and inefficient. This type of influence is seen in one way or another in several areas of the profession.

The American Psychological Association, for instance, represented primarily by clinicians, has actively resisted the adoption of standards, sanctions, and mandates which would better ensure that practitioners implement effective treatments (e.g., Giles, 1990b; Hayes, 1987). (The *American Psychologist* also has been a principal sounding board for advocates of the equivalence of therapies hypothesis; see Giles, 1990a.) The representative bodies for licensed social workers and board-certified psychiatrists have similarly failed to mandate efficacy standards for the psychotherapeutic practices of these practitioners. There is also a dearth of such requirements—across practitioners—attempting to pass state examinations for licensure or certification.

Although there have been forces countervailing the implementation of comparatively ineffective techniques, these have provided only modest deterrence to date. The ongoing pressure of research, for example, has provided, over the last 30 years, a slow but steady impetus for professional change. The American Psychological Society, formed by the break of Division 25 psychologists from the American Psychological Association, was also an interesting and potentially useful development in that it resulted primarily from the reactance of scientists and scientist-practitioners to the antiempirical bias of the APA (Hayes, 1987). Another development of interest has been the emergence of litigation against clinicians who have implemented comparatively ineffective psychotherapeutic techniques (see Giles, 1990b, for a review).

While these and other developments made a positive impact on the utilization problem, progress, as indicated, remained inadequate. A potentially more effective development, however, may be occurring with the advent of managed mental health care. The remainder of this chapter will detail the history of this development and provide reasons why managed care may soon cause many more psychotherapists to provide empirically validated techniques.

Inflationary Influences

As stated, the fee-for-service payment system contributed in large measure to the cost-containment crisis. Under this arrangement, physicians' earnings are directly related to the provision of more, not less, health care services. This in turn has led in some cases to the overprescription of services, especially those available on an inpatient-only basis. Patients covered by indemnity based (and other) insurance plans also become less likely to make cost-conscious decisions about health care, a phenomenon known as "moral hazard" in the health economics literature (Robinson, 1991).

Fee-for-service encourages overbilling as well. Chrysler Corporation's review of its health claims found that 25% of diagnostic and treatment procedures were inappropriate, due either to incompetence, inefficiency, or "deliberate fraud." The Department of Health, Education and Welfare tagged 47,000 physicians and pharmacists for submitting fraudulent Medicare/Medicaid claims (Califano, 1986).

Economists have long recognized that health care services provide dramatic exception to the law of supply and demand: As the number of providers, on both an inpatient and outpatient basis, increases, so do the aggregate costs of the services they provide. In 1985, for example, there were 30 psychologists and psychiatrists per 1,000 population, ten times greater than in 1950. The total number of licensed mental health professionals (M.D.'s, Ph.D.'s, M.S.W.'s, and R.N.'s) increased from 23,000 in 1947 to 121,000 in 1977 (Mechanic, 1980). Correspondingly, between 1950 and 1976 the number of people in the United States seeking mental health treatment increased by 25% (Kiesler & Morton, 1988).

Robinson and Luft (1987) examined general hospital competition in the United States in 1982. After controlling for wage rates, state regulations, and teaching requirements, these researchers found that hospitals with the greatest competition charged 26% more—for equivalent services—than hospitals which were relatively competition-free. The elimination of the certificate of need for new hospitals during the Reagan administration led to an explosion of hospital beds, both psychiatric and medical, and a consequent rise in inpatient per diem costs. The National Center for Health Statistics reported that 33% of the escalation in health care costs was a result of such increases in services (VandenBos, 1983).

Insurance representatives allege that state mandates for health services also have been inflationary to the extent that they have required coverage of "unnecessary" services such as hair transplants, electrolysis, acupuncture, and excessively long hospital stays. Other contributors include the significant rise in the frequency of medical malpractice claims, leveling off in the mid-1980s to $15 billion per year; an increase in the number of elderly people; technological advances; and an emphasis in the United States upon "catastrophic" (versus preventative) medical care coverage (see Kiesler & Morton, 1988). It is only within the context of such factors, combined with their cost consequences, that the takeover of the provision of mental health services by corporate giants can be adequately understood.

Health Care Costs

Many of the underpinnings of the present crisis began with the introduction of Medicare in 1965, establishing the federal government as a principal payer for a substantial portion of the population. The continued rise in health care costs added heavily to a burden already made enormous by the national debt. In 1965, national health care costs were 6% of the gross national product ($38 billion). By 1982 they had risen to 11% of the GNP ($355 billion) and have since redoubled (Flinn, McMahon, & Collins, 1987). The private sector also bore an enormous burden of health care expenditure during the last 30 years: American corporations currently spend almost 40% of pre-tax profits for health insurance benefits (Califano, 1986).

Health care costs increased by two to three times the national inflation rate over the past decade. Chain hospital beds increased by 37% in the year ending July

1, 1985. In 1986—in the Los Angeles area alone—hospital costs increased by 88% (Cummings, 1987).

The number of Americans seeking health care has increased more than 1,000% over the last 30 years. The top three U.S. automakers spent $3.5 billion in 1984 on health costs, a figure exceeding that which most states received from tax revenues (Ludwigsen & Enright, 1988).

For the decade ending in 1983, cost of inpatient beds rose 20% annually, accounting for more than two-thirds of the Medicare expense alone. In 1967, the U.S. government spent $3 billion on Medicare, an amount which would have lasted only 20 days in 1982 (English *et al.*, 1986). More than one-third of the national health expense is currently paid by the federal government (Flinn, McMahon, & Collins, 1987). Health costs are projected to escalate to 17% of the GNP by the year 2000 (Davies & Felder, 1990).

Health costs are increasing not only as a function of the relative share of the GNP but also at a rate relatively faster than that of other categories of federal spending. The federal government's health expenditures grew 20% from 1987 to 1989. This was faster than Social Security increases (12.4%), interest on the national debt (17.8%), and military spending (5.7%; see Giles, 1993).

The Foster Higgins survey (Foster Higgins, 1989) of more than 1,600 companies found that the mean employee cost for health in 1984 was $1,645, $1,724 in 1986, and $2,354 in 1988. Only small variations in costs were due to geography, type of industry, or size of employer group. (For further review of the implications of this crisis, see Giles, 1993.)

Mental Health Care Costs

Mental health expenditures comprise the third most expensive category of health costs in the United States (Mechanic, 1980). They have also tended to rise more quickly than health costs over the past 10 years: 40% increases per annum have not been uncommon (Cummings, 1987; Giles, 1992).

Approximately one in four hospital days in the United States are utilized by patients with psychiatric disorders (Kiesler & Sibulkin, 1987). The fee-for-service indemnity system, combined with the usual counterincentives provided by this system for outpatient care, accounts in part for this alarming figure.

The Foster Higgins report mentioned above indicated that the cost of mental health and substance abuse benefits increased in 1989 by nearly 50% among companies with more than 5,000 employees. This percentage increase was greater than for mid- and small-sized employer groups; however, increases were consistent and significant across the type as well as the size of industry surveyed.

Such increases in health and mental health care, if sustained, will consume the entirety of the U.S. GNP by the year 2015 (Jane Herfkens, William Mercer, Inc., personal communication, 1991).

The Managed Care Alternative

The growth in health care costs forced the federal government, despite a number of political obstacles (Inglehart, 1985) to consider the development of alternative delivery systems for cost-containment. This led to the passage of the Health Maintenance Act in 1973, followed by the passage of the Tax Equity and Fiscal Responsibility Act (TEFRA), allowing the federal government to contract with and promote HMOs. These and other cost-related factors (Kiesler & Morton, 1988) led to substantial growth of the managed health care system. HMO membership increased 300% to more than 28 million covered lives between 1982 and 1987 (Rundle, 1987). HMOs increased to a current coverage of more than 50 million lives. This figure does not include coverage by managed care variants such as self-funded employer groups or preferred provider organizations (Giles, 1993).

The means by which HMOs reduce or contain health care costs have been discussed in detail elsewhere (e.g., Davis, Anderson, Rowland, and Steinberg, 1990; Kongstvedt, 1989). Although HMO efforts to contain health costs have achieved only modest success (Giles, 1993), they have actually *reduced* mental health care costs via the purchase of specialized vendors. Traveler's purchased U.S. Behavioral Health; Aetna purchased Human Affairs International; United Health Care purchased United Behavioral Systems; and Cigna purchased MCC Managed Behavioral Care, Inc. Although these and other (see Giles, 1993) managed mental health care companies vary considerably from one another, they tend to have the following three characteristics in common which work effectively to contain costs: (1) they rely upon variable (and typically brief) lengths of inpatient stay; (2) they direct services as much as possible toward brief, goal-directed outpatient care; and (3) their services are typically reimbursed on a prepaid (capitated) basis.

Capitation is a fiscal arrangement antipodean to the traditional fee-for-service system. Under capitation, the managed mental health care firm is reimbursed by the payer (typically an insurance plan) in advance for services on a fixed-fee basis per covered life per month. This "caps" the amount of incoming revenue to the firm: As opposed to fee-for-service, *expenditures* (vs. incoming revenues) increase with greater use.

Critics of these systems (e.g., Armenti, 1991) worry that capitation motivates managed care firms to deny appropriate care. Although this concern is valid (Giles, 1989a), it should be noted that the denial of appropriate mental health services is likely to be associated with a number of serious consequences. These include malpractice suits, consumer complaints, investigations by state regulatory agencies such as the Office of the Insurance Commissioner or the Board of Psychologist Examiners, deterioration of the relationship between the managed mental health care vendor and the HMO, increasingly stringent state and/or federal legislation, and vocal protests by inpatient and outpatient providers in the community (Giles, 1989a).

With traditional indemnity plans, inpatient costs typically exceed 70% of gross revenues. Efficient inpatient management by managed care firms, however, combined with benefit disincentives to the overuse of inpatient care, usually reduces inpatient costs by at least 30%. These cost savings, however, have been offset to a degree by the consequent rise in outpatient mental health care use. It is this increase in outpatient costs—in the context of capitation—that makes managed mental health care controllers particularly motivated to deliver psychotherapeutic services which maximize efficiency and effectiveness.

Source descriptions from a number of the most prominent managed mental health care companies (e.g., American PsychManagement, MCC Managed Behavioral Care, Inc., American Biodyne, U.S. Behavioral Health, and so forth; see Giles, 1993) describe a number of management techniques for the containment of outpatient costs. These include ongoing utilization review, referral preference to practitioners specializing in brief, empirically validated treatments, development of management information systems capable of tracking providers with the highest efficiency and customer satisfaction ratings, and, perhaps most importantly, the use of outcome research to direct the provision of care.

MCC Managed Behavioral Care, Inc., for example, has completed an extensive literature search of comparative outcome data across a number of prevalent disorders. Contrary to the equivalence literature, and consistent with the findings and recommendations of the chapters in this handbook, preferred practices—that is, interventions which yield superior outcome compared to placebo and to traditional psychotherapies—have been identified for bulimia nervosa, the anxiety disorders, conduct/oppositional disorder, attention deficit disorder, psychotic disorders, chemical dependency, and so forth (e.g., Giles, 1989b, 1989c). Clinicians internal to the system are expected to practice by these guidelines once the appropriate diagnoses have been made. Clinicians external to the system who practice by these outcome standards gain a substantial referral advantage (Giles, 1990b).

MCC is currently responsible for more than 4 million lives and is expected to triple its capacity within the next 5 years. This is just one of several managed mental health care firms with national presence. Should HMOs thrive as expected during the Clinton Administration, then the fiscal systems motivating clinical standards may be expected to promote outcome literature—for perhaps the first time in the history of psychotherapy—to the position of primary arbiter of choice of care. Thus a major step will finally have been made toward the extensive implementation of comparatively effective therapy techniques.

References

American Psychiatric Association. (1989). *Treatment of psychiatric disorders, volume I.* Washington, DC: American Psychiatric Association.

Armenti, N. (1991). The provider network in managed care. *Behavior Therapist, 14*, 123–128.

Backer, T., Liberman, R., & Kuehner, T. (1986). Dissemination and adoption of innovative psychosocial interventions. *Journal of Consulting and Clinical Psychology, 54*, 111–118.

Barlow, D. (1981). On the relation of clinical research to clinical practice: Current issues, new directions. *Journal of Consulting and Clinical Psychology, 49*, 147–155.

Califano. (1986). A corporate Rx for America: Managing runaway health costs. *Issues in Science and Technology, 2*, 81–90.

Cummings, M. (1987). The future of psychotherapy: One psychologist's perspective. *American Journal of Psychotherapy, 61*, 349–360.

Davies, N., & Felder, L. (1990). Applying brakes to the runaway American health care system. *Journal of the American Medical Association, 263*, 73–76.

Davis, K., Anderson, G., Rowland, D., & Steinberg, E. (1990). *Health care cost containment.* Baltimore: Johns Hopkins University Press.

Dickerson, F. (1989). Behavioral therapy in private hospitals: A national survey. *Behavior Therapist, 12*, 158.

English, J., Sharfstein, S., Sherl, D., Strazhan, B., & Miszynsky, I. (1986). Diagnosis-related groups and general hospital psychiatry: The APA study. *American Journal of Psychiatry, 143*, 131–139.

Flinn, D., McMahon, T., & Collins, M. (1987). Health maintenance organizations and their implications to psychiatry. *Hospital and Community Psychiatry, 38*, 255–262.

Foster Higgins & Co. (1989). *Mental health and substance abuse benefits survey*. Princeton, NJ.

Garfield, S. (1980). *Psychotherapy: An eclectic approach*. New York: Wiley.

Garfield, S. (1989). *The practice of brief psychotherapy*. New York: Pergamon Press.

Garfield, S., & Kurtz, R. (1976). Clinical psychologists in the 1970s. *American Psychologist, 31*, 1–9.

Giles, T. (1983). Probable superiority of behavioral interventions-I: Traditional comparative outcome. *Journal of Behavior Therapy and Experimental Psychiatry, 14*, 29–32.

Giles, T. (1989a, August). Ethical considerations in managed mental health care systems. Paper presented at the American Psychological Association convention, New Orleans.

Giles, T. (1989b). *Preferred practices for eating disorders*. Unpublished monograph, MCC Managed Behavioral Care, Inc., Minneapolis.

Giles, T. (1989c). *Preferred practices for anxiety disorders*. Unpublished monograph, MCC Managed Behavioral Care, Inc., Minneapolis.

Giles, T. (1990a). Bias against behavior therapy in outcome reviews: Who speaks for the patient? *Behavior Therapist, 19*, 86–90.

Giles, T. (1990b). Underutilization of effective psychotherapy: Managed mental health care and other forces of change. *Behavior Therapist, 19*, 107–110.

Giles, T. (1993). *Managed mental health care: A guide for practitioners, employers, and hospital administrators*. New York: Allyn and Bacon.

Hayes, S. (1987). Bracing for change. *Behavior Analysis, 32*, 7–10.

Ingelhart, J. (1985). Medicare turns to HMOs. *New England Journal of Medicine, 312*, 132–136.

Kiesler, C., & Sibulkin, A. (1987). *Mental hospitalization: Myths and facts about a national crisis*. Newbury Park, CA: Sage.

Kiesler, C., & Morton, T. (1988). Psychology and public policy in the "health care revolution." *American Psychologist, 43*, 993–1003.

Kongstvedt, P. (1989). *The managed health care handbook*. Rockville, MD: Aspen Publishing, Inc.

Ludwigson, K., & Enright, M. (1988). The health care revolution: Implications for psychology and hospital practice. *Psychotherapy, 25*, 424–428.

Mechanic, D. (1980). *Mental health and social policy*. Englewood Cliffs, NJ: Prentice-Hall.

Meredith, R., & Milby, J. (1980). Obsessive–compulsive disorders. In R. Daitzman (Ed.), *Clinical behavior therapy and behavior modification*. New York: Garland.

Miller, W. (1982). Treating problem drinkers: What works? *Behavior Therapist, 5*, 15–18.

Norcross, J., Prochaska, J,. & Gallagher, K. (1989). Clinical psychologists in the 1980s: Theory, research and practice. *Clinical Psychologist, 12*, 42–53.

Robinson, C., & Luft, H. (1987). Competition and the cost of hospital care, 1972–1982. *Journal of the American Medical Association, 257*, 3241–3245.

Robinson, J. (1991). *Perspectives on managed care*. Presentation at the Annual Residents' Seminar, Colorado Health Sciences Center, Denver.

Rundle, R. (1987, October 6). Medical debate: Doctors who oppose the spread of HMOs are losing their fight. *Wall Street Journal*, pp. 22–23.

Smith, D. (1982). Trends in counseling and psychotherapy. *American Psychologist, 37*, 802.

VandenBos, G. (1983). Health financing, service utilization, and national policy: A conversation with Stan Jones. *American Psychologist, 38*, 948–955.

Wilson, G., & Rachman, S. (1983). Meta-analysis and the evaluation of psychotherapy outcome: Limitations and liabilities. *Journal of Consulting and Clinical Psychology, 51*, 54–64.

Wolpe, J. (1959). Psychotherapy by reciprocal inhibition: A reply to Dr. Glover. *British Journal of Medical Psychology, 32*, 232–235.

Wolpe, J. (1990). *The practice of behavior therapy* (4th ed.). Oxford: Pergamon Press.

Index